The Johns Hopkins
Internal Medicine
Board Review

The Johns Hopkins
Internal Medicine
Board Review

Certification and Recertification

FOURTH EDITION

Bimal H. Ashar, MD, MBA
The Johns Hopkins University School of Medicine,
Baltimore, Maryland

Redonda G. Miller, MD, MBA
The Johns Hopkins University School of Medicine,
Baltimore, Maryland

Stephen D. Sisson, MD
The Johns Hopkins University School of Medicine,
Baltimore, Maryland

ELSEVIER
SAUNDERS

1600 John F. Kennedy Blvd.
Ste 1800
Philadelphia, PA 19103-2899

Notice

Knowledge and best practice in this field are constantly changing. As new research and experience broaden our understanding, changes in research methods, professional practices, or medical treatment may become necessary.

Practitioners and researchers must always rely on their own experience and knowledge in evaluating and using any information, methods, compounds, or experiments described herein. In using such information or methods they should be mindful of their own safety and the safety of others, including parties for whom they have a professional responsibility.

With respect to any drug or pharmaceutical products identified, readers are advised to check the most current information provided (i) on procedures featured or (ii) by the manufacturer of each product to be administered, to verify the recommended dose or formula, the method and duration of administration, and contraindications. It is the responsibility of practitioners, relying on their own experience and knowledge of their patients, to make diagnoses, to determine dosages and the best treatment for each individual patient, and to take all appropriate safety precautions.

To the fullest extent of the law, neither the Publisher nor the authors, contributors, or editors, assume any liability for any injury and/or damage to persons or property as a matter of products liability, negligence or otherwise, or from any use or operation of any methods, products, instructions, or ideas contained in the material herein.

Library of Congress Cataloging-in-Publication Data

The Johns Hopkins Internal Medicine Board review: certification and recertification/ [edited by] Bimal H. Ashar, Redonda G. Miller, Stephen D. Sisson. – 4th ed.
    p. ; cm.
Internal medicine board review
Includes bibliographical references and index.
ISBN 978-1-4557-0692-1 (pbk. : alk. paper)
I. Ashar, Bimal H. II. Miller, Redonda G. III. Sisson, Stephen D. IV. Johns Hopkins University. V. Title: Internal medicine board review.
[DNLM: 1. Internal Medicine–Examination Questions. 2. Internal Medicine–Outlines. WB 18.2]
616.0076–dc23   2011041216

Senior Content Strategist: Kate Dimock
Content Developer: Joan Ryan
Publishing Services Manager: Pat Joiner-Myers
Senior Project Manager: Joy Moore
Designer: Steven Stave

Printed in China

Last digit is the print number: 9 8 7 6 5 4 3 2 1

Working together to grow
libraries in developing countries

www.elsevier.com | www.bookaid.org | www.sabre.org

ELSEVIER   BOOK AID International   Sabre Foundation

CONTRIBUTOR

Shabina R. Ahmed, MD
Fellow, Division of Endocrinology and Metabolism,
The Johns Hopkins University School of Medicine,
Baltimore, Maryland
Thyroid Disease

Deborah K. Armstrong, MD
Associate Professor of Oncology, Sidney Kimmel
Comprehensive Cancer Center at Johns Hopkins;
Associate Professor of Gynecology and Obstetrics,
The Johns Hopkins University School of Medicine,
Baltimore, Maryland
Breast and Ovarian Cancer

Bimal H. Ashar, MD, MBA
Associate Professor of Medicine, and Clinical Director,
Division of General Internal Medicine, The Johns Hopkins
University School of Medicine, Baltimore, Maryland
*Anemia; Complementary and Alternative Medicine;
Immunization and Prevention*

John N. Aucott, MD
Instructor in Medicine, Division of General Internal
Medicine, The Johns Hopkins University School of
Medicine, Baltimore, Maryland
Selected Topics in Infectious Disease II

Paul G. Auwaerter, MD
Associate Professor of Medicine and Clinical Director,
Division of Infectious Diseases, The Johns Hopkins
University School of Medicine, Baltimore, Maryland
Respiratory Infections

Wendy L. Bennett, MD, MPH
Assistant Professor of Medicine, Division of General
Internal Medicine, The Johns Hopkins University
School of Medicine; Assistant Professor, Population,
Family, and Reproductive Health, The Johns Hopkins
Bloomberg School of Public Health, Baltimore, Maryland
Selected Topics in Women's Health

Gail Berkenblit, MD, PhD
Assistant Professor of Medicine, Division of General
Internal Medicine; Associate Program Director, Osler
Medicine Residency Program, The Johns Hopkins
University School of Medicine, Baltimore, Maryland
Human Immunodeficiency Virus Infection

Dionne Blackman, MD
Assistant Professor of Medicine, Division of General
Internal Medicine, University of Chicago Pritzker
School of Medicine, Chicago Illinois
*Maximizing Test Performance: Effective Study and Test-Taking
Strategies*

Roger S. Blumenthal, MD
Professor of Medicine, Division of Cardiology; Director,
Johns Hopkins Ciccarone Center for the Prevention of
Heart Disease, The Johns Hopkins University School of
Medicine, Baltimore, Maryland
Lipid Disorders

L. Ebony Boulware, MD, MPH
Associate Professor of Medicine, Division of General
Internal Medicine; Associate Professor of Epidemiology,
The Johns Hopkins Bloomberg School of Public Health,
Baltimore, Maryland
Clinical Epidemiology

Todd T. Brown, MD, PhD
Associate Professor of Medicine, Division of Endocrinology
and Metabolism, The Johns Hopkins University,
Baltimore, Maryland
Reproductive Endocrinology

Michael A. Carducci, MD
AEGON Professor in Prostate Cancer Research and
Professor of Oncology and Urology, The Johns Hopkins
University School of Medicine, Baltimore, Maryland
Genitourinary Cancer

Amina A. Chaudhry, MD, MPH
Assistant Professor of Medicine, Division of General
Internal Medicine, The Johns Hopkins University
School of Medicine, Baltimore, Maryland
Substance Use Disorders

Michael J. Choi, MD
Associate Professor of Medicine and Clinical Director,
Division of Nephrology, The Johns Hopkins University
School of Medicine, Baltimore, Maryland
Selected Topics in Nephrology

Grant V. Chow, MD
Fellow, Division of Cardiology, The Johns Hopkins
University School of Medicine, Baltimore, Maryland
Arrhythmias

Colleen Christmas, MD
Assistant Professor of Medicine, Division of Geriatric
Medicine and Gerontology, The Johns Hopkins University
School of Medicine; Residency Program Director, Johns
Hopkins Bayview Medical Center, Baltimore, Maryland
Selected Topics in Geriatric Medicine

John O. Clarke, MD
Assistant Professor of Medicine, Division of Gastroenterology
and Hepatology, and Director of Gastrointestinal Motility,
The Johns Hopkins University, Baltimore, Maryland
*Peptic Ulcer Disease and Gastrointestinal Bleeding; Esophageal
Disease*

Geoffrey R. Connors, MD
Assistant Professor, Division of Pulmonary and Critical Care, Yale University School of Medicine, New Haven, Connecticut
Critical Care Medicine

David S. Cooper, MD
Professor of Medicine, Division of Endocrinology and Metabolism; Director, Thyroid Clinic, The Johns Hopkins University School of Medicine, Baltimore, Maryland
Thyroid Disease

Mary Corretti, MD
Associate Professor of Medicine, Division of Cardiology; Medical Director, Adult Echocardiography Laboratory, The Johns Hopkins University School of Medicine, Baltimore, Maryland
Pericardial Disease

David Cosgrove, MD
Assistant Professor of Oncology, Sidney Kimmel Comprehensive Cancer Center at Johns Hopkins, The Johns Hopkins University School of Medicine, Baltimore, Maryland
Colorectal Cancer; Selected Topics in Oncology; Lung Cancer and Head and Neck Cancer

Andrew P. DeFilippis, MD, MSc
Assistant Professor of Medicine, Division of Cardiology, University of Louisville, Louisville, Kentucky
Lipid Disorders

Susan E. Dorman, MD
Associate Professor of Medicine and International Health, Division of Infectious Diseases, The Johns Hopkins University, Baltimore, Maryland
Mycobacterial Infections

M. Bradley Drummond, MD, MHS
Assistant Professor of Medicine, Division of Pulmonary and Critical Care Medicine, The Johns Hopkins University School of Medicine, Baltimore, Maryland
Obstructive Lung Disease

Kerry B. Dunbar, MD
Assistant Professor of Medicine, University of Texas Southwestern Medical Center; Staff Physician, VA North Texas Healthcare System – Dallas VA Medical Center, Dallas, Texas
Pancreatic and Biliary Disease

James P. Dunn, MD
Associate Professor of Ophthalmology, The Johns Hopkins University School of Medicine, Baltimore, Maryland
Ophthalmology for the Internist

Michelle M. Estrella, MD, MHS
Assistant Professor of Medicine, Division of Nephrology, The Johns Hopkins University School of Medicine, Baltimore, Maryland
Selected Topics in Nephrology

Derek M. Fine, MD
Associate Professor of Medicine and Fellowship Director, Division of Nephrology, The Johns Hopkins University School of Medicine, Baltimore, Maryland
Glomerular Disease; Chronic Kidney Disease and End-Stage Renal Disease

April S. Fitzgerald, MD
Instructor of Medicine, Division of General Internal Medicine, The Johns Hopkins University School of Medicine, Baltimore, Maryland
Headaches

John A. Flynn, MD, MBA, MEd
Professor of Medicine, Division of General Internal Medicine, Medical Director, Spondyloarthritis Program, and Co-Director, The Osler Center for Clinical Excellence at Johns Hopkins, The Johns Hopkins University School of Medicine, Baltimore, Maryland
Office Orthopedics

Matthew Foy, MD
Fellow, Division of Nephrology, The Johns Hopkins University School of Medicine, Baltimore, Maryland
Selected Topics in Nephrology

Allan C. Gelber, MD, MPH, PhD
Associate Professor of Medicine and Fellowship Director, Division of Rheumatology, The Johns Hopkins University School of Medicine, Baltimore, Maryland
Arthritis

Jonathan M. Gerber, MD
Assistant Professor of Medicine, Division of Hematology, The Johns Hopkins University School of Medicine, Baltimore, Maryland
Blood Smear and Bone Marrow Review

Khalil G. Ghanem, MD, PhD
Associate Professor of Medicine, Division of Infectious Diseases, The Johns Hopkins University School of Medicine; Director of STD, HIV, TB Clinical Services, Baltimore City Health Department, Baltimore, Maryland
Genitourinary Infections

Michael Goggins, MD
Professor of Medicine, Division of Gastroenterology and Hepatology, The Johns Hopkins University School of Medicine, Baltimore, Maryland
Disorders of the Small and Large Intestine

Sherita H. Golden, MD, MHS
Associate Professor of Medicine, Division of Endocrinology, The Johns Hopkins University School of Medicine; Director, Inpatient Diabetes Management Service, and Chairperson, Glucose Steering Committee, The Johns Hopkins Hospital, Baltimore, Maryland
Diabetes Mellitus

Elizabeth A. Griffiths, MD
Assistant Professor of Medicine, Roswell Park Cancer Institute, Buffalo, New York
Platelet Disorders

Thomas B. Habif, MD
Adjunct Professor of Medicine, Dartmouth Medical School, Hanover, New Hampshire
Dermatology for the Internist

Robert W. Hallowell, MD
Fellow, Division of Pulmonary and Critical Care, The Johns Hopkins University School of Medicine, Baltimore, Maryland
Interstitial Lung Disease

James P. Hamilton, MD
Assistant Professor of Medicine, Division of Gastroenterology and Hepatology, The Johns Hopkins University School of Medicine, Baltimore, Maryland
Acute and Chronic Liver Disease; Complications of Liver Disease

Hans Hammers, MD, PhD
Assistant Professor of Oncology, Sidney Kimmel Comprehensive Cancer Center at Johns Hopkins, The Johns Hopkins University School of Medicine, Baltimore, Maryland
Genitourinary Cancer

Maureen R. Horton, MD
Associate Professor of Medicine, Division of Pulmonary and Critical Care, The Johns Hopkins University School of Medicine, Baltimore, Maryland
Interstitial Lung Disease

Carol Ann Huff, MD
Associate Professor of Oncology and Medicine, and Director, Myeloma Program, The Johns Hopkins University School of Medicine, Baltimore, Maryland
Plasma Cell Dyscrasias

Mark T. Hughes, MD, MA
Assistant Professor of Medicine, Division of General Internal Medicine, The Johns Hopkins University School of Medicine; Core Faculty, Johns Hopkins Berman Institute of Bioethics, Baltimore, Maryland
Medical Ethics

Yvette L. Kasamon, MD
Associate Professor of Oncology, Sidney Kimmel Comprehensive Cancer Center at Johns Hopkins, The Johns Hopkins University School of Medicine, Baltimore, Maryland
Lymphoma and Chronic Lymphocytic Leukemia

Rebecca A. Kazin, MD
Assistant Professor of Dermatology, The Johns Hopkins University, Baltimore, Maryland; Medical Director, Johns Hopkins Dermatology and Cosmetic Center at Green Spring Station, Lutherville, Maryland
Dermatology for the Internist

Sabiha Khan, MD
Johns Hopkins Community Physicians, Bethesda, Maryland
Office Orthopedics

Thomas W. Koenig, MD
Assistant Professor of Psychiatry and Behavioral Sciences; Associate Dean for Student Affairs, The Johns Hopkins University School of Medicine, Baltimore, Maryland
Psychiatry for the Internist

Sophie M. Lanzkron, MD, MHS
Associate Professor of Medicine, Division of Hematology, The Johns Hopkins University School of Medicine, Baltimore, Maryland
Platelet Disorders

Linda A. Lee, MD
Assistant Professor of Medicine, and Clinical Director, Division of Gastroenterology and Hepatology, The Johns Hopkins University School of Medicine, Baltimore, Maryland
Peptic Ulcer Disease and Gastrointestinal Bleeding; Esophageal Disease

Anne Marie Lennon, MB, PhD, MRCPI
Assistant Professor of Medicine, Division of Gastroenterology and Hepatology, The Johns Hopkins University School of Medicine, Baltimore, Maryland
Disorders of the Small and Large Intestine

Howard Levy, MD, PhD
Assistant Professor, Division of General Internal Medicine, The Johns Hopkins University School of Medicine, Baltimore, Maryland
Genetics for the Internist

Hyung M. Lim, MD
Instructor of Medicine, Division of Nephrology, The Johns Hopkins University School of Medicine, Baltimore, Maryland
Acute Kidney Injury

Tara Lin, MD
Assistant Professor of Medicine, University of Kansas School of Medicine, Kansas City, Kansas
Acute and Chronic Leukemias; Myelodysplastic Syndrome

Rafael H. Llinás, MD
Associate Professor of Neurology, The Johns Hopkins University School of Medicine; Neurology Vice-Chair, Clinical Services and Quality, The Johns Hopkins Hospital/Johns Hopkins Bayview Medical Center, Baltimore, Maryland
Cerebrovascular Disease and Seizure Disorders; Selected Topics in Neurology

Joseph E. Marine, MD
Associate Professor of Medicine, Division of Cardiology, The Johns Hopkins University School of Medicine; Associate Director of Electrophysiology, Johns Hopkins Health System, Baltimore, Maryland
Arrhythmias

Meredith C. McCormack, MD, MHS
Assistant Professor of Medicine, Division of Pulmonary and Critical Care Medicine, The Johns Hopkins University School of Medicine, Baltimore, Maryland
Pulmonary Function Testing

Vishal C. Mehra, MD, PhD
Fellow, Division of Cardiology, The Johns Hopkins University School of Medicine, Baltimore, Maryland
Coronary Artery Disease

Christian A. Merlo, MD, MPH
Assistant Professor of Medicine, Division of Pulmonary and Critical Care, The Johns Hopkins University School of Medicine, Baltimore, Maryland
Chest Radiograph Review

Redonda G. Miller, MD, MBA
Associate Professor of Medicine, Division of General Internal Medicine, The Johns Hopkins University School of Medicine; Vice President for Medical Affairs, The Johns Hopkins Hospital, Baltimore, Maryland
Calcium Disorders and Metabolic Bone Disease; Selected Topics in Women's Health

David B. Pearse, MD
Professor of Medicine, Division of Pulmonary and Critical Care, The Johns Hopkins University, Baltimore, Maryland
Venous Thromboembolic Disease

Brent G. Petty, MD
Associate Professor of Medicine, Division of Clinical Pharmacology, The Johns Hopkins University School of Medicine, Baltimore, Maryland
Electrocardiogram Review

Albert J. Polito, MD
Assistant Professor of Medicine, Division of Pulmonary and Critical Care Medicine, Department of Medicine, The Johns Hopkins University School of Medicine; Chief, Division of Pulmonary Medicine, and Director, The Lung Center at Mercy, Department of Medicine, Mercy Medical Center, Baltimore, Maryland
Selected Topics in Pulmonary Medicine; Pleural Disease

Gregory P. Prokopowicz, MD, MPH
Assistant Professor of Medicine, Division of General Internal Medicine, The Johns Hopkins University School of Medicine, Baltimore, Maryland
Hypertension

Rosanne Rouf, MD
Assistant Professor, Division of Cardiology, The Johns Hopkins University School of Medicine, Baltimore, Maryland
Heart Failure

Sarbjit S. Saini, MD
Associate Professor of Medicine, Division of Allergy and Clinical Immunology, The Johns Hopkins University School of Medicine, Baltimore, Maryland
Allergy and Immunology for the Internist

Roberto Salvatori, MD
Associate Professor of Medicine, Division of Endocrinology and Metabolism, The Johns Hopkins University School of Medicine; Medical Director, Pituitary Center, The Johns Hopkins Hospital, Baltimore, Maryland
Neuroendocrine and Adrenal Disease

Joseph M. Savitt, MD, PhD
Assistant Professor of Neurology, The Johns Hopkins University School of Medicine, Baltimore, Maryland
Movement Disorders

Paul J. Scheel, Jr., MD, MBA
Director, Division of Nephrology, The Johns Hopkins University School of Medicine, Baltimore, Maryland
Chronic Kidney Disease and End-Stage Renal Disease

Cynthia L. Sears, MD
Professor of Medicine and Oncology, The Johns Hopkins University School of Medicine, Baltimore, Maryland
Infectious Diarrhea

Philip Seo, MD, MHS
Associate Professor of Medicine, Division of Rheumatology; Director, Johns Hopkins Rheumatology Fellowship Program; Director, Johns Hopkins Vasculitis Center, The Johns Hopkins University School of Medicine, Baltimore, Maryland
Vasculitis

Jonathan Sevransky, MD, MHS
Assistant Professor of Medicine, Emory University; Director, Medical ICU, Emory University Hospital; Assistant Director for Medicine, Emory Center for Critical Care, Atlanta, Georgia
Critical Care Medicine

Tariq Shafi, MBBS, MHS
Assistant Professor of Medicine, Division of Nephrology, The Johns Hopkins University School of Medicine, Baltimore, Maryland
Glomerular Disease; Chronic Kidney Disease and End-Stage Renal Disease

Mary Sheu, MD
Assistant Professor and Associate Residency Director, Department of Dermatology, The Johns Hopkins University School of Medicine, Baltimore, Maryland
Dermatology for the Internist

Stephen D. Sisson, MD
Associate Professor of Medicine and Vice-Chair for Clinical Operations, Department of Medicine, The Johns Hopkins University School of Medicine, Baltimore, Maryland
Acid-Base Disorders and Renal Tubular Acidosis; Preoperative Evaluation

B. Douglas Smith, MD
Associate Professor of Oncology, Sidney Kimmel Comprehensive Cancer Center at Johns Hopkins, The Johns Hopkins University School of Medicine, Baltimore, Maryland
Acute and Chronic Leukemias; Myelodysplastic Syndrome

Shawn F. Smyth, MD
Fellow, Department of Neurology, The Johns Hopkins University School of Medicine, Baltimore, Maryland
Movement Disorders

C. John Sperati, MD, MHS
Assistant Professor of Medicine, Division of Nephrology, The Johns Hopkins University School of Medicine, Baltimore, Maryland
Electrolyte Disorders

Michael B. Streiff, MD
Associate Professor of Medicine, Division of Hematology; Medical Director, Johns Hopkins Anticoagulation Management Service, The Johns Hopkins University School of Medicine, Baltimore, Maryland
Coagulation Disorders

Aruna K. Subramanian, MD
Assistant Professor, Division of Infectious Diseases, The Johns Hopkins University School of Medicine, Baltimore, Maryland
Selected Topics in Infectious Disease I

Lori M. Tam, MD
Fellow, Division of Cardiology, The Johns Hopkins University School of Medicine, Baltimore, Maryland
Lipid Disorders

Peter B. Terry, MD, MA
Professor of Medicine, Division of Pulmonary and Critical Care, The Johns Hopkins University School of Medicine, Baltimore, Maryland
Chest Radiograph Review

Thomas A. Traill, MD, FRCP
Professor of Medicine, Division of Cardiology, The Johns Hopkins University School of Medicine, Baltimore, Maryland
Valvular Heart Disease

Rainer von Coelln, MD, PhD
Resident, Department of Neurology, University of Maryland Medical Center, Baltimore, Maryland
Movement Disorders

Robert A. Wise, MD
Professor of Medicine, Division of Pulmonary and Critical Care Medicine, The Johns Hopkins University School of Medicine, Baltimore, Maryland
Obstructive Lung Disease; Pulmonary Function Testing

Ilan S. Wittstein, MD
Assistant Professor of Medicine, Division of Cardiology, The Johns Hopkins University School of Medicine, Baltimore, Maryland
Coronary Artery Disease

Robert J. Wityk, MD
Associate Professor of Neurology, The Johns Hopkins University School of Medicine, Baltimore, Maryland
Cerebrovascular Disease and Seizure Disorders

Tao Zheng, MD
Associate Professor of Medicine, Division of Allergy and Clinical Immunology, The Johns Hopkins University School of Medicine, Baltimore, Maryland
Allergy and Immunology for the Internist

Carol M. Ziminski, MD
Associate Professor of Medicine, Division of Rheumatology, The Johns Hopkins University School of Medicine, Baltimore, Maryland
Selected Topics in Rheumatology

With the assistance of our publisher, Elsevier, we are pleased to offer the fourth edition of *The Johns Hopkins Internal Medicine Board Review*. The strength of any book of this type ultimately hinges on the quality of its contributors; in this regard, we are quite fortunate, as each chapter has been written by an accomplished faculty member with extensive knowledge of the topic discussed. The book is divided into sections weighted according to the level of emphasis on the American Board of Internal Medicine certifying examination, with additional coverage of the related (and also tested) fields of psychiatry, dermatology, and ophthalmology. Our format is unique in that it features comparative tables and decision algorithms, which lend themselves to ease of study and quick review. The book also includes a link to an exclusive website that provides practice questions and answers that are patterned after those seen on the actual board examination and that stress important "take home" points and allow self-assessment of knowledge retention.

In many ways, this book is the product of more than a century of medical teaching at Johns Hopkins. In the late nineteenth century, Sir William Osler developed the modern concept of an internal medicine training program during his tenure as the first Chair of Medicine at The Johns Hopkins Hospital. He became famous for his bedside teaching and instituted the practice of "rounds," which remains the principal method of clinical instruction in use today. Among Dr. Osler's many achievements during his remarkable life was the completion of his magnum opus, *The Principles and Practice of Medicine*, which was the first textbook to systematically categorize and describe disease with a measure of precision and clarity that had not previously been seen. In the words of Osler, "Books are tools, doctors are craftsmen, and so truly as one can measure the development of any particular handicraft by the variety and complexity of its tools, so we have no better means of judging the intelligence of a profession than by its general collection of books."

We hope you find the text to be a worthy addition to your preparation materials.

The Editors

CONTENTS

Maximizing Test Performance: Effective Study and Test-Taking Strategies

DIONNE BLACKMAN, MD

Research has identified a number of factors that affect test performance:
- Study skills
- Content knowledge
- Practice of questions in the same format as the test
- Test-taking skills
- Anxiety
- Fatigue and sleep deprivation

By reading this book, the exam taker will improve content knowledge and have the opportunity to test this knowledge with many case-based practice questions. This chapter, however, addresses the three topics not related to content knowledge: study skills, test-taking skills, and anxiety. The strategies provided will make studying for the Board Examination more effective and optimize test performance on the exam.

Strategies for More Effective Studying

Anticipate Test Content

A strategic approach to studying such as what follows has been found to lead to better performance on examinations (McManus et al., 1998; Ward, 2011).
- Review the examination blueprint to understand the percentage of questions derived from each content area (available on the Web site for the American Board of Internal Medicine [ABIM] at *www.abim.org*)
- Complete the tutorial on taking the computer-based exam, which you can download from the ABIM Web site. The tutorial sample questions will explain how to use exam functions and provide a practice test to familiarize you with the different types of exam questions and format. Specifically, you will preview how to
  - Answer questions
  - Change answers
  - Make notes electronically
  - Access the table of normal laboratory values, calculator, and electronic calipers
  - View figures and video clips
  - Mark questions for review
  - Use the Progress Indicator and Time Remaining functions to keep track of item completion and time remaining for the test session

  - Use the Navigation button or Review Screen to view item completion status, items you have marked for review, or items with an electronic note, and to move quickly to items within the test
- Board Examination questions are derived using the following criteria and will
  - **Be focused on patient care**
  - Address important clinical problems for which medical intervention has a significant effect on patient outcomes
  - Address commonly overlooked or mismanaged clinical problems
  - Pose a challenging management decision
  - Assess ability to make optimal clinical decisions
- Maintenance of Certification examination questions will not address clinical problems that are typically referred to specialists or recent clinical advances before they are widely used in practice
- Clinical decision-making can be broken down into different tasks; the Board Examination is meant to test your ability to perform these tasks:
  - Identify characteristic clinical features of diseases
  - Identify characteristic pathophysiologic features of diseases
  - Choose the most appropriate diagnostic tests
  - Determine the diagnosis
  - Determine the prognosis or natural history of diseases
  - Select the best treatment or management strategy
  - Choose risk-appropriate prevention strategies
- **Board Examination questions will never address an area in which there is no consensus of opinion among experts in the field**
- Carefully review visual information, as this is frequently used in Board Examination questions regarding disorders with characteristic skin lesions or findings on blood smear, bone marrow, electrocardiogram, radiograph, and other visual diagnostic tests

Time Management

- **Use the Residency In-Training Examination or a full-length practice test (as on the Web site accompanying this book) to identify your areas of weakness**
- Complete practice tests in your weaker subjects first to identify specific gaps in content knowledge to address by a focused review of these subjects

- Use a "question drill–to-content" review ratio of 2:1 or greater to review subjects, as this has been shown to be more successful than traditional review using the reverse ratio (see McDowell, 2008)
- After addressing your weaker subjects, conduct a focused review of other subjects as discussed earlier
- Create a realistic study schedule and stick to it!
- Using the examination blueprint, budget your study time to cover all of the examination content areas without last-minute cramming
- **Plan to complete your study several days before the examination**
- **Plan a question drill period for the last few days before the examination. Use answers to incorrectly answered practice questions for targeted content review.**

Effective Approaches to Studying

- The Survey, Question, Read, Recite, Review (SQ3R) study method has proven effective in improving reading efficiency, comprehension, and material retention
  - It provides a useful way to study for the Board Examination, regardless of study resource used
  - Steps in the method are outlined in Table 1-1
- Studying with a small group can enhance study effectiveness by providing social support and increased confidence as individuals assume responsibility to review and teach particular areas to the group

Strategies for More Effective Test Taking

The following strategies will only be effective if practiced, so plan to practice them in your question drill sessions; the Web site accompanying this book allows exam takers to practice answering questions in a timed test format.

Strategies for Time Use

- Know the examination schedule for the computer-based examination (see *www.abim.org*)
- **Return from breaks 10 minutes early. You must check in after breaks, and the examination clock restarts at the end of the break regardless of your return time**
- Know the time allotted per exam question (i.e., exam time in minutes divided by number of exam questions). This is about 2 minutes per question based on the maximum 60 questions allowed per 2-hour board exam session.

TABLE 1-1	SQ3R Study Method	
Step	**Description**
Survey	Survey section headings and summaries first
Question	Convert headings, legends, and board examination tasks into "questions"
Read	Read to answer your "questions"
Recite	Recite answers and write down key phrases and cues
Review	Review notes, paraphrase major points, draw diagrams, and make flashcards for material that is difficult to recall

- Budget your time; unfinished questions are lost scoring opportunities
- Keep track of your use of time by checking time targets at each quarter of the total exam time
- To fully use other test-taking strategies, use less than the allotted time per question (we suggest 15 to 30 seconds less per question)
- **To focus on pertinent data, read the question and the answer options before reading the question stem (the stem is the part of the test item that precedes the question and answer options and is usually case-based)**
- Answer questions you know first and quickly guess on those you don't know

Strategies for Guessing and Reasoning

- Identify key words or phrases that affect the question's intent (e.g., *at this time, now, initially, most, always, never, except, usually, least*)
- Determine whether the following factors limit your thinking to certain disease categories:
  - Patient factors
    - Age, sex, race, or ethnicity
    - Habits (e.g., smoking, alcohol or illicit drug use)
    - Exposures due to occupation, travel, or residence
    - Immune status
  - Factors related to illness presentation
    - Time course of illness (i.e., acute, subacute, or chronic)
    - Symptoms or findings present or stated to be absent
    - Pattern of diagnostic data (e.g., presence of a known symptom triad, pathognomic finding)
- Eliminate answer options likely to be incorrect. Remember that incorrect options are usually written to be plausible or even partially correct.
- Examine similarities and differences between answer options (e.g., mutually exclusive options)
- Answer questions based on established standards of care, not anecdotal experiences (many current guidelines are available at National Guideline Clearinghouse at *www.guideline.gov*)
- Do not be afraid to use partial knowledge to eliminate answers
- When unsure of an answer, enter your best guess (research shows it is often correct) and flag the question on the computer for later review
- **Answer all questions—there is no penalty for wrong answers**
  - **Please note that, once you click the "End Session" button, you cannot go back to review or change responses for that test session**
  - **Be sure to check that you have completed any review or changing of answers and have entered a response for all questions before you click "End Session"**

Strategies for Changing Answers

- Spending less than the allotted time per exam question allows you to finish exams early; this extra time allows you to benefit from answer changing
- **Despite "conventional wisdom," research shows most test-takers benefit from answer changing**

- You are more likely to change from a wrong to a right answer if you
  - Reread and better understand the test item
  - Rethink and conceptualize a better answer
  - Gain information from another test item
  - Remember more information
  - Correct a clerical error (e.g., the intended answer was not the entered answer)

Strategies for Error Avoidance

- Read each question and all answer options carefully. Be certain you understand the intent of the question before answering (e.g., questions stating "all of the following are correct except …").
- Do not "read into a question" information or interpretations that are not there
- Check that the answer entered is the answer you intended

Strategies for Anxiety Reduction

- Anxiety is a natural part of taking an examination, but high test anxiety will adversely affect test performance
- Consider formal counseling if you have had problems with high test anxiety in the past
- Consider writing about your negative thoughts and worries about the examination for 10 minutes on the day of the test, as this has been found to significantly improve test performance for those with high test anxiety (Ramirez and Beilock, 2011)
- Actively manage anxiety by decreasing the effect of unknowns on your anxiety level:
  - **Test drive the travel route and time to the test site;** locate parking and the site itself if it is in a building with other businesses
  - **Bring a sweater or dress in layers to prepare for examination room temperature variations**
  - **Bring a snack for unexpected hunger and medications for potential illness symptoms**

- Allow a minimum of 30 minutes before your test appointment for check-in procedures (see www.abim.org for details regarding check-in)
- Avoid overly anxious test takers; they heighten your anxiety level, which can hurt your test performance
- Use relaxation techniques:
  - Deep muscle relaxation is an effective relaxation technique; it involves tensing and relaxing each muscle group until all muscles are relaxed
  - To reduce anxiety further, engage in exercise during the period when you are preparing for the examination
- Being well-rested is imperative

SUGGESTED READINGS

Frierson HT, Hoband D: Effect of test anxiety on performance on the NBME Part I Examination, *J Med Educ* 62:431–433, 1987.
Frierson HT, Malone B, Shelton P: Enhancing NCLEX-RN performance: assessing a three-pronged intervention approach, *J Nurs Educ* 32:222–224, 1993.
Harvill LM, Davis G III: Test-taking behaviors and their impact on performance: medical students' reasons for changing answers on multiple choice tests, *Acad Med* 72:S97–S99, 1997.
Hembree R: Correlates, causes, effects, and treatment of test anxiety, *Rev Educ Res* 58:47–77, 1988.
McDowell BM: KATTS: a framework for maximizing NCLEX-RN performance, *J Nurs Educ* 47:183–186, 2008.
McManus IC, Richards P, Winder BC, Sproston KA: Clinical experience, performance in final examinations, and learning style in medical students: prospective study, *BMJ* 316:345–350, 1998.
Ramirez G, Beilock SL: Writing about testing worries boosts exam performance in classroom, *Science* 331:211–213, 2011.
Robinson FP: *Effective study*, rev ed, New York, 1961, Harper & Row.
Seipp B: Anxiety and academic performance: a meta-analysis of findings, *Anxiety Res* 4:27–41, 1991.
Waddell DL, Blankenship JC: Answer changing: a meta-analysis of the prevalence and patterns, *J Cont Educ Nurs* 25:155–158, 1994.
Ward PJ: First year medical students' approaches to study and their outcomes in a gross Anatomy Course, *Clin Anat* 24:120–127, 2011.

Cardiology

Hypertension

GREGORY P. PROKOPOWICZ, MD, MPH

Hypertension is present in more than 25% of the general population and, with the aging of the population and the increase in obesity, its prevalence is expected to increase. Hypertension is an important risk factor for many common diseases including stroke, end-stage renal disease, congestive heart failure, and myocardial infarction, and it is the most common modifiable cardiac risk factor. Aggressive control of blood pressure (BP) results in a significant decline in morbidity and mortality.

Basic Information

- Definition of hypertension
  - **Hypertension is defined as a BP of 140/90 mm Hg or higher (i.e., a systolic BP of ≥140 mm Hg, a diastolic BP of ≥90 mm Hg, or both) (Table 2-1).**
    - The classification of BP applies to patients not taking antihypertensives and without acute illness (which may raise or lower BP); patients taking antihypertensive medication are considered to have hypertension
  - BP of 140–159/90–99 mm Hg is designated as stage 1 hypertension, and BP greater than or equal to 160/100 mm Hg as stage 2 hypertension
    - If the systolic and diastolic BPs fall in different stages, the higher stage is used (e.g., a BP of 182/95 mm Hg is categorized as stage 2)
  - **BP of 120–139/80–89 mm Hg is designated as prehypertension**
    - Prehypertension is a risk category, not a disease— patients in this category are at high risk of progressing to actual hypertension and should be targeted for lifestyle modification
  - **Hypertensive urgency refers to severe hypertension without acute end-organ dysfunction**
    - There is no agreed-upon BP that defines hypertensive urgency, although some sources use 180/120 mm Hg
    - Headache, anxiety, or medication nonadherence often contribute to elevated blood pressure in such patients
  - **Hypertensive emergency implies elevated BP with acute end-organ dysfunction (Table 2-2)**
    - Although hypertensive emergency is not defined by any specific level of BP, most patients have BPs greater than or equal to 160/120 mm Hg
- Epidemiology
  - Hypertension affects more than 60 million Americans and is the most common modifiable cardiac risk factor
  - Hypertension is more prevalent among African Americans, who also suffer more end-organ damage
  - There is a graded relationship between the level of BP and the incidence of stroke, end-stage renal disease, congestive heart failure, and ischemic heart disease

- **Under age 50, diastolic BP is the most important predictor of cardiovascular outcomes; above age 50, systolic BP is the most important predictor**
- BP and the prevalence of hypertension rise with age (Fig. 2-1).
  - Systolic BP rises continuously; diastolic BP rises until approximately age 50 years and then declines
  - Isolated systolic hypertension (i.e., systolic >140 mm Hg and diastolic <90 mm Hg) is common among the elderly and is an important cardiovascular risk factor
  - Patients with prehypertension have an increased risk of progression to hypertension with aging
- Pathophysiology
  - **Most patients (>90%) do not have an identifiable cause of hypertension; this is commonly referred to as essential hypertension**
  - BP is the product of cardiac output and peripheral vascular resistance; although increased cardiac output may play a role in the initiation of hypertension, most patients with long-standing hypertension have increased peripheral resistance with normal or diminished cardiac output
  - Certain persons respond more strongly to changes in sodium intake and extracellular fluid status and are described as salt sensitive; salt sensitivity occurs more commonly among African Americans and the elderly
  - End-organ damage from hypertension affects the kidneys, heart, vasculature, brain, and eyes (Table 2-3)

Clinical Presentation

- Most patients are asymptomatic
- Some may already have evidence of target organ damage at first presentation (see Table 2-3)
- Occasionally, patients may present with hypertensive urgencies or emergencies (see Table 2-2)

Diagnosis and Evaluation

- Measurement of BP
  - **Use appropriate cuff size. The bladder of the cuff should encircle 80% or more of the arm without overlapping; use of a cuff that is too small may cause falsely elevated readings**
  - The patient should refrain from smoking or consuming caffeine for 30 minutes and sit quietly for 5 minutes before measurement
  - The arm in which BP is being measured should be supported and relaxed at the level of the heart
  - At each clinical visit, the BP should be taken at least twice, or until successive readings are within 5 mm Hg of each other

TABLE 2-1	Classification of Blood Pressure (BP)			
Category	**Systolic BP (mm Hg)**		**Diastolic BP (mm Hg)**	
Normal	<120	and	<80	
Prehypertension	120–139	or	80–89	
Hypertension				
Stage 1	140–159	or	90–99	
Stage 2	≥160	or	>100	

Adapted from The Seventh Report of the Joint National Committee on Prevention, Detection, Evaluation, and Treatment of High Blood Pressure, *JAMA* 289:2560–2572, 2003.

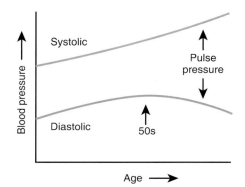

FIGURE 2-1   Blood pressure and age.

TABLE 2-2	Manifestations of Acute End-Organ Damage in Hypertensive Emergency
Hypertensive encephalopathy	Headache Altered mental status Seizures Nausea, vomiting Papilledema (see Fig. 2-2) Abnormalities on brain MRI
Intracranial hemorrhage	Headache Altered mental status Focal neurologic abnormalities Hemorrhage on brain CT
Unstable angina	Chest pain ECG abnormalities
Acute myocardial infarction	Chest pain ECG abnormalities Cardiac enzyme elevation
LV failure with pulmonary edema	Dyspnea Hypoxia Pulmonary congestion on chest radiograph
Acute aortic dissection	Chest pain Syncope End-organ ischemia
Eclampsia	Proteinuria Seizures

CT, computed tomography; ECG, electrocardiographic; LV, left ventricular; MRI, magnetic resonance imaging.

TABLE 2-3	Clinical Manifestations of Chronic Target Organ Damage in Hypertension

Heart	Left ventricular hypertrophy
	  Enlarged PMI or S_4 gallop
	  Evidence of LVH on ECG or echo
	Left ventricular dysfunction
	  Signs/symptoms of CHF
	  Enlarged PMI or S_4 gallop
	  Systolic or diastolic dysfunction on echo
	Coronary artery disease
	  Angina
	  History of MI, PTCA, or CABG

Brain	Cerebrovascular disease
	  History of stroke
	  Carotid bruit

Eyes	Retinovascular disease
	  Arteriolar narrowing
	  Arteriovenous nicking
	  Hemorrhage
	  Exudates

Vasculature	Atherosclerosis
	  Claudication
	  Diminished or absent pulses
	  Renal or femoral bruits

Kidneys	Hypertensive nephrosclerosis, ESRD
	  Proteinuria or microalbuminuria
	  Elevated serum creatinine

CABG, coronary artery bypass graft; CHF, congestive heart failure; ECG, electrocardiography; echo, echocardiography; ESRD, end-stage renal disease; LVH, left ventricular hypertrophy; MI, myocardial infarction; PMI, point of maximum impulse; PTCA, percutaneous transluminal coronary angioplasty.

- BP should be measured in both arms, and the higher of the two readings used
- By the auscultatory method, systolic BP is defined as the first appearance of sounds and diastolic pressure as the disappearance of sounds; automatic BP measuring devices use the oscillometric method, which is also acceptable
- Two or more readings on each of two separate clinical visits should be obtained before classifying a patient as hypertensive; multiple sequential readings may be obtained during a visit using an automated oscillometric device
- In elderly patients, or when orthostatic hypotension is suggested, standing BP measurements should be taken

- For home BP monitoring, BPs above 135/85 mm Hg are considered hypertensive. For 24-hour ambulatory BP monitoring, an average BP above 130/80 mm Hg is considered hypertensive.
- Goals in initial evaluation of the hypertensive patient
  - Assessment of target organ damage (Fig. 2-2; see also Table 2-3)
  - Identification of comorbidities
    - Diabetes mellitus (DM)
    - Chronic kidney disease (CKD)
    - Ischemic heart disease and cardiomyopathy

FIGURE 2-2 Papilledema in hypertension. *(From Yanoff M: Ophthalmology, ed 2, Philadelphia, Mosby, 2004, Fig. 113-7.)*

- Other cardiac risk factors: cigarette smoking, dyslipidemia, older age, obesity, physical inactivity, family history
  - Identification of identifiable (secondary) causes of hypertension (see following discussion)
- Recommended laboratory tests for initial evaluation
  - Serum creatinine, sodium, potassium, fasting glucose
  - Urinalysis with microscopic examination
  - Electrocardiogram (or echocardiogram)
  - Fasting lipid profile
  - Optional: serum calcium, thyroid-stimulating hormone
- Identifiable (secondary) causes of hypertension (Table 2-4)
  - **When to consider secondary hypertension**
    - **Sudden onset of hypertension in a previously normotensive patient**
    - **Age, history, physical examination, severity of hypertension, or initial laboratory findings suggestive of a specific cause (see Table 2-4)**
    - **Recurrence of hypertension in a previously well-controlled patient (nonadherence should also be considered)**
    - **Hypertension that is resistant to three or more drugs, including a diuretic**
  - Substances that may cause or worsen hypertension
    - Alcohol (use or withdrawal)
    - Amphetamines, cocaine
    - Over-the-counter medications (decongestants, diet pills, nonsteroidal anti-inflammatory drugs)

- Prescription medications (nonsteroidal anti-inflammatory drugs, oral contraceptives, cyclosporine, erythropoietin)
  - Supplements (ephedra)
  - Licorice (inhibits metabolism of endogenous cortisol to cortisone)
- Other correctable causes of hypertension
  - Acute pain or stress in hospitalized or institutionalized patients
  - Obstructive sleep apnea
  - Hyperthyroidism or hypothyroidism
  - Chronic kidney disease (due to renin oversecretion and impaired sodium excretion)
  - Coarctation of the aorta (very uncommon in adults)
    - Delayed femoral pulses, diminished BP in the legs, and rib notching on chest radiograph suggest the diagnosis, which is confimed with computed tomography (CT) or magnetic resonance imaging (MRI)
    - Treatment is with surgery or angioplasty

Treatment

- Initial follow-up of BP
  - The timing of follow-up for elevated BP depends on the degree of elevation (Table 2-5)
  - The suggested follow-up intervals may need to be shortened if important risk factors (e.g., diabetes) or target organ damage is present
- Risk stratification, goal BP, and therapy
  - Choice of therapy depends on the stage of hypertension and the presence of risk factors or target organ damage (Table 2-6)
  - Guidelines in the Seventh Report of the Joint National Committee on Prevention, Detection, Evaluation, and Treatment of High Blood Pressure (JNC 7) recommend initiation of two drugs for stage 2 hypertension
  - **Goal BP is 130/80 mm Hg for DM, CKD, or coronary artery disease (CAD) and 120/80 mm Hg for congestive heart failure (CHF); otherwise, the goal is 140/90 mm Hg**
  - DM, CKD, or clinical cardiovascular disease mandates drug therapy (in addition to lifestyle modification) for hypertension of any stage
- Lifestyle modification
  - **Always start with lifestyle modification even if drug therapy is also needed**
  - Weight reduction of 10 pounds or more
  - 30 minutes or more of moderately intense physical activity (e.g., brisk walking) four or more times a week
  - Moderation of alcohol intake (1 ounce or less of alcohol per day in men, ½ ounce in women)
  - Low sodium intake (100 mmol/day, i.e., 6 g NaCl or 2.4 g Na$^+$, or less)
  - Adoption of diet high in fruits, vegetables, and low-fat dairy products: Dietary Approaches to Stop Hypertension (DASH) eating plan
  - Smoking, caffeine acutely raise BP, but have not been demonstrated to cause chronic hypertension; smoking cessation and lipid modification are important for decreasing overall cardiovascular risk

TABLE 2-4	*Major Causes of Secondary Hypertension*		
Pathophysiology	**Clinical Presentation**	**Diagnosis**	**Treatment**
Renal Artery Stenosis			
Underperfused kidney produces excess renin, which increases angiotensin II (vasoconstriction) and aldosterone (sodium retention and volume expansion) Usually due to atherosclerosis, especially in older patients May also be caused by FMD, usually in younger patients	Sudden onset of significant hypertension at older (>55 yr) or younger (<30 yr) age Abdominal bruit Patient with peripheral vascular disease Unexplained deterioration in renal function Consider FMD in young females Unusually large drop in BP with ACE inhibitors or ARBs may also suggest the diagnosis	Magnetic resonance angiography—highly sensitive, no contrast required CT angiography—highly sensitive, contrast is required Doppler ultrasound—sensitivity dependent on operator skill, no contrast required Captopril radionuclide scan—less sensitive, requires discontinuation of antihypertensive medications prior to test Renal artery angiography—gold standard, invasive, may be performed with CO_2 to avoid use of iodinated contrast	Goal is to improve HTN control and preserve renal function Revascularized patients usually still require medication for BP control Statin therapy decreases progression The longer stenosis has been present, the less likely intervention will help (kidney becomes atrophic) Options Angioplasty ± stent (lesions at ostia of renal arteries often not amenable to angioplasty) Surgical bypass Surgical excision of kidney if size <8 cm Medical therapy may be best option if recovery of renal function is unlikely
Pheochromocytoma			
Tumors that originate in the adrenal medulla or sympathetic ganglia and release catecholamines periodically Most are sporadic Familial forms (20–35%) MEN IIA and IIB Neurofibromatosis von Hippel-Lindau disease (with retinal angiomas, cerebellar hemangioblastomas, and renal cell carcinoma)	Headache Sweating Palpitations Pallor Anxiety Weight loss Orthostatic hypotension Hypertension may be episodic or sustained	Screen with plasma free metanephrines, confirm with 24-hr urine for catecholamines, VMA, metanephrines Certain drugs may cause false-positive or false-negative screens If screen is positive, localize with MRI (or MIBG if MRI negative)	Surgical resection Preoperatively, patients should receive phentolamine or phenoxybenzamine to prevent crisis
Hyperaldosteronism (see Chapter 42)			
Adenoma that produces aldosterone vs. bilateral hyperplasia (zona granulosae) Rarely, aldosterone-producing carcinoma	Spontaneous hypokalemia in a hypertensive patient (may cause cramps, muscle weakness) Severe hypokalemia induced by diuretics Mild metabolic alkalosis	Screen with plasma aldosterone and renin serum—ratio of aldosterone to renin >20 suggests disease Confirm by measuring 24-hr urine aldosterone after 3 days of salt loading: >12 μg confirms disease If screen positive, localize with CT or MRI; adrenal vein sampling	Surgical resection of adenoma May try spironolactone for hyperplasia
Hypercortisolism (see Chapter 42)			
Several possible causes ACTH-secreting pituitary tumor (Cushing's disease) Adrenal adenomas Ectopic ACTH secretion Iatrogenic steroid administration	Truncal obesity Moon facies Purple striae Proximal weakness Hirsutism Hyperglycemia Osteoporosis	Screen with 24-hr urinary free cortisol, salivary cortisol, or 1-mg overnight dexamethasone suppression test If positive, perform high-dose dexamethasone suppression test and measure plasma ACTH Localize with imaging of adrenals or pituitary	Surgical resection of tumor or discontinuation of steroid therapy

ACTH, adrenocorticotropic hormone; ACE inhibitors, angiotensin-converting enzyme inhibitors; ARB, angiotensin receptor blocker; BP, blood pressure; CT, computed tomography; FMD, fibromuscular dysplasia; HTN, hypertension; MEN, multiple endocrine neoplasia; MIBG, iodine-131 metaiodobenzylguanidine; MRI, magnetic resonance imaging; VMA, vanillylmandelic acid.

2

- Relaxation therapy and stress management are of uncertain benefit in lowering BP
- Drug therapy: General principles
  - **If possible, choose agents with 24-hour duration of action and once-daily dosing**
  - **Use of two or more drugs is often necessary to attain goal BP**
- Specific agents: see Table 2-7
- Therapeutic strategy
  - **Thiazide diuretics are the agents of choice for most patients with uncomplicated hypertension**
  - **Certain comorbidities mandate the use of particular agents (see below)**
  - β-Blockers are increasingly seen as third-line agents in uncomplicated hypertension, to be used only after diuretics, calcium channel blockers, and angiotensin-converting enzyme (ACE) inhibitors or angiotensin receptor blockers (ARBs) have been tried
  - **If there is a partial but inadequate response to the first drug, either increase the dose of the first drug or add a second agent from a different class (Fig. 2-3)**

TABLE 2-5 | *Initial Management of Blood Pressure*

INITIAL BP (mm Hg)		
Systolic	**Diastolic**	**Recommended Follow-up**
<120	<80	Recheck in 2 yr
120–139	80–89	Recheck in 1 yr*
140–159	90–99	Confirm within 2 mo*
160–179	100–109	Evaluate or refer within 1 mo
≥180	≥110	Evaluate and treat immediately or within 1 wk, depending on clinical situation and complications

*Provide advice about lifestyle modification.
Adapted from The Seventh Report of the Joint National Committee on Prevention, Detection, Evaluation, and Treatment of High Blood Pressure: Hypertension, *JAMA* 42:1206, 2003.

- **Low-dose combination therapy may be preferable to higher doses of a single agent, because dose-dependent side effects are minimized**
- Formulations combining two drugs may offer improved convenience or lower cost
  - Low-dose diuretics with ACE inhibitors, β-blockers, or ARBs
  - Thiazides with potassium-sparing diuretics
  - Calcium antagonists with ACE inhibitors or ARBs
  - Three-drug combinations containing a calcium antagonist, ACE inhibitors or ARB, and diuretic are available
- If there is no response to the first drug or if the drug is not tolerated, substitute a drug from a different class
- **A diuretic should be part of any regimen containing three or more drugs**
- Short-acting loop diuretics (furosemide, bumetanide) should be dosed twice daily, or replaced with a long-acting diuretic (e.g., torsemide)
- Compelling indications for selection of initial antihypertensive agent
  - Chronic renal disease: ACE inhibitor, ARB
  - CHF: ACE inhibitor, ARB, diuretic, β-blocker, aldosterone antagonist
  - Myocardial infarction (MI): β-blocker, ACE inhibitor, aldosterone antagonist
- Other disease-specific indications
  - Migraines: β-blockers, calcium channel antagonists
  - Benign prostatic hypertrophy: α-blockers
  - Essential tremor: β-blockers
  - Hyperthyroidism: β-blockers
- Contraindications to certain antihypertensives
  - **Pregnancy: Avoid ACE inhibitors and ARBs (absolute contraindication)**
  - Asthma, chronic obstructive pulmonary disease (COPD), peripheral vascular disease: caution with β-blockers
  - Gout: avoid or minimize dose of diuretics
  - First or second degree heart block: avoid β-blockers, verapamil, or diltiazem

TABLE 2-6 | *Treatment Recommendations by Risk Group*

Blood Pressure Classification	Lifestyle Modification	INITIAL DRUG THERAPY	
		No Compelling Indication	**Compelling Indication(s) Present**
Normal (<120/80 mm Hg)	Encourage	None	None
Prehypertension (120–139/80–89 mm Hg)	Yes	None	Appropriate drug(s) for DM, CKD, or CAD if BP >130/80 mm Hg, for CHF if BP >120/80 mm Hg
Stage 1 (140–159/90–99 mm Hg)	Yes	Thiazide diuretic for most; may consider other drug classes	Appropriate drug(s) for compelling indication
Stage 2 (≥160/>100mm Hg)	Yes	Two-drug combination for most, including thiazide diuretic	Two-drug combination for most, usually including appropriate drug(s) for compelling indication

BP, blood pressure; CAD, coronary artery disease; CHF, congestive heart failure; CKD, chronic kidney disease; DM, diabetes mellitus.
Adapted from The Seventh Report of the Joint National Committee on Prevention, Detection, Evaluation, and Treatment of High Blood Pressure, *JAMA* 289:2561, 2003.

TABLE 2-7	*Antihypertensive Agents*		
Class	**Examples**	**Side Effects**	**Comments**
Thiazide diuretics	Hydrochlorothiazide Chlorthalidone Indapamide Metolazone	Hypokalemia Hyponatremia Alkalosis Hyperuricemia Dehydration Hypercalcemia	Thiazides not effective if GFR <30 mL/min Side effects rarely a problem at low doses
Loop diuretics	Furosemide Torsemide Bumetanide	As for thiazide diuretics except for hypercalcemia	Furosemide has a short half-life—dose twice a day for HTN Sodium restriction should accompany diuretics
Potassium-sparing diuretics	Distal tubule sodium channel blockers: triamterene, amiloride Aldosterone antagonists: spironolactone, eplerenone	Hyperkalemia Hyponatremia Dehydration	Often given in combination with thiazides (to prevent hypokalemia) Avoid or use with caution in renal insufficiency
β-Adrenergic antagonists (β-blockers)	β_1-selective: atenolol, metoprolol Non–β_1-selective: propranolol, nadolol α_1 and β_1 blockade: carvedilol, labetalol ISA: pindolol, acebutolol, penbutolol	Bradycardia Fatigue Insomnia Erectile dysfunction Bronchospasm in asthma and COPD patients	ISA β-blockers useful for patients with bradycardia May mask hypoglycemic symptoms in diabetics Do not use alone in cases of catecholamine excess (cocaine intoxication, pheochromocytoma) as unopposed α_1 vasoconstriction without β_2 vasodilation may increase BP precipitously
ACE inhibitors	Benazepril Captopril Enalapril Fosinopril Lisinopril Moexipril Perindopril Quinapril Ramipril Trandolapril	Cough Angioedema Hyperkalemia Decrease in CKD, renovascular disease, CHF, or dehydration	Inhibit the renin-angiotensin-aldosterone system by blocking conversion of angiotensin I to angiotensin II Dilate renal efferent arterioles Also inhibit degradation of bradykinin, which may lead to cough Avoid in pregnancy; teratogenic
ARBs	Azilsartan Candesartan Eprosartan Irbesartan Losartan Olmesartan Telmisartan Valsartan	Minimal	Inhibit the renin-angiotensin-aldosterone system by blocking the angiotensin II receptor Avoid in pregnancy; teratogenic
α-Adrenergic antagonists	Doxazosin Prazosin Terazosin	Orthostatic hypotension	Block postsynaptic α_1 receptors, causing vasodilation Favorable effect on lipid profile and glucose level May increase CHD mortality if used as a single agent
Non-dihydropyridine calcium antagonists	Verapamil Diltiazem	Bradycardia, heart block Decreased cardiac contractility Constipation	Verapamil may increase cyclosporine and digoxin levels
Dihydropyridine calcium antagonists	Amlodipine Felodipine Isradipine Nicardipine Nifedipine Nisoldipine	Headache Flushing Tachycardia Pedal edema	Dilate arterioles Possible increased heart rate Short-acting nifedipine causes marked reflex tachycardia and is *not* recommended for HTN Nifedipine increases cyclosporine levels

TABLE 2-7	Antihypertensive Agents (continued)		
Class	Examples	Side Effects	Comments
Direct vasodilators	Minoxidil Hydralazine	Headache Tachycardia Fluid retention Minoxidil Hirsutism Pericardial effusion Hydralazine Drug-induced lupus	Considered third-line agents

Central adrenergic inhibitors	Clonidine
	Guanfacine
	Methyldopa
	Reserpine
		Clonidine, guanfacine
		Sedation
		Dry mouth
		Withdrawal hypertension
		Methyldopa
		Coombs-positive hemolytic
		  anemia
		Liver toxicity
			Inhibit sympathetic outflow
			  from CNS
			Clonidine also available in patch
			Methyldopa safe in pregnancy

ACE inhibitors, angiotensin-converting enzyme inhibitors; ARBs, angiotensin receptor blockers; BP, blood pressure; CHD, coronary heart disease; CHF, congestive heart failure; CKD, chronic kidney disease; CNS, central nervous system, COPD, chronic obstructive pulmonary disease; GFR, glomerular filtration rate; HTN, hypertension; ISA, intrinsic sympathomimetic activity.

FIGURE 2-3 Hypertension treatment algorithm. (ACEI, angiotensin-converting enzyme inhibitor; ARB, angiotensin receptor blocker; BB, β-blocker; CCB, calcium channel blocker.)

TABLE 2-8	*Drugs Used in Treatment of Hypertensive Emergency*	
Drug	**Indication**	**Precaution**
Nitroprusside	Most emergencies	Thiocyanate toxicity
Nitroglycerin	Angina, MI	Headache, tolerance
Nicardipine	Most emergencies	Tachycardia
Labetalol	Most emergencies	CHF, bradycardia
Fenoldopam	Most emergencies	Tachycardia
Enalaprilat	CHF	Rapid, unpredictable BP drop
Esmolol	Perioperative, aortic dissection	Nausea

BP, blood pressure; CHF, congestive heart failure; MI, myocardial infarction.

- Treatment of hypertensive urgency and emergency
  - Hypertensive urgency (severely elevated BP without acutely progressive end-organ damage):
    - Gradual control of BP using oral agents and outpatient follow-up is appropriate
    - Short-acting nifedipine or clonidine is not indicated
  - Hypertensive emergency (severely elevated BP with acutely progressive end-organ damage):
    - BP must be brought down immediately via admission to an intensive care unit and administration of intravenous medication
    - Intravenous medication is used for rapid effect and ability to titrate (Table 2-8)

- Initial goal is to lower mean arterial BP by approximately 25%, but not more, within 2 hours
- Subsequent goal is to lower BP to approximately 160/100 mm Hg over next 2 to 24 hours (reduce BP further as tolerated for aortic dissection)

Prevention

- Patients with prehypertension (BP <140/90 mm Hg and >120/80 mm Hg) should be provided counseling for lifestyle modification to decrease their risk of progression to hypertension

REVIEW QUESTIONS

For review questions, please go to www.expertconsult.com.

SUGGESTED READINGS

Izzo JL, Black HR, editors: *Hypertension primer: the essentials of high blood pressure*, ed 3, Baltimore, 2003, Lippincott Williams & Wilkins.

Kaplan NM: *Clinical hypertension*, ed 9, Baltimore, 2006, Lippincott Williams & Wilkins.

Oparil S, Weber MA, editors: *Hypertension: a companion to Brenner and Rector's the kidney*, ed 2, Philadelphia, 2005, WB Saunders.

The Seventh Report of the Joint National Committee on Prevention: Detection, Evaluation, and Treatment of High Blood Pressure: Hypertension, JAMA 42:1206–1252, 2003. [The comprehensive, unabridged version of the JNC 7 report.].

The Seventh Report of the Joint National Committee on Prevention: Detection, Evaluation, and Treatment of High Blood Pressure, JAMA 289:2560–2572, 2003. [The "express," or abbreviated, version of the JNC 7 report.]

CHAPTER 3

Lipid Disorders

LORI M. TAM, MD; ANDREW P. DeFILIPPIS, MD, MSc; and
ROGER S. BLUMENTHAL, MD

Lipid disorders (dyslipidemias) are important risk factors for the development of atherosclerotic vascular disease. Many of the disorders result from both genetic and environmental factors. The Adult Treatment Panel III report and 2004 modification of the treatment algorithm summarize guidelines for cholesterol testing and management and provide a useful resource for clinicians.

Basic Information

- Cholesterol
  - Involved in vital functions such as cell membrane biogenesis, steroid synthesis, and bile acid formation
  - Liver is the primary producer of endogenous cholesterol and the main processor of dietary cholesterol
  - Cholesterol is produced when 3-hydroxy-3-methyl-glutaryl coenzyme A (HMG-CoA) is converted to mevalonic acid by HMG-CoA reductase
- Lipoproteins
  - Spherical complexes of lipid core and outer protein monolayer that transport lipids such as cholesterol and triglyceride in the circulation
  - **Most common classification divides lipoprotein particles according to increasing density;** a patient's cholesterol levels are most commonly expressed as the concentration of cholesterol in each of the individual lipoprotein particle groups as follows:
    - Chylomicrons
    - Very-low-density lipoprotein (VLDL)
    - Intermediate-density lipoprotein (IDL)
    - Low-density lipoprotein (LDL)
    - High-density lipoprotein (HDL)
- Chylomicrons
  - Intestinal triglyceride-rich lipoproteins responsible for transporting dietary fat and cholesterol to the body
  - Synthesized by the intestinal epithelial cells from fatty acids
  - Increased fat consumption during meals leads to increased chylomicrons in the blood
  - Lipoprotein lipase hydrolyzes free fatty acids from chylomicrons, leaving chylomicron remnants
- VLDL
  - Synthesized in the liver from free fatty acids obtained from chylomicron catabolism (dietary fat) and from endogenously produced triglycerides (generated from excess dietary protein and carbohydrate)
  - Hydrolyzed by lipoprotein lipase and converted to smaller particles (IDL) and then into LDL
- LDL
  - **Principal cholesterol-containing lipoprotein and a major atherogenic lipoprotein**

- Approximately 25% of LDL is cleared by the peripheral tissues
- Approximately 75% of LDL is returned to the liver, primarily via the LDL receptors
- LDL receptor expression by hepatic cells regulates cholesterol homeostasis
  - Decreased level of cholesterol in hepatocytes leads to an increase in LDL receptor density, causing a greater clearance of LDL
  - Increased dietary saturated fatty acids decrease the production of hepatic LDL receptors, which can contribute to hypercholesterolemia
  - Dietary cholesterol inhibits the production of endogenous cholesterol, but once endogenous cholesterol production is fully suppressed, additional dietary cholesterol may result in increased serum cholesterol
- HDL
  - Small lipoprotein that participates in reverse cholesterol transport from the arteries back to the liver
  - **Levels are generally inversely associated with the risk of atherosclerotic vascular disease**
- Apolipoproteins
  - Major structural protein components of lipoproteins embedded in the surface monolayer
  - Affect the metabolism of lipoproteins by activating enzymes and aiding receptor-mediated processes
  - Are divided into five classes (apo A–apo E)
    - apo A–containing lipoproteins are associated with a reduction in atherosclerosis
    - apo B–containing lipoproteins are associated with an increased risk of atherosclerosis
- Lipoprotein(a) [Lp(a)]
  - Assembled from an LDL particle and apolipoprotein (a) [apo(a)]
  - Elevated levels of Lp(a) are associated with an increased risk of vascular disease

Clinical Presentation

- Many patients are asymptomatic until coronary heart disease (CHD) develops
- Physical signs
  - Minority of patients with lipid disorders have physical signs that suggest a diagnosis (Table 3-1 and Figs. 3-1 and 3-2)
  - Tendinous xanthomas
    - Nontender, firm nodules that appear on the extensor surfaces of various tendons, including Achilles tendon, extensor tendons of the hands, patellar tendons
    - More prominent as subjects age

TABLE 3-1			*Characteristics of Various Lipid Disorders*		
Name	**Phenotype**	**Abnormal Lipid**	**Defect**	**Possible Clinical Findings**	**Risk of CHD**
Familial hypercholesterolemia	IIa	↑ LDL	Defective LDL receptor or apo B-100; heterozygous and homozygous forms	Tendinous xanthomas Xanthelasma Planar xanthomas Corneal arcus	+++
Familial lipoprotein lipase deficiency	I	↑ Chylomicrons	Lipoprotein lipase deficiency	Eruptive xanthomas Lipemia retinalis Abdominal pain Hepatosplenomegaly	0
Familial hypertriglyceridemia	IV	↑ VLDL	Reduction of activity of lipoprotein lipase	Often asymptomatic	+
	V	↑ VLDL, chylomicrons	Acquired lipoprotein, lipase dysfunction, and chylomicronemia	Often asymptomatic	+
Combined hyperlipidemia	IIb	↑ VLDL, LDL	Excessive secretion of apo B containing particles	Often asymptomatic except for CHD	+++
Familial dysbetalipoproteinemia	III	↑ VLDL, IDL	apo E polymorphism	Tuberoeruptive xanthomas Hyperuricemia Glucose intolerance Corneal opacities Yellow-orange discoloration of palmar creases	+++
Lecithin-cholesterol acetyltransferase (LCAT) deficiency	N/A	↓ HDL	Reduced ability to esterify cholesterol	Renal insufficiency Hemolytic anemia "Fish-eye disease" in mild form	+
Tangier disease	N/A	↓ HDL	Reduced ability to esterify cholesterol	Corneal opacities Polyneuropathy Orange tonsils	+
Gain of function of proprotein convertase subtilisin-like kexin type 9 (PSCK9)	N/A	↑ LDL	Increase in LDL receptor degradation	None	0

apo, apolipoprotein; CHD, coronary heart disease; HDL, high-density lipoprotein; IDL, intermediate-density lipoprotein; LDL, low-density lipoprotein; VLDL, very low-density lipoprotein; ↑, increase; ↓, decrease.

- Xanthelasma (palpebral xanthomas)
  - Soft, off-white plaques
  - Originate near the eyelids
- Corneal arcus (arcus senilis)
  - Arcus is composed of cholesterol ester deposited in the peripheral cornea
  - Appears as a normal variant in white patients older than 40 years but a sign of hypercholesterolemia in white adults younger than 40 years
- Tuberous xanthomas
  - Raised, yellowish nodules about 0.5 to 1 cm in diameter
  - Found in areas of pressure such as elbows and knees
- Lipemia retinalis
  - Pink discoloration of the retinal vessels
  - May be seen on funduscopic examination
- Eruptive xanthomas
  - Small, light yellow papules on a reddish base
  - May be present on arms, thighs, and buttocks

Diagnosis and Evaluation

- Phenotyping—describing the clinical lipid profile
  - Often classified into types I through V based on levels of LDL and VLDL

- Several familial (hereditary) forms of primary hyperlipidemia exist (see Table 3-1)
- Many patients have primary idiopathic hyperlipidemia
  - Secondary dyslipidemia (caused by a concomitant disorder)
  - Sedentary lifestyle with caloric excess and excessive consumption of saturated and *trans*–fatty acids and the lack of consumption of foods rich in fiber and nutrients (fruits, vegetables, whole grains) and mono- and polyunsaturated fatty acids (fish, nuts, seeds, olive and canola oil) is by far the most common cause of dyslipidemia in industrialized countries, but other causes need to be considered in all patients
  - Elevated LDL differential diagnosis: hypothyroidism, chronic liver disease, cholestasis, nephrotic syndrome
  - Hypertriglyceridemia differential diagnosis: alcohol consumption, obesity, pregnancy, diabetes mellitus, hypothyroidism, chronic renal failure, medications (nonselective β-blockers, high-dose diuretics, oral estrogen replacement therapy, oral contraceptives)

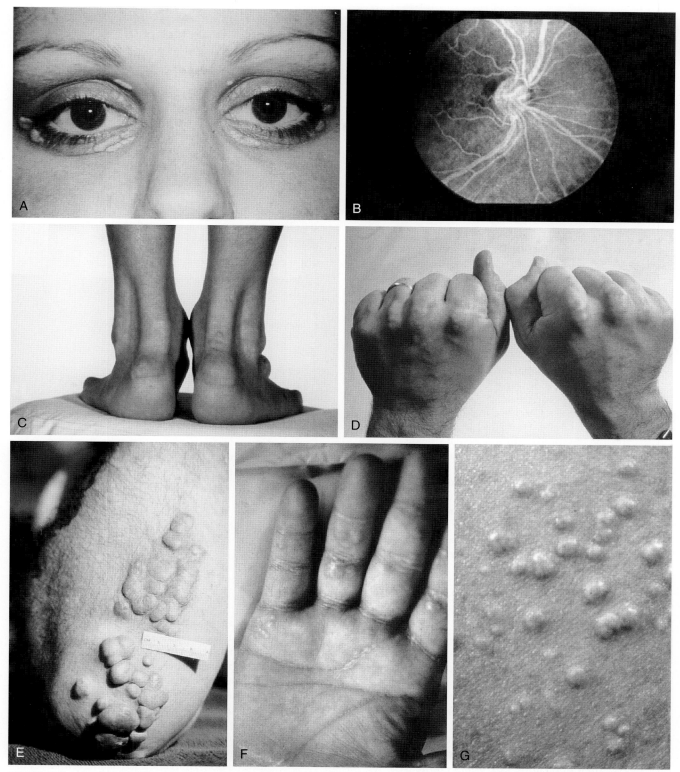

3

FIGURE 3-1 Physical findings of hyperlipidemia. **A,** Xanthelasma. **B,** Lipemia retinalis. **C,** Achilles tendon xanthomas. Note the marked thickening of the tendons. **D,** Tendon xanthomas. **E,** Tuberous xanthomas. **F,** Palmar xanthomas. **G,** Eruptive xanthomas. (A and B courtesy of Dr. Mark Dresner and Hospital Practice [May 1990, p 15]. C to F courtesy of Dr. Tom Bersot. G, Courtesy of Dr. Alan Chait. From Larsen PR, Kronenberg HM, Melmed S, et al: Williams textbook of endocrinology, ed 10, Philadelphia, WB Saunders, 2003, Fig. 34-26.)

FIGURE 3-2 Corneal arcus (arcus senilis). Corneal arcus in an elderly man. (From Yanoff M, Fine BS: Ocular pathology, ed 5, St. Louis, Mosby, 2002, Fig. 60-4.)

TABLE 3-2	Adult Treatment Panel III Classification of LDL, Total, and HDL (mg/dL)
LDL	
<100	Optimal
100–129	Near or above optimal
130–159	Borderline high
160–189	High
≥190	Very high
Total Cholesterol	
<200	Desirable
200–239	Borderline high
≥240	High
HDL	
<40	Low
≥60	High

HDL, high-density lipoprotein; LDL, low-density lipoprotein.

- Low HDL differential diagnosis: smoking, diabetes mellitus, obesity, sedentary lifestyle, hypertriglyceridemia, medications (progestins, anabolic steroids, corticosteroids)
- Type B pattern
  - Apolipoprotein B measurement numerically greater than the LDL, indicating the presence of small, dense atherogenic particles
  - These patients often have impaired fibrinolysis, endothelial dysfunction, and an accelerated progression of atherosclerotic vascular disease
  - This pattern is typical of the metabolic syndrome
- CHD risk assessment
  - **Adults age 20 years or older should have fasting lipoprotein analysis (total cholesterol [TC], LDL, HDL, and triglycerides) at least once every 5 years**
  - **In nonfasting sample, only the values for TC, HDL, and non-HDL cholesterol are generally accurate**
  - Adult Treatment Panel III (ATP III) guidelines suggest the intensity of risk reduction therapy; should be adjusted to a person's absolute risk of developing CHD
  - ATP III classification (Table 3-2)
- Risk categories, Framingham Risk Score (FRS), and LDL goals
  - ATP III recommends assessment of the CHD risk status of a person without CHD or other forms of atherosclerotic vascular disease
  - **Assess number of risk factors for heart disease (Box 3-1)**
  - **If two or more risk factors are present, estimate 10-year risk of myocardial infarction (MI) or CHD death, then determine LDL goals (Table 3-3)**
  - Ten-year risk assessment uses revised FRS with risk factors of age, TC, HDL, blood pressure, and cigarette smoking (details in ATP III guidelines)
  - **Zero to 1 risk factor**
    - **Minimal LDL goal of less than 160 mg/dL**
    - Patients typically have a 10-year risk of CHD less than 10%
  - Two or more risk factors

BOX 3-1	Major Risk Factors (Exclusive of LDL) That Modify LDL Goals

Cigarette smoking

Hypertension (BP ≥140/90 mm Hg or prescription of an antihypertensive medication)

Low HDL (≤40 mg/dL)

Family history of premature CHD (CHD in father, brother, or son <55 yr of age; CHD in mother, sister, or daughter <65 yr of age)

Age (men ≥45 yr; women ≥55 yr)

An HDL ≥60 mg/dL is a negative risk factor, and its presence removes one risk factor from the total count

BP, blood pressure; CHD, coronary heart disease; HDL, high-density lipoprotein; LDL, low-density lipoprotein.

- **10-year CHD risk less than 10%**
  - LDL goal of less than 130 mg/dL
- **10-year CHD risk 10% to 20%**
  - LDL goal of less than 130 mg/dL with optional goal of less than 100 mg/dL
  - Optional LDL goal of less than 100 mg/dL should be strongly considered for patients in this risk category with more than two risk factors, severe risk factors (e.g., significant family history of CHD), advanced age, elevated triglyceride with elevated non-HDL cholesterol and low HDL, or the metabolic syndrome
  - Emerging risk factors may also be considered (electron beam computed tomography [EBCT] or multidetector computed tomography [MDCT] showing high coronary calcium burden [>75th percentile for age and sex] or high-sensitivity C-reactive protein (hs-CRP) >2 mg/L)

TABLE 3-3	*LDL Goals and Cutpoints for Drug Therapy*	
Risk Category	**LDL Goal**	**LDL Level at Which to Consider Drug Therapy**
CHD or CHD risk equivalents	<100 mg/dL (Optional: <70 mg/dL)	≥100 mg/dL (>70 mg/dL: consider treatment)
2 or more risk factors	<130 mg/dL (Optional: <100 mg/dL)	10-year risk of 10–20%: ≥130 mg/dL (≥100 mg/dL: consider treatment) 10-year risk of <10%: ≥160 mg/dL
0–1 risk factor	<160 mg/dL	≥190 mg/dL (160–189 mg/dL: drug therapy optional)

CHD, coronary heart disease; LDL, low-density lipoprotein.
Adapted from Grundy SM, Cleeman JL, Merz CN, et al: Implications of recent clinical trials for the National Cholesterol Education Program Adult Treatment Panel III guidelines, *Circulation* 110:227–239, 2004.

- Known CHD (MI or >50% stenosis by angiography) and CHD equivalents
  - CHD equivalents refer to a risk for major coronary events equal to that of established CHD (>20% per 10 years of developing CHD death or nonfatal MI), and include
    - Other forms of atherosclerotic disease
    - Peripheral arterial disease
    - Abdominal aortic aneurysm
    - Carotid artery disease—transient ischemic attack or stroke of carotid origin or greater than 50% obstruction of a carotid artery
    - Diabetes
      - Confers a high risk of new CHD events within 10 years
      - Diabetic patients who experience an MI have a significantly worse prognosis than nondiabetics of similar age
    - Multiple risk factors that confer a greater than 20% 10-year risk for CHD
- Metabolic syndrome (Table 3-4)
  - **A condition associated with a constellation of factors related to insulin resistance, including**
    - **Abdominal obesity**
    - **Atherogenic/type B dyslipidemia (low HDL, elevated triglycerides, small LDL particles)**
    - **Increased blood pressure**
    - **Glucose intolerance**
    - **Prothrombotic and proinflammatory states**
  - The abnormal findings in the metabolic syndrome are secondary targets of risk-reduction therapy
  - Metabolic syndrome may be considered a "prediabetic" state, increasing CHD risk
    - Fulfillment of diagnostic criteria may warrant reevaluation of a person's ATP III risk classification
  - Lifestyle modification is initial, primary therapy for persons with metabolic syndrome
- Limitations of Framingham-based ATP III risk categorization
  - **Although clinically valuable, the FRS may underestimate a person's true atherosclerotic vascular disease risk, especially for women (this includes risk for angina requiring revascularization, stroke, and congestive heart failure)**
  - Based on published guidelines, it is difficult for women to qualify for statin and aspirin therapy (i.e., FRS ≥10% over 10 years)

TABLE 3-4	*Clinical Identification of the Metabolic Syndrome**
Risk Factor	**Defining Level**
Abdominal obesity (waist circumference) In men In women	 >40 inches >35 inches
Triglycerides	≥150 mg/dL
HDL In men In women	 <40 mg/dL <50 mg/dL
Blood pressure	≥130/85 mm Hg
Fasting glucose	≥100 mg/dL

HDL, high-density lipoprotein.
*Three or more risk factors are required for the diagnosis.

- Women are less likely than men to present with an MI as the initial manifestation of cardiovascular disease
- The latest American Heart Association (AHA) Prevention Guidelines in women suggests using a cardiovascular disease (CVD) (MI/CHF/cerebrovascular accident [CVA] and peripheral artery disease [PAD]) risk ≥10% to designate higher risk status given the higher prevalence of CVA in women
- Several factors not considered by the FRS should be considered to reassess and refine CHD risk prediction
  - Is there a family history of premature cardiovascular disease?
  - Diagnosis of the metabolic syndrome, in particular, those with elevated triglycerides, increased waist circumference, and sedentary lifestyle
  - Extent of smoking history
- Emerging risk factors
  - An elevated hs-CRP above 2 mg/dL is generally associated with a doubling of predicted relative risk
  - Consider measuring hs-CRP or coronary calcium burden (EBCT or MDCT) if FRS 10-year risk is 6 to 20% to refine intensity of risk-factor reduction
- Screening in asymptomatic adults (Class IIa recommendations)
  - Measurement of coronary artery calcium is reasonable for cardiovascular risk assessment in asymptomatic patients at intermediate risk (10–20% 10-year risk).

- Measurement of hs-CRP may be reasonable for cardio-vascular risk assessment in intermediate-risk men ≤50 years of age or women ≤60 years of age.
- Measurement of hs-CRP can be considered to help select patients for statin therapy in men greater than 50 years of age or women greater than 60 years of age with LDL less than 130 mg/dL who are not on lipid-lowering, hormone replacement, or immunosuppressant therapy; without clinical CHD, diabetes, chronic kidney disease, severe inflammatory conditions, or contraindications to statins
- Measurement of carotid artery intimal-medial thickness is reasonable for cardiovascular risk assessment in intermediate-risk asymptomatic patients. The test should be performed in compliance with published recommendations on required equipment, technical approach, and operator training and experience to achieve high-quality results.
- Measurement of lipoproteins, apolipoproteins, and particle size and density is not recommended in asymptomatic patients, with an exception for patients with metabolic syndrome to assess the adequacy of lipid-lowering therapy (goal apo B level is <90)

Treatment

- **Lifestyle modification is the cornerstone of lipid management**
  - Therapeutic lifestyle changes
    - Weight reduction if overweight
    - Increased physical activity
      - Daily energy expenditure should include at least moderately brisk physical activity, contributing at least 200 kcal/day
      - **Brisk aerobic activity should be undertaken for at least 30 minutes, three to four times per week (>10,000 steps per day)**
    - Implement a diet that is rich in fruits, vegetables, whole grains, fish, lean meats; and low saturated fat or nonfat dairy products and low in simple carbohydrates, sugars, *trans* and saturated fatty acids
      - Recommended intake of saturated fat less than 7% of total calories, and recommended cholesterol intake less than 200 mg/day
      - Majority of carbohydrates should be from foods rich in complex carbohydrates such as whole grains, fruits, and vegetables
    - For primary prevention: Consume fish (preferably fatty fish) a minimum of twice per week and include foods and oils rich in alpha-linolenic acid in the diet
    - For secondary prevention: Consume approximately 1 g of eicosapentaenoic acid (EPA) + docosahexaenoic acid (DHA) every day, preferably from fatty fish
    - EPA + DHA (fish oil) supplements could be considered in consultation with a physician
  - Pharmacologic options
    - Statins
      - Cholesterol is produced when HMG-CoA is converted into mevalonic acid by HMG-CoA reductase

- Statins work by inhibiting this conversion and by promoting up-regulation of LDL receptors on the surface of hepatocytes
- Options: atorvastatin, fluvastatin, lovastatin, pravastatin, simvastatin, rosuvastatin, pitavastatin
- **Lower LDL by 20% to 60% (more than most other agents)**
- Raise HDL by 5% to 15%
- Lower triglyceride levels by 10% to 35%
- **Statins have been shown to decrease total mortality rates, decrease CHD events, slow progression of CHD, and decrease recurrent episodes of unstable angina requiring hospitalization**
- Side effects: Myositis and increased liver enzymes occur less than 3% of the time and often resolve without intervention or dose reduction
- Myalgias are a more common side effect in statin- than placebo-treated patients (5–10%); the frequency depends on a person's age and the number of and type of concomitant medications
- Beware of increased incidence of rhabdomyolysis (very rare at <1% but potentially fatal), especially when used in combination with gemfibrozil and macrolide antibiotics
- Lipid and hepatic profiles should be repeated 6 to 12 weeks after initiation or dose titration
  - Once goals achieved, lipid and hepatic profiles should generally be checked about every 12 months
- Ezetimibe
  - Inhibits cholesterol absorption at the brush border of the small intestine
  - Decreases delivery of cholesterol to the liver, reducing hepatic stores and increasing hepatic uptake from the blood
  - Lowers LDL by 15% to 25%
  - May be given as monotherapy or in conjunction with a statin to lower LDL cholesterol
  - Side effects: abdominal and back pain, diarrhea, fatigue
  - Not yet proven to reduce CVD events, and it has shown variable effects on carotid intimal-medial thickness in trials
- Resins (cholestyramine, colestipol, colesevelam)
  - Also known as bile acid sequestrants
  - Lower LDL by 10% to 25%, depending on the dose and agent used
  - Work synergistically with statins
  - Some types of resins decrease the absorption of other drugs
  - Resins may raise triglycerides
  - Side effects: gastrointestinal symptoms (bloating, cramping, flatulence)
  - Small but statistically significant reduction in CVD events as monotherapy
- Nicotinic acid (niacin)
  - Lowers LDL by 5% to 25%
  - **Raises HDL by 15% to 35% (more than most other agents)**

- Lowers triglyceride levels by 20% to 40%
- Extended-release niacin has been shown to slow progression of carotid intimal-medial thickness, but no data yet on clinical events to show benefit of statin + niacin vs. niacin alone
- Side effects: flushing, hyperuricemia, hyperglycemia (in high doses), gastrointestinal distress, and hepatotoxicity
  - Flushing may be ameliorated by premedication with aspirin
- Modest long-term decrease in mortality rates in patients following MI
- Fibrates (gemfibrozil, fenofibrate)
  - **Lower triglycerides by 25% to 50% (more than most other agents)**
  - Raise HDL by 10% to 20%
  - Lower LDL by 5% to 20%
  - **Persons with type 2 diabetes: Reduce CHD events, but do not reduce CHD mortality rate**
    - Effects on triglycerides and HDL useful in managing atherogenic dyslipidemia seen in diabetes
    - Should not be used as a substitute for statins in the lowering of LDL (for which decreased mortality rates have been observed)
  - Side effects: dyspepsia, myalgias, and gallstones
  - No proven benefit to adding fibrates to statin therapy in patients with diabetes who do not have high triglycerides

Approach to the Patient

Figure 3-3 illustrates a management algorithm for LDL.
- Measurement of lipids
  - Fasting lipid profile beginning at age 20 years
    - If nonfasting, only TC and HDL values are accurate
    - If normal, repeat measurement in 5 years
    - If abnormal, pursue appropriate therapy
  - **All patients hospitalized for a suggested coronary event should have lipid profile within 24 hours**
  - Emerging risk factors not routinely measured: Lp(a), hs-CRP, apo B, LDL particle number, prothrombotic and proinflammatory factors
- Drug therapy to achieve LDL goals:
  - Goals and LDL levels at which to consider therapy are per updated ATP III guidelines (see Table 3-3)
  - **LDL goal of less than 100 mg/dL with optional goal of less than 70 mg/dL for CHD and CHD equivalents**
  - This optional LDL goal of less than 70 mg/dL should be considered for very high-risk patients, which includes patients with established CHD and other severe risk factors such as diabetes, the metabolic syndrome, or resistant hypertension

- Trial of diet therapy for 4 to 6 months is reasonable first-line therapy in most patients with moderately elevated LDL and no known atherosclerotic vascular disease
- If not successful, statins are often first-line choice
- If LDL goal not achieved, a higher dose of the medication or an additional type of medication should be considered
  - Ezetimibe, fibrates, niacin, and resins may be considered for combination therapy
- Management of triglyceride disorders
  - Classification
    - Normal triglycerides: less than 150 mg/dL
    - Borderline high: 150 to 199 mg/dL
    - High: 200 to 499 mg/dL
    - Very high: greater than 500 mg/dL
  - Triglyceride levels above 150 mg/dL are associated with smaller, denser LDL particles
  - Weight reduction, increased physical activity, and decreased alcohol intake (if relevant) are important lifestyle modifications
  - Ingestion of omega-3 fatty acids can be beneficial
    - When triglyceride levels are greater than 500 mg/dL, a fibrate is often the preferred initial drug choice
  - The sum of LDL plus VLDL cholesterol is termed non-HDL cholesterol and represents the majority of atherogenic (apo B) lipoproteins in the serum
    - Is a secondary target of therapy in persons with high triglycerides
    - Measured as "TC minus HDL"
    - **Goal for non-HDL in person with high triglycerides is 30 mg/dL higher than for LDL, in that a VLDL less than 30 mg/dL is normal (Table 3-5)**
    - The non-HDL can be lowered by lifestyle changes, as well as through more aggressive drug therapy to lower triglycerides and/or LDL
- Management of low HDL
  - Exercise may raise HDL
  - **Nicotinic acid is the most effective drug for raising HDL**
  - Certain statins may be somewhat more effective than others in raising HDL

Acknowledgment

We are grateful to Dr. J. Gabriel Schneider for his help in preparing the initial draft of this chapter.

REVIEW QUESTIONS

For review questions, please go to www.expertconsult.com.

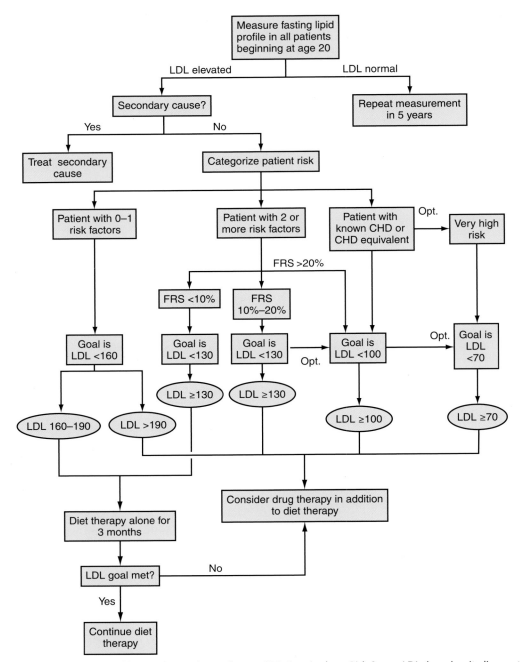

FIGURE 3-3 Approach to the patient. (CHD, coronary heart disease; FRS, Framingham Risk Score; LDL, low-density lipoprotein; Opt., optional.)

TABLE 3-5	Comparision of LDL and Non-HDL Goals for Three Risk Categories	
Risk Category	**LDL-C Goal (mg/dL)**	**TC minus HDL-C Goal (mg/dL)**
CHD and CHD risk equivalent	<100 (Optional: <70)	<130 (<100)
2+ risk factors and 10-year risk ≤20%	<130 (Optional: <100)	<160 (<130)
0–1 risk factor	<160	<190

CHD, coronary heart disease; HDL, high-density lipoprotein; LDL, low-density lipoprotein; TC, total cholesterol.

SUGGESTED READINGS

Ashen MD, Blumenthal RS: Clinical practice: low HDL cholesterol levels, *N Engl J Med* 353:1252–1260, 2005.

Ballantyne CM, O'Keefe JH Jr, Gotto A Jr: *Dyslipidemia essentials*, Houston, 2005, Physicians' Press.

Brunzell JD, Davidson M, Furberg CD, et al: Lipoprotein management in patients with cardiometabolic risk, *J Am Coll Cardiol* 51:1512–1524, 2008.

Cui Y, Blumenthal RS, Flaws JA, et al: Non-high-density lipoprotein cholesterol level as a predictor of cardiovascular disease mortality, *Arch Intern Med* 161:1413–1419, 2001.

Expert Panel on Detection, Evaluation, and Treatment of High Blood Cholesterol in Adults: executive summary of the third report of the National Cholesterol Education Program (NCEP) Expert panel on Detection, Evaluation, and Treatment of High Blood Cholesterol in Adults (Adult Treatment Panel III), *JAMA* 285:2486–2497, 2001.

Ginsberg HN, Elam MB, Lovato LC, et al: for the ACCORD study group: Effects of combination lipid therapy in type 2 diabetes mellitus, *N Engl J Med* 362:1563–1574, 2010.

Gluckman TJ, Baranowski B, Ashen MD, et al: A practical and evidence-based approach to cardiovascular disease risk reduction, *Arch Intern Med* 164:1490–1500, 2004.

Greenland P, Alpert JS, Beller GA, et al: 2010 ACCF/AHA Guideline for the Assessment of Cardiovascular Risk in Asymptomatic Adults: a report of the American College of Cardiology Foundation/American Heart Association Task Force on Practice Guidelines, *Circulation* 122:e584–e636, 2010.

Lakoski SG, Greenland P, Wong ND, et al: Coronary artery calcium scores and risk for cardiovascular events in women classified as "low risk" based on Framingham risk score: the Multi-Ethnic Study of Atherosclerosis (MESA), *Arch Intern Med* 167:2437–2442, 2007.

Mosca L, Benjamin EJ, Berra K, et al: Effectiveness-based guidelines for the prevention of cardiovascular disease in women—2011 update, *Circulation* 123:1243–1262, 2011.

Mudd JO, Borlaug BA, Johnston PV, et al: Beyond low-density lipoprotein cholesterol: defining the role of low-density lipoprotein heterogeneity in coronary artery disease, *J Am Coll Cardiol* 50:1735–1741, 2007.

Ridker PM, Danielson E, Fonseca FA, et al: Rosuvastatin to prevent vascular events in men and women with elevated C-reactive protein, *N Engl J Med* 359:2195–2207, 2008.

Scandinavian Simvastatin Survival Study Group: Randomized trial of cholesterol lowering in 4444 persons with coronary heart disease: the Scandinavian Simvastatin Survival Study (4S), *Lancet* 44:1383–1389, 1994.

Smith SC Jr, Allen JA, Blair SN, et al: AHA/ACC guidelines for secondary prevention for patients with coronary and other atherosclerotic vascular disease: 2006 update, *Circulation* 113:2363–2372, 2006.

Coronary Artery Disease

VISHAL C. MEHRA, MD, PhD; and ILAN S. WITTSTEIN, MD

In the United States, over 12 million people suffer from coronary artery disease (CAD), and the cost of caring for these patients is over $120 billion per year. Despite great advances in treatment, CAD remains the leading cause of death for both men and women in the United States, with approximately 1 million people dying from it each year; roughly 25% of these deaths occur suddenly.

Chronic Coronary Artery Disease

Basic Information

- Atherogenesis
  - The endothelial cells lining the coronary arteries have two major roles
    - Regulation of vascular tone by vasodilation (e.g., nitric oxide) and vasoconstriction (e.g., endothelin, angiotensin-converting enzyme [ACE])
    - Prevention of intravascular thrombosis (e.g., prostacyclin, plasminogen)
  - Numerous insults can impair normal endothelial function
    - Insults can be hemodynamic (e.g., shear stress, hypertension); chemical (e.g., low-density lipoprotein [LDL], modified LDL, homocysteine); or even biologic (e.g., viruses, bacteria, immune complexes)
    - Insults can affect both epicardial vessels and microvessels
  - Atherosclerotic plaque formation
    - Begins with interruption of endothelial cell integrity
    - Leukocytes, mostly macrophages, are attracted to the site of injury, where they collect lipids and coalesce to form the soft lipid core of a growing plaque
    - Earliest lesion of atherosclerosis is the fatty streak, made up mostly of lipid-laden macrophages containing cholesterol ester droplets
    - Chemoattractants (e.g., platelet-derived growth factor) cause smooth muscle cells to migrate to the site of the atheroma, where they produce collagen and fibrous tissue that contribute to plaque formation
    - The atherosclerotic plaque is covered by a layer of connective tissue called the fibrous cap
    - Most acute coronary syndromes (ACSs) occur when the fibrous cap ruptures, leading to thrombus formation (see the later section on Acute Coronary Syndromes)

- **It is the characteristics of a plaque, not its size, that determine its vulnerability; a large, fibrotic plaque with a thick cap is often more stable and less prone to rupture than a small plaque with a soft lipid core and a thin fibrous cap**
- Pathophysiology of chronic CAD or chronic stable angina
  - **Fundamental problem is an imbalance between myocardial oxygen supply and demand**
  - Symptoms occur during periods of exercise or stress when increased myocardial oxygen demand (e.g., from an increase in heart rate, contractility, afterload, or wall stress) is inadequately met because of impaired coronary blood flow
  - Insufficient coronary flow can occur in one of two major ways:
    - Impaired from stenotic plaque
    - Impaired flow in the absence of severe luminal narrowing because of inadequate coronary flow reserve due to endothelial dysfunction (i.e., insufficient vasodilatory response during exercise)

Clinical Presentation

- **Risk factors for coronary atherosclerosis (Table 4-1)**
- **Special considerations**
  - **A low high-density lipoprotein (HDL) level is an independent risk factor for CAD (see Chapter 3)**
  - **Small, dense LDL has the lowest affinity for the LDL receptor and is therefore cleared to the least degree from plasma by the liver; it may be the most atherogenic type of LDL**
    - Fenofibrate is probably best treatment
  - Homocystinuria is a rare homozygous genetic disorder of impaired homocysteine metabolism that results in severe premature atherosclerosis
    - The heterozygous form has a 1% to 2% prevalence and may account for up to 30% of cases of premature atherosclerosis
    - Though elevated homocysteine levels are associated with increased vascular events, moderate reduction in homocysteine levels by treating with folate, vitamin B_6, and vitamin B_{12} did not reduce the risk of myocardial infarction (MI) or death in a large clinical trial
  - Lipoprotein(a) [Lp(a)] is an LDL particle that contains the large glycoprotein apoprotein (a); it has a higher density than LDL and is more atherogenic
    - Higher levels have been associated with increased CAD

TABLE 4-1	*Risk Factors for Coronary Artery Disease (CAD)*		
Strong Epidemiologic Evidence	**Moderate Epidemiologic Evidence**	**Association with CAD**	
Older age	High triglycerides	Lipoprotein(a)	
Male	Small dense LDL	*Chlamydia*	
Postmenopausal	Elevated	*pneumoniae*	
Elevated LDL	homocysteine		
Low HDL	Stress or depression		
Cigarette smoking	Inflammatory		
Hypertension	markers		
Diabetes mellitus	(C-reactive		
Obesity or sedentary	protein,		
lifestyle	fibrinogen)		
Family history of early			
CAD			

HDL, high-density lipoprotein; LDL, low-density lipoprotein.

- Niacin, estrogen, fenofibrate, and benzafibrate all reduce Lp(a) levels
- One should screen for Lp(a) when statin therapy does not lower LDL
- Elevated C-reactive protein (CRP) and fibrinogen levels are associated with an increased risk of MI; it is unclear whether they cause CAD or are simply markers of an associated inflammatory process
- *Chlamydia pneumoniae* has been isolated from atheromas and may contribute to plaque inflammation. In a recent randomized clinical trial, however, patients hospitalized with an ACS who received long-term treatment with the antibiotic gatifloxacin had no reduction in cardiovascular events.
- Clinical symptoms
  - Symptoms typically occur during physical exertion and gradually resolve with cessation of the exercise
  - Symptoms can also be elicited by conditions that stress the system and increase oxygen demand (e.g., anemia, fever, sepsis, thyrotoxicosis)
    - Typical symptoms include substernal chest pressure or burning and are less commonly characterized by sharp pain
    - May radiate to the upper extremities (left arm more often than right arm), neck, jaw, or face
    - May be accompanied by dyspnea, diaphoresis
    - Symptoms may be atypical, particularly in women, diabetics, and the elderly

Diagnosis and Evaluation

- **The Framingham Risk Score**
  - **Scoring system used to calculate a patient's risk of coronary events**
  - Uses the following risk factors to assess cumuluative risk: age, smoking status, systolic blood pressure, treatment for hypertension, total cholesterol, and HDL cholesterol
  - The cumulative score classifies the patients:
    - Low risk (<10% coronary heart disease [CHD] risk at 10 years)
    - Intermediate risk (10–20% risk of coronary event at 10 years)
    - High rish (>20% risk of coronary event at 10 years)

- Resting electrocardiogram (ECG)
  - Approximately 50% of patients with chronic stable angina have a normal resting ECG
  - The presence of Q waves and conduction system abnormalities (e.g., left bundle branch block [LBBB], left anterior fascicular block) increases the likelihood of having underlying CAD
- Stress tests
  - Rationale
    - Because stress tests can yield both false-negative and false-positive results (the sensitivity of an exercise treadmill test is around 70%, the specificity around 80%), the presence of CAD can never be definitively ruled in or out through stress testing alone
    - **A better rationale for performing a stress test is to risk-stratify the patient: Use the information obtained from the test to determine the patient's risk for future cardiovascular events and death (see the following examples)**
  - Pretest probability
    - Refers to the prevalence of CAD in the population being tested (i.e., the likelihood that the patient has CAD)
    - The likelihood of a patient having CAD increases with age, with having other coronary risk factors, and with a history that is typical of exertional angina
    - The clinician should be able to determine from history and physical examination alone whether a patient has a low, medium, or high pretest probability of CAD
      - Example: A 25-year-old woman with atypical symptoms and no risk factors for CAD has a very low pretest probability
      - Example: A 75-year-old man with exertional angina and a history of hypertension (HTN), diabetes mellitus (DM), high cholesterol, and cigarette use has a high pretest probability
    - Considering pretest probability will help interpret a patient's stress test results
      - Example 1: A healthy 25-year-old woman presents with atypical symptoms of chest pain and no CAD risk factors. She exercises for 15 minutes on a Bruce protocol and has no symptoms, but her ECG shows 1- to 2-mm ST-segment depression, and the test is read as positive.
        - *Interpretation:* This patient has a low pretest probability, and at her age, with atypical symptoms and no risk factors, it is extremely unlikely that she has CAD. This is reinforced by her high treadmill performance without symptoms. The ECG changes almost certainly represent a false positive.
      - Example 2: For the past several months, a 75-year-old man with DM, HTN, and high cholesterol has been having substernal chest pain when he walks up a hill. His symptoms resolve quickly with rest. On a treadmill, he exercises for 6 minutes on a Bruce protocol and develops chest pain at peak exercise. The ECG shows only nonspecific changes, and the test is read as negative.

BOX 4-1	*Features of a High-Risk Stress Test*

Angina or ischemic ECG changes at low workload (<6 min or <4 METS on Bruce protocol)

ST-segment depression >2 mm

ST-segment elevation

ST-segment depression persisting >6 min into recovery period

Exercise-induced hypotension

Ventricular arrhythmias

If thallium or echocardiogram used
  Reversible defects in multiple territories
  Left ventricular cavity dilation

ECG, electrocardiogram; METS, metabolic equivalents.

- *Interpretation:* This man is elderly, has a classic story for exertional angina, and has several major risk factors. His pretest probability is very high, and it is almost a certainty that he has CAD. The stress test is likely a false negative.
  - **Stress tests add little diagnostic information in patients with either high or low pretest probabilities for CAD**
  - **Stress tests are most useful for diagnosing CAD in patients with intermediate pretest probability**
- Determining risk with stress testing
  - Stress test results should be categorized as
    - Inadequate
    - Negative
    - Positive—low risk
    - Positive—high risk
  - Features of a stress test that make it high risk (Box 4-1)
  - Duke Treadmill Score
    - A scoring system that can be used to assess long-term risk
    - (Duration of exercise in minutes) – (5 × maximal ST-segment deviation in mm) – (4 × treadmill angina index)
    - Treadmill angina index: 0 = no symptoms, 1 = angina that does not limit exercise, 2 = angina that limits exercise
    - Score: Less than −10: 79% 4-year survival; −10 to +4: 95% 4-year survival; +5 or greater: greater than 99% 4-year survival
  - **Patients with positive stress tests who have no high-risk features are often best treated medically**
  - **Positive tests with high-risk features suggest higher-risk coronary anatomy (e.g., left main disease, proximal left anterior descending [LAD] artery disease, three-vessel disease); the best approach here is often cardiac catheterization with the ultimate goal of revascularization**
- Types of stress tests (Table 4-2)
  - To decide which stress test is best for a given patient, the clinician must ask two questions:
    1. Can the patient exercise?

    - If yes, a treadmill test is the best choice; allows you to assess your patient's functional capacity, and several studies have demonstrated a good correlation between how long a patient can exercise on the treadmill and overall long-term survival
    - If the patient cannot exercise (e.g., severe chronic obstructive pulmonary disease [COPD], peripheral vascular disease, arthritis), pharmacologic stress (e.g., persantine, dobutamine) with an accompanying imaging modality is required
    2. Does the resting ECG have ST-segment abnormalities?
    - In patients who have baseline ST-segment abnormalities (e.g., left ventricular hypertrophy with strain, paced rhythm, LBBB, ST-segment depression on resting ECG), the ECG alone may not permit an accurate diagnosis of ischemia, and an imaging modality will be required
- Stress testing is very safe
  - 1 to 2 deaths per 10,000 tests
  - **Should be avoided in patients with active symptoms of unstable angina (UA), severe aortic stenosis, possible aortic dissection**
  - **Pharmacologic testing with dipyridamole should be avoided in patients with severe COPD**
- Noninvasive imaging of coronary arteries
  - Electron beam computed tomography (EBCT)
    - Provides a noninvasive and quantitative assessment of coronary artery calcification
    - Higher coronary artery calcium scores are associated with increased risk of MI and death
    - In asymptomatic patients:
      - High coronary artery calcium scores (>75th percentile for age and sex) suggest extensive atherosclerosis and may help to identify high-risk patients who would benefit from aggressive lipid-lowering therapy
      - Has a very high negative predictive value so it can be used to reliably rule out CAD; a calcium score of 0 is associated with a very low (<1%) risk of coronary events
      - Calcium scoring, when added to the Framingham Risk Score, further risk stratifies patients; its use is recommended in asymptomatic subjects with intermediate Framingham Risk Score (10–20% risk of coronary events in 10 years) to identify subjects who would most benefit from aggressive medical intervention
  - **Multidetector row computed tomography (MDCT)**
    - **Can also measure coronary calcification**
    - Improved temporal resolution of these scanners allows for direct coronary artery visualization of a beating heart with little motion artifact
    - MDCT is the most accurate noninvasive modality to diagnose obstructive CAD with a very high negative predictive value (>95%)
    - However, its inability to reliably differentiate between degrees of stenosis greater than 50% makes it more difficult to interpret if it is positive; the positive predictive value is only 60%

TABLE 4-2	*Types of Stress Tests*		
	Agent	**Advantages**	**Disadvantages**
Options for Stress			
Exercise	N/A	Mimics physiologic increases in O_2 demand Provides useful clinical information (e.g., exercise capacity) Inexpensive	Not all patients can exercise adequately ECG alone without imaging modality has higher rates of false positives and false negatives
Pharmacologic	Dobutamine: β-agonist that ↑ heart rate and myocardial contractility (and thus O_2 demand) Adenosine: vasodilates coronary vascular bed and ↑ myocardial blood flow; dilation greater in normal arteries than diseased arteries resulting in steal phenomenon from diseased vascular beds Dipyridamole: coronary dilator that blocks reabsorption of adenosine	Helpful in patients who cannot exercise	More expensive Drugs can cause symptoms of chest pain, nausea, and hypotension, making test interpretation more difficult
Options for Imaging			
Nuclear isotope	Thallium-201: potassium analogue taken up by myocardial cells; hypoperfused myocardium initially shows decreased uptake; tracer redistributes overall several hours Technetium-99m (sestamibi): also taken up by myocardial cells but binds irreversibly—no late washout makes it ideal for imaging MI and unstable angina	Helpful in distinguishing ischemia from infarcted myocardium Technetium-99m has higher proton energy—better agent for imaging obese patients Increases sensitivity and specificity of test	More expensive More invasive Requires radiation
Echocardiography	N/A	Direct visualization of ventricular function Can quantify and localize ischemia Noninvasive Increases sensitivity and specificity of test	More expensive Imaging may be limited in obese patients Can yield false positives in patients with LBBB

ECG, electrocardiogram; LBBB, left bundle branch block; MI, myocardial infarction.

- Coronary angiography
  - Considered the gold standard for the diagnosis of coronary atherosclerosis
  - Three major indications to refer for cardiac catheterization:
    - Failure of medical therapy to relieve symptoms
    - Suggested high-risk coronary anatomy (usually determined by history and stress test)
    - To confirm or exclude CAD

Treatment of Chronic Coronary Disease

- Address modifiable risk factors (e.g., lipid lowering, cigarette cessation)
- Correct illnesses that can precipitate or exacerbate angina (e.g., anemia, infection, thyroid disease)
- Medications that relieve symptoms of angina
  - **β-Blockers**
    - Reduce myocardial O_2 demand by decreasing heart rate, blood pressure (BP), and contractility
    - **Considered first-line therapy for symptoms of exertional angina**
    - Have not been shown to reduce MI or death in patients with chronic stable angina
  - Nitrates
    - Very good at relieving angina and improving exercise tolerance

- Major effect comes from venodilation, which decreases preload, thereby decreasing wall stress and O_2 demand
- Contraindicated in patients using sildenafil
- Calcium channel blockers
  - Considered second-line agents for chronic stable angina
  - Whereas the short-acting dihydropyridines may increase mortality rates in patients with acute ischemic syndromes (see later discussion), long-acting agents can be used safely in patients with chronic stable angina
- Medications that decrease risk of MI and death
  - Aspirin
    - Reduces risk of MI and death in patients with CAD
    - **All patients with CAD should be on aspirin unless there is a clear contraindication**
  - Lipid-lowering agents
    - 3-Hydroxy-3-methylglutaryl coenzyme A **(HMG-CoA) reductase inhibitors (statins) reduce risk of MI and death in patients with CAD**
    - Gemfibrozil decreases MI and death risk in patients with low HDL levels and normal LDL and triglyceride levels
    - National Cholesterol Education Program (NCEP) guidelines recommend lipid-lowering therapy in

patients with CAD to achieve LDL below 100 mg/dL (see Chapter 3)
- ACE inhibitors
  - Conflicting data: The largest and most recent trial showed no decrease in mortality rate in patients with coronary disease who had good left ventricular (LV) function and no heart failure
  - **Clear decrease in mortality rate in patients with CAD who have LV dysfunction and heart failure**
- Revascularization of chronic CAD
  - **Three major indications for revascularization**
    - **Relief of anginal symptoms**
    - **Prevention of nonfatal cardiac events (e.g., MI, congestive heart failure, ventricular tachycardia)**
    - **Decrease mortality**
  - Two methods of revascularization
    - Percutaneous coronary intervention (PCI)
      - PCI refers to percutaneous transluminal coronary angioplasty (PTCA) plus stent deployment
      - With PTCA, a balloon is used to split the atheromatous plaque and stretch the artery
      - Two classes of stents used:
        - Bare metal stents
        - Drug-eluting stents: Coated with a drug that blocks cell proliferation, thus decreasing restenosis rate
      - Because the drug also inhibits re-endothelialization of the stent, there is an increased risk of in-stent thrombosis
      - To decrease this risk, patients should be on aspirin for life and clopidogrel for at least 1 year following stent placement
      - Major benefits: Highly successful (>90%); decreases the need for bypass surgery
      - When compared to bare metal stents, drug-eluting stents do not provide a survival advantage or reduction in reinfarction rates but do reduce risk of repeat revascularization of the target vessel
      - Bare metal stents are used in patients who cannot tolerate long-term dual antiplatelet therapies
      - Antiplatelet agents commonly used during PCI
        - Aspirin: An irreversible cyclooxygenase inhibitor
        - Clopidogrel: Inhibits adenosine diphosphate (ADP)-mediated platelet activation; helps to prevent acute stent thrombosis; side effects include rash and gastrointestinal (GI) upset; can rarely cause thrombotic thrombocytopenic purpura
        - Prasugrel: Mechanism of action is similar to clopidogrel but has a more rapid onset of action and more effective inhibition of platelet activation; lower rate of death and reinfarction in patients treated with prasugrel compared to clopidogrel but a slightly higher rate of bleeding (risk of bleeding is higher in patients with prior stroke/transient ischemic attack [TIA], body weight <60 kg and age >75 years)
        - Ticlopidine: Inhibits ADP-mediated platelet activation; because of associated neutropenia, it has been largely replaced by clopidogrel
        - Glycoprotein IIb/IIIa inhibitors: Abciximab and eptifibatide; reduce cardiovascular complications of PCI in the acute setting
      - Risks and complications
        - Restenosis: Renarrowing of the arterial lumen following PCI; mechanism incompletely understood but likely involves neointimal thickening because of smooth muscle cell proliferation as well as shrinkage of the dilated segment of artery; incidence of restenosis peaks between 3 and 6 months after PCI; restenosis rates have decreased significantly with the use of intracoronary stents
        - Other: 1% to 2% risk of emergent bypass, 2% to 4% risk of MI, 1% risk of death; risks increase with long, tubular, eccentric, calcified lesions
      - **Although PCI is quite effective in reducing symptoms of angina in patients with stable CAD, it does not reduce the risk of death, MI, or other major cardiovascular events when compared with optimal medical therapy alone**
      - The use of PCI guided by measurement of fractional flow reserve (FFR) in stable angina patients is associated with better outcomes; FFR less than 0.8 is considered abnormal and suggests a significant coronary stenosis
    - Coronary artery bypass grafting (CABG)
      - Excellent for relieving anginal symptoms
      - Need for repeated revascularization procedures is less than with PCI
      - Complications include sternal wound infection, MI, stroke, postoperative arrhythmias, and death
      - **Select groups of patients derive mortality benefit from CABG**
        - **Left main disease**
        - **Three-vessel CAD and decreased LV function**
        - **Three-vessel CAD and ischemia at low workload**
        - **Two- or three-vessel disease with proximal LAD involvement**
        - **Patients with DM—higher 5-year survival with CABG than with PTCA**
      - The role of CABG in three-vessel disease with decreased LV function has been called into question by recent data that suggest no significant difference in all-cause mortality between medical management and CABG
      - Following CABG, treatment with a statin has been shown to reduce disease progression in grafts (even in patients with only mild LDL elevation)
      - How does multivessel PCI compare with CABG in patients with left main or three-vessel CAD?
        - At 1 year, rates of major adverse cardiac events are higher in the PCI group, largely due to an increased rate of repeat revascularization
        - At 1 year, rates of death and MI are the same in both groups, but stroke is more likely to occur with CABG

Primary Prevention of Coronary Artery Disease and Myocardial Infarction

- Risk factor modification
  - Smoking cessation
    - Smoking cessation results in 60% reduction in CHD risk by 3 years
    - Behavior and pharmacologic intervention should be considered
  - Blood pressure control
    - A 5- to 6-mm Hg reduction in BP results in 16% reduction in cardiovascular disease
    - Approach should include lifestyle changes, weight loss, exercise, and medical management if necessary
  - Cholesterol lowering
    - Reduction in serum cholesterol by 10% reduces cardiovascular events by 18% and cardiovascular death by 10%
    - Management should include dietary modification, exercise, and lipid-lowering therapy (see NCEP III guidelines)
  - Tight glycemic control
    - Diabetes mellitus increases risk of heart disease by two- to fourfold in men and three- to sevenfold in women
    - Data suggest that tight glycemic control reduces microvascular disease and may reduce risk of cardiovascular events
    - Patients with metabolic syndrome are at increased risk of cardiovascular disease; aggressive risk factor modification is warranted in these patients (diet, exercise, weight loss, lipid and glucose management)
  - Weight loss
    - Obesity and physical inactivity are risk factors for CAD
    - Though data are limited, trials suggest that maintaining ideal body weight and staying physically active may reduce risk of MI by 50%
- Pharmacologic therapy
  - Aspirin
    - In men, pooled data suggest a 33% reduction in first MI
    - In a recent large clinical trial, aspirin reduced the risk of stroke in women 65 years or older but had no effect on risk of MI or death from cardiovascular causes
  - Statins
    - Several large trials have shown that statins reduce the risk of first MI, even in patients with only moderately elevated cholesterol
  - Hormone therapy
    - Though cardiovascular risk increases in postmenopausal women, evidence from large trials suggests that hormone therapy may increase the risk of cardiovascular disease in the first 1 to 2 years of use; routine use for primary prevention should be avoided
- Diet and exercise
  - Though trial data are limited, maintaining ideal body weight and a physically active lifestyle may reduce risk of MI by 50%
- The consumption of fish and omega-3 fatty acids has been associated with reduced risk of coronary disease in both men and women
- Moderate alcohol intake (one drink per day) decreases risk of MI by 30% to 50%; decision to recommend moderate intake should be based on risk-benefit ratio in setting of comorbidities (e.g., liver disease, peptic ulcer disease)
- Trials with antioxidants have been disappointing; in a large study of patients with vascular disease, administration of folic acid and vitamins B_6 and B_{12} did not reduce the risk of cardiovascular death, MI, or all-cause mortality

Acute Coronary Syndromes

Basic Information

- Epidemiology
  - In the United States, over 1 million people annually suffer an MI; death results in one third of these patients.
  - Fifty percent of the deaths from MI occur within the first hour
- Pathophysiology
  - Acute coronary syndromes (ACSs) include unstable angina (UA), non–ST-segment elevation MI (NSTEMI), and ST-segment elevation MI (STEMI)
  - **The common pathophysiology of all three syndromes is rupture of a vulnerable plaque that leads to platelet activation and aggregation resulting in the formation of intracoronary thrombus (Fig. 4-1)**
  - The vulnerable plaque
    - Larger, fibrotic plaques with thicker caps are less prone to rupture than are smaller plaques, which often have soft atherogenic lipid cores and thinner caps
    - Inflammation is important in plaque instability and rupture; elevated serum levels of certain inflammatory markers (e.g., CRP, fibrinogen, interleukin-6, tumor necrosis factor) correlate with an increased incidence of acute coronary events
    - Numerous factors, including inflammation, weakening of the cap from shear stress, and enzymatic degradation of the cap, can contribute to plaque vulnerability and rupture
  - Formation of thrombus
    - Following plaque rupture, the atherogenic lipid core is exposed to the bloodstream
    - Platelets adhere to the vessel wall when platelet glycoprotein binds to von Willebrand factor
    - Exposure of tissue factor activates the coagulation cascade and leads to thrombin formation, the most potent platelet activator
    - The final common pathway of platelet activation is exposure of the platelet glycoprotein IIb/IIIa receptor, which binds fibrinogen, causing platelets to stick to one another
  - Not all thrombi have the same composition
    - Red thrombi are richer in fibrinogen and red blood cells; they are seen more commonly in STEMI

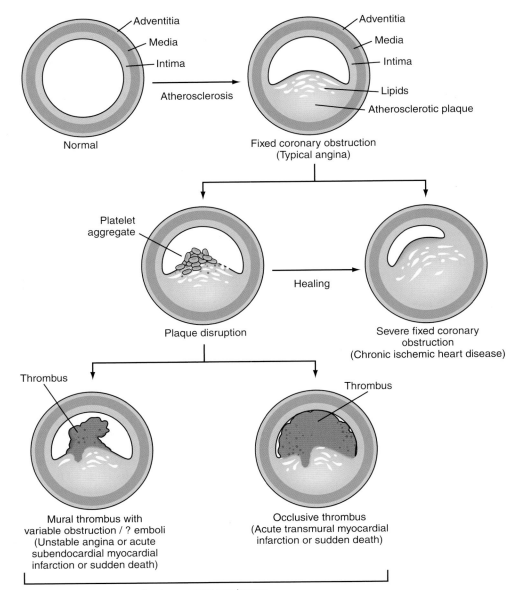

FIGURE 4-1 Schematic representation of sequential progression of coronary artery lesion morphology, beginning with stable chronic plaque responsible for typical angina and leading to the various acute coronary syndromes. *(Modified and redrawn from Schoen FJ: Interventional and surgical cardiovascular pathology: clinical correlations and basic principles, Philadelphia, WB Saunders, 1989, p 63, and from Zipes DP, Libby P, Bonow RO, Braunwald E [eds]: Braunwald's heart disease: a textbook of cardiovascular medicine, ed 7, Philadelphia, WB Saunders, 2005, Fig. 12-12.)*

- White thrombi are more platelet-rich; they are more common in UA and NSTEMI
- Definitions
  - *Unstable angina (UA):* Defined as either rest angina (usually prolonged >20 minutes), new-onset exertional angina at least class III in severity (i.e., angina with only mild exertion), or preexisting angina that has increased in frequency or duration or that is now brought on with less exertion than before
  - *Non–ST-segment elevation MI (NSTEMI):* Can be similar clinically to UA, but is distinguished by evidence of myocardial necrosis (i.e., an elevation in serum cardiac enzymes); ECG does not show ST-segment elevation
  - *ST-segment elevation MI (STEMI):* This type of MI is defined by the presence of elevated cardiac enzymes and ECG criteria that include greater than 1 mm ST-segment elevation in two or more contiguous limb leads, or greater than 2 mm ST-segment elevation in two or more contiguous precordial leads, or a new or presumed new LBBB
    - **The presence of ST-segment elevation on ECG suggests total occlusion of the infarct artery by thrombus; in contrast, most patients presenting with UA or NSTEMI do not have a totally occluded infarct artery**
  - Other differences between NSTEMI and STEMI: see Table 4-3

Clinical Presentation

- Unlike chronic stable angina, in which symptoms occur with exertion, an ACS is often characterized by abrupt symptom onset while at rest
- Symptoms can include chest pain or pressure, shortness of breath, nausea, vomiting, diaphoresis, and radiation of pain to the left arm, neck, or jaw

TABLE 4-3	Comparison of Non-ST Segment Elevation MI and ST Segment Elevation MI	
	NSTEMI	**STEMI**
ECG findings	ST-segment depressions; T-wave inversions; nonspecific ST-T changes	ST-segment elevation
Vessel at time of catheterization	Only 30–40% totally occluded	>80% totally occluded
Type of clot	Rich in platelets (white)	Rich in fibrin (red)
Extent of disease	More likely multivessel with collaterals	More commonly single vessel
Treatment	Thrombolysis not recommended; GP IIb/IIIa inhibitors indicated	Thrombolysis beneficial; GP IIb/IIIa inhibitors usually not indicated (unless PCI performed)
Hospital mortality	Lower	Higher
Reinfarction rate	Higher after hospital discharge	Lower after hospital discharge
Long-term prognosis	Higher 1-yr mortality rate after discharge	Lower 1-yr mortality rate after discharge

GP, glycoprotein; MI, myocardial infarction; NSTEMI, non–ST-segment elevation myocardial infarction; PCI, percutaneous coronary intervention; STEMI, ST-segment elevation myocardial infarction; ST-T, ST segment and T wave.

- Symptoms can be atypical, particularly in women, diabetics, and the elderly
- Some 20% to 30% of ACSs may be clinically silent

Diagnosis and Evaluation

- ECG findings
  - UA and NSTEMI
    - A number of ECG patterns may be seen, including a normal ECG, ST-segment depression, T-wave inversions, or nonspecific ST-segment and T-wave changes
  - STEMI
    - This type of MI is defined electrocardiographically by the presence of more than 1 mm ST-segment elevation in two or more contiguous limb leads, or more than 2 mm ST-segment elevation in two or more contiguous precordial leads, or a new or presumed new LBBB
    - Patients who meet these ECG criteria require rapid reperfusion (with either thrombolytic therapy or PCI)
- Cardiac enzymes used to diagnose NSTEMI and STEMI (Fig. 4-2)
  - *Creatine phosphokinase myocardial band (CPK-MB):* First measurable in the bloodstream at 6 to 10 hours; peaks at 24 hours; baseline by 48 to 72 hours
  - *Troponin T and I:* Greater sensitivity than CPK-MB; appear at 4 to 6 hours; peak at 24 to 48 hours and decline slowly; remain detectable for up to 7 to 10 days
  - *Lactate dehydrogenase:* Increases at 24 to 48 hours and remains elevated for 10 days; used less commonly now that troponins are available
- Risk stratification of UA and NSTEMI
  - Patients presenting with UA and NSTEMI should be risk-stratified to determine if they are at low, intermediate, or high risk for subsequent adverse cardiac events
  - ECG and cardiac enzymes
    - The presence of ST-segment depression greater than 1 mm in two or more contiguous limb leads (or >2 mm in two or more contiguous precordial leads) is a predictor of an increased risk for adverse cardiac events

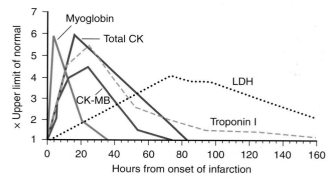

FIGURE 4-2 Timing of various cardiac enzymes after myocardial infarction. (CK, creatine kinase; CK-MB, creatine kinase myocardial band; LDH, lactate dehydrogenase.) *(From Antman EM: General hospital management. In Julian DG, Braunwald E [eds]: Management of acute myocardial infarction, London, WB Saunders, 1994.)*

- An elevation of cardiac troponin I or T is a strong predictor of subsequent cardiac events
- Patients with both ST-segment depression and elevated cardiac enzymes are considered to be at high risk; those with only one of the two factors are intermediate risk; patients with neither of the two factors are considered low risk
- The Thrombolysis In Myocardial Infarction (TIMI) risk score for UA/NSTEMI (Box 4-2)
  - A scoring system that uses seven clinical factors to help physicians predict the risk of subsequent adverse cardiac events (defined as MI, persistent ischemia, or cardiac-related death) in patients presenting with UA or NSTEMI
  - A score of 0 to 2 is considered low risk, 3 to 4 is intermediate risk, 5 to 7 is high risk
- **As a general rule, it is often most appropriate to treat low-risk patients conservatively (i.e., noninvasive testing, medical management); more aggressive treatment (e.g., catheterization, PCI) is often the best choice for intermediate- and high-risk patients**

TIMI Risk Score for Unstable Angina and Non–ST-Segment Elevation MI

Risk Factors

Age >65 yr
Three or more coronary artery risk factors
Prior coronary stenosis ≥50%
Two or more anginal events in past 24 hr
Aspirin use in past 7 days
ST-segment changes
Positive cardiac markers
TIMI Score = Sum of Applicable Risk Factors

Risk of Adverse Cardiac Event by TIMI Score

0–1: 4.7%

2: 8.3%   } Low Risk

3: 13.2%

4: 19.9%   } Intermediate Risk

5: 26.2%

6–7: 41%   } High Risk

MI, myocardial infarction; TIMI, Thrombolysis In Myocardial Infarction.

TABLE 4-4 **TIMI Risk Score for ST-Segment Elevation MI**

Clinical Risk Factors	Points
History	
≥75 yr old	3
65–74 yr old	2
History of diabetes, hypertension, or angina	1
Physical examination	
Systolic blood pressure <100 mm Hg	3
Heart rate >100 beats/min	2
Killip class II–IV	2
Weight <67 kg	1
Presentation	
Anterior STEMI or left bundle branch block	1
Time to reperfusion therapy >4 hr	1
Total possible points	14

MI, myocardial infarction; STEMI, ST-segment elevation myocardial infarction; TIMI, Thrombolysis In Myocardial Infarction.
Data from Morrow DA, Antman EM, Parsons L, et al: Application of the TIMI risk score for ST-elevation MI in the National Registry of Myocardial Infarction 3, *JAMA* 286:1356–1359, 2001.

- Risk stratification of STEMI (Table 4-4)
  - The TIMI risk score for STEMI assesses risk based on history, exam, and clinical presentation; there is an increased risk in 30-day mortality rates, ranging from 1.1% to 30% for scores ranging from 0 to greater than 8, respectively
- Differential diagnosis (diagnoses that can mimic an ACS)
  - **Always consider other conditions presenting with chest pain and ECG changes that mimic an acute MI, as the management of these conditions is often very different**
  - Aortic dissection
    - Clinical clues include "tearing" pain that radiates to the back, unequal pulses or BP in the upper extremities, new murmur of aortic regurgitation
    - ECG can reveal ST-segment elevations if the dissection involves one or more of the coronary arteries
    - Thrombolytics are contraindicated
  - Acute pericarditis
    - Clinical clues include chest pain that may be pleuritic or that is relieved by sitting up; friction rub may be present
    - ECG may reveal diffuse ST-segment elevation and P–R interval depression
    - Heparin and thrombolytics contraindicated
  - Pulmonary embolism (PE)
    - Clinical clues include risk factors for PE (e.g., sedentary or immobile, history of deep venous thrombosis, leg trauma, oral contraceptive use); sudden-onset chest pain and shortness of breath

- ECG may show only sinus tachycardia, but classic findings include S wave in lead I, Q wave in lead III, and T-wave inversion in lead III; or possibly a new right bundle branch block or right axis deviation

Treatment of Acute Coronary Syndromes
- Management of UA and NSTEMI (Fig. 4-3)
  - Medical therapy
    - Antiplatelet therapy
      - *Aspirin:* More than 50% reduction in risk of MI and death in patients with UA/NSTEMI; **ideally, aspirin should be continued indefinitely**
      - *Clopidogrel:* Has been shown in a large clinical trial to reduce adverse cardiac events in patients with UA/NSTEMI when given in addition to aspirin; it should be continued for at least 12 months if PCI with drug-eluting stent is performed, 1 month if PCI with bare metal stent is performed, and for at least 9 months if no PCI is done
      - *Prasugrel:* Is associated with lower rates of death and cardiovascular morbidity compared to clopidogrel, but is associated with a slightly higher risk of bleeding and should be avoided in subjects who may be potential candidates for CABG
      - *Glycoprotein IIb/IIIa inhibitors:* Clear benefit demonstrated in both UA and NSTEMI; the greatest benefit seen in patients who have positive troponins and who are going to the catheterization lab for PCI
        - *Abciximab:* Fab fragment of a monoclonal antibody directed at the IIb/IIIa receptor; clear benefit for patients undergoing PCI; no benefit seen in patients with UA/NSTEMI who do not require PCI

4

FIGURE 4-3 Approach to the patient with a non–ST-segment elevation acute coronary syndrome. The Thrombolysis In Myocardial Infarction (TIMI) risk score calculation appears in Box 4-2. (ACS, acute coronary syndrome; ASA, aspirin; ECG, electrocardiogram; GP IIB/IIIA inhibitor, glycoprotein IIb/IIIa inhibitor; LMWH, low-molecular-weight heparin; NSTEMI, non–ST-segment elevation myocardial infarction; UA, unstable angina.) *(Modified with permission from Yang EH, Ardehali H, Achuff SC: Acute coronary syndromes: non-ST elevation. In Cheng A, Zaas A [eds]: The Osler medical handbook, St. Louis, Mosby, 2003, pp 95–110.)*

- *Eptifibatide:* A synthetic peptide; benefit demonstrated in UA/NSTEMI as well as PCI
- *Tirofiban:* A nonpeptide molecule; benefit demonstrated in UA/NSTEMI
- Antithrombotic therapy
  - Unfractionated heparin (UFH)
  - Low-molecular-weight heparin (LMWH): Compared to UFH, has less nonspecific binding and causes less thrombocytopenia; can be dosed by body weight without need to follow activated partial thromboplastin time (aPTT)
    - *Enoxaparin:* Superior to UFH in reducing death, MI, and recurrent ischemic events
    - *Fondaparinux:* Acts through antithrombin to neutralize factor Xa; can be used both with conservative strategy as well as invasive strategy in patients with UA/NSTEMI; preferable to UFH or enoxaparin in patients with increased risk of bleeding
  - Direct thrombin inhibitor
    - *Bivalirudin:* This is an option only in patients where an early invasive approach is planned

- β-Blockers: In UA, β-blockers reduce ischemia and have been shown to reduce subsequent infarction; in NSTEMI, they decrease ischemia, reduce infarct size, help prevent reinfarction, and decrease mortality
- Nitrates: Decrease O_2 demand; quite effective in relieving anginal symptoms; have not been shown to improve survival
- Calcium channel blockers: Should not be considered first-line for UA or NSTEMI; the short-acting dihydropyridines have been associated with increased mortality in ACSs; non-dihydropyridine calcium channel blockers may be used to treat ischemia refractory to β-blockers and nitrates
- Statins: In addition to lipid-lowering ability, these agents have been shown to have antiplatelet and antioxidant properties as well; there is evidence to support their use during the acute presentation with UA/NSTEMI
- **Thrombolytics are not indicated in UA and NSTEMI**
- Cardiac catheterization in UA/NSTEMI

- Indications for emergent catheterization
  - Persistent ischemia despite medical therapy
  - Hemodynamic instability
  - Ventricular tachycardia, ventricular fibrillation, sudden death
- Indications for catheterization in the patient with UA/NSTEMI who has been stabilized with medication
  - Early positive stress test
  - Large territory of ischemia on ECG
  - High risk as determined by ST-segment depression on ECG and elevated cardiac enzymes
  - High or intermediate risk as determined by TIMI risk score
  - **Although stable patients with NSTEMI can be treated conservatively, data from large clinical trials suggest that these patients derive benefit (e.g., improved survival, fewer adverse cardiac events) if referred early for catheterization/PCI (i.e., during first 48 to 72 hours of hospitalization)**
- Management of STEMI (Fig. 4-4)
  - **Rapid recognition of a STEMI and immediate initiation of reperfusion therapy are crucial; the faster normal flow can be restored in the occluded artery, the better the prognosis**
  - Two major reperfusion strategies
    - Thrombolytic therapy
      - About 60% success rate of opening the occluded artery
      - **Thrombolytics have the most benefit when given in the first 6 hours, but can be given up to 12 hours after onset of chest pain; after 12 hours, the benefit decreases and the risk of rupture increases**
      - **Indications and contraindications: see Table 4-5**
      - Patients receiving thrombolytics who are at the highest risk of stroke include elderly, female, hypertensive, and diabetic patients as well as those who have a history of prior stroke or are on warfarin
      - Commonly used thrombolytics
        - Streptokinase: derived from group C streptococcus; inexpensive; can cause allergic reactions
        - Tissue plasminogen activator (tPA): faster and more clot-specific; more expensive; no allergic potential
        - The latest generation of lytics (e.g., reteplase [recombinant tPA], tenecteplase [TNK-tPA]): mutants of tPA and tend to be even more clot-specific
    - PCI
      - Major advantages over thrombolytics include higher reperfusion rate (>90% success rate of opening the occluded artery) and decreased incidence of stroke
      - More effective than thrombolytics in patients with CHF, cardiogenic shock, and prior bypass surgery
      - Major disadvantage is that it is not available in all hospitals, and it may take too much time to get the patient to the appropriate facility

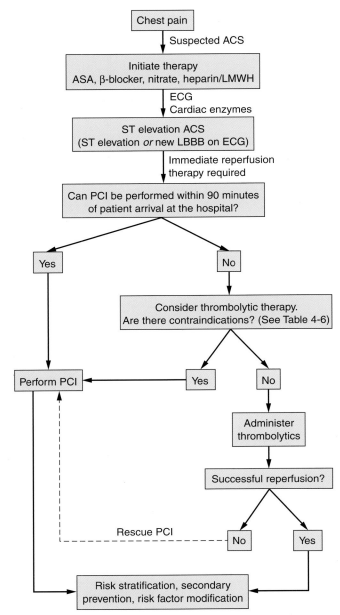

FIGURE 4-4 Approach to the patient with ST-segment elevation acute coronary syndrome. (ACS, acute coronary syndrome; ASA, aspirin; ECG, electrocardiogram; LBBB, left bundle branch block; LMWH, low-molecular-weight heparin; PCI, percutaneous coronary intervention.)

- Terminology
  - *Primary PCI:* Patient with STEMI is taken directly to the catheterization lab for PCI instead of receiving thrombolytics
  - *Rescue PCI:* Urgent PCI after failure to reperfuse with thrombolytics
- Approximately 20% to 30% of patients receiving thrombolytics fail to reperfuse and have a high mortality rate; recent data show that patients who fail to reperfuse with thrombolytics have better outcomes if they are then sent for rescue PCI

TABLE 4-5 *Thrombolytic Therapy in STEMI*

Indication	Absolute Contraindications	Relative Contraindications
In a patient presenting with chest pain, the ECG criteria are ≥1 mm ST-segment elevation in two contiguous leads *or* A new or presumed new left bundle branch block Duration of symptoms <12 hr	Any history of intracranial bleed Known cerebral vascular lesion (e.g., AVM) Known malignant intracranial neoplasm Ischemic stroke within 3 mo Suspected aortic dissection Active bleeding or bleeding diathesis (excluding menses) Closed-head or facial trauma within 3 mo	Systolic BP >180 mm Hg or diastolic BP >110 mm Hg at presentation History of ischemic stroke >3 mo prior Prolonged CPR (>10 min) Major surgery within <3 wk Recent internal bleeding (within 2–4 wk) Pregnancy Active peptic ulcer For streptokinase/anistreplase: Prior exposure >5 days ago or prior allergic reaction

AVM, arteriovenous malformation; BP, blood pressure; CPR, cardiopulmonary resuscitation; ECG, electrocardiogram; STEMI, ST-segment elevation myocardial infarction.

- General strategy for managing STEMI
  - Reperfusion therapy with either PCI or thrombolytics should be performed as quickly as possible
  - **PCI is usually the first choice for reperfusion if it can be performed in less than 90 minutes after patient arrival**
  - If PCI cannot be performed within 90 minutes of patient arrival, thrombolytics should be given if there are no contraindications; **thrombolytics should be given within 30 minutes of patient arrival.**
  - If a patient receives thrombolytics and fails to reperfuse, he/she should be referred for rescue PCI
- Other pharmacologic therapy for STEMI
  - **Aspirin: proven to prevent recurrent infarction and decrease mortality**
  - Clopidogrel: Improved outcomes when used in combination with aspirin; use of prasugrel compared to clopidogrel is associated with better outcomes with slightly higher bleeding risk
  - β-Blockers: Decrease ischemia, reduce infarct size, help prevent reinfarction, decrease mortality
  - ACE inhibitors: Proven benefit, particularly in patients with impaired LV function and heart failure; particular benefit in anterior wall MI to help prevent remodeling; angiotensin receptor blocker (ARB) should be used if there is an ACE inhibitor intolerance
  - Nitroglycerin: Good for relieving pain and ischemia; typically used for 24 to 48 hours after STEMI but can be used longer for persistent ischemia, hypertension, or heart failure
  - Heparin: Should be used unless there is a bleeding contraindication
    - Indicated for patients going for PCI
    - Should be given to patients receiving tPA (continued for at least 48 hours)
    - Patients receiving a nonselective thrombolytic (e.g., streptokinase) should receive heparin after coagulation factors have normalized (usually after 6 hours); typically given to keep aPTT 50 to 70 seconds for at least 48 hours
  - Statins: Have been shown to have benefit even in the acute infarct setting; can be started even before a lipid profile has been obtained
- Medications not recommended for STEMI

- Calcium channel blockers: Short-acting dihydropyridines should be avoided; diltiazem should be avoided in patients with LV dysfunction
- Empirical antiarrhythmics: Prophylactic antiarrhythmic use can actually increase mortality in the peri-MI setting
- Glycoprotein IIb/IIIa inhibitors: Not of proven benefit to use in conjunction with thrombolytics
- Complications of acute MI: see Table 4-6

Care Following Myocardial Infarction and Secondary Prevention

- Risk factor modification (e.g., diet and weight loss, BP control, control of blood glucose, lipid lowering, smoking cessation)
- Physical rehabilitation and exercise
- Long-term medications
  - **Aspirin: Reduces rate of second MI and improves survival; should be taken indefinitely following infarct**
  - Clopidogrel
    - In patients presenting with an acute MI, clopidogrel should be taken in combination with aspirin for at least 1 month, and ideally up to 12 months if patient is not at high risk for bleeding; should be used indefinitely in patients who have an intolerance or allergy to aspirin
    - In patients who undergo placement of a drug-eluting stent at the time of infarct, clopidogrel should be used in combination with aspirin for at least a year
  - β-Blockers: Improve survival; should be used indefinitely in most patients following MI
  - ACE inhibitors (or ARBs): Decrease reinfarction rate and improve survival; should clearly be used in all patients with LV dysfunction; help prevent remodeling in patients with anterior wall infarcts
  - Aldosterone blockers: Should be used long term for patients who do not have significant renal dysfunction or hyperkalemia, who are already on therapeutic doses of ACE inhibitor or ARB, have ejection fraction less than 40%, and have either symptomatic heart failure or DM
  - Statins: Reduce reinfarction rates and improve survival in patients with both high and average cholesterol levels; should be used indefinitely to keep LDL cholesterol less than 100 mg/dL

TABLE 4-6   *Complications of Myocardial Infarction*

Complication	Type of MI	Timing and Presentation	Treatment
Bradyarrhythmias			
Mobitz type I block (Wenckebach)	Mobitz I: Usually seen with IMI; caused by ischemia or increased vagal tone; conduction block usually in AV node	Usually in first 24–48 hr for all types Asymptomatic or hypotension	Mobitz I: Responds to atropine and usually resolves in 2–3 days
Mobitz type II block	Mobitz II: Usually AMI; block typically infranodal		Mobitz II: Temporary pacer because high risk for progression to complete block; many will require permanent pacer
Third degree block (complete heart block)	Third degree: AMI or IMI		Third degree: Permanent pacer usually required with AMI; often resolves spontaneously with IMI
Bundle branch block	Usually AMI	First 24–48 hr	Temporary pacer indicated for alternating left and right BBB; RBBB with alternating LAFB and LPFB; LBBB or RBBB with first degree AV block BBB associated with higher mortality
Premature ventricular contractions	Any MI	First 24–72 hr Usually asymptomatic	Treatment usually not required Avoid lidocaine (can ↑ mortality) Can use β-blockers
Ventricular tachycardia or fibrillation	Any territory, but commonly AMI	VT in first 24 hr—usually transient and benign Late VT—consider recurrent ischemia Most VF occurs in first 48 hr	Defibrillation for VF and hemodynamically significant VT For hemodynamically tolerated VT, meds can be tried before cardioversion (e.g., lidocaine, procainamide, amiodarone) β-blockers decrease incidence of lethal VF peri-infarct
Papillary muscle rupture	Usually IMI	2–10 days after MI Sudden-onset CHF and hypotension caused by mitral regurgitation Large V waves on Swan-Ganz tracing	IABP to help stabilize Urgent surgery required
Ventricular septal rupture	Both AMI and IMI	1–20 days after MI Pansystolic murmur and palpable thrill Hypotension Increased pulmonary artery O_2 saturation by Swan-Ganz	IABP to help stabilize Urgent surgery required
Ventricular free wall rupture	Both AMI and IMI	2–14 days after STEMI Sudden PEA, tamponade, or death Elderly women at greatest risk	Emergency surgery Very high mortality
Right ventricular infarct	IMI	Classic triad: ↑ JVP, clear lungs, hypotension ECG: ST ↑ in V_4 with right-sided leads	Aggressive IV fluids Avoid agents that decrease preload (e.g., nitrates, morphine) May require inotrope support (e.g., dobutamine)
Pericarditis	AMI or IMI	2–14 days after MI "Dressler's syndrome" Pericardial rub ECG may show diffuse ST-segment elevation and P–R interval depression	Nonsteroidal anti-inflammatory agents Avoid anticoagulation

AMI, anterior myocardial infarction; AV, atrioventricular; BBB, bundle branch block; CHF, congestive heart failure; ECG, electrocardiogram; IABP, intra-aortic balloon pump; IMI, inferior myocardial infarction; IV, intravenous; JVP, jugular venous pressure; LAFB, left anterior fascicular block; LBBB, left bundle branch block; LPFB, left posterior fascicular block; MI, myocardial infarction; PEA, pulseless electrical activity; RBBB, right bundle branch block; STEMI, ST-segment elevation myocardial infarction; VF, ventricular fibrillation; VT, ventricular tachycardia.

- Warfarin: Indicated in patients who have severe LV dysfunction or evidence of apical thrombus; no proven survival benefit
- **Implantable defibrillators**
  - **Shown to improve survival in patients with ischemic cardiomyopathy and low ejection fraction (even in the absence of ventricular arrhythmias)**
  - **Indicated for patients with ejection fraction ≤30% measured at least 40 days after the acute infarction**

REVIEW QUESTIONS

For review questions, please go to www.expertconsult.com.

SUGGESTED READINGS

Antman EM, Anbe DT, Armstrong PW, et al: ACC/AHA guidelines for the management of patients with ST-elevation myocardial infarction–executive summary: a report of the American College of Cardiology/American Heart Association Task Force on Practice Guidelines (Committee to Revise the 1999 Guidelines for the Management of Patients with Acute Myocardial Infarction), *J Am Coll Cardiol* 4:E1–E211, 2004.

Antman EM, Cohen M, Bernink PJ, et al: The TIMI risk score for unstable angina/non-ST elevation MI: a method for prognostication and therapeutic decision making, *JAMA* 284:835–842, 2000.

Boden WE, O'Rourke RA, Teo KK, et al: Optimal medical therapy with or without PCI for stable coronary disease, *N Engl J Med* 356:1503–1516, 2007.

Morrow DA, Antman EM, Parsons L, et al: Application of the TIMI risk score for ST-elevation MI in the National Registry of Myocardial Infarction 3, *JAMA* 286:1356–1359, 2001.

Morrow DA, Gersh BJ, Braunwald E: Chronic coronary artery disease. In Zipes DP, Libby P, Bonow RO, Braunwald E, editors: *Braunwald's heart disease: a textbook of cardiovascular medicine*, ed 7, Philadelphia, 2005, WB Saunders, pp 1281–1354.

Moss AJ, Zareba W, Hall WJ, et al: Prophylactic implantation of a defibrillator in patients with myocardial infarction and reduced ejection fraction, *N Engl J Med* 346:877–883, 2002.

Mudd JO, Waters R, Keleman M: Acute coronary syndromes: ST elevation. In Cheng A, Zaas A, editors: *The Osler medical handbook*, St. Louis, 2003, Mosby, pp 111–122.

Velazquez EJ, Lee KL, et al: Coronary artery bypass surgery in patients with left ventricular dysfunction, *N Engl J Med* 364:17, 2011.

Wright RS, et al: 2011 AHA Focused Update of the Guidelines for the management of unstable angina/non ST elevation myocardial infarction, *Circulation* 123:2022, 2011.

Yang EH, Ardehali H, Achuff SC: Acute coronary syndromes: non-ST elevation. In Cheng A, Zaas A, editors: *The Osler medical handbook*, St. Louis, 2003, Mosby, pp 95–110.

CHAPTER 5

Arrhythmias

GRANT V. CHOW, MD; and JOSEPH E. MARINE, MD

Arrhythmias are a diverse group of disorders that account for significant morbidity and mortality affecting all age groups. They are classified as brady- or tachyarrhythmias based on heart rate. Bradyarrhythmias (heart rates <60 bpm) can occur at any point along the conduction path, and result from depressed automaticity, conduction delay, or block. Tachyarrhythmias (heart rates >100 bpm) are typically classified as supraventricular or ventricular based on their site of origin. Current treatment options for arrhythmias vary according to the underlying cause and may encompass pharmacotherapy, electrical conversion, pacemaker or defibrillator insertion, or catheter or surgical ablation.

Bradyarrhythmias

Basic Information

Bradyarrhythmias arise from three sites: sinoatrial node, atrioventricular node, or infranodal (Table 5-1).
- Sinoatrial (SA) node
  - Sinus node dysfunction
    - Usually manifested as sinus pauses
    - Another form (chronotropic incompetence) manifested by inability to raise sinus rate appropriately in response to exercise
    - Often coexists with atrial fibrillation (i.e., "tachy-brady" syndrome)
    - **Brief asymptomatic sinus pauses are common; treatment is generally indicated only in the presence of symptoms. Symptomatic patients usually require a permanent pacemaker.**
- Atrioventricular (AV) node and His-Purkinje system
  - First degree AV block
    - P–R interval prolongation greater than 200 ms
  - Second degree AV block
    - Mobitz I: Progressive P–R interval prolongation followed by single blocked P wave
    - Mobitz II: No progressive P–R interval prolongation before blocked P wave
  - Third degree (complete) AV block
    - No association between P waves and QRS complexes
    - Narrow QRS (junctional) escape rhythm: Usually block in AV node
    - Wide QRS (ventricular) escape rhythm: Suggests block in His bundle or below

Clinical Presentation

- Some patients are asymptomatic
- May present with fatigue, dyspnea on exertion, presyncope, or syncope

- Often better tolerated than tachyarrhythmias due to slow progression, except for infranodal AV block, which may present with syncope or cardiac arrest

Diagnosis and Evaluation

- Clues often obtained from electrocardiogram (ECG) (Table 5-2)
- Event recorders allow correlation of symptoms with the bradyarrhythmia

Treatment

- Acute management of bradyarrhythmias (see Table 5-1)
- Permanent pacemaker implantation for chronic management of bradyarrhythmias
  - **Indicated for**
    - **Sinus node dysfunction and Mobitz I second degree AV block in the presence of symptoms that correlate with bradycardia**
    - **Mobitz II second degree AV block and third degree AV block, even when asymptomatic**
  - Device types
    - Dual-chamber pacemaker (DDD, senses and paces right atrium and ventricle) unless permanent atrial fibrillation is present, in which case single-chamber ventricular (VVI) pacing is most appropriate
    - Biventricular pacemaker providing cardiac resynchronization therapy (CRT) is increasingly used for patients with chronic systolic heart failure who require ventricular pacing

Supraventricular Tachyarrhythmias (SVTs)

AV NODAL RE-ENTRANT TACHYCARDIA (AVNRT)

Basic Information (Table 5-3)

- Mechanism of arrhythmia: re-entrant pathway within the AV node complex (Fig. 5-1)
- Dual AV nodal physiology
  - Two functionally and anatomically distinct pathways
    - Slow-conducting path with short refractory period
    - Fast-conducting path with long refractory period
- **Typical form (90%) conducts antegrade down slow pathway; retrograde up the fast**
- **Atypical form conducts antegrade down fast pathway; retrograde up the slow**

TABLE 5-1	*Bradyarrhythmias*		
Arrhythmia	**Location of Conduction Defect**	**Features**	**Acute Management**
Sinus node dysfunction	Sinus node	Common with advanced age, coronary artery disease, and in association with atrial fibrillation. Very rare in young, healthy patients	Treat only if symptomatic Atropine Isoproterenol Rarely, temporary pacer (if symptomatic)
First degree AV block	Slowed conduction within AV node	PR interval ≥210 msec May limit medical therapy for other cardiac conditions	None required
Second degree AV block Mobitz I (Wenckebach)	AV node dysfunction	Progressive prolongation of the P–R interval until a P wave is blocked May occur with high vagal tone in healthy individuals at rest or during sleep Usually progresses slowly	Rarely, temporary pacer (if symptomatic)
Mobitz II	Lower conduction system (His-Purkinje) defect	Nonconducted P waves without progressive P–R prolongation Often associated with LBBB or bifascicular block Often associated with prior MI cardiomyopathy, hypertension, or diabetes mellitus	Consider temporary pacemaker
Third degree (complete) AV block	Either within or below AV node conduction system defect	Complete dissociation of P waves and QRS complexes	Level of urgency depends on symptoms, QRS width, and escape rate If asymptomatic with narrow QRS: atropine or observation If symptomatic or with wide QRS: temporary pacer

AV, atrioventricular; LBBB, left bundle branch block; MI, myocardial infarction.

TABLE 5-2	*Electrocardiogram Examples of Common Bradyarrhythmias*

First degree AV block

Second degree AV block Mobitz I

Second degree AV block Mobitz II

Third degree AV block

AV, atrioventricular.

TABLE 5-3	Narrow QRS Complex Tachycardias			
Arrhythmia	**Atrial Rate (beats/min)**	**Ratio of Number of Atrial Waves (A) to QRS Complexes (V)**	**P-Wave Morphology**	**Response to Carotid Sinus Pressure**
Sinus tachycardia	100–200	1:1	Sinus	Slowing
AVNRT	150–250	1:1	Retrograde	Termination
ORT*	150–250	1:1	Eccentric	Termination
Atrial flutter	240–320	A > V	Sawtooth flutter waves	↑ AV block
Atrial fibrillation	350–500	A >> V	Fib (F) waves	↓ Ventricular rate
Atrial tachycardia	100–250	A ≥ V	Eccentric	↑ AV block
Junctional tachycardia	60–120	1:1	Retrograde	Slight slowing
MAT	100–180	A ≥ V	3 or more different types	Usually none

*In Wolff-Parkinson-White syndrome.
AV, atrioventricular; AVNRT, atrioventricular nodal re-entrant tachycardia; MAT, multifocal atrial tachycardia; ORT, orthodromic reciprocating tachycardia.

FIGURE 5-1 Re-entrant pathways in atrioventricular (AV) nodal re-entrant tachycardia (AVNRT). The AV node and perinodal tissue have dual physiology: slow-conducting pathway with a short refractory period (S) and fast-conducting pathway with a long refractory period (F). **A,** A normal sinus beat conducts through fast pathway, but conduction through slow pathway is blocked when it hits refractory period of fast pathway. **B,** A premature atrial beat cannot traverse the fast pathway because it remains refractory after prior (normal) beat. Rather, it conducts down slow pathway. **C,** In the typical form of AVNRT, conduction occurs down slow pathway, then retrograde up the fast pathway, with delivery of an echo beat (retrograde P wave immediately following or buried in the QRS complex on electrocardiogram) back up to the atrium. If slow pathway has recovered, the impulse re-enters and re-entrant tachycardia is established. **D,** In the atypical form of AVNRT, conduction occurs down the fast pathway and then retrograde up the slow pathway. The echo atrial beat appears significantly later than the QRS complex because of slow retrograde conduction (R–P > P–R interval).

Clinical Presentation

- **Notable for abrupt onset and termination of rapid regular heartbeat**
- Heart rate usually 150 to 220 beats/min
- Age of onset may range from childhood to old age
- May occasionally be associated with syncope or near-syncope, but usually well tolerated

Diagnosis and Evaluation

- Typical AVNRT findings on ECG (Table 5-4)
  - 1:1 relationship of P wave to QRS complex
  - R–P interval less than P–R interval ("short RP" tachycardia), if P wave can be seen

  - Retrograde P wave at end of QRS complex (pseudo-R′ in V_1; pseudo-S in II)
- Atypical AVNRT findings on ECG
  - R–P interval greater than P–R interval ("long RP" tachycardia)
- Event monitor may be useful in patients with intermittent palpitations

Treatment

- Acute management
  - **May respond to vagal maneuvers**
    - Carotid sinus pressure
    - Valsalva maneuver
  - IV adenosine (6–12 mg rapid push) usually highly effective (90% conversion)
  - IV verapamil (2.5–10 mg) also highly effective
- Chronic management
  - **Catheter ablation (AV node modification, with ablation of slow AV nodal pathway)**
    - **First-line treatment**
    - **Permanent elimination of arrhythmia in more than 95% of patients**
  - Medications—if not a candidate for ablation (Table 5-5)
    - Suppress AV node: verapamil, diltiazem, β-blocker
    - Slow conduction within the re-entrant circuit: flecainide

WOLFF-PARKINSON-WHITE (WPW) SYNDROME

Basic Information

- Definition: WPW syndrome is a term reserved for patients with both pre-excitation on ECG and tachyarrhythmias
  - Most common tachyarrhythmia is AV reciprocating tachycardia (AVRT)
  - Atrial fibrillation is the next most common arrhythmia, and may be life-threatening in this setting, due to rapid conduction down the accessory pathway
- The accessory pathway is a congenital muscle fiber that connects the myocardium of atrium to ventricle across AV groove outside of the AV node (Fig. 5-2)

TABLE 5-4   *Electrocardiogram Examples of Common Supraventricular Tachyarrhythmias*

| AV nodal reentrant tachycardia |
| Atrial flutter |
| Atrial fibrillation |
| Wolff-Parkinson-White (ventricular pre-excitation) |
| Multifocal atrial tachycardia |

TABLE 5-5   *Common Antiarrhythmic Drugs*

Class	Action	Examples	Notable Side Effects
I	Block sodium channels; varying effects on maximal velocity of depolarization and duration of action potential	Class IA: quinidine, procainamide, disopyramide Class IB: lidocaine, mexiletine Class IC: flecainide, propafenone	Class: nausea, vomiting Quinidine: hemolytic anemia, thrombocytopenia, tinnitus Procainamide: drug-induced lupus Lidocaine: dizziness, confusion, seizures, coma Mexiletine: tremor, ataxia, rash Flecainide: proarrhythmic toxicity, nausea, dizziness
II	β-Blockers; ↓ SA node automaticity and ↓ AV node conduction	Propranolol, metoprolol	Class: CHF, bronchospasm, bradycardia, hypotension
III	Prolong action potential duration	Amiodarone, sotalol, dronedarone, ibutilide	Amiodarone: hepatitis, pulmonary toxicity, hypo- and hyperthyroidism, peripheral neuropathy Sotalol: bronchospasm Ibutilide: 1–2.5% risk of inducing polymorphic VT, requiring telemetry during use and at least 4 hr afterward
IV	Calcium channel blockers; ↓ AV nodal conduction	Verapamil, diltiazem	Class: AV block, hypotension, bradycardia, constipation

AV, atrioventricular; CHF, congestive heart failure; SA, sinoatrial; VT, ventricular tachycardia.

- Accessory pathway may be:
  - Manifest: Accessory pathway conducts in antegrade direction (atrium to ventricle) and usually retrograde (ventricle to atrium) as well. Baseline ECG shows pre-excitation (short P–R interval and delta wave, a slurred upstroke of the QRS complex)
  - Concealed: Accessory pathway conducts only in retrograde direction; baseline ECG appears normal
- Age of symptom onset is childhood through middle age

Clinical Presentation

- Some patients with accessory pathways may never develop symptomatic tachycardia (technically do not have WPW *syndrome*, but rather have a WPW ECG)
- Patients may present with tachycardia: AVRT (70%) or atrial fibrillation (30%)
- AVRT in WPW (see Fig. 5-2)
  - Classified into orthodromic or antidromic depending on direction of conduction over the AV node
    - Orthodromic AV reciprocating tachycardia (ORT): Tachycardia conducts antegrade down AV node and retrograde up accessory pathway
      - Most common form of AVRT (95%)
      - May occur with manifest or concealed accessory pathways
    - Antidromic AV reciprocating tachycardia (ART): Tachycardia conducts antegrade down the accessory pathway and retrograde up the AV node or a second accessory pathway
      - Less common (5%)
      - Wide-complex tachycardia on ECG; may be mistaken for ventricular tachycardia (VT)
- **Atrial fibrillation in WPW**
  - **May be life-threatening**
  - **Manifest accessory pathways often conduct rapidly with short refractory period; may result in extremely rapid transmission of atrial fibrillation to ventricles**
  - **Wide, irregularly irregular QRS complex morphologies on ECG**
  - **May degenerate to ventricular fibrillation and cardiac arrest**

FIGURE 5-2 Re-entrant tachycardia in Wolff-Parkinson-White syndrome. In orthodromic re-entrant tachycardia, the impulse conducts down the atrioventricular (AV) node and then retrograde up the accessory pathway. ECG during tachycardia shows a narrow QRS complex without the delta wave. In antidromic re-entrant tachycardia, the opposite circuit is established (conduction down the accessory pathway and up through the AV node). ECG shows a wide, bizarre QRS complex.

Diagnosis and Evaluation

- ECG findings with manifest accessory pathway (see Table 5-4)
  - **Short P–R interval (<120 ms)**
  - **Delta wave with widened QRS complex**
    - Caused by dual ventricular activation through both the accessory pathway and the normal AV node/His-Purkinje conduction system

Treatment

- Asymptomatic patients
  - **Risk of sudden death is generally low**
  - Usually do not benefit from electrophysiologic (EP) testing, except those in high-risk occupations (e.g., pilot, competitive athletes). Some studies support prophylactic EP testing in younger asymptomatic individuals (<35 years) as well.
- Symptomatic patients
  - **Acute management of AVRT: vagal maneuvers, IV nodal blockers (adenosine, β-blockers, verapamil)**
  - **Acute management of atrial fibrillation with pre-excitation**
    - **First-line therapy: IV procainamide or IV amiodarone (both slow accessory pathway and AV nodal conduction)**
    - **Avoid use of digoxin or calcium channel blockers, which may cause even more rapid ventricular response via selective nodal blockade and shortening of atrial refractoriness**
    - **Emergent electrical cardioversion if patient hypotensive or otherwise unstable**
- Chronic management
  - Catheter ablation: first-line therapy in symptomatic patients
    - 2- to 4-hour procedure to localize and ablate (cauterize) the accessory pathway
    - Success rates 90% to 95% depending on the site of the accessory pathway
  - Flecainide and β-blockers used to prevent further episodes of AVRT in patients with prior episodes while awaiting catheter ablation, or if ablation contraindicated or not accepted by the patient

ATRIAL FIBRILLATION AND ATRIAL FLUTTER

Basic Information

- Atrial fibrillation (AF) and atrial flutter are distinct arrhythmias that often occur in the same patient population
- Atrial fibrillation
  - Most common sustained arrhythmia
  - Sustained by multiple re-entrant wavelets within the atria; the role of triggering atrial ectopy from pulmonary veins has been increasingly recognized
  - Increasing incidence with advancing age and with hypertension, diabetes, and structural heart disease
  - May be paroxysmal (episodes lasting <7 days) or persistent (>7 days)
    - Paroxysmal form often initiated by premature atrial contractions (PACs) or bursts of ectopic atrial activity (often originating in pulmonary veins); often no structural heart disease present

- Persistent form often associated with one or more of the following:
  - Structural heart disease (mitral stenosis and other valvular disease, atrial enlargement, hypertension)
  - Hyperthyroidism (about 1% of AF cases)
- Atrial flutter
  - Macro re-entrant circuit usually confined to the right atrium, typically proceeds counterclockwise around the tricuspid valve annulus in the left anterior view
  - Age of onset: Usually age 40 years or older, similar to AF

Clinical Presentation

- Atrial fibrillation: palpitations, fatigue, exertional dyspnea, dizziness
- Atrial flutter: palpitations, exertional dyspnea; may present with syncope or presyncope with 1:1 AV conduction

Diagnosis and Evaluation (see Table 5-3)

- ECG in AF (see Table 5-4)
  - **Fibrillatory (F) waves instead of P waves; atrial rate 350 to 500 beats/min**
  - **Irregularly irregular and often rapid ventricular response**
- ECG in atrial flutter (see Table 5-4)
  - **"Sawtooth" P-wave pattern in the inferior leads**
  - **Atrial rate typically 300 beats/min with 2:1 AV conduction**
  - Carotid sinus massage or adenosine will slow AV conduction and may reveal flutter waves previously hidden
  - 1:1 AV conduction may occur in younger patients when atrial flutter rate is relatively slow and excellent AV conduction is present

Treatment

- Acute management of AF and atrial flutter
  - Rate control with β-blocker, calcium channel blocker (verapamil, diltiazem)
  - Digoxin less potent but useful if heart failure present or if single-agent therapy inadequate. Digoxin is not effective for paroxysmal AF.
  - Rate-controlling drugs do not terminate the arrhythmia or prevent recurrence
  - Cardiovert if hemodynamically unstable (hypotension, congestive heart failure, angina, etc.)
- Chronic management options for AF
  - Rate control as in preceding section (β-blockers, calcium channel blockers, digoxin)
  - **Suppression with antiarrhythmic agents (if symptomatic despite rate controlling agents)**
    - Class IC antiarrhythmic agents (flecainide, propafenone) often used first-line in patients with structurally normal heart
    - Amiodarone generally used in patients with systolic heart failure and in patients with severe left ventricular hypertrophy
    - Sotalol, dofetilide (class III agents) are acceptable alternatives in patients with coronary disease who cannot take class I agents
    - Dronedarone is a new class III agent with clinical action similar to amiodarone. It appears to be safer though less efficacious than amiodarone.

- Electrical cardioversion may be attempted to achieve sinus rhythm in symptomatic patients
  - Before cardioversion, patients with AF or flutter continuously present for over 36 to 48 hours should receive either:
    - Anticoagulation (therapeutic for at least 4 weeks before conversion and 4 weeks after conversion)
    - Transesophageal echocardiogram to exclude atrial thrombus before conversion, followed by 4 weeks of continuous anticoagulation after conversion
- "Ablate and pace": In selected patients with refractory symptoms due to rapid ventricular response, AV node ablation prevents conduction of rapid impulses to ventricle
  - Atria still fibrillate—therefore, chronic anticoagulation remains necessary
  - Requires permanent ventricular pacemaker placement for subsequent AV block
  - Generally reserved for older patients with symptoms refractory to other therapies
- Paroxysmal or short-duration persistent AF may be palliated by pulmonary vein isolation (a catheter ablation procedure that does not involve AV node ablation) in symptomatic individuals refractory to or intolerant of antiarrhythmic medications
- Chronic anticoagulation (generally with warfarin or dabigatran) to prevent stroke in both paroxysmal and persistent AF based primarily on stroke risk factors
  - Antithrombotic therapy is recommended for all patients with AF except lone AF, unless contraindications exist
  - Choice of antithrombotic agent is based on risk of stroke versus risk of bleeding
  - Risk assessment and indications for antithrombotic agents: see Box 5-1
  - Patients initiated on warfarin should have international normalized ratio (INR) checked weekly until a stable goal INR of 2 to 3 is achieved
  - Dabigatran, an oral direct-acting thrombin inhibitor, has recently emerged as an alternative to warfarin for many patients with non-valvular AF and preserved renal function

---

BOX 5-1 | *Indications for Antithrombotic Agents in Atrial Fibrillation*

Low risk: Aspirin 81–325 mg/day

Moderate risk: Warfarin or dabigatran for patients with one or more risk factors
  Age >75
  Diabetes
  Hypertension
  Heart failure
  Impaired left ventricular systolic function (EF ≤35%)

High risk: Warfarin*
  Mechanical heart valves
  Prior thromboembolism (stroke/TIA or systemic embolization)
  Rheumatic mitral stenosis

EF, ejection fraction; TIA, transient ischemic attack.
*Dabigatran acceptable if prior thromboembolism is only high-risk feature.

- Chronic management of atrial flutter
  - Cardioversion (electrical or chemical)
  - Catheter ablation of re-entrant circuit: More than 90% to 95% permanent elimination of atrial flutter
  - **Anticoagulation**
    - **Thromboembolic risk probably similar to that in AF; strong consideration should be given to anticoagulant therapy (same guidelines as for AF; see Box 5-1)**

OTHER SUPRAVENTRICULAR TACHYCARDIAS

- Sinus tachycardia
  - Almost always caused by physiologic stimulus (e.g., fever, hypotension, infection, hemodynamic stress, endocrine disorder)
  - Features: see Table 5-3
  - Treatment
    - Critical to identify and treat the underlying cause
    - **β-Blockade helpful if caused by thyrotoxicosis, inappropriate sinus tachycardia, or if associated with cardiac ischemia**
- Focal atrial tachycardia
  - Mechanism is usually enhanced automaticity or triggered activity
  - May be caused by digoxin toxicity
  - Features: see Table 5-3
  - Acute management: Rate control or suppression with β-blocker or verapamil
  - Chronic management: Rate control; suppression with flecainide, sotalol, or amiodarone; catheter ablation can eliminate arrhythmia in most patients
- Multifocal atrial tachycardia
  - Arises from multiple automatic or triggered foci in one or both atria
  - Occurs with elevated sympathetic tone, pulmonary disease (e.g., chronic obstructive pulmonary disease), hypoxemia, stimulant use
  - **ECG: Three or more P-wave morphologies present, usually with varying P–R intervals (see Table 5-4)**
  - **Treatment: Treat underlying cause (e.g., hypoxemia); rate control**
  - Generally not amenable to catheter ablation
- Junctional tachycardia
  - Automatic rhythm arising in AV node

- Occurs with enhanced automaticity (elevated sympathetic tone), after cardiac surgery, myocardial ischemia, digoxin toxicity
- Features: see Table 5-3
- Acute management: Treat underlying cause
- Chronic management: Usually none required
  - Rare cases require antiarrhythmic therapy; catheter ablation may to lead to AV block

Ventricular Tachyarrhythmias

VENTRICULAR TACHYCARDIA

Basic Information

- Characterized by wide QRS complex (Table 5-6)
- Majority (85%) of wide-complex tachycardias are ventricular; remainder are supraventricular with aberrant conduction
- Helpful clues to distinguish supraventricular versus ventricular origin (Box 5-2)
- Several forms of ventricular tachycardia (VT) (see Table 5-6)
  - May be nonsustained (3 beats to 30 sec) or sustained (>30 sec), monomorphic, or polymorphic
  - Prognosis and therapeutic approach are dependent on presence of underlying structural heart disease (Fig. 5-3)
  - Several forms of generally benign idiopathic VT may occur in otherwise healthy patients with structurally normal hearts; RVOT VT is most common

Clinical Presentation

- **Nonsustained VT: May be asymptomatic or cause occasional palpitations**
- Sustained VT: More likely to cause lightheadedness, near-syncope, syncope, or cardiac arrest

Diagnosis and Evaluation

- ECG findings (Table 5-7)
- Evaluation for structural heart disease: Should always include echocardiography; additional studies may include exercise/stress testing, nuclear imaging, or cardiac magnetic resonance imaging
- Monitoring: Depending on frequency of symptoms, may include 24- to 48-hour Holter monitor, 30-day event monitor, or long-term implantable loop recorder (ILR)

TABLE 5-6	Ventricular Tachyarrhythmias				
Arrhythmia	**Ventricular Rate (bpm)**	**QRS Morphology**	**Substrate**	**Drug Therapy**	**Ablatable**
Sustained monomorphic VT	140–250	Any	Post-MI, cardiomyopathy	Procainamide, amiodarone	Yes
Idiopathic RVOT VT	140–220	LBBB	Normal	β-Blockers, verapamil	Yes
Ventricular fibrillation	>300	Polymorphic	Ischemia, cardiomyopathy	Lidocaine, amiodarone	No
Torsades de pointes	200–300	Polymorphic	Long QT	β-Blockers	No

LBBB, left bundle branch block; MI, myocardial infarction; RVOT, right ventricular outflow tract; VT, ventricular tachycardia.

- Electrophysiologic study: Most useful in evaluation of monomorphic (rather than polymorphic) VT

Treatment

- Medications: see Table 5-6
- If acutely hemodynamically unstable—emergent cardioversion/defibrillation
- Chronic treatment of most VTs based on underlying presence of ischemic heart disease
  - Patients with monomorphic VT and no underlying structural heart disease (i.e., idiopathic VT) have a good prognosis
    - Medical treatment: β-blockers, verapamil, flecainide, sotalol, amiodarone

BOX 5-2	*Characteristics Suggestive of Ventricular Origin (vs. Supraventricular Origin) of Wide-Complex Tachycardias*

History of structural or ischemic heart disease
Absence of an RS complex in all precordial leads
Peak of R wave to nadir of S interval >100 ms in one precordial lead
Presence of AV dissociation (P waves unrelated to QRS complexes)
Presence of fusion complexes (sinus QRS complex fuses with VT beats) or capture beats (sinus QRS complex appears between VT beats)
QRS duration >0.16 sec

- Catheter ablation highly effective (80–90%) for long-term elimination of idiopathic VT
- Patients with underlying heart disease and depressed left ventricular function (EF ≤35%) are at increased risk of sudden death
  - Implantable cardioverter-defibrillator (ICD) shown to prolong survival in patients with:
    - Ischemic heart disease and left ventricular ejection fraction (LVEF) ≤30%
    - Ischemic or nonischemic cardiomyopathy (LVEF ≤35%), and New York Heart Association (NYHA) class II or III heart failure
  - EP study may be useful for risk stratification of some patients with milder forms of cardiomyopathy who have nonsustained VT or symptoms possibly related to VT (i.e., palpitations, syncope)
  - Catheter ablation provides useful adjunctive therapy for recurrent VT in patients with ICDs to prevent symptoms and recurrent ICD shocks

VENTRICULAR FIBRILLATION

Basic Information

- Characterized by irregular, chaotic wide QRS complex (see Table 5-6) with rate greater than 300 beats/min
- Causes
  - Acute myocardial infarction
  - Myocardial ischemia
  - Cardiomyopathy

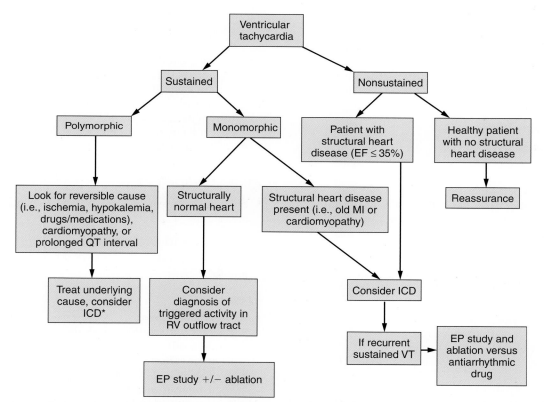

FIGURE 5-3 Approach to ventricular tachycardia. (EF, ejection fraction; EP, electrophysiology; ICD, implantable cardioverter-defibrillator; MI, myocardial infarction; RV, right ventricular; VT, ventricular tachycardia.) *Polymorphic VT due to congenital long QT syndrome or irreversible cardiomyopathy usually requires ICD implantation.

TABLE 5-7	*Electrocardiogram Examples of Common Ventricular Tachyarrhythmias*

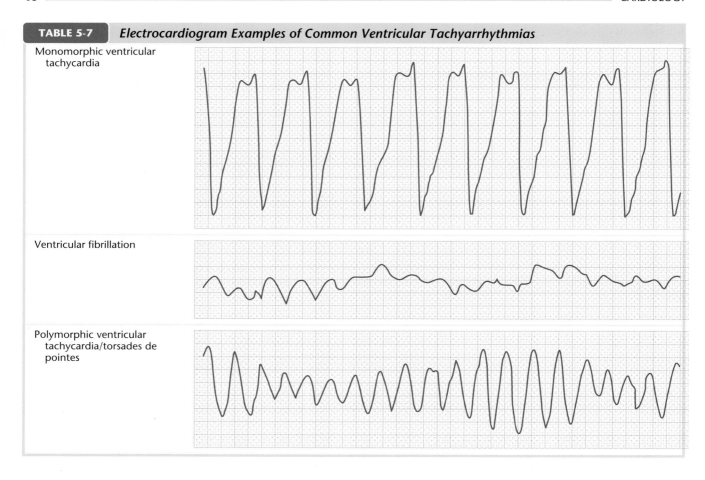

Monomorphic ventricular tachycardia

Ventricular fibrillation

Polymorphic ventricular tachycardia/torsades de pointes

- Metabolic disturbance (i.e., hypokalemia, acidosis)
- Drugs (i.e., digoxin, tricyclic antidepressants, cocaine)

Clinical Presentation
- Cardiac arrest or sudden death

Diagnosis and Evaluation
- ECG findings: see Table 5-7

Treatment
- Medications: see Table 5-6
- **Immediate electrical defibrillation is essential**
- ICD for secondary prevention in most patients, unless VF due to transient or reversible cause (i.e., intoxication, acute myocardial infarction)

TORSADES DE POINTES
Basic Information
- A form of polymorphic VT associated with prolonged ventricular repolarization, manifested as prolonged QT interval on ECG
- May be seen in congenital or acquired long QT syndromes
  - Congenital long QT syndrome (LQTS) usually due to mutations in cardiac ion channels that affect ventricular repolarization (most commonly cardiac potassium or sodium channels)

- A mutation can be identified in 60% to 70% of affected individuals
- Acquired LQTS most commonly associated with certain medications (see www.qtdrugs.org; Box 5-3) or electrolyte disturbance (i.e., hypokalemia, hypomagnesemia)
- Tachycardia usually precipitated by a premature ventricular contraction (R-on-T wave), which may occur in a bigeminal pattern

Clinical Presentation
- Sudden death, syncope, presyncope, or may be asymptomatic

Diagnosis and Evaluation
- ECG: Often with prolonged QT interval (see Tables 5-6 and 5-7)

Treatment
- **Acute management**
  - **Correct underlying metabolic abnormality or remove offending medication**
  - **IV magnesium**
  - IV lidocaine (1–1.5 mg/kg over 2 min)
  - Increase heart rate to decrease QT duration:
    - IV isoproterenol (Isuprel)
    - Temporary overdrive pacing to 90 to 100 beats/min
- Chronic management

BOX 5-3	Select Drugs Associated with Torsades de Pointes (see www.qtdrugs.org)

Class IA antiarrhythmics (quinidine, procainamide, disopyramide)
Class III antiarrhythmics (sotalol, dofetilide, ibutilide, amiodarone, dronedarone)
Methadone
Erythromycin
Ketoconazole
Haloperidol
Cisapride
Pentamidine

- Avoidance of QT-prolonging drugs in all patients
- Avoidance of hypokalemia and hypomagnesemia in all patients
- β-Blockers for congenital LQTS
- ICD in selected patients with congenital LQTS (recurrent syncope or torsades on β-blockers, personal/family history of cardiac arrest, other high-risk markers)

Syncope

Basic Information

- Syncope is common, with approximate lifetime prevalence of 20% to 25% of the population
- Differential diagnosis categorized into cardiac, neurally mediated, and orthostatic etiologies (Box 5-4)
- A cause is never identified in up to 25% to 40% of cases

Clinical Presentation

- **Characterized by transient, unintentional loss of consciousness and postural tone (seconds to minutes in duration) due to cerebral hypoperfusion, followed by full spontaneous recovery**
  - Does *not* include seizure, hypoglycemia, cataplexy, etc.
- History and physical examination
  - Ascertain history, symptoms, or signs of cardiac or neurologic disease
  - Characterize episode: Precipitating factors, prodromal and recovery symptoms
  - Evaluate for possible offending medications
  - Obtain orthostatic vital signs

Diagnosis and Evaluation

- History and physical examination often provide most important clues in diagnosis
- Careful review of a 12-lead ECG is essential in all patients
- Echocardiogram often useful to assess for structural heart disease
  - **Arrhythmia is most likely cause in presence of structural heart disease** (see management in preceding sections)
    - Refer for EP evaluation
  - **Vasovagal syncope is most likely cause in absence of structural heart disease**

BOX 5-4	Causes of Syncope

Cardiogenic syncope
Anatomic: Aortic stenosis, atrial myxoma, acute myocardial infarction, hypertrophic cardiomyopathy
Arrhythmic: Bradycardia, tachycardia
Extracardiac obstructive: pericardial constriction or tamponade, pulmonary embolism, aortic dissection
Neurally-mediated (reflex) syncope
Vagally-mediated/vasovagal
Carotid sinus sincope
Situational: cough, sneeze, micturition, postexercise
Orthostatic syncope
Volume depletion
Drug-induced: antihypertensives, alcohol, antidepressants
Primary autonomic failure: idiopathic dysautonomia, Lewy body dementia, multiple system atrophy, Parkinson's disease with autonomic involvement
Secondary autonomic failure: diabetes, amyloidosis, spinal injury
Conditions with altered consciousness commonly *miscategorized* **as syncope:**
Metabolic: hyperventilation, hypoglycemia, hypoxemia
Neurologic: seizures, migraines

- Consider tilt-table test to evaluate autonomic system (more useful in recurrent episodes)

Treatment

- Treat the underlying condition; remove nonessential medications that may contribute
- Vasovagal syncope
  - Hydration and liberalization of salt consumption
  - Educate about standing slowly from sitting position
  - Eliminate any offending medications if possible
  - Midodrine in refractory cases
  - Pacemakers in exceptional cases associated with prolonged asystole

Sudden Cardiac Death

Basic Information

- "Sudden cardiac death" is defined as sudden unexpected death that occurs within 1 hour of symptoms due to documented or presumed cardiac cause
- Ventricular fibrillation or pulseless VT is responsible for 30% to 60% of events, depending on the setting, with a majority of events in patients with structural heart disease
- May represent the first manifestation of ischemic heart disease

Diagnosis and Evaluation

- ECG for evidence of myocardial infarction or ischemia, accessory pathway (WPW syndrome), prolonged QT interval, Brugada syndrome
- Laboratory data to rule out reversible causes, such as cardiac enzymes, electrolytes, drug levels, and urine toxicology screen

BOX 5-5 · *Indications for ICD Implantation*

- Documented VT/VF cardiac arrest not due to transient or reversible cause (i.e., MI, intoxication)
- Documented familial or inherited conditions with high risk of life-threatening arrhythmia, such as LQTS, HCM
- Documented prior MI (>40 days), LVEF <40%, inducible sustained VT or VF at EP study (MADIT-1 criteria)
- Documented prior MI, LVEF ≤30% either 40 days following MI or 3 mo following revascularization
  Patients must *not* have:
  - NYHA class IV symptoms
  - Cardiogenic shock while in a stable baseline rhythm
  - CABG or PTCA within past 3 months
  - Enzyme-positive MI within past 40 days
  - Symptoms or findings that indicate candidacy for coronary revascularization
  - Coexisting disease with expected survival <1 yr
- Patients with ischemic cardiomyopathy, documented prior MI, measured LVEF ≤35%, and NYHA class II or III CHF
- Patients with nonischemic dilated cardiomyopathy >3 mo on appropriate medical therapy and measured LVEF ≤35% and NYHA class II or III CHF
- Patients with NYHA class IV CHF who meet other requirements for cardiac resynchronization therapy

CABG, coronary artery bypass grafting; CHF, congestive heart failure; EP, electrophysiology; HCM, hypertrophic cardiomyopathy; LQTS, long QT syndrome; LVEF, left ventricular ejection fraction; MADIT-1, Multicenter Automatic Defibrillator Implantation Trial 1; MI, myocardial infarction; NYHA, New York Heart Association; PTCA, percutaneous transluminal coronary angioplasty; VF, ventricular fibrillation; VT, ventricular tachycardia.

- Continuous telemetry to monitor for recurrent event until definitive therapy is in place
- Echocardiogram to evaluate for structural heart disease
- Coronary angiography in most cases to exclude coronary disease or congenital coronary anomaly

Treatment

- Treat underlying causes
  - Eliminate proarrhythmic medications
  - Coronary revascularization for ischemic heart disease

- IV amiodarone or lidocaine useful in acute management of repeated arrhythmia
- ICD for most patients with VT or ventricular fibrillation causing cardiac arrest not due to transient or reversible cause (Box 5-5)

REVIEW QUESTIONS

For review questions, please go to www.expertconsult.com.

SUGGESTED READINGS

A comparison of antiarrhythmic-drug therapy with implantable defibrillators in patients resuscitated from near-fatal ventricular arrhythmias: The Antiarrhythmics Versus Implantable Defibrillators (AVID) Investigators, *N Engl J Med* 337:1576–1583, 1997.

Bardy GH, Lee KL, Mark DB, et al: Amiodarone or an implantable cardioverter-defibrillator for congestive heart failure, *N Engl J Med* 352:225–237, 2005.

Bristow MR, Saxon LA, Boehmer J, et al: Cardiac-resynchronization therapy with or without an implantable defibrillator in advanced chronic heart failure, *N Engl J Med* 350:2140–2150, 2004.

Buxton AE, Lee KL, Fisher JD, et al: A randomized study of the prevention of sudden death in patients with coronary artery disease. Multicenter Unsustained Tachycardia Trial Investigators, *N Engl J Med* 341:1882–1890, 1999.

Calkins H, Yong P, Miller JM, et al: Catheter ablation of accessory pathways, atrioventricular nodal reentrant tachycardia, and the atrioventricular junction: final results of a prospective, multicenter clinical trial. The Atakr Multicenter Investigators Group, *Circulation* 99:195–197, 1999.

Epstein AE, Dimarco JP, Ellenbogen KA, et al: ACC/AHA/HRS 2008 guidelines for device-based therapy of cardiac rhythm abnormalities, *Heart Rhythm* 5:e1–e62, 2008.

Haissaguerre M, Jais P, Shah DC, et al: Spontaneous initiation of atrial fibrillation by ectopic beats originating in the pulmonary veins, *N Engl J Med* 339:659–666, 1998.

Moss AJ, Zareha W, Hall WJ, et al: Prophylactic implantation of a defibrillator in patients with myocardial infarction and reduced ejection fraction, *N Engl J Med* 346:877–883, 2002.

Moya A, Sutton R, Ammirati F, et al: Task Force for the Diagnosis and Management of Syncope; European Society of Cardiology (ESC); European Society Heart Rhythm Association (EHRA); Heart Failure Association (HFA); Heart Rhythm Society (HRS)Guidelines for the diagnosis and management of syncope (version 2009), *Eur Heart J* 30:2631–2671, 2009.

Heart Failure

ROSANNE ROUF, MD

Heart failure (HF) is a common health problem that leads to significant morbidity and mortality. In the United States, approximately 5 million people have HF, and up to 550,000 cases are newly diagnosed each year. The condition exists when the heart can no longer meet the metabolic needs of the body. It can result from any disorder that impairs the ability of the ventricle to fill with or pump blood. It has been estimated that HF causes or contributes to about 290,000 deaths per year. Survival is poor, with only 50% of patients surviving longer than 5 years. Identification of the cause, followed by aggressive treatment, is crucial to improve survival.

Basic Information

- **Definition: HF is a complex clinical syndrome that occurs when the heart or circulation is unable to meet the metabolic demands of peripheral tissue at normal cardiac filling pressures; it can occur in patients with normal or depressed systolic function**
- Commonly divided into systolic and nonsystolic heart failure (Table 6-1)
  - Systolic: Left ventricle (LV) contracts poorly and empties inadequately, leading to depressed systolic function and ejection fraction (EF)
    - Often leads to right ventricular failure
    - Over time, the LV dilates, increasing wall stress and oxygen demand
    - More common (60% of patients)
    - Can result from pressure, volume overload, or myocardial damage
  - Nonsystolic: Elevated diastolic filling pressure despite normal diastolic volumes and normal systolic function and EF
    - Poor LV filling may produce low cardiac output state and poor perfusion
    - Occurs in 40% of patients
    - Can result from high output or diastolic function impairment
- Clinical signs and symptoms: dyspnea, fatigue, fluid retention, effort intolerance, inadequate organ perfusion, and arrhythmias
- Caused by a variety of conditions, some unrelated to the heart
- High output: Results from a persistent need for high cardiac output; normal systolic function
  - Increased metabolic demands (thyrotoxicosis, Paget disease, beriberi)
  - Severe anemia
  - Arteriovenous fistula
  - Persistent tachycardia

- Pressure or volume overload
  - Hypertension
  - Valvular heart disease (aortic stenosis, mitral regurgiration)
  - Intracardiac shunting (ventricular septal defect, atrial septal defect, patent ductus arteriosus)
  - Myocyte damage or abnormality
  - Myocardial infarction, ischemia
  - Drugs (chemotherapeutic agents)
  - Toxins (alcohol, cocaine)
  - Infection/inflammation
  - Inherited/familial (dilated cardiomyopathy, muscular dystrophy, glycogen storage diseases)
- Impaired diastolic function
  - Aging
  - Hypertension
  - Ischemia
  - Constrictive pericarditis
  - Infiltrative disease (amyloid, sarcoid, hemochromatosis)
  - Inherited/familial (hypertrophic cardiomyopathy [HCM])
- **Most common causes are coronary artery disease, myocardial infarction, and hypertension**
- **In the elderly, 50% of cases may be caused by nonsystolic dysfunction, particularly with concurrent hypertension**
- Causes of acute HF
  - Decompensation of preexisting chronic HF from a precipitating factor (see next list)
  - Myocardial infarction or ischemia, especially if (1) the papillary muscle is involved, leading to mitral regurgitation; (2) if ventricular septum rupture occurs; or (3) a right ventricular infarct results in a low cardiac output state
  - Hypertensive crisis
  - Acute arrhythmia
  - Valvular heart disease
  - Acute endocarditis (with aortic or mitral regurgitation)
  - Acute dilated cardiomyopathy (myocarditis, cocaine, toxins)
  - Cardiac tamponade
  - High-output HF (Paget disease, thyrotoxicosis, beriberi)
- Factors precipitating decompensated HF in preexisting chronic HF
  - Natural course of disease
  - Dietary indiscretion (excessive fluid or salt intake)
  - Noncompliance with medications

TABLE 6-1	*Comparison of Systolic Versus Nonsystolic Heart Failure*	
	Systolic Dysfunction	**Nonsystolic Dysfunction**
Incidence	60% of heart failure patients	40% of heart failure patients
Mechanism	Impaired ejection	Impaired filling
Physical findings	S_3 and/or S_4 Weak carotid upstroke Displaced apical impulse	S_4 more common Normal carotid upstroke Forceful apical impulse Hypertrophic cardiomyopathy Rapid, strong carotid upstroke S_4 more common Outflow murmur Ventricular heave
Causes	Coronary artery disease Idiopathic cardiomyopathy Valvular heart disease Hypertension Myocarditis Drug-induced Toxin-induced Systemic disease	Hypertension Diabetes mellitus Ischemia Aging Pericardial disease Restrictive cardiomyopathy Hypertrophic cardiomyopathy Amyloidosis

- Infection
- New myocardial ischemia
- Metabolic stress (e.g., anemia, hyperthyroidism)
- Medications such as nonsteroidal anti-inflammatory medications (leads to sodium retention)
- **Cardiomyopathy: Primary heart muscle disease usually classified into three types**
  - **Dilated cardiomyopathy (Fig. 6-1)**
    - **Ventricular dilation associated with decreased contractility (left ventricular ejection fraction [LVEF] <45%)**
    - **Most common type of cardiomyopathy**
    - Multiple causes (Box 6-1)
    - Most commonly caused by coronary artery disease, followed by idiopathic causes
    - Commonly presents as decompensated HF; can also see angina, systemic emboli, syncope, and sudden death as initial presentation
    - Most forms worsen after an initial period of compensation, leading to eventual death or transplantation
    - Prognosis depends on cause; some improve spontaneously (15–20%)
      - The more symptomatic, the worse the prognosis
      - New York Heart Association (NYHA) class IV: 1-year mortality is 50%
      - For any given EF, ischemic cause always has worse prognosis
      - Predictors of bad prognosis: hyponatremia, high filling pressures, and low cardiac index
  - **Hypertrophic cardiomyopathy (see Fig. 6-1)**
    - **Hypertrophy of left, right, or both ventricles**

- **Hypertrophy may be generalized or focal; if localized to septum, old term was idiopathic hypertrophic subaortic stenosis (IHSS) or asymmetrical septal hypertrophy (ASH)**
- Most cases are caused by mutations in genes involved in contractile apparatus
  - Beta-myosin heavy chain (most common)
  - Others include troponin T and tropomyosin
  - Clinical course may depend on genotype
- Histologically characterized by myofibril disarray
- Differential diagnosis is hypertrophy resulting from hypertension (called hypertensive HCM), renal failure, or Fabry disease
- Pathophysiology
  - May cause left ventricular outflow tract obstruction, sometimes dynamic—made worse by increased contractility and decreased ventricular volume
  - Results in a high-pressure apical region and a low-pressure subaortic region—a gradient results in a contact point between the septum and the anterior leaflet of the mitral valve during systole
  - Gradient defined as a greater than 30 mm Hg difference at rest or with stimulation (exercise, post–ventricular premature beat)
  - Ventricular volumes are small and EF is *increased*
- Presentation
  - Hypertrophy almost always presents by age 20s and symptoms by age 30s
  - **May be obstructive or nonobstructive (more common)**
  - Many never develop obstruction or symptoms
  - **Symptoms: dyspnea, palpitations, syncope, and sudden death**
  - Outflow murmur may be augmented with maneuvers that decrease preload (Valsalva, squat-to-stand) or medications that decrease afterload (amyl nitrite, vasodilators)
  - Carotid upstroke is rapid (versus delayed in aortic stenosis)
  - Variable prognosis; some patients die suddenly, often young and during organized sports (most common cause of death in a young athlete during competition); others develop HF
  - A few patients will evolve into a dilated cardiomyopathy
  - **Familial screening of first-degree relatives with echocardiogram and electrocardiogram (ECG) mandatory**
- **Restrictive cardiomyopathy**
  - **Most uncommon form of cardiomyopathy in developed world**
  - **Characterized by restrictive filling of left or right ventricle, yet normal or near-normal ventricular function**
  - Hallmark is diastolic dysfunction
  - Ventricular wall thickness normal or increased; biatrial enlargement
  - May see square root sign on cardiac catheterization (dip and plateau signifying rapid, early filling)
    - Usually presents clinically as right-sided HF
    - Multiple causes

FIGURE 6-1 Gross pathology of hypertrophic and dilated cardiomyopathies. **A,** Hypertrophic cardiomyopathy showing marked hypertrophy especially of the interventricular septum. **B,** Normal heart. **C,** Dilated cardiomyopathy with increased chamber size and spherical shape of left ventricle. *(From Seidman JG, Seidman C: The genetic basis for cardiomyopathy: from mutation identification to mechanistic paradigms, Cell 104:557, 2001.)*

BOX 6-1 *Selected Causes of Dilated Cardiomyopathy*

Coronary artery disease
Alcohol
Peripartum
Infections (viral, Chagas disease)
Myocarditis
Hypertension
Drugs (doxorubicin, cyclophosphamide, cocaine)
Familial
Storage disease
Thyroid disease
Vasculitis (lupus)
Pheochromocytoma
Neuromuscular diseases (Duchenne muscular dystrophy)
Uremia
Idiopathic

- Usually unknown (idiopathic)
- Infiltrative diseases
- Amyloid: Usually caused by primary (AL) form; echo often shows a hyper-refractile ground-glass appearance of the myocardium; low voltage on ECG; frequent arrhythmias
- Sarcoid: Many have subclinical heart involvement; conduction disturbances common
- Hemochromatosis: 15% may present with cardiac involvement; arrhythmias may occur; rapid progression to death if untreated
- Fabry disease
- Endocardial fibroelastosis
- Löffler syndrome
- Variable prognosis that depends on cause
  - Idiopathic variety almost always a slow, progressive decline
  - Amyloid associated with high mortality in patients with congestive HF (almost 90% mortality in 6 months)
- Pathophysiology of HF
  - Neurohormonal mechanisms

- Neurohormonal activation often initially compensatory but detrimental long term, leading to further ventricular dysfunction
- Norepinephrine, renin-angiotensin-aldosterone, endothelin, atrial natriuretic peptide, vasopressin, cytokines, nitric oxide, and others are involved (Fig. 6-2)
- Leads to vasoconstriction and increases systemic and pulmonic vascular resistance and decreases renal blood flow
- Enhances the vasopressin and renin-angiotensin-aldosterone system
- Induces ventricular hypertrophy and changes in interstitium
- Induces ischemia and possibly programmed cell death (apoptosis)
- This process leads to further dilation termed *remodeling*; ventricular shape becomes more spherical
- Renin-angiotensin-aldosterine-vasopressin system (RAA system)
  - Poor renal blood flow activates the RAA system, increasing sodium and water retention
  - Angiotensin II enhances aldosterone production, which enhances sodium resorption and produces myocardial collagen deposition and fibrosis
  - Angiotensin II also enhances vasopressin, which decreases renal excretion of free water contributing to hyponatremia in HF

Clinical Presentation

- Symptoms and signs of HF—usually caused by fluid retention or poor cardiac output (or both) (Table 6-2)
- NYHA classification—a measure of severity of symptoms (Table 6-3)
- It is often difficult to differentiate dilated cardiomyopathy from HCM on history or physical examination
  - S4 more common in HCM (because of atrial contraction against a stiff ventricle)
  - Outflow tract murmur may be present in HCM and pulse may be bisferiens (two humps)

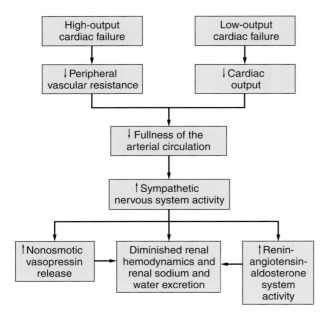

FIGURE 6-2 Pathophysiology of heart failure. Mechanism of high-output and low-output heart failure leading to activation of neurohormonal vasoconstrictor systems and renal sodium and water retention. *(From Schrier RW, Abraham WT: Hormones and hemodynamics in heart failure, N Engl J Med 341:577, 1999.)*

TABLE 6-3	New York Heart Association Classification	
Class	**Severity of Symptoms**	**Description**
I	None to mild	No symptoms
II	Mild to moderate	Symptoms with moderate exertion
III	Moderate to severe	Symptoms with minimal exertion
IV	Severe	Symptoms at rest

TABLE 6-2	Symptoms and Signs of Congestive Heart Failure	
Symptoms	**Signs**	
Dyspnea	Increased jugular venous pressure	
Cough (especially when recumbent)	Crackles (rales)	
	Hepatojugular reflux	
Anorexia and weight loss	S_3 and/or S_4	
Orthopnea	Pedal edema and/or ascites	
Paroxysmal nocturnal dyspnea	Hepatomegaly	
	Tachycardia	
RUQ abdominal pain (hepatic congestion)	Decreased pulse pressure	
	Cachexia	
Fatigue and poor exercise tolerance	Mitral or tricuspid regurgitation	
	Hypotension	
Nocturia	Cool extremities	

RUQ, right upper quadrant.

- Outflow murmur is harsh, crescendo-decrescendo, located at lower sternal border
  - Increased by standing, post-extrasystole, hypovolemia, Valsalva maneuver (during strain) (decreased preload increases the obstruction)
  - Decreased by squatting, isometric handgrip (increased afterload decreases the obstruction)
  - Ventricular heave
- Restrictive cardiomyopathy and pericardial disease (tamponade, constrictive pericarditis) often present with predominately right-sided findings; findings of infiltration often present in other organs in systemic disorders (e.g., amyloid also causes enlarged tongue and liver).

Diagnosis and Evaluation

- **Good history and physical examination: Severity and duration of symptoms, alcohol/cocaine use, angina, family history of HF or sudden cardiac death**
- **Diagnosis of HF based on clinical history and exam**
- **Strictly a clinical diagnosis**
- ECG to evaluate for ischemia, evidence of old infarction, or tachyarrhythmia
- **Echocardiogram: Most cost-effective way to evaluate systolic versus nonsystolic dysfunction**
- Labs: electrolytes, liver profile, urinalysis to evaluate possible renal or hepatic disease
- Brain natriuretic peptide (BNP) may be useful in distinguishing between cardiac and pulmonary causes of dyspnea
  - A cutoff of 100 pg/mL most commonly used; higher cutoff values improve specificity at the expense of sensitivity
  - Most patients with acutely decompensated heart failure have BNP values greater than 400 pg/mL; an important exception is patients with morbid obesity, who tend to have normal BNP levels even in HF
- Chest radiograph: Usually shows cardiomegaly and pulmonary venous redistribution; with acute failure, chest film may also show enlarged hilar vessels and Kerley B lines (Fig. 6-3)
- Thyroid function tests if patient is in atrial fibrillation, if the patient's age is greater than 60 years, or if the patient has symptoms of thyroid disease
- Stress testing is not usually done for the diagnosis of coronary artery disease; more commonly done for reasons of prognosis
- Cardiac catheterization should be done if patient has angina, shows evidence of ischemia or infarction on ECG, or has multiple risk factors

Treatment

- Treatment of acutely decompensated HF
  - Oxygen (to treat hypoxemia and promote diuresis)
  - Morphine sulfate (to decrease patient anxiety and increase arterial and venous dilation)
  - Diuretics (loop diuretics are first line)
  - Nitroglycerin (to decrease preload and pulmonary capillary wedge pressure)
  - Sodium nitroprusside (useful in hypertensive crisis)
  - Nesiritide— recombinant human BNP; works as a vasodilator
    - Questionable association with increased mortality—limit use to severe acute HF
    - Delivered as a continuous IV infusion

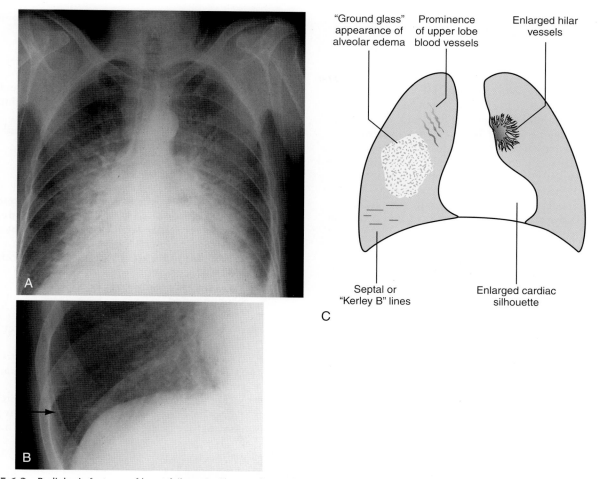

FIGURE 6-3   Radiologic features of heart failure. **A,** Chest radiograph of a patient with pulmonary edema. **B,** Enlargement of lung base showing Kerley B lines (*arrow*). **C,** Schematic highlighting the radiologic features of heart failure. (*From Haslett C, Chilvers ER: Davidson's principles and practice of medicine, ed 19, Philadelphia, Churchill Livingstone, 2003, Figs. 12.22A, 12.22B, and 12.22C.*)

- Monitor for hypotension and worsening renal function during use
- Inotropic agents (use if peripheral signs of hypoperfusion present)
  - Dobutamine, milrinone
  - Beware of increase in ventricular arrhythmias with these agents
- **Treatment of chronic systolic HF: goal is to delay onset of symptoms if asymptomatic, ameliorate symptoms when present, and prevent sudden death**
  - **Angiotensin-converting enzyme inhibitors (ACEIs)**
    - **Indicated in all patients with systolic dysfunction whether symptomatic or not**
    - Start with low dose and titrate upward; monitor potassium and creatinine
    - Titrate to highest tolerated dose or doses used in clinical trials
    - Patients with hyponatremia, hypotension, diabetes mellitus are most prone to problems with renal insufficiency
    - Side effects: Cough, angioedema, renal dysfunction are class effects
    - Contraindications to ACEI: Bilateral renal artery stenosis, previous angioedema with use of an ACEI;

chronic kidney disease relative contraindication depending on creatinine clearance
  - Angiotensin II receptor blocker (ARB) is an alternative, especially if patient develops cough with ACEI
- **β-Blockers**
  - Indicated in all patients with systolic dysfunction whether symptomatic or not
  - Agents of choice are carvedilol or long-acting metoprolol (succinate)
  - Do not start when patient is volume overloaded
  - Start at low dose and titrate upward to highest tolerated dose or doses used in clinical trials
- **Both ACEI and β-blockers increase survival in patients with HF due to systolic dysfunction**
- Diuretics for volume overload if present
- Teach patient about low-salt diet (3–4 g daily), daily weights, symptoms of HF, flexible diuretic regimen
- Loop diuretics most effective at sodium excretion
  - Thiazides used sparingly for booster effect
  - Aldosterone inhibitor (spironolactone, eplerenone) has mortality benefit in patients with severe (NYHA class IV) HF, normal renal function, and normal potassium

- Watch potassium carefully as risk of hyperkalemia exists
- Digoxin for those still symptomatic on ACEI, β-blocker, and loop diuretic
  - No effect on mortality
  - Decreases hospitalization for HF
  - Use low dose (0.125 mg/dL) and be careful in elderly, those with renal failure, and when starting amiodarone (amiodarone decreases excretion)
  - Symptoms of toxicity include heart block, atrial and ventricular tachycardia, visual disturbances (blurred or yellow vision), nausea, vomiting, dizziness
    - Toxicity exacerbated by hypokalemia
    - Treatment may require digoxin immune antibody, atropine, temporary pacer, and potassium repletion
- Hydralazine and isosorbide dinitrate
  - Recommended for African American patients who continue to be symptomatic despite optimal therapy with ACEI and β-blocker
  - Should not be a substitute for ACEI or ARB
  - Combination can be used as an alternative to ACEI if patient is intolerant to ACEI and ARB
- Drugs to avoid: Nonsteroidal anti-inflammatory agents, calcium channel blockers (only vasoselective ones do not negatively affect survival), antiarrhythmic drugs (only amiodarone and dofetilide do not negatively affect survival), alcohol, cocaine, tobacco
- Warfarin: Advocated for those in atrial fibrillation, with previous embolic event, or with visible cardiac clot on echocardiography; controversial in dilated cardiomyopathy without history of embolic events
- Cardiac resynchronization therapy (CRT or biventricular pacing): Use to promote mechanical synchrony if LVEF less than 35%, QRS duration greater than or equal to 120 ms, in normal sinus rhythm, and NYHA class III or IV HF on maximal medical therapy
- **Internal cardioverter-defibrillator (ICD): To prevent sudden cardiac death for patients with LVEF less than or equal to 35% and NYHA class II or III HF on maximal medical therapy**
- Transplantation: Associated with 90% 1-year survival and 70% 5-year survival rates
  - Strict criteria for eligibility given organ shortage
  - Major early problems are infection and rejection
  - Major late problem is transplant vasculopathy, which affects coronary arteries
  - Mechanical circulatory support:
    - Can be used for short-term support, "bridge" to transplantation, or "destination" (permanent) therapy for non–transplantation candidates
- Treatment of chronic nonsystolic HF is less evidence-based than treatment for systolic dysfunction
  - Treat hypertension aggressively
  - Consider myocardial ischemia as potential cause
  - Diuretics to control fluid
  - Candesartan (ARB) is the only agent to be studied in a large trial of patients with nonsystolic HF; no difference in mortality but fewer hospital admissions for HF
  - Avoid digoxin and positive inotropic drugs
  - Avoid atrial fibrillation—shortens diastolic filling time

- Treatment of chronic HCM: goal is to ameliorate symptoms and prevent sudden death
  - Usually either a β-blocker or verapamil to slow heart rate, decrease inotropy, and treat hypertension
    - Verapamil may occasionally worsen gradient in patients with high resting gradient (>50 mm Hg) and severe symptoms
    - Avoid in such patients and use disopyramide instead
  - Avoid digoxin and positive inotropic drugs
  - Avoid atrial fibrillation
  - Avoid drugs that reduce preload or afterload
  - **ICD for history of sudden death or syncope, family history of sudden death or syncope, sustained ventricular tachycardia, extreme hypertrophy, or a high-risk genotype**
  - **Screen family for HCM with echocardiogram and ECG**
  - **Endocarditis prophylaxis is no longer recommended**
  - Treat as if patient has systolic HF if patient evolves into dilated cardiomyopathy (see previous discussion)
  - Myectomy rarely necessary and only for obstructive HCM with severe drug-refractory symptoms and a gradient greater than 50 mm Hg
  - Alcohol ablation of proximal septum—an alternative therapy for obstructive HCM with severe drug-refractory symptoms and a gradient greater than 50 mm Hg
- Treatment of restrictive cardiomyopathy
  - Poor options
  - Cautious use of diuretics as noncompliant ventricle is preload dependent
  - Attempt to treat underlying cause
  - Avoid digoxin, especially in patients with amyloid (high local cardiac digoxin levels lead to increased arrhythmias)
  - Transplantation is an option
  - Avoid atrial fibrillation
  - **Make sure the patient does not have constrictive pericarditis, which is surgically correctable**

REVIEW QUESTIONS

For review questions, please go to www.expertconsult.com.

SUGGESTED READINGS

Hunt SA, Abraham WT, Chin MH, et al: Guidelines for the diagnosis and management of heart failure in adults: a report of the American College of Cardiology Foundation/American Heart Association Task Force on Practice Guidelines (Writing Committee to Update the 2005 Guidelines for the Evaluation and Management of Heart Failure), *J Am Coll Cardiol* 53:e1–e90, 2009.

Kushwaha SS, Fallon JT, Fuster V: Restrictive cardiomyopathy, *N Engl J Med* 336:267–276, 1997.

Maron BJ, McKenna WJ, Danielson GK, et al: ACC/ESC clinical expert consensus document on hypertrophic cardiomyopathy: a report of the American College of Cardiology Task Force on Clinical Expert Consensus Documents and the European Society of Cardiology Committee for Practice Guidelines, *J Am Coll Cardiol* 43:1687–1713, 2003.

Valvular Heart Disease

THOMAS A. TRAILL, MD, FRCP

Valvular heart disease is recognized by finding a heart murmur. Here, even more than elsewhere in cardiology, the physical findings are all-important to making a diagnosis and assessing severity. Often they trump the results of special testing. Murmurs may first be detected in a symptomless patient, perhaps a young would-be athlete at a high school physical, or they may be the clue in someone with dyspnea and fluid retention that valvular disease is the reason for their cardiac failure.

Aortic Stenosis

Basic Information

- Causes and etiology
  - Congenital unicuspid valve
    - Usually severe
    - Presents in children
  - Congenital bicuspid valve
    - Murmur present from childhood
    - Common cause of aortic regurgitation (AR), as well as aortic stenosis (AS)
    - **AS develops in middle age with calcification**
  - Degenerative calcific disease
    - Develops usually in late middle age or later in a previously normal, trileaflet valve
    - Earliest manifestation is aortic sclerosis, defined as thickening of the leaflets, presence of a heart murmur, and gradient less than 25 mm Hg
    - Progression of aortic sclerosis to stenosis is biologically similar to that of atherosclerosis and has been linked to the same risk factors
    - Hence, interest exists in the possibility that lipid lowering will slow progression of AS (unproven)

Clinical Presentation

- Physical signs
  - Slow-rising carotid upstroke (*parvus et tardus*)
  - May be difficult to detect in older patients with stiff vessels and wide pulse pressure; should be obvious in patients younger than 70 years
  - **Systolic ejection murmur**
    - **Synonyms: crescendo-decrescendo, diamond-shaped**
    - **Intensity is no guide to severity**
    - **Murmur of severe disease sounds "late-peaking"**
    - May be conducted to the apex with a musical quality ("Gallavardin murmur")
  - Reduced intensity of A_2 (aortic closure sound) in calcific disease

- Ejection sound (close after S_1) signals bicuspid valve
- See Table 7-1 for effects of various maneuvers
- Natural history
  - Excellent prognosis in presymptomatic patients
  - **50% 3-year mortality in patients with symptoms**
    - Classic symptoms: angina, dyspnea, dizziness/syncope
    - Outflow tract velocity on Doppler echocardiography helps to anticipate onset of symptoms
    - Greater than 4 m/sec (corresponds to gradient >64 mm Hg); implies likely symptoms (hence referral for surgery) within 3 years
  - Poor prognosis in patients with left ventricular (LV) dysfunction (in whom the outflow velocity and gradient may also be misleadingly low)

Diagnosis and Evaluation

- Role of testing
  - Electrocardiogram (ECG)
    - Usually shows LV hypertrophy
    - Severe AS requiring operation is unusual with normal ECG
  - Echocardiography
    - Shows morphology of the valve
    - Allows Doppler measurement of outflow tract velocity
    - Velocity allows gradient and valve area calculations, but these have limited additional role over the raw velocity
      - Surgery for a high gradient in the absence of symptoms is not routine
    - Demonstrates aortic ectasia in 30% to 50% of patients with bicuspid aortic valve

Treatment

- Timing of surgery
  - Asymptomatic patients are followed, often for years
  - **Symptoms of angina, dyspnea, fluid retention, syncope, or exertional dizziness require prompt surgical referral**
  - Poor cardiac function requires prompt surgical referral (even if the gradient is low)
- Medical issues
  - **Nitrates contraindicated (dangerous to lower preload)**
  - Antibiotic prophylaxis for dental work and other potentially contaminated procedures
- Surgical options
  - Mechanical prosthetic valves require lifelong anticoagulation, but should obviate need for future surgery

TABLE 7-1 *Effects of Maneuvers on Valvular Murmurs*

Valve Abnormality	MANEUVERS: EFFECT ON MURMUR INTENSITY*			
	Valsalva (during Continuous Strain)	Amyl Nitrite	Handgrip	Squatting
Aortic stenosis	↓	↑	↓	↑
Hypertrophic cardiomyopathy (see Chapter 6)	↑	↑	↓	↓
Chronic aortic regurgitation	↓	↓	↑	↑
Chronic mitral regurgitation	↓	↓	↑	↑
Mitral valve prolapse	Moves click and murmur onset closer to S_1	Moves click and murmur onset closer to S_1	Moves click and murmur onset closer to S_2	Moves click and murmur onset closer to S_2
Mitral stenosis	↓	↑	↑	↑

*Valsalva maneuver: During continuous strain, increases intrathoracic pressure, thereby decreasing venous return and preload. After strain, arterial pressure drops and venous return subsequently increases.
Amyl nitrite inhalation: Systemic vasodilator causing a drop in blood pressure followed by a reflex increase in heart rate and myocardial contractility.
Handgrip (isometric exercise): Increases systemic pressure and increases afterload.
Squatting: Increases peripheral resistance and thus increases venous return.

- Biologic prostheses offer 15 to 20 years' use before degenerating
  - Less time to degeneration in the young, in patients with kidney disease, and in those on corticosteroids
  - Biologic prostheses do not need anticoagulant treatment
- Pulmonary autograft procedures are rarely used
- Growing interest in percutaneous stent-valve implants for the very old or very frail

Chronic Aortic Regurgitation

Basic Information

- Etiology and differential diagnosis
  - AR has a broad differential diagnosis, and it is critical to identify the underlying cause before determining management; AR demands a diagnosis
  - Diseases of the valve
    - Bicuspid aortic valve
    - Following endocarditis
    - Rheumatic valve disease
  - Diseases of the aorta
    - Connective tissue disorders
      - Marfan syndrome (Box 7-1 and Fig. 7-1)
      - Familial aortic ectasia
      - Other rare, inherited vascular disorders
    - Aortic dissection
    - Inflammatory disorders
      - Vasculitis (Takayasu disease)
      - Giant-cell arteritis
      - Syphilis
  - Diseases affecting aorta and valve
    - Spondyloarthropathies
      - Ankylosing spondylitis
      - Reiter syndrome
      - Psoriatic arthropathy

BOX 7-1 *Marfan Syndrome*

Etiology: Dominant mutations in fibrillin 1, but genetic diagnosis not yet applicable to most cases
Clinical features
    Skeleton
        Height
        Wingspan >105% of height
        Arachnodactyly
        Pectus carinatum
        Pectus excavatum
        Scoliosis
        Thumb and wrist signs
        Joint laxity
    Ocular
        Ectopia lentis
        Myopia
    Cardiovascular
        Aortic ectasia
        Mitral valve prolapse
    Other
        Dural ectasia
        Spontaneous pneumothorax
        Emphysema
Management of aortic involvement
        Periodic (every 6–12 months) evaluation of aortic dimension by echo
        β-Blocker therapy to slow progression
        Losartan may reduce aortic involvement
        Aortic root replacement for ectasia >5 cm

Clinical Presentation

- Physical signs and assessing severity
  - Abnormal pulses, LV enlargement, and a diastolic murmur
  - Pulses
    - **Bounding pulses reflect wide pulse pressure due to runoff from the aorta**

FIGURE 7-1 External phenotype of patient with Marfan syndrome, showing long extremities and digits, tall stature, and pectus carinatum. *(From Zipes DP: Braunwald's heart disease: a textbook of cardiovascular medicine, ed 7, Philadelphia, Saunders, 2005, Fig. 70-7.)*

| TABLE 7-2 | *Peripheral Pulse Findings in Chronic Aortic Regurgitation* | |

Sign	Description
Quincke's sign	Nail bed pulsation
Corrigan's pulse	Visible carotid pulsation
de Musset's sign	Head bobbing to pulse
Müller's sign	Uvula bobbing to pulse
Duroziez's sign	Diastolic bruit with compression of the femoral artery at the groin
Hill's sign	Systolic pressure in the leg >10 mm Hg higher than the measurement at the brachial artery; reflects large stroke volume
Traube's sign	Pistol-shot sounds best heard over the femoral artery

- Associated disease of other valves
  - Mitral valve prolapse—connective tissue disorder
  - Mitral stenosis—rheumatic disease
  - Left ventricular cavity size and function

Treatment

- Natural history and timing of surgery
  - Chronic AR is well tolerated for many years by most patients, in contrast to acute and subacute AR; if uncorrected, eventually leads to irreversible dilation of the LV and poor systolic function
    - The largest LVs seen are those of long-standing chronic AR (*cor bovinum*)
  - Surgery recommended for:
    - First hint of symptoms: dyspnea, fatigue
      - Angina unusual in AR; may reflect coronary ostial involvement by aortitis or unrelated coronary artery atherosclerosis
    - Enlarging LV cavity
    - LV end-systolic dimension more than 5.5 cm (such a figure for dimension at end-systole implies combination of large cavity and some reduction in systolic function)
    - Aortic ectasia
    - Aortic root measurement more than 5 cm in Marfan or Loeys-Dietz syndromes, more than 5.5 cm with other diagnoses

Chronic Mitral Regurgitation

Basic Information

- Differential diagnosis
  - Myxomatous (floppy) valve (i.e., mitral valve prolapse)
  - Ruptured chordae tendineae
  - Following endocarditis
  - Papillary muscle dysfunction
  - Mitral annulus calcification
  - Rheumatic
  - "Functional" (i.e., from annulus or LV dilation)
  - Rarities (e.g., Libman-Sacks endocarditis in lupus)

- Differential diagnosis of such pulses includes persistent ductus arteriosus (PDA), arteriovenous fistula, and hypertrophic cardiomyopathy
  - Various eponyms attached to AR pulses (Table 7-2)
- The water-hammer pulse refers to the slapping quality when the hand is held up and the arterial diastolic pressure is below approximately 25 mm Hg
- Other peripheral findings (see Table 7-2)
- Auscultatory findings
  - Early diastolic murmur starts at the instant of aortic closure, usually medium frequency
    - Longest and loudest when AR is chronic and the patient is doing well
    - When the LV diastolic pressure rises because of failure or a torrential leak, or in the acute setting, the murmur is less conspicuous
  - Austin Flint described a second murmur, beginning in mid- or late diastole, caused by turbulent flow through the mitral orifice
    - It reflects high LV diastolic pressure, thus an adverse hemodynamic situation
    - Often indicates the need for surgical valve replacement
  - Effects of various maneuvers on murmur intensity: see Table 7-1

Diagnosis and Evaluation

- Role of laboratory testing: as needed to investigate for underlying cause/condition
- Echocardiography
  - Site of the problem: Valve or aortic wall
  - Morphology of valve: Bicuspid versus other
  - Vegetation, perforation

Clinical Presentation

- Physical signs and assessing severity
  - Hyperkinetic left ventricle
  - Pansystolic murmur
    - In acute, severe mitral regurgitation (MR), murmur may be shortened by high left atrial pressure
    - In mitral valve prolapse, late systolic murmur implies mild regurgitation
    - **In general, loudness correlates with severity**
    - Effects of maneuvers on murmur: see Table 7-1
  - Third heart sound

Diagnosis and Evaluation

- Role of testing
  - Chest radiography: cardiomegaly, left atrial size, pulmonary congestion, pulmonary artery enlargement
  - ECG: May see atrial fibrillation

Treatment

- Natural history and timing of surgery
  - Chronic MR is tolerated even better than AR; hence, there has been a tendency to operate too late, at a point when the LV is irremediably damaged
  - **It is important, therefore, to follow LV size carefully and be alert to even subtle changes in effort tolerance, stamina, and energy level**
  - **Atrial fibrillation often an indication of the time to operate**
  - Enlarging LV may be reflected by end-systolic dimension of 4.5 cm
- Mitral valve repair generally preferred over replacement

Mitral Valve Prolapse

Basic Information

- Etiology
  - Mitral valve prolapse (MVP) is the bulging of the mitral leaflets past the plane of the annulus into the left atrium
    - May be accompanied by MR, not necessarily severe
    - Is normally the result of myxomatous change, but can occur in a normal valve under certain conditions (e.g., a hyperkinetic circulation with excessive sympathetic stimulation or an underfilled left ventricle)

Clinical Presentation

- **Physical signs**
  - **Mid-systolic click**
  - **Late systolic murmur heard best at the apex**
- Natural history and complications
  - Generally benign
  - Infrequent complications
    - Endocarditis; thus, some recommend antibiotic prophylaxis in patients with late systolic murmurs
    - Progressive valve degeneration leading to severe regurgitation (~10% of patients)
    - Atrial and ventricular arrhythmias
    - Sudden death—extremely rare; hence, virtually unpredictable
    - Stroke—very rare; thus, no routine antiplatelet or anticoagulant prophylaxis

Acute Valvular Regurgitation

Basic Information

- Causes
  - Endocarditis
  - Chordal rupture
  - Aortic dissection

Clinical Presentation

- Pathophysiology and presentation
  - Acute AR and MR present differently from their chronic counterparts, because the LV and left atrium are of normal size
  - Acute AR causes LV diastolic pressure to rise abruptly during diastole, so aortic diastolic pressure is not much reduced; pulse pressure is narrow and patients present with cardiogenic shock, small-volume pulses, and an unimpressive or absent murmur
  - Acute MR causes a very abrupt tall V wave in the left atrium; hence, acute pulmonary edema, low cardiac output, and a murmur that is unimpressive and may sound like an ejection murmur

Treatment

- Natural history and management
  - Acute AR
    - Natural history is poor, and early surgery is almost always advised
    - **Surgery should not be delayed pending completion of antibiotic treatment**
    - Antibiotic treatment should be continued after operation to finish full course
  - Acute MR
    - Natural history better than acute AR
    - Surgery advised for patients with acute pulmonary edema

Mitral Stenosis

Basic Information

- Causes
  - **Acquired mitral stenosis (MS) is invariably from rheumatic fever; clinically recognized in about 50% of patients**
  - Congenital MS is recognized but rare

Clinical Presentation

- Symptoms
  - Mobile valve
    - Loud S_1
    - Opening snap (follows S_2)
    - Mid-diastolic rumble
  - Calcified valve
    - Normal or soft S_1, dull or absent snap
    - Soft but long murmur
  - Effect of various maneuvers: see Table 7-1

Diagnosis and Evaluation

- Symptoms and management
  - Young patient, mobile valve

- Symptoms include dyspnea, paroxysmal nocturnal dyspnea, hemoptysis, paroxysmal atrial fibrillation
  - Balloon commissurotomy if there is pure MS (without MR) and no thrombus
- Older patient; calcified, immobile valve; or subvalve chordal disease
  - Valve replacement for symptoms or findings of fatigue, dyspnea, atrial fibrillation, pulmonary hypertension, right-heart failure, edema
- Role of laboratory studies
  - Chest radiography
    - Left atrial enlargement
    - Pulmonary artery and right-heart enlargement
  - Echocardiography
    - Valve morphology
    - Involvement of other valves
    - Transesophageal echocardiography (TEE) before balloon commissurotomy to examine left atrium for clot

Treatment

- **Mitral stenosis and pregnancy**
  - **Ostensibly well young women with MS may tolerate pregnancy poorly because of combined effects of blood volume increase and high cardiac output**
  - Careful preconception assessment indicated
  - In a pregnant woman with new-onset pulmonary edema, consider
    - Mitral stenosis
    - Peripartum cardiomyopathy

Antibiotic Prophylaxis

Diagnosis and Evaluation

- Goal is to prevent infective endocarditis
- Recent updated guidelines (American Heart Association, 2007) contain major changes based on current evidence
- **Patients for whom prophylaxis is indicated (only patients at highest risk):**
  - **Prosthetic heart valves (including bioprosthetics)**
  - **Personal history of infective endocarditis**
  - **Unrepaired congenital cyanotic heart disease**
  - **Incompletely repaired cyanotic heart disease or repaired using prosthetic material**
  - **Cardiac valvulopathy in a transplanted heart**
- **No longer indicated in relatively low-risk valvular disorders such as mitral valve prolapse, bicuspid aortic valve, acquired aortic and mitral valve disorders, hypertrophic cardiomyopathy, and others**
- Procedures for which prophylaxis is indicated
  - Dental procedures that involve manipulation of gingival tissue or periapical tooth region or mucosal perforation
  - Respiratory tract procedures that involve incision or biopsy
  - Procedures in patients with gastrointestinal or genitourinary tract infections
  - Procedures on infected skin or tissue
  - Surgery to implant prosthetic valves or prosthetic intravascular or intracardiac materials

Treatment

- Standard regimen for most dental and respiratory procedures: amoxicillin 2 g given 30 to 60 minutes before procedure
- Alternatives for penicillin-allergic patients: cephalexin, azithromycin, clarithromycin, or clindamycin
- For other procedures, need to tailor antibiotic to likely organisms

Artificial Valves

Treatment

- Choosing a prosthesis
  - Repair preferred over replacement, but generally only available for mitral valve disease
  - **Bioprostheses last roughly 5 to 20 years—shorter lifespan than mechanical prostheses**
  - Consider biologic valves rather than the more durable mechanical prostheses when
    - Prepregnancy condition exists (and anticoagulants undesirable)
    - Anticoagulation undesirable or risky
    - Patient is in atrial fibrillation and will be on anticoagulants
    - Patients are older than 60 years (bioprosthesis should last long enough)
    - In setting of high endocarditis risk, as it is less likely to require removal in event of endocarditis
  - Bioprostheses deteriorate more rapidly in young patients, those with kidney disease, or those on corticosteroids
- Follow-up of prostheses
  - Prosthetic malfunction
    - Produces the same murmurs as in native valves (exception is paraprosthetic MR, which can be silent)
    - Consider in a patient with hemolysis
    - TEE often required for confirmation and assessing severity
  - Interrupting anticoagulants
    - Relatively safe in patients with aortic prostheses
    - Should generally use heparin (usually low-molecular-weight) for patients with mitral prostheses

REVIEW QUESTIONS

For review questions, please go to www.expertconsult.com.

SUGGESTED READINGS

Bonow RO, Carabello BA, Chatterjee K, et al: ACC/AHA 2006 guidelines for the management of patients with valvular heart disease, *J Am Coll Cardiol* 48:1–148, 2006.

Lung B, Gohlke-Barwolf C, Tornos P, et al: for the Working Group on Valvular Heart Disease: Recommendations on the management of the asymptomatic patient with valvular heart disease, *Eur Heart J* 23:1252–1266, 2002.

Otto CM: Evaluation and management of chronic mitral regurgitation, *N Engl J Med* 345:740–746, 2001.

Otto CM: Valvular aortic stenosis: disease severity and timing of intervention, *J Am Coll Cardiol* 47:2141–2151, 2006.

Pericardial Disease

MARY CORRETTI, MD

Pericardial disease is a group of disorders that may manifest as an asymptomatic effusion, tamponade, acute pericarditis, or chronic constriction. Possible causes are quite varied. A thorough history and physical examination often provide clues to the underlying cause.

Acute Pericarditis

Basic Information

- Function and anatomy of normal pericardium
  - Visceral and parietal pericardial layers separated by a potential space, the pericardial cavity
  - Normally contains 15 to 50 mL of straw-colored serous pericardial fluid, an ultrafiltrate of plasma; the fluid acts as a lubricant to reduce interlayer friction during cardiac contraction
- Three main functions of pericardium
  - Suspends the heart in place—keeping the position of the heart relatively constant
  - Serves as a physical barrier to prevent spread of infection and malignancy from contiguous structures
  - Prevents acute cardiac dilation
- Pericarditis can manifest as acute, subacute, or chronic
  - Acute pericarditis occurs when there is inflammation of the pericardium and is defined as signs or symptoms from pericardial inflammation of no more than 1 to 2 weeks' duration
- Pericarditis is relatively common in patients presenting to emergency departments, with up to 5% of those with nonischemic chest pain and 1% with ST-segment elevation on electrocardiogram (ECG)
- Major causes are idiopathic, infectious, neoplastic, autoimmune disorders; uremia; cardiac surgery; irradiation; traumatic events; and infarction (Table 8-1)
- Most common cause is viral or idiopathic

Clinical Presentation

- Clinical features
  - Chest pain can be severe
    - Sudden onset, sharp, and worse with inspiration, cough, and body movements
    - May radiate to neck, back, left shoulder, or trapezius muscle ridge
    - Is variable: May be persistent or may wax and wane
    - Pain is typically substernal or localized to left chest; left arm radiation is not typical
    - **Pain may be positional in nature: worse when patient is supine and relieved with sitting up and leaning forward**

- Patient may also complain of dyspnea
- Less common symptoms: cough, dysphagia, hiccups
- An antecedent history of fever and symptoms of a viral syndrome are common
- Physical examination
  - 85% of patients have an audible friction rub (high-pitched scratchy or squeaky sound best heard at the left sternal border at end-expiration with the patient leaning forward)
    - Rub may be evanescent—disappearing and returning over short periods of time
    - **Rub may have three components, related to movement of the heart during the cardiac cycle: atrial systole, ventricular systole, and ventricular diastole**
    - **In reality, the rub is triphasic in about half the patients, biphasic in a third, and monophasic in the remainder**
  - Performance of a complete, careful examination of the patient with acute pericarditis is essential to delineate specific diagnoses and to assess for the presence of coexistent myocarditis
- Special syndromes
  - Dressler syndrome
    - Occurs weeks to months after myocardial infarction
    - Consists of fever, malaise, serositis, pulmonary infiltrates, and pleural effusion in addition to pericardial effusion
    - Due to an immunologic reaction
  - Postpericardiotomy syndrome
    - Pericarditis occurs weeks to months after cardiac surgery
    - Possibly due to hypersensitivity of injured myocardial tissue

Diagnosis and Evaluation

- Diagnosis
  - ECG findings: Classically evolves through four stages over time (Fig. 8-1)
    - Stage I: Diffuse ST-segment elevation with concomitant P–R iinterval depression in almost all leads (except aVR)
    - Stage II: Normalization of the ST segment and P–R interval
    - Stage III: Widespread T-wave inversions
    - Stage IV: Normalization of the T waves
  - Most common ECG changes of myocarditis are diffuse T-wave inversions without abnormality of the ST segment unless there is concurrent pericarditis

TABLE 8-1	*Causes of Acute Pericarditis*
Process	**Examples**
Infectious	Viral Bacterial Mycobacterial Fungal Protozoal HIV

Neoplastic	Primary (mesothelioma—rare,
	   sarcomas, fibroma, lipoma)
	Secondary (breast, lung, melanoma,
	   sarcoma, lymphoma, leukemia,
	   ovarian)

Immune/
  Inflammatory
	Autoimmune and connective tissue
	   disorders (e.g., SLE, RA, ankylosing
	   spondylitis, scleroderma, sarcoidosis,
	   dematomyositis, polyarteritis
	   nodosa, Wegener's granulomatosis,
	   Sjögren syndrome)
	IBD
	Löffler syndrome
	Stevens-Johnson syndrome
	Myocardial infarction
	Dressler syndrome
	Postpericardiotomy syndrome
	Post-traumatic
	Pleural and pulmonary diseases

Metabolic	Uremia Dialysis-associated Myxedema Gout

Iatrogenic	Radiation injury
	Related to cardiac catheterization or
	   placement of implantable cardioverter-
	   defibrillators and pacemakers

Traumatic	Blunt trauma Penetrating trauma Chylopericardium
Drug-induced	Hydralazine, procainamide, minoxidil isoniazide, anticoagulants

HIV, human immunodeficiency virus; IBD, inflammatory bowel disease;
RA, rheumatoid arthritis; SLE, systemic lupus erythematosus.

A

B

C

FIGURE 8-1 ECG changes associated with pericarditis. **A,** Acute pericarditis. Note the raised ST segment, concave upward (*arrow*). **B,** Chronic phase of pericarditis associated with a pericardial effusion. Note the T-wave flattening and inversion and the alternation of the QRS amplitude (QRS alternans). **C,** The same patient after evacuation of the pericardial fluid. Note that the QRS voltage has increased and the T waves have returned to normal. *(From Kumar P, Clark M: Clinical medicine, ed 5, Philadelphia, Saunders, 2005, Fig. 13.96.)*

- Chest radiography: May be normal in uncomplicated acute idiopathic pericarditis
  - Occasionally pleural effusions are present
  - Pulmonary vascular congestion may indicate severe concomitant myocarditis
- Echocardiography: Typically normal in most patients with acute idiopathic pericarditis (Fig. 8-2)
  - Most do not have effusions or have ones that are very small and inconsequential
  - Echocardiography is also useful to determine whether the effusion is loculated or diffuse, or contains elements of blood, fibrinous, or inflammatory material
  - Can assess for tamponade or constrictive pericarditis physiology (see later discussion)
- Laboratory studies
  - Nonspecific markers of inflammation (i.e., erythrocyte sedimentation rate, C-reactive protein, and white blood cell count) usually only modestly increased

- In the patient with concomitant myocardial inflammation, there may be a modest elevation of cardiac enzymes—creatine phosphokinase myocardial band (CPK-MB) fraction or troponin I (or both)
- Complete blood count
  - Serum creatinine, blood urea nitrogen, antinuclear antibodies, serologic test for HIV
  - Other laboratory tests should be aimed at diagnosing the underlying cause as guided by the history and physical exam
- Evaluation
  - Guided by the history and physical exam, but usually includes
    - ECG (frequent to detect evolutionary changes)
    - Chest radiography
    - Laboratory tests as previously described
    - Tuberculin skin test
    - Transthoracic echocardiogram
  - Pericardiocentesis rarely provides diagnosis in the patient with a small or moderate effusion

FIGURE 8-2 **A,** Echocardiogram of a large pericardial effusion with findings of tamponade physiology. Diastolic compression of the RV on two-dimensional images. **B,** Marked variation of mitral inflow velocity by Doppler. (EXP, expiration; INS, inspiration.)

Treatment

- **Acute idiopathic or viral pericarditis is usually a benign, self-limited disease that resolves within 2 to 6 weeks**
- **Treatment is primarily supportive: Bed rest and non-steroidal anti-inflammatory drugs (NSAIDs)**
  - Aspirin (2–4 g/day), indomethacin (75–225 mg/day), and ibuprofen (1600–3200 mg/day) prescribed most often
  - Anti-inflammatory agents may be tapered after 1 to 2 weeks
  - Severe pain that does not respond to NSAIDs within 48 hours may be treated by adding colchicine (0.6 mg twice daily) or administering high doses of corticosteroids (60–80 mg of prednisone per day in divided doses) to be tapered slowly over a period of several months.
- Additional therapy is aimed at treating the underlying cause of pericarditis
- Avoid anticoagulants in the acute phase to reduce the risk of intrapericardial hemorrhage and tamponade
- Routine hospitalization usually not necessary
- Hospitalize patients with temperature greater than 38°C; subacute onset (symptoms developing over several weeks); immunosuppressed state; trauma; on oral anticoagulant therapy; myopericarditis (pericarditis with clinical or serologic evidence of myocardial involvement); large pericardial effusion (an echo-free space >20 mm in width); cardiac tamponade; or myocardial infarction

Pericardial Effusion and Cardiac Tamponade

Basic Information

- Pericardial effusion
  - Accumulating fluid in the pericardium may be transudative or exudative
  - May occur with acute pericarditis or may accumulate in fluid-retentive states (heart failure, renal failure, or cirrhosis)
  - Features that determine whether an effusion will cause increased intrapericardial pressure and hemodynamic compromise
    - The rate of accumulation of fluid
    - The volume of the fluid
    - The physical characteristics of the pericardium itself
  - **Gradual accumulations of up to 1 to 2 L of fluid may be well tolerated, whereas the rapid addition of even 80 to 200 mL will result in markedly increased intrapericardial pressure**
- Cardiac tamponade
  - Occurs when pericardial fluid increases intrapericardial pressure, exceeding intracardiac pressures and resulting in compression of the cardiac chambers
    - Limits diastolic filling of the heart
    - Results in decreased stroke volume, cardiac output, and systemic blood pressure, and elevated venous pressures
  - Any cause of acute pericarditis and pericardial effusion may lead to tamponade, but the most common causes are neoplastic, uremic, and viral/idiopathic pericarditis
  - Occurs in 15% of acute pericarditis cases

Clinical Presentation

- Symptoms of pericardial effusion
  - May be asymptomatic even if effusion is large and there is no tamponade
  - With large effusions, patients may experience dull chest pain, pressure, or a nonspecific sense of discomfort
  - Other symptoms related to mechanical compression of adjacent structures include dysphagia, cough, hoarseness (left recurrent laryngeal nerve compression), hiccups (phrenic nerve compression), nausea, or abdominal fullness
- Physical examination findings with a pericardial effusion
  - Pericardial effusions that are small or moderate may present with normal physical examination
  - Muffled heart sounds
    - Ewart's sign: Dullness to percussion and bronchial breath sounds beneath the left scapula caused by compressive atelectasis in the left lower lung field
- Symptoms of tamponade
  - Symptoms result from decreased cardiac output and elevated filling pressures
  - Fatigue, lightheadedness, and dyspnea; patients may feel more comfortable sitting forward
- Physical examination findings in tamponade

TABLE 8-2	Characteristic Features of Constrictive Pericarditis and Cardiac Tamponade	
	Constrictive Pericarditis	**Cardiac Tamponade**
Equalization of end-diastolic pressures	Yes (within 5 mm Hg)	Yes (within 5 mm Hg)
Right atrial pressure waveform	Prominent X and Y descent (X = Y or Y > X)	Blunted or absent Y descent (X > Y)
Pericardium	Thickened (>3–4 mm)	Normal
Kussmaul's sign	Present	Absent
Pulsus paradoxus	Absent	Present

- Classically presents with Beck's triad: (1) elevated jugular venous pressure, (2) arterial hypotension, and (3) quiet "muffled" heart sounds
- Other manifestations of tamponade related to reduced cardiac output include: tachypnea, diaphoresis, depressed sensorium, cool extremities, peripheral cyanosis
- With gradual accumulation of fluid, blood pressure may be maintained and signs of right-heart failure (hepatomegaly, ascites, and lower extremity edema) may be present
- Pulsus paradoxus: Greater than 10 mm Hg decrease in systolic blood pressure with inspiration
- Kussmaul's sign: Paradoxical rise in jugular venous pressure with deep inspiration

Diagnosis and Evaluation

- Characteristic features of cardiac tamponade are shown in Table 8-2
- **ECG: Voltage may be reduced, nonspecific T-wave flattening, and electrical alternans (change in QRS voltage from beat to beat)**
- Chest radiography: Cardiac silhouette may be enlarged
- Echocardiography
  - Most useful imaging modality for demonstrating pericardial effusion and tamponade
  - Effusion is visualized as an echo-free space (black) between the pericardial layers
  - Right atrial (RA) (late diastolic) and right ventricular (RV) (early diastolic) collapse is observed when tamponade occurs
  - RV diastolic collapse is more specific (85–100%) than RA collapse for contributing evidence of tamponade physiology
  - An increase in RV volume with inspiration shifts the septum toward the left ventricle in diastole, and toward the right ventricle in systole. A decrease in RV volume occurs with expiration. This pattern of motion corresponds to the physical finding of pulsus paradoxus.
  - Marked respiratory variation in Doppler echocardiography inflow velocities across the mitral and tricuspid valves (flow velocity paradox) is seen in tamponade, as well as in constrictive pericarditis

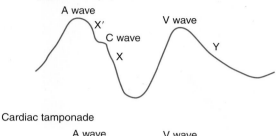

Right atrial pressure tracings—obtained from right heart catheterization (Swan-Ganz catheter)

Normal jugular venous pressure wave

Cardiac tamponade

Blunted Y descent

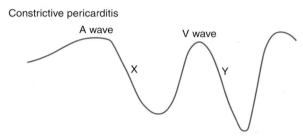

Constrictive pericarditis

Left ventricular pressure tracing—obtained with catheter in the left ventricle

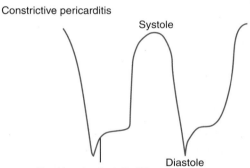

Constrictive pericarditis

Rapid early diastolic filling followed by plateau phase— the "square root" sign

FIGURE 8-3 Typical catheterization findings in pericardial disease.

- Computed tomography (CT) or magnetic resonance imaging (MRI): Can detect an effusion, but less useful than echocardiography; pericardial thickness can be measured with both CT and MRI, allowing for the severity and chronicity of inflammation and other pericardial disease entities
- Right-heart catheterization (RHC)
  - RA pressure tracings normally composed of a series of waveforms (Fig. 8-3)
    - The A wave represents atrial contraction (and follows the P wave on ECG)
    - The X descent follows the A wave and represents atrial relaxation

FIGURE 8-4 Aspiration of pericardial fluid. A wide-bore needle is inserted into the epigastrium below the xiphoid process and advanced in the direction of the medial third of the right clavicle. If the needle is connected to the V lead of an ECG monitor, ST-segment elevation is usually seen if the needle touches the epicardium. This can be useful in distinguishing a bloody pericardial effusion from accidental puncture of the heart. Other complications of the procedure may include arrhythmias, vasovagal attack, and pneumothorax. *(From Forbes C, Jackson W: Color atlas and text of clinical medicine, St. Louis, Mosby, 2003, Fig. 5.140.)*

- The V wave represents passive filling of the right atrium beginning after ventricular systole has closed the tricuspid valve
- The Y descent follows the V wave and represents the rapid flow of blood from the atrium into the ventricle in early diastole
- In tamponade, RHC findings can be diagnostic, although this modality is not usually required to make the diagnosis
  - Because increased intrapericardial pressures cause equalization of RA and RV pressures in diastole, there is a minimal pressure gradient pushing blood from the right atrium to ventricle during diastole
  - Equalization of RA, RV diastolic, and pulmonary capillary wedge pressures occurs
  - **The Y descent is blunted or absent (see Fig. 8-3)**
  - The X descent, which corresponds to atrial relaxation, is preserved

Treatment

- Pericardial effusion
  - Indications for drainage of pericardial effusion by pericardiocentesis (Fig. 8-4)
    - **Evidence of hemodynamic compromise**
    - **Examination of fluid required to establish a diagnosis**
    - **Suggested purulent pericarditis**
  - Asymptomatic effusions, even large ones, may be followed indefinitely with serial echocardiograms and clinical assessments
  - As with the management of pericarditis, anticoagulation should be avoided
- Cardiac tamponade
  - Cardiac tamponade is potentially life-threatening and should be treated as a medical emergency
  - Definitive treatment for tamponade is removal of the pericardial fluid via pericardiocentesis

- Medical management
  - Temporizing until pericardiocentesis performed
  - Expansion of intravascular volume with fluids
- Recurrent episodes of pericardial effusion and tamponade may be treated with repeated pericardiocenteses, balloon pericardiotomy, surgical creation of a pericardial window, or pericardiectomy
- Another option is injection of a sclerosing agent into the pericardial space to cause adherence of the visceral and parietal pericardium

Constrictive Pericarditis

Basic Information

- Thickened (and often calcified) pericardium that may occur following any form of acute pericarditis; constrictive pericarditis is the end stage of such inflammatory process involving the pericardium
- **Most common causes are viral/idiopathic, uremic, postsurgical, tuberculous, or radiation-induced**
- Other causes include neoplastic, autoimmune, posttrauma, sarcoid, methysergide therapy, and implantable cardioverter-defibrillator patches
- Typically occurs months to years after the initial episode of pericarditis
  - Pericardial effusion undergoes organization (instead of resorption) with deposition of fibrin
  - Progresses to a chronic stage with fibrous scarring and thickening of the pericardium with obliteration of the pericardial space
  - Calcium deposition may contribute to the stiffening of the pericardium
- The primary pathophysiologic feature is impaired diastolic filling caused by the presence of a rigid pericardium
  - Conceptually, constrictive pericarditis can be thought of as a normally contracting heart confined in a small box
  - Rigid pericardium impairs diastolic filling, resulting in increased and equal diastolic filling pressures in all the cardiac chambers
  - During early to mid-diastole, ventricular filling ceases abruptly when the intracardiac blood volume reaches the limit set by a stiff pericardium
  - Most ventricular filling occurs in diastole, and systemic venous congestion results
  - The myocardium may be involved in the chronic inflammatory process, leading to intrinsic contractile dysfunction as well

Clinical Presentation

- Signs and symptoms of constrictive pericarditis are the result of decreased cardiac output and increased venous pressures manifesting as right-heart failure
- Clinical features
  - Abdominal fullness (due to hepatic congestion and ascites) and peripheral edema
  - Symptoms of decreased cardiac output such as fatigue, weight loss, and muscle weakness
  - Less commonly, pulmonary congestion with orthopnea, dyspnea, and cough

- Physical examination
  - Elevated jugular venous pressure; signs of passive liver congestion (icterus, ascites); lower extremity edema
  - **Kussmaul's sign**
    - An increase in jugular venous pressure with inspiration (normally decreases with inspiration)
    - Occurs because the rigid pericardium insulates the heart from the decreased intrathoracic pressure that occurs with inspiration
  - **Pericardial knock:** Extra heart sound heard in early diastole (mimics an S_3), coinciding with abrupt cessation in ventricular filling due to the rigid pericardium

Diagnosis and Evaluation

- ECG: Usually nonspecific findings such as T-wave flattening or inversion
- Chest radiography: May show calcified pericardium
- Echocardiogram: two-dimensional and M-mode may demonstrate abnormal diastolic ventricular septal motion due to interventricular interdependence, marked respiratory variation in ventricular size/filling (>25%), plethoric inferior vena cava, and at times, thickened pericardium (>4 mm)
- CT or MRI: Most useful in identifying thickened (>4 mm) and calcified pericardium
- Right-heart catheterization (RHC)
  - Important for establishing or confirming the diagnosis of constrictive pericarditis
  - Reveals elevation and equalization of RA, RV diastolic, pulmonary capillary wedge, and left ventricular diastolic pressures
  - Prominent X and Y descents result in an **M** or **W** configuration of the RA pressure tracing (see Fig. 8-3)
  - The early diastolic filling of the right and left ventricles shows a characteristic "dip and plateau" pattern, or square root sign, caused by early rapid diastolic filling of the ventricle and then its abrupt halt (see Fig. 8-3)

Treatment

- **Total pericardiectomy (surgical removal of the pericardium) is the treatment of choice**
  - With complete pericardiectomy, 90% of patients are symptomatically improved and 50% have complete relief of symptoms
  - These results may take up to 6 months to be clinically apparent
  - Pericardiectomy is less effective when constrictive pericarditis is due to irradiation, as an underlying restrictive cardiomyopathy is often also present
  - Surgical mortality is between 5% and 19%
- Prior to pericardiectomy, calcium channel blockers and β-blockers should be avoided, because sinus tachycardia is a compensatory mechanism

REVIEW QUESTIONS

For review questions, please go to www.expertconsult.com.

SUGGESTED READINGS

Ariyarajah V, Spodicak DH: Acute pericarditis: diagnostic cues and common electrocardiographic manifestations, *Cardiol Rev* 15:24–30, 2007.

Imazio M, Spodick DH, Brucato A, et al: Controversial issues in the management of pericardial diseases, *Circulation* 210:916–928, 2010.

Lange RA, Hillis LD: Acute pericarditis, *N Engl J Med* 351:2195–2202, 2004.

Libby P, Bonow R, editors: *Braunwald's heart disease: a textbook of cardiovascular medicine*, ed 8, Philadelphia, 2008, WB Saunders.

Little WC, Freeman GL: Pericardial disease, *Circulation* 113:1622–1632, 2006.

Myers RB, Spodick DH: Constrictive pericarditis: clinical and pathophysiologic characteristics, *Am Heart J* 138:219–232, 1999.

Spodick DH: Acute cardiac tamponade, *N Engl J Med* 349:684–690, 2003.

Spodick DH: Acute pericarditis: current concepts and practice, *JAMA* 289:1150–1153, 2003.

Electrocardiogram Review

BRENT G. PETTY, MD

The electrocardiogram (ECG) is an important tool in diagnosing a variety of cardiac conditions. A systematic approach to ECG interpretation involves evaluating heart rate, rhythm, axis, intervals, and waveforms. Putting this ECG interpretation together with the patient's clinical picture can aid in formulating a diagnosis and treatment plan.

Fundamental Features to Assess When Reading an Electrocardiogram

Rate

- Normal is 60 to 100 beats/min
- Estimate rate by dividing 300 by the R–R interval (as measured by number of large boxes from R to R)
- Measure R–R interval to nearest 0.01 second and divide into 60 to calculate the rate more accurately

Rhythm

See also Chapter 4 on coronary artery disease.
- Too fast or too slow?
- Regular or irregular?
- Ventricular or supraventricular?

Axis

- Normal is 0° to +90°
- Leftward axis, between 0° and up to −30°, is "borderline" but not necessarily pathologic; axis more negative than −30° is abnormal
- Determine axis quadrant by evaluating positive or negative deflection of the QRS complex in leads I and aVF (Table 9-1)

Intervals

Figure 9-1 illustrates intervals and waveforms of surface ECGs.
- P–R interval: Normal is 0.12 to 0.2 seconds
- QRS duration: Normal is less than 0.12 seconds
- Q–T interval varies with heart rate
  - Q–T interval is inversely proportional to heart rate
  - Corrected Q–T (Q–T$_{corrected}$, or Q–T$_c$) adjusts for the heart rate
  - Calculated as: Q–T divided by the square root of R–R interval
  - Normal Q–T$_c$ is 0.36 to 0.41 seconds

Waveform

- Pathologic Q waves (indicative of prior transmural ST-segment elevation myocardial infarction)
  - **To be considered "pathologic," Q waves must be 1 small box wide and 1 small box deep (1 small box in width equals 0.04 sec at correct paper speed of 25 mm/sec)**
- ST segments (elevation or depression >1 mm)
- T-wave abnormalities (inversion or pseudonormalization)

Selected Electrocardiogram Abnormalities

Low Voltage

- Definition
  - No R or S wave in limb leads greater than 5 mm
  - No R or S wave in precordial leads greater than 15 mm
- Causes
  - Obesity
  - Chronic obstructive pulmonary disease
  - Pericardial effusion
  - Hypothyroidism
  - Addison disease
  - Infiltrative diseases (e.g., amyloidosis, hemochromatosis, sarcoidosis)

Atrioventricular Block

- First degree
  - P–R interval greater than 0.2 seconds
  - By itself, of no clinical consequence
- **Second degree**
  - **Mobitz I (also called Wenckebach block)**
    - Gradually increasing P–R interval until a P wave is not followed by a QRS complex
    - Usually self-limited and not clinically significant, so no treatment required
  - **Mobitz II**
    - **Higher degree of block, where only a fraction of the P waves are followed by QRS complexes (e.g., 3:1)**
    - **Usually caused by disease of the His bundle system rather than the atrioventricular (AV) node itself**
- **Third degree**
  - Also known as complete heart block

TABLE 9-1 *Determination of Axis Quadrant on Electrocardiogram*

	Lead I	Lead AVF	Axis	Common Causes
Normal			0° to +90°	Normal
Left axis deviation			−30° to −90°	LVH Left anterior hemiblock Inferior MI
Right axis deviation			+90° to +180°	Right ventricular hypertrophy Left posterior hemiblock Acute pulmonary disease (PE, pneumothorax)
Extreme axis deviation			−90° to −180° (or +180° to +270°)	Combination of left and right axis deviation causes

LVH, left ventricular hypertrophy; MI, myocardial infarction; PE, pulmonary embolism.

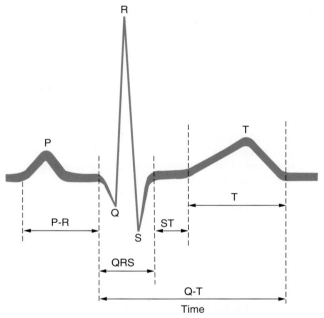

FIGURE 9-1 Intervals and waveforms of surface electrocardiogram.

- **Characterized by AV dissociation, where the P–P interval and the R–R interval are different and P waves are not responsible for the QRS complexes**
  - The QRS complexes are usually at a slow rate ("escape"), arising from intrinsic depolarization of the AV node (usually around 45–55 beats/min and with a narrow [<0.12-second] QRS complex) or the ventricle (usually around 35–45 beats/min and with a wide [≥0.12-second] QRS complex)

Left Ventricular Hypertrophy

- The gold standard for diagnosing left ventricular hypertrophy (LVH) is echocardiogram

- ECG may be suggestive of LVH; many different ECG criteria exist
- **Common ECG standard: Increased QRS voltage plus evidence of either "strain," left axis deviation, or left atrial abnormality**
  - Increased QRS voltage, as evidenced by one of the following:
    - R or S wave greater than 20 mm in any limb lead
    - S wave in V_{1-3} or R wave in V_{4-6} greater than 30 mm
    - (R wave in V_5 + S wave in V_1) greater than 35 mm
    - R wave in aVL greater than 11 mm
    - "Strain": Nonspecific ST-T changes (usually mild, downward-sloping ST depression and T-wave inversion or biphasic T waves) associated with voltage criteria for LVH
    - Left axis deviation (see Table 9-1)
  - **Left atrial abnormality: Net negative P wave in V_1 and P wave in V_2 at least slightly biphasic**
- Major causes
  - Hypertension
  - Aortic valve disease, either insufficiency or stenosis
  - Mitral insufficiency
  - Hypertrophic cardiomyopathy

Wide QRS Complex

- Definition: QRS complex greater than or equal to 0.12 second
- Primary causes
  - Bundle branch block
  - Ventricular rhythm
  - Hyperkalemia
  - Wolff-Parkinson-White syndrome

Bundle Branch Block

Figure 9-2 provides a bundle branch block algorithm.
- Can determine by ECG (Table 9-2; see Fig. 9-2)
- Causes
  - Myocardial infarction

FIGURE 9-2 Bundle branch block (BBB) algorithm. AV, atrioventricular.

- Infiltrative diseases (e.g., amyloidosis, hemochromatosis, sarcoidosis)
- Degenerative diseases of the conduction system

Trifascicular Block

- Can manifest in three ways (in order of decreasing frequency):
  - Bifascicular block and prolonged P–R interval
  - Complete heart block
  - Alternating right and left bundle branch block

Other Electrocardiogram Findings

- **Osborn waves**
  - **Positive deflection off declining shoulder of R wave**
  - Gives a "notched" appearance to the R wave
  - **Often seen with hypothermia**
- ST-segment elevation
  - **Consider myocardial infarction if**
    - **ST-segment elevation in anterior (I, aVL, V_{1-4}), inferior (II, III, aVF), or lateral (V_{4-6}) pattern**
    - **ST-segment elevation tends to be convex upward (sharp angle of takeoff from QRS complex) or horizontal**
    - Common sequential ECG changes in myocardial infarction (Fig. 9-3)
    - Diffuse concave upward ST-segment elevation (as may be seen in early repolarization) does not rule out infarction
  - **Early repolarization has previously been considered benign, but more recent research suggests that it may have pathologic implications,**
particularly if present in the inferior leads (II, III, and aVF). This pattern was associated with an increased risk of death from cardiac causes in middle-aged subjects.
  - Consider ventricular aneurysm if "acute" sharp-angled ST-segment elevation persists after an ST-segment elevation myocardial infarction
  - Consider pericarditis if
    - ST-segment elevation is diffuse and tends to be concave upward (smooth, curved takeoff from QRS complex)
    - Rarely may have P–R interval depression
- **Possible ECG findings with pulmonary embolus**
  - **Sinus tachycardia is most common ECG association**
  - T-wave inversions in inferior and precordial leads
  - Deep S wave in lead I (right axis elevation) with a Q-wave and T-wave inversion in lead III ($S_1Q_3T_3$)
- Electrical alternans
  - Alternating amplitude or direction of QRS complexes
  - Often seen with a pericardial effusion
  - May be caused by the "to-and-fro" motion of the heart swinging in a pericardial sac filled with fluid
- Diffusely inverted T waves
  - Nonspecific finding, potentially related to intracranial catastrophies (hemorrhage or stroke) or evolving pericarditis
  - Also associated with "broken heart syndrome," an acute, temporary but profound cardiomyopathy frequently following sudden fear or surprise

TABLE 9-2   *Examples of Bundle Branch Block*

Type of Bundle Branch Block	Description	Example Electrocardiogram
Right bundle branch block (RBBB)	Terminal S in I and V_6 + rSR' or tall R in V_1	
Left bundle branch block (LBBB)	Tall broad R in I and V_6 + QS or rS in V_1	
Bifascicular block	RBBB + left axis deviation beyond −30° (shown to right) *or* RBBB + right axis deviation at least +120° *or* LBBB	
Trifascicular block	Bifascicular block (at right, LBBB) + prolonged P–R interval	

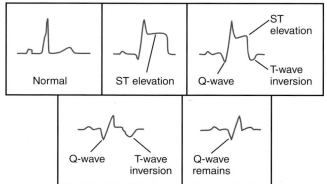

(in leads recording the area of MI)

FIGURE 9-3   Sequential electrocardiographic changes occurring in ST-segment elevation myocardial infarction (MI).

REVIEW QUESTIONS

For review questions, please go to www.expertconsult.com.

SUGGESTED READINGS

Anguera I, Vallis V: Giant waves in hypothermia, *Circulation* 101: 1627–1628, 2000.

Sakata K, Yoshino H, Houshaku H, et al: Myocardial damage and left ventricular dysfunction in patients with and without persistent negative T waves after Q-wave anterior myocardial infarction, *Am J Cardiol* 87:510–515, 2001.

Taylor GJ, Petty BG: Electrocardiogram. In Taylor GJ, editor: *Primary care and management of heart disease*, St. Louis, 2000, Mosby, pp 54–68.

Tikkanen JT, Anttonen O, Junttila MJ, et al: Long-term outcome associated with early repolarization on electrocardiography, *N Engl J Med* 361:2529–2537, 2009.

Wittstein IS, Thiemann DR, Lima JAC, et al: Neurohumoral features of myocardial stunning due to sudden emotional stress, *N Engl J Med* 352:539–548, 2005.

SECTION TWO

Infectious Disease

Respiratory Infections

PAUL G. AUWAERTER, MD

Infections of the respiratory tract result in more antibiotic prescriptions than any other group of medical disorders in the outpatient setting. **In many cases, respiratory tract infections do not require administration of antibiotics for cure.** The inappropriate prescription of antibiotics contributes to antibiotic resistance, particularly of concern in *Streptococcus pneumoniae*.

Bacterial Sinusitis

Basic Information

- **Acute bacterial sinusitis (ABS) is often preceded by viral upper respiratory tract infection (URTI), allergy flare, trauma, or dental manipulation**
- Symptoms often mimicked by common cold or allergies
- Diagnosis best made on clinical grounds, although history and physical findings are not specific
- Nasal passages also commonly involved (Fig. 10-1); thus some view this as rhinosinusitis
- Chronic sinusitis is a poorly understood entity, diagnosed after at least 12 weeks of sinus symptoms and signs, resulting from chronic obstruction of sinus passages. The role of bacterial pathogens in this disorder is debated.
- Microbiology of ABS shows that respiratory pathogens predominate (in order of decreasing frequency):
  - *S. pneumoniae*
  - *Haemophilus influenzae*
  - *Moraxella catarrhalis*
- Antibacterial resistance among these organisms is increasingly common (>40% of *H. influenzae* and 100% of *M. catarrhalis* are now β-lactamase producers, meaning they are resistant to amoxicillin); high-level pneumococcal resistance to penicillin (defined as mininimum inhibitory concentration [MIC] ≥8 mg/dL) for nonmeningeal isolates is uncommon, accounting for approximately 4% of isolates in the United States. The clinical importance of resistant bacteria in sinus conditions is debated.
- Other pathogens, such as anaerobes, other streptococci, and *Staphylococcus aureus*, account for small percentages of isolates in ABS
- **In chronic sinusitis, *S. aureus*, *Staphylococcus epidermidis*, and anaerobes predominate. Whether antibiotic treatment helps this condition is unclear, but it is often used.**

Clinical Presentation

- **ABS most commonly follows viral URTI**
- **Change in color or character of nasal discharge is not specifically indicative of bacterial infection**

- **ABS (as opposed to viral or allergic sinusitis) is unlikely if symptoms are less than 7 days' duration**
- History or physical findings suggestive of ABS include
  - Persisting or worsening of symptoms after 7 to 10 days
  - Unilateral sinus pain or tenderness
  - Purulent nasal discharge
  - Maxillary tooth or facial pain (particularly unilateral)

Diagnosis

- Gold standard is culture from sinus puncture (not commonly done)
- Best made on clinical grounds, usually only after symptoms have lasted more than 7 days, although sensitivity and specificity of history and physical examination are poor
- **Imaging studies not recommended for uncomplicated cases of ABS because findings are no more sensitive or specific than clinical evaluation**

Treatment

- Many patients, even with true ABS, will resolve without antimicrobial therapy; use of decongestants, analgesics, antipyretics possibly helpful but not well studied
- **Patients with moderate or severe symptoms should receive antibiotics (Fig. 10-2)**
- Goals of ABS treatment: Avoid acute complications (e.g., brain abscess, meningitis, or osteomyelitis—all rare; Fig. 10-3) and chronic complications (e.g., chronic sinusitis)
- Antibiotic choice dictated by local sensitivities, cost, drug allergy history. Preferred drug: Amoxicillin—no other antibiotic has been shown to work better for uncomplicated ABS; need to treat approximately seven patients for one to benefit.
- **True, recurrent ABS may indicate obstruction or immunodeficiency (e.g., HIV, hypogammaglobulinemia)**
- Attempts to treat chronic sinusitis with antibiotics may result in little improvement; treatments should focus on relieving obstruction
- For chronic sinusitis, decrease mucosal swelling, exudates, and crusting by using nasal saline irrigation, topical nasal corticosteroids, antihistamines, decongestants, leukotriene antagonists
- **Sinus computed tomography (CT) scan helpful in chronic sinusitis suspects to document obstruction (e.g., polyps) in patients not responding to initial therapy; otolaryngology consultation is recommended**
- If a patient with chronic sinusitis has an acute flare, treatment with antibiotics against *S. pneumoniae* and *H. influenzae* should be given

Otitis Media

Basic Information

- Acute otitis media is infection of middle ear. It needs to be distinguished from otitis media with effusion (noninfectious).
- Often initiated by either URTI or allergies blocking the eustachian tube, resulting in pressure imbalance of inner ear with subsequent bacterial infection
- **Uncommon in adults; less than 0.25% incidence**

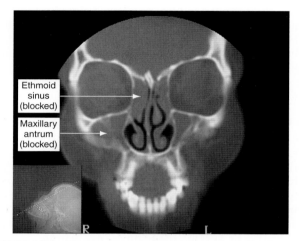

FIGURE 10-1 Coronal computed tompgraphy scan showing ethmoid, labyrinth, and maxillary antral opacification in a patient with sinusitis. *(From Swash M: Hutchison's clinical methods, ed 21, Philadelphia, WB Saunders, 2002, Fig. 13.10.)*

- Intensively studied in children; less known about infection in adults
- *S. pneumoniae* and *H. influenzae* common isolates; unclear frequency of viral and allergic inflammation

Clinical Presentation

- Commonly follows URTI or history of allergies
- **Otalgia and fever are most frequent symptoms**
- Severe cases may be complicated by meningitis, mastoiditis, or brain abscess (all rare)

Diagnosis

- Physical examination in children imprecise, but accuracy increases with insufflation demonstrating decreased mobility of tympanic membrane
- **Examination findings in adults have not been studied, but typical presentation is bulging, red tympanic membrane (Fig. 10-4)**
- Perforation of tympanic membrane may occur and lead to drainage or crusting within ear canal

Treatment

- Antimicrobial therapy not well defined; amoxicillin/clavulanate, cefuroxime axetil, azithromycin possible options

Pharyngitis

Basic Information

- Outpatient visits for pharyngitis account for 1% to 2% of all office visits

FIGURE 10-2 Management of acute bacterial sinusitis. *If patient is diabetic, immunocompromised, or in an iron-overload state and/or critically ill, consider rhinocerebral mucormycosis. (CT, computed tomography; TMP-SMX, trimethoprim-sulfamethoxazole.)

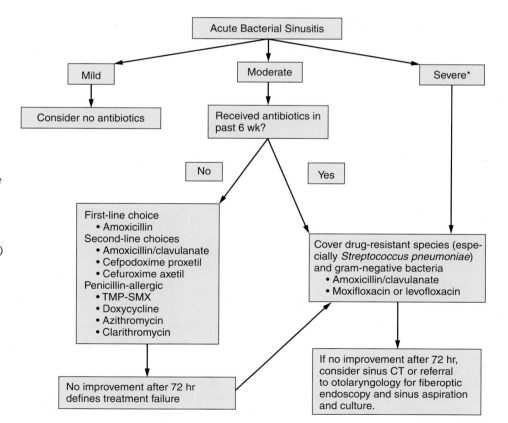

- **Most common cause is viral in adults, with a much higher incidence of group A streptococci in children**
- Some cases may be associated with evidence of more systemic infection (Epstein-Barr virus [EBV], acute HIV infection); severe pharyngitis (*Neiserria gonorrohoeae* or group A β-hemolytic streptococci [GABHS]); adult patients with a history of rheumatic fever managed differently, with lower threshold for prescription of antibiotics
- Viral infection causes most adult cases (~80%)
  - Rhinovirus (20%) is most common viral cause
  - Coronavirus (5–10%), adenovirus (5%), herpes simplex (2–4%) less common
- Uncommon causes include parainfluenza (2%), influenza (1%), EBV (<1%), cytomegalovirus (<1%), acute HIV type 1 (<1%), coxsackievirus (<1%)
- Bacterial infection less common in adults than children
- ***Streptococcus pyogenes* most common bacterial cause in adults (5–10%)**
  - Other streptococci less common, usually group G or C
  - Rare bacterial causes include *N. gonorrhoeae* (<1%), *Corynebacterium diphtheriae* (<1%), *Arcanobacterium haemolyticum* (often associated with rash, <1%), *Chlamydophila pneumoniae* (1%), *Mycoplasma pneumoniae* (<1%)
- Many cases unknown and presumed viral

Clinical Presentation

- Typical presentations include sore throat and malaise with possible fever or cervical lymphadenopathy
- Severe sore throat with inability to swallow secretions or associated dyspnea should be evaluated in an emergency department setting; may indicate epiglottitis
- Dehydration in severe cases may require IV hydration
- Red, beefy tonsils with exudates may have either bacterial or viral causes (i.e., presence of exudate is not specific for bacterial cause; Fig. 10-5)
- **Primary infection with EBV (infectious mononucleosis) may present with fever, sore throat, and lymphadenopathy (anterior and posterior cervical lymph nodes—may be generalized and include splenomegaly) and is easily confused with GABHS**
  - In infectious mononucleosis, laboratory abnormalities may include predominance of lymphocytes or atypical lymphocytes. In 90% of adult cases, the aspartate aminotransferase, alanine aminotransferase, or lactate deyhydrogenase level is elevated to at least two to three times normal.
  - **Prescription of amoxicillin for mistakenly believed or secondary concurrent GABHS predictably yields diffuse, pruritic, maculopapular rash in 95% to 100% of patients (rash does not mean patient is amoxicillin allergic for future dosing; Fig. 10-6)**

FIGURE 10-3 Cerebral abscess secondary to sinusitis. Right frontal abscess is demonstrated in a patient who had ethmoid sinusitis. An orbital abscess is also demonstrated. *(From Forbes C, Jackson W: Color atlas and text of clinical medicine, ed 3, St. Louis, Mosby, 2003, Fig. 11.63.)*

FIGURE 10-4 Acute left otitis media. *(From Behrman RE: Nelson textbook of pediatrics, ed 16, Philadelphia, WB Saunders, 2003, Fig. 630-3.)*

FIGURE 10-5 Acute streptococcal pharyngitis. Note purulent discharge in tonsillar crypts. A similar appearance may be seen with pharyngitis caused by infectious mononucleosis. *(From Forbes C, Jackson W: Color atlas and text of clinical medicine, ed 3, St. Louis, Mosby, 2003, Fig. 1.82.)*

Diagnosis

Because the signs and symptoms of group A streptococcal and other viral presentations overlap, physicians are generally unable to include or exclude the diagnosis of streptococcal pharyngitis on epidemiologic and clinical grounds; therefore, laboratory testing should be done to determine whether group A streptococci are present in the pharynx (Fig. 10-7).
- Throat culture gold standard (90% sensitive)
  - False positives may result from carrier state
- Rapid strep tests
  - Throat swab detecting carbohydrate antigen
  - Sensitivity 80% to 90% in adults but highly specific
  - **If positive test, treat as GABHS; no further culture required**
  - In children and adolescents, negative tests should be confirmed by standard culture. It is unclear whether this is necessary in adults.

FIGURE 10-6 Generalized erythematous papular eruption of infectious mononucleosis precipitated by oral penicillin intake. *(From Shah BR, Laude TA: Atlas of pediatric clinical diagnosis, Philadelphia, WB Saunders, 2000, Fig. 3-32.)*

- Sensitivity and specificity of clinical presentation 50% to 75% for GABHS (Fig. 10-8)
- The production of heterophile antibodies used to diagnose infectious mononucleosis (that are not directed against EBV but agglutinate either horse or sheep red blood cells [RBCs]) occurs in 90% of cases and is detected by blood testing with commercial kits (e.g., Monospot, Meridian Bioscience, Cincinnati, OH)
  - **Detection of anti-EBV capsid immunoglobulin M (IgM) antibodies typically done if heterophilic antibodies are negative but EBV still suspected (~10% of cases)**
  - Anti-EBV immunoglobulin G (IgG) may be present at presentation in new infection or with preexisting infection and has less clinical utility in diagnosis of acute infection

Treatment

- Viral: Generally benign, self-limited illness remedied by rest, hydration, nonsteroidal drugs for pain or fever, and saltwater gargles
- GABHS: Historically, treatment is given to avoid complications of acute rheumatic fever and may prevent suppurative complications such as tonsillar abscess. However, acute rheumatic fever is now rare in adults, and the main use of antibiotics offers shorter duration of illness (16–24 hours) if given within 72 hours of symptom onset.
  - **All GABHS strains remain penicillin sensitive**
  - Penicillin (PCN) V standard for adults, 250 mg four times daily or 500 mg twice daily orally; long-acting intramuscular PCN given as one dose (1.2 million units benzathine ± procaine PCN G)
  - Erythromycin 250 mg four times daily or 500 mg twice daily orally for PCN-allergic patients

Acute Bronchitis

Basic Information
- **Most common cause of acute cough in the outpatient setting**
- Clinical challenge is to distinguish bronchitis from pneumonia

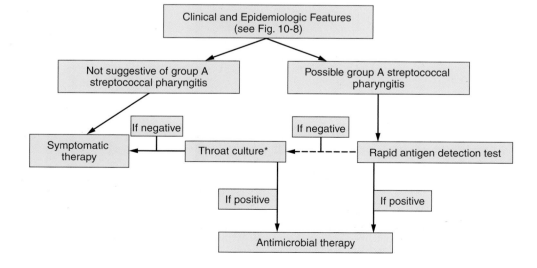

FIGURE 10-7 Diagnosis and management of pharyngitis. *Considered optional in adults.

- **90% of cases are from nonbacterial cause in healthy nonsmokers**
  - Purulent sputum may or may not indicate bacterially induced process
  - Viral causes predominate, especially coronaviruses, paramyxoviruses, rhinoviruses, and also, in season, influenza (A or B)

FIGURE 10-8 Differentiation of streptococcal (group A β-hemolytic streptococci [GABHS]) pharyngitis from viral causes. (LN, lymph nodes.)

- **Pertussis is an uncommon cause of bronchitis but is more likely if cough is severe or persists longer than 3 weeks**

Clinical Presentation

- Acute respiratory infection with cough with or without phlegm for less than 3 weeks
- Wheezing may be present, including in those without asthma

Diagnosis

- **Diagnosis based on history and physical examination; sputum cultures are not recommended**
- **Pneumonia is uncommon if vital signs and chest examination are normal**

Treatment

- Symptomatic support; antibiotics not recommended regardless of cough duration, and prescription represents antibiotic abuse (Table 10-1; see notes on pertussis that follow)
- 50% will experience resolution of cough at 14 days; 90% will experience resolution at 21 days
- **Albuterol inhalation may decrease cough; most beneficial in those with documented reductions in peak airflow**
  - Antitussives often prescribed, but few data to clarify role
  - Consider antiviral therapy for influenza if early in course of illness (<48 hours) for ambulatory patients

TABLE 10-1	**Treatment of Bronchitis**			
Basic Clinical State	**Symptoms/Risk Factors**	**Likely Pathogens**	**First-Line Treatment**	**Alternatives/ Treatment Failure**
Acute tracheobronchitis	Cough and sputum without previous pulmonary disease	Usually viral	None	Macrolide or tetracycline if symptoms >10–14 days
Acute flare of chronic bronchitis without risk factors (group I)	Increased cough and sputum, sputum purulence, and increased dyspnea	*Haemophilus influenzae* *Haemophilus* spp. *Moraxella catarrhalis* *Streptococcus pneumoniae*	2nd-generation macrolide 2nd- or 3rd-generation cephalosporin Amoxicillin Doxycycline TMP-SMX	Fluoroquinolone or β-lactam/ β-lactamase inhibitor
Acute flare of chronic bronchitis with risk factors (group II)	Symptoms as in group I *plus* at least 1 of the following: FEV₁ <50% predicted >4 exacerbations/yr Cardiac disease Use of home oxygen Chronic oral steroid use Antibiotic use in past 3 mo	Organisms as in group I, *plus* *Klebsiella* spp. Other gram-negative pathogens Increased probability of β-lactam resistance	Fluoroquinolone β-lactam/β-lactamase inhibitor	May require parenteral therapy; consider referral to a specialist or hospital
Acute flare of chronic suppurative bronchitis (group III)	Symptoms as in group II, but with constant purulent sputum Some have bronchiectasis FEV₁ <35% predicted Multiple risk factors (e.g., frequent exacerbations and FEV₁ <50% predicted)	Organisms as in group II, *plus* *Pseudomonas aeruginosa* Multiresistant Enterobacteriaceae	Ambulatory patients Tailor treatment to airway pathogen (*P. aeruginosa* common; use ciprofloxacin) Hospitalized patients Parenteral therapy usually required	

FEV₁, forced expiratory volume in 1 second; TMP-SMX, trimethoprim-sulfamethoxazole.
Adapted from Balter MS, LaForge J, Low DE, et al: Canadian guidelines for the management of acute exacerbations of chronic bronchitis, *Can Respir J* 10(suppl B):3B–32B, 2003.

at high risk for severe infection (comorbidities, pregnancy) or for all hospitalized patients with suspected or confirmed influenza
- **Pertussis should be suspected if cough persists beyond 3 weeks; treatment with azithromycin or tetracycline is done more for public health reasons to limit the potential for transmission because treatment initiation after 7 to 10 days of cough onset does not lead to reduction in cough duration, which can persist for 6 to 10 weeks regardless**
- Patient education essential: Patients not receiving an antibiotic are happier if told they have a "chest cold" rather than "bronchitis"

Acute Exacerbations of Chronic Bronchitis

Basic Information
- Part of the clinical spectrum of chronic obstructive pulmonary disease (COPD)
- Cigarette smoking is major contributor to COPD, with less than 10% of patients with COPD having disease from other reasons such as occupational or environmental exposure
- Accounts for 5% of all deaths in United States
- Viral or bacterial infections may cause acute exacerbations of chronic bronchitis
- Bacterial causes
  - *H. influenzae* is most common cause (~22%), particularly in smokers
  - *M. catarrhalis* (9–15%)
  - *S. pneumoniae* (10–12%)
  - *Pseudomonas aeruginosa* or other gram-negative bacteria (up to 15%) seen in those with recent prior antibiotic use or hospitalizations and in those with frequent flares
- Many cases without predominant bacterial species are presumed viral

Clinical Presentation
- **Patients with COPD flare may have a combination of worsening dyspnea, increased sputum purulence and/or volume**
- Winnipeg criteria may be used to stratify severity of flares (Box 10-1)
  - Type 1 or type 2 flares require hospitalization and are associated with increased mortality (3–4%) that increases to 11% to 24% in-hospital mortality if care in the intensive care unit is required
- Chest radiograph (CXR) abnormalities are common
- Consider deep venous thrombosis leading to pulmonary embolus as cause of exacerbation

Diagnosis
- Diagnosis made on clinical grounds
- **CXR, pulse oximetry, and arterial blood gas tests are beneficial to either rule out pneumonia or gauge severity**
- May be difficult to differentiate from pneumonia if CXR has baseline abnormalities
- **Acute spirometry considered unhelpful**
- Sputum culture not routinely recommended but may be helpful in severe cases

BOX 10-1	*Winnipeg Criteria for Stratifying Severity of Acute Exacerbation of Chronic Bronchitis*

Symptoms
Increasing dyspnea
Increasing purulence of sputum
Increasing volume of sputum

Classification
Type 1: Severe, all three symptoms
Type 2: Moderate, two or three symptoms
Type 3: Mild, at least one symptom along with
    Upper respiratory tract infection within last 5 days
    Fever without other apparent cause
    Increased wheezing
    Increased nonproductive cough
    Increased respirations or pulse >20% over baseline

Treatment
- Few good data to guide recommendations (see Table 10-1)
- **Bronchodilators and corticosteroids helpful**
- **Antibiotics useful for more severe flares, but data using amoxicillin and tetracycline are more than 30 years old; unclear role of emerging antimicrobial resistance and newer antibiotics**
- Mucolytics and chest physiotherapy without clear benefit
- Oxygen helpful with hypoxemia but may heighten risk of respiratory failure

Influenza

Basic Information
- **Two major virus subtypes: influenza A and influenza B**
- Antigenic characteristics determined by surface-spike glycoproteins that have either hemagglutinin activity (HA) or neuraminidase activity (NA) (Fig. 10-9)
  - Hemagglutinin attaches to erythrocytes and is responsible for initiation of infection
  - Neuraminidase cleaves hemagglutinin protein, allowing viral release from infected cells
  - Significant antigenic variation of HA or NA bypasses prior immune memory in the host infected with influenza in the past
    - Antigenic drift: Minor changes in HA or NA and minor changes in immunogenicity
    - Antigenic shift: Major changes in HA or NA resulting in completely new immunogenicity with risk of pandemic infection
  - Avian influenza (H5N1) is a concern because of similarity to 1918 influenza severity; however, few cases to date in humans with limited human-to-human transmissibility
  - The pandemic H1N1 strain arising in 2009 behaved similarly to seasonal influenza with the exception that children and young adults were more often affected than the customary elderly populations; increased mortality was seen more often in those with comorbidities

FIGURE 10-9 Schematic drawing of influenza A, demonstrating hemagglutinin and neuraminidase. Hemagglutinin is responsible for attachment to cells; neuraminidase is responsible for viral release. Figure demonstrates antigenic shifts that have caused major influenza outbreaks. *(From Roitt I, Brostoff J, Male D [eds]: Immunology, ed 6, St Louis, Mosby, 2001, Fig. 14.9.)*

Clinical Presentation

- Seasonal influenza outbreaks typically in epidemic pattern, peaking at 2 to 3 weeks after introduction and completed after 5 to 6 weeks in any given community
- Seasonal peaks usually occur in winter, but may occur from early fall to late spring. Influenza is uncommon in the summertime
- **Symptoms for individual often begin abruptly with fever, rigors, malaise, headache, myalgia, and arthralgia**
- Fever, rigors, and myalgia peak at 3 days, after which respiratory symptoms (cough) and nasal congestion predominate
- **Major complication is pneumonia**
  - Viral pneumonia from influenza occurs early and may be severe
  - **Postinfectious bacterial pneumonia often follows a period of recovery from influenza and is most often caused by *S. pneumoniae, S. aureus, S. pyogenes,* or *H. influenzae***
- Other complications may include rhabdomyolysis, myocarditis, or Guillain-Barré syndrome

Diagnosis

- **Clinical presentation in an individual during community outbreak is most common method and is 70% specific for influenza based on abrupt onset of cough and fever in an adult**
- Seasonal strains of influenza may be detected from sputum, nasal, or throat swab or from nasopharyngeal aspirate by rapid antigen test (70% specific), polymerase chain reaction (PCR) assay (90–100% specific), or culture (90–100% specific but slow)

Treatment

- Optimal treatment is prevention, with influenza vaccine now universally recommended for all people over the age of 6 months
- **Amantadine and rimantadine block ion channel function only in influenza A virus and *should only be used if circulating strains are known to be susceptible;* these drugs have no role in treatment of influenza B**
- Neuraminidase inhibitors (zanamivir and oseltamivir) prevent infection of cells by inhibiting influenza NA for both influenza A and influenza B. Both must be administered within first 48 hours of infection to shorten the duration of influenza symptoms in ambulatory patients, but severely ill or hospitalized patients may benefit from administration during any phase of their acute illness.
  - **Since 2009, neuraminidase inhibitors have been the preferred treatment for influenza since circulating strains have been resistant to amantadines.** Resistance profiles of circulating virus may change with every season, hence check for up-to-date recommendations [*http://www.cdc.gov/flu/about/season/index.htm*]
  - Oseltamivir is administered orally and may result in nausea
  - **Zanamivir is administered by inhalation and is well tolerated but may result in bronchospasm and should be avoided in susceptible patients, such as those with asthma or COPD**

Pneumonia

Basic Information

- Remains leading cause of infectious death in United States; seventh overall cause of death
- Mortality highest in older patients and in those with multiple comorbidities
- ***S. pneumoniae* and *Legionella pneumophila* are the leading bacterial causes of pneumonia death**
- Microbiology is altered by host factors (e.g., age, immunosuppression, alcohol use) and geography
  - *S. pneumoniae* remains the most commonly diagnosed etiologic agent in studies of community-acqired pneumonia
    - *S. pneumoniae* with high-level penicillin resistance is less frequent than previously stated as a result of revised resistance breakpoints for nonmeningeal isolates (about 4% in recent U.S. studies)
    - Clinical significance of antibiotic-resistant organisms in pneumonia is debated
- **Atypical agents account for 15% to 20% of community-acquired pneumonias and include infections with *L. pneumophila, M. pneumoniae,* and *C. pneumoniae***
- *H. influenzae, S. aureus,* and gram-negative bacilli each account for 3% to 10% of community-acquired pneumonias
- **Viral pneumonia uncommon** in adults
  - Influenza A and B most common viral causes
  - Cytomegalovirus causes pneumonia only in immunosuppressed patients
  - Adenovirus, varicella-zoster virus, and EBV are rare causes of viral pneumonia in adults

TABLE 10-2	*Fungal Infections of the Lung*		
Organism	**Presentation**	**Diagnosis**	**Treatment**
Histoplasma capsulatum	Up to 60% asymptomatic; endemic to Ohio and Mississippi River valleys Acute infection: Includes fever, infiltrates, pleurisy, hilar and mediastinal adenopathy ARDS: If inoculum sufficiently large, fulminant respiratory failure may result Progressive disseminated histoplasmosis: May result from primary infection or reactivation; more common in immunocompromised; diffuse lymphadenopathy, hepatosplenomegaly, and adrenal insufficiency may result Chronic pulmonary histoplasmosis: Usually in setting of COPD; resembles tuberculosis with cavitation	Culture is gold standard, but takes 4–6 wk *Histoplasma* antigen may be detected in serum and urine of patients with disseminated disease; may cross-react with blastomycosis and coccidioidomycosis Complement fixation of antibody to *H. capsulatum* may be used, including those with acute pulmonary infection (fourfold rise in titer consistent with acute infection)	Acute infection does not typically require treatment Chronic pulmonary infections may require treatment with itraconazole Disseminated infections treated with itraconazole or amphotericin High index of suspicion should be held for adrenal insufficiency in disseminated disease
Blastomyces dermatitidis	Endemic to region between Dakotas and Louisiana Disease may be self-limited or require treatment Pulmonary presentations include infiltrates, nodules, or cavitation Skin, bone, and genitourinary tract (prostate and epididymis) most common extrapulmonary sites of infection	Culture is gold standard Visualization of fungi in appropriate clinical setting used to initiate antimicrobial treatment Complement fixation is currently neither sensitive nor specific	Itraconazole in immunocompetent with mild to moderate disease Amphotericin in immunocompromised or with CNS involvement
Coccidioides immitis	Endemic to dry regions of southwestern United States Acute pulmonary infection: Most common presentation, with fever, cough, and extensive alveolar infiltrates; may be accompanied by massive hilar and mediastinal adenopathy; cavitation may occur, with hemoptysis; erythema nodosum Dissemination may be widespread, with skin, muscle, bone, and CNS involvement	Stain and culture of infected fluid or tissues Elevated complement fixation titers to *C. immitis;* these may be followed as markers of disease, with rising titers a poor prognostic sign	Itraconazole Fluconazole Fluconazole used if CNS involvement or refractory disease
Aspergillus fumigatus	ABPA: A hypersensitivity reaction characterized by asthma and fleeting infiltrates accompanied by eosinophilia Aspergilloma (fungal ball or mycetoma): Most common noninvasive form, occurring in old scars, cavities, or blebs Invasive aspergillosis: Usually occurs in immunocompromised, with organ transplant and hematologic malignancies common predisposers; presents as acute pneumonia with cavitation, then invades locally along with hematogenous dissemination	Diagnosis of ABPA by positive sputum culture, elevated total IgE, elevated specific antibodies to *Aspergillus,* and cutaneous reaction to *Aspergillus* immunogen Aspergilloma diagnosed by clinical presentation Invasive aspergillosis diagnosed by clinical microbiologic and radiographic presentation and CT scan; biopsy with culture usually suggested to distinguish from colonization; serum galactomannan may be elevated	ABPA: Corticosteroids; role of antifungal treatment unclear Aspergilloma may require embolization or resection for control of hemoptysis; otherwise no antifungal treatment necessary Invasive aspergillosis: Voriconazole is treatment of choice

ABPA, allergic bronchopulmonary aspergillosis; ARDS, acute respiratory distress syndrome; CNS, central nervous system; COPD, chronic obstructive pulmonary disease; CT, computed tomography; IgE, immunoglobulin E.

- Hantavirus, seen mostly in the southwestern United States, is a rare cause of viral pneumonia that quickly evolves to acute respiratory distress in previously health individuals and is associated with a high mortality rate
- Fungal infections
  - Rarely a cause of acute, community-acquired pneumonia
  - More than 300 fungi capable of causing lung infection, mostly in immunocompromised patients, with *Aspergillus* spp. and zygomycete organisms (*Rhizopus,* *Mucor* spp.) the leading causes of serious clinical pulmonary infection
  - Endemic fungi (*Histoplasma capsulatum, Blastomyces dermatitidis, Coccidioides immitis,* and *Cryptococcus neoformans*) can infect normal hosts and cause lung disease, but greater than 60% of infections are asymptomatic and only a small percentage are not self-limiting (Table 10-2)
  - **Candida spp. are a very rare cause of pneumonia and should be considered as the causative**

FIGURE 10-10 Right upper lobe pneumonia. On this postero-anterior chest radiograph, note that the right cardiac border is well seen. The alveolar infiltrate is seen in the right midlung. *(From Mettler FA: Essentials of radiology, ed 2, Philadelphia, WB Saunders, 2005, Fig. 3-44.)*

FIGURE 10-11 Chest radiograph of a patient with *Pneumocystis jiroveci* pneumonia. *(From Haslett C, Chilvers ER, Boon NA, Colledge NR [eds]: Davidson's principles and practice of medicine, ed 19, Edinburgh, Elsevier Science, 2002, Fig. 1.86.)*

agent only in the profoundly immunosuppressed or neutropenic patient. Positive sputum cultures otherwise merely represent upper airway colonization.

Clinical Presentation

- Cough, fever, and new pulmonary infiltrate constitute the classic triad
- Other common symptoms include pleurisy, dyspnea, malaise, headache, nausea, vomiting, abdominal pain, and diarrhea
- **Although no reliable clinical indicators have been established to differentiate "typical" pneumonia from "atypical" pneumonia, purulent sputum without predominant organisms heightens suspicion for *Legionella*, *Mycoplasma*, and *Chlamydophilia* spp.**
- Some presentations are associated with etiologic agent
    - **S. *pneumoniae* classically presents with sudden rigor, fever, and cough productive of rust-colored sputum (Fig. 10-10)**
    - **Legionella, which may be sporadic or cluster in an outbreak associated with aerosol spread of a contaminated water system, presents as a severe pneumonia with high-spiking fevers, classically accompanied by diarrhea and, in some cases, relative bradycardia in spite of high fevers. Hyponatremia may be more common with *Legionella* than with other etiologic agents.**
    - The hallmark of *Mycoplasma* infection is a paroxysmal, nonproductive cough, often with minimal findings on CXR; however, CXR may demonstrate diffuse pulmonary infiltrates and even effusions
        - Bullous myringitis, contrary to lore, is *not* a usual finding in *Mycoplasma* infection
        - The production of cold agglutinins (IgM produced in *Mycoplasma* infection that reversibly agglutinates RBCs when blood is cooled) may lead to Raynaud's phenomenon and even digital necrosis (particularly in patients with sickle cell anemia)

- *C. pneumoniae* results in a typically mild pneumonia that is slowly progressive and only rarely severe; it may follow URTI symptoms (pharyngitis, sinus infection) by 1 or 2 weeks
    - There is little clinically to differentiate *C. pneumoniae* from other causes of pneumonia
- Pneumonia is the most common initial AIDS-defining illness, with *Pneumocystis jiroveci* (Fig. 10-11) and *S. pneumoniae* the leading etiologies
- Infiltrates with cavitation or subacute pneumonia, especially in an immunocompromised patient, demand consideration of tuberculosis (1–2% of all cases of community-acquired pneumonia)

Diagnosis

- CXR is critical to establish infiltrate and to decrease administration of antibiotics given mistakenly for acute bronchitis
- Chest physical examination is unreliable to include or to exclude pneumonia diagnosis
- Abnormal vital signs heighten the likelihood of positive CXR (see Acute Bronchitis section)
- **Sputum with more than 25 polymorphonuclear neutrophils and fewer than 10 epithelial cells per high-powered field considered purulent specimen that may adequately reflect pathogen of pneumonia (Fig. 10-12)**
- Blood cultures are considered an optional study but should be obtained in certain patients, including those with severe pneumonia, cavitary infiltrates, leukopenia, active alcohol abuse, chronic severe liver disease, asplenia, positive pneumococcal urinary antigen test, or pleural effusion
- **If significant pleural effusion is seen at presentation, thoracentesis with analysis and culture should be performed**

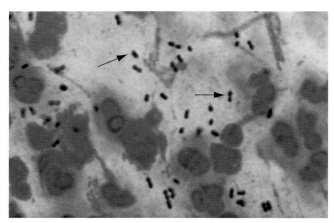

FIGURE 10-12 Purulent sputum in a patient with pneumococcal pneumonia. Gram stain shows gram-positive diplococci characteristic of *Streptococcus pneumoniae* (arrows). (From Haslett C, Chilvers ER, Boon NA, Colledge NR [eds]: Davidson's principles and practice of medicine, ed 19, Edinburgh, Elsevier Science, 2002, Fig. 13.30.)

- Cause of pneumonia is considered definitive only if bacteria are isolated from normally sterile space (blood, pleura)
- Cause is considered probable but not definitive if only cultured from sputum unless sputum grows *Legionella*, tuberculosis, or some fungi
  - *Legionella* urinary antigen detects only type 1
  - *L. pneumophila*; sputum direct fluorescent antibody less reliable for *Legionella* spp.
- **Chlamydophila and Mycoplasma infections best diagnosed by PCR assay of respiratory specimen; serologic tests unreliable**

Treatment

Table 10-3 summarizes the initial therapy for suspected bacterial community-acquired pneumonia.
- First decision is whether to manage as outpatient or whether hospitalization appropriate
  - Pneumonia severity index or CURB-65 score may help guide hospitalization decision (Tables 10-4 and 10-5)
  - **Usually patients who are elderly or with comorbidities, highly abnormal vital signs, hypoxemia, or laboratory abnormalities should be treated in hospital**
- Initial antibiotic choice typically empirical and should cover *S. pneumoniae* but should also cover atypical agents and drug-resistant *Pneumococcus* if patient is severely ill (see Table 10-3)
- Timely antibiotic administration (within 6 hours of initial encounter) correlates with decreased mortality and now considered standard of care

TABLE 10-3	*Recommended Empirical Antibiotics for Community-Acquired Pneumonia*

Outpatient Treatment

1. Previously healthy and no use of antimicrobials within previous 3 mo
   A macrolide (azithromycin, clarithromycin) (strong recommendation)
   Doxycycline (weak recommendation)
2. Presence of comorbidities such as chronic heart, lung, liver, or renal disease; diabetes mellitus; alcoholism; malignancies; asplenia; immunosuppressing conditions or use of immunosuppressing drugs; or use of antimicrobials within the previous 3 mo (in which case an alternative from a different class should be selected)
   A respiratory fluoroquinolone (moxifloxacin or levofloxacin) (strong recommendation)
   A β-lactam (amoxicillin/clavulanate, high-dose amoxicillin 1 g tid, cefpodoxime, or cefuroxime) plus a macrolide
3. In regions with a high rate (>25%) of infection with high-level (MIC ≥16 μg/mL) macrolide-resistant *Streptococcus pneumoniae*, consider use of alternative agents listed above in (2) for patients without comorbidities (moderate recommendation)

Inpatients, Non-ICU Treatment
A respiratory fluoroquinolone (strong recommendation)
A β-lactam (ceftriaxone, cefotaxime, ertapenem) plus a macrolide (strong recommendation)

Inpatients, ICU Treatment
A β-lactam (cefotaxime, ceftriaxone, or ampicillin/sulbactam) plus either azithromycin or a respiratory fluoroquinolone (strong recommendation) (for penicillin-allergic patients, a respiratory fluoroquinolone and aztreonam are recommended)

Special Concerns
If *Pseudomonas* is a consideration
   An antipneumococcal, antipseudomonal β-lactam (piperacillin/tazobactam, cefepime, imipenem, or meropenem) plus either ciprofloxacin or levofloxacin (750 mg)

or

The above β-lactam plus an aminoglycoside and a respiratory fluoroquinolone (for penicillin-allergic patients, substitute aztreonam for above β-lactam) (moderate recommendation)
If CA-MRSA is a consideration, add vancomycin or linezolid (moderate recommendation)

CA-MRSA, community-acquired methicillin-resistant *Staphylococcus aureus;* ICU, intensive care unit; MIC, minimum inhibitory concentration.
Adapted from Mandell LA, Wunderink RG, Anzueto A, et al: Infectious Diseases Society of America/American Thoracic Society consensus guidelines on the management of community-acquired pneumonia in adults, *Clin Infect Dis* 44:S27–S73, 2007.

- Many guidelines exist with slight variations; consider unusual factors

REVIEW QUESTIONS

For review questions, please go to www.expertconsult.com.

TABLE 10-4	*Pneumonia Severity Index**

Step 1. Is the patient at low risk (class I) based on the history and physical examination and not a resident of a nursing home?
  Age ≤50 yr
  and
  None of the coexisting conditions or physical examination findings listed in step 2
  No: Go to step 2
  Yes: Outpatient treatment is recommended
Step 2. Calculate risk score for classes II to V

Patient Characteristics	Points Assigned	Patient's Points
Demographic factors		
Age (yr)		
Males	Age	_____
Females	Age −10	_____
Nursing home resident	+10	_____
Coexisting conditions		
Neoplastic disease	+30	_____
Liver disease	+20	_____
Congestive heart failure	+10	_____
Cerebrovascular disease	+10	_____
Renal disease	+10	_____
Initial physical examination findings		
Altered mental status	+20	_____
Respiratory rate ≥30 breaths/min	+20	_____
Systolic blood pressure <90 mm Hg	+20	_____
Temperature <35°C (95°F) or ≥40°C (104°F)	+15	_____
Pulse ≥125 beats/min	+10	_____
Initial laboratory findings (score zero if not tested)		
pH <7.35	+30	_____
Blood urea nitrogen >30 mg/dL (10.5 mmol/L)	+20	–
Sodium <130 mEq/L (130 mmol/L)	+20	_____
Glucose ≥250 mg/dL (13.9 mmol/L)	+10	_____
Hematocrit <30% (0.30)	+10	_____
Arterial Po_2 <60 mm Hg or O_2 saturation <90%	+10	_____
Pleural effusion	+10	_____
Total score (sum of patient's points):		

30-DAY MORTALITY DATA BY RISK CLASS

Total Score	Risk Class	Recommended Site of Treatment	Mortality Range Observed in Validation Cohorts (%)
None (see step 1)	I	Outpatient	0.1
≤70	II	Outpatient	0.5
71–90	III	Outpatient	0.9–2.8
91–130	IV	Inpatient	8.2–9.3
>130	V	Inpatient	27.0–29.2

O_2, oxygen; Po_2, partial pressure of oxygen.

*Step 1 identifies patients in risk class I on the basis of age ≤50 years and the absence of all comorbid conditions and vital sign abnormalities listed in step 2. For all patients who are not classified as risk class I, the laboratory data listed in step 2 should be collected to calculate a pneumonia severity score. Risk class and recommended site of care based on the pneumonia severity score are listed in the final portion of the table. Thirty-day mortality data are based on two independent cohorts of 40,326 patients.

From Metlay JP, Fine MJ: Testing strategies in the initial management of patients with community-acquired pneumonia, *Ann Intern Med* 138:115, 2003.

TABLE 10-5	*Clinical Feature Points (CURB-65) (score one point for each variable present)*
Confusion (defined as a mental test score ≤8, or disorientation in person, place, or time)	1
Uremia: Blood urea ≥7 mmol/L (~19 mg/dL)	1
Respiratory rate: ≥30 breaths/min	1
Blood pressure: systolic ≤90 mm Hg or diastolic ≤60 mm Hg	1
Age > **65** yr	1
Total points	

MORTALITY RISKS AND TREATMENT RECOMMENDATIONS BASED ON CURB-65 SCORE

Score	Group
0 or 1	Mortality risk low (1.5%), consider home treatment
2	Mortality risk moderate (9.2%), consider hospital-supervised treatment
3	Mortality risk high (22%), manage in hospital
4 or 5	Consider admission to intensive care unit

From Lim WS, van der Eerden MM, Laing R, et al: Defining community acquired pneumonia severity on presentation to hospital: an international derivation and validation study, *Thorax* 58:377–382, 2003.

SUGGESTED READINGS

Alcaide ML, Bisno AL: Pharyngitis and epiglottitis, *Infect Dis Clin North Am* 21:449–469, 2007.

Bisno AL, Gerber MA, Gwaltney JM Jr, et al: Practicse guidelines for the diagnosis and management of group A streptococcal pharyngitis. Infectious Diseases Society of America, *Clin Infect Dis* 35:113–125, 2002.

Butorac-Petanjek B, Parnham MJ, Popovic-Grle S: Antibiotic therapy for exacerbations of chronic obstructive pulmonary disease (COPD), *J Chemother* 22:291–297, 2010.

Centers for Disease Control and Prevention: Effects of new penicillin susceptibility breakpoints for *Streptococcus pneumoniae*—United States, 2006–2007, *MMWR Morb Mortal Wkly Rep* 57:1353–1355, 2008.

Centers for Disease Control and Prevention: *Seasonal influenza, antiviral drugs.* (Available at: *http://www.cdc.gov/flu/professionals/antivirals/index. htm*).

Fiore AE, Shay DK, Broder K, et al: Prevention and control of seasonal influenza with vaccines: recommendations of the Advisory Committee on Immunization Practices (ACIP), 2009, *MMWR Recomm Rep* 58:1–52, 2009. erratum in *MMWR Recomm Rep* 58:896–897, 2009.

Gonzales R, Bartlett JG, Besser RE, et al: Principles of appropriate antibiotic use for treatment of uncomplicated acute bronchitis: background, *Ann Intern Med* 134:521–529, 2001.

Liñares J, Ardanuy C, Pallares R, Fenoll A: Changes in antimicrobial resistance, serotypes and genotypes in *Streptococcus pneumoniae* over a 30-year period, *Clin Microbiol Infect* 16:402–410, 2010.

Mandell LA, Wunderink RG, Anzueto A, et al: Infectious Diseases Society of America/American Thoracic Society consensus guidelines on the management of community-acquired pneumonia in adults, *Clin Infect Dis* 44(Suppl 2):S27–S72, 2007.

Piccirillo JF: Clinical practice: acute bacterial sinusitis, *N Engl J Med* 26:902–910, 2004.

Pratter MR, Brightling CE, Boulet LP, et al: An empiric integrative approach to the management of cough: ACCP evidence-based guidelines, *Chest* 129(Suppl 1):S222–S231, 2006.

CHAPTER 11

BOARD REVIEW

Genitourinary Infections

KHALIL G. GHANEM, MD, PhD

Sexually transmitted diseases (STDs) may be classi-fied according to syndromes. These include genital ulcer diseases, urethritis, cervicitis, pelvic inflammatory disease, epididymitis, vaginal discharge, genital warts, proctitis, and ectoparasite infestations. Updated treatment guidelines for STDs are available on the Centers for Disease Control and Prevention (CDC) Web site: www.cdc.gov. Urinary tract infections (UTIs) may involve the lower genitourinary tract or both the upper and lower tract. Updated guidelines for the management of uncomplicated cystitis and pyelone-phritis are available (see Suggested Readings).

Genital Ulcer Diseases

Table 11-1 provides a summary of the presentation and causes of urogenital ulcer diseases. Routine diagnostic tests include the following: culture, antigen test, nucleic acid amplification test or serology for herpes simplex virus (HSV); darkfield examination and serology for *Treponema pallidum*; culture, serology, and nucleic acid amplification tests for lymphogranuloma venereum (LGV); culture for *Haemophilus ducreyi*; and skin biopsy with histopathology for donovanosis.

HERPES SIMPLEX VIRUS

Figure 11-3 shows an example of primary genital herpes.

Basic Information

- **Common sites of HSV infection are skin and mucous membranes**
- Genital infections are caused by both HSV-2 and HSV-1; HSV-1 now predominates among young people
- Seroprevalence of HSV-2 in adults in the United States is 23%
- **Most cases of genital herpes are asymptomatic and unrecognized**
- Incubation period is 2 to 7 days
- Viral shedding occurs even in the absence of lesions

Clinical Presentation

- Primary genital herpes lesions are classically painful, multiple, and grouped on erythematous base, beginning as macules and papules, evolving to vesicles and ulcers
- Local symptoms may include pain, itching, dysuria, and tender inguinal adenopathy
- Primary lesions may be accompanied by fever, headache, malaise, and myalgias. Recurrent disease is less severe than primary disease but may be severe in immunosup-pressed individuals.

- Primary infections with HSV-1 and 2 are similar; recur-rent infections with HSV-1 tend to be less severe and less frequent than recurrent infections with HSV-2
- Extragenital complications include aseptic meningitis and urinary retention

Diagnosis

- Clinical diagnosis can be confirmed by cell culture (low sensitivity), detection of viral antigen, polymerase chain reaction (PCR), and serology (type-specific glycoprotein G1 and G2). Serology is the preferred method when no active lesions are present.
- Tzanck preparation may show multinucleated giant cells (low sensitivity)
- Serologic testing may be negative in primary infection; serologic false positives may occur, particularly if the pretest probability of having HSV is low; there are no universal screening recommendations

Treatment

- **Systemic antiviral drugs (e.g., acyclovir, famciclovir, or valacyclovir) can be used as episodic or suppres-sive therapy and they are all equally efficacious**
- Episodic treatment does not eradicate the virus or reduce frequency of recurrences
- **Daily suppressive therapy among patients with six or more recurrences per year can reduce the fre-quency by up to 80% and prevents recurrences in 25% to 30% of patients; frequency of episodes may diminish over time**
- Suppressive therapy does not eliminate subclinical viral shedding
- Prevention: Once-daily valacyclovir in the infected partner, in addition to consistent condom use, may help decrease transmission to an uninfected partner by ~50%

SYPHILIS

Basic Information

- Systemic illness with protean manifestations caused by *T. pallidum*
- Major routes of transmission are via sexual intercourse and from mother to fetus

Clinical Presentation

- Primary syphilis (Fig. 11-4)
  - **Begins as a chancre (a single, painless papule) at the site of inoculation 2 to 3 weeks after initial exposure**

TABLE 11-1	*Urogenital Ulcer Disease*			
Ulcerative Disease	**Causative Agent**	**Clinical Presentation**	**Diagnosis**	**Treatment**
Genital herpes	HSV-2 > HSV-1	Cluster of vesicles on erythematous base **Painful** and pruritic Dysuria Tender lymphadenopathy	Tzanck preparation, multinucleated giant cells (low sensitivity) Viral culture (70% sensitivity) PCR Glycoprotein G–based serologies	Acyclovir or famciclovir or valacyclovir
Syphilitic chancre	*Treponema pallidum*	Single, **painless** papule at the site of inoculation Erodes into clean base and raised, firm borders Painless rubbery lymphadenopathy	Darkfield examination Serology Nontreponemal (RPR, VDRL) Treponemal (FTA-ABS, MHA-TP, TP-PA, EIAs)	Penicillin
Chancroid (Fig. 11-1)	*Haemophilus ducreyi*	**Painful** ulcer Tender inguinal adenopathy Hallmark is suppurative adenopathy Occurs in outbreaks	Clinical diagnosis Culture available but not widely used	Azithromycin or ceftriaxone or ciprofloxacin
Donovanosis or granuloma inguinale	*Klebsiella granulomatis*	**Painless** papule or nodule erodes into beefy-red granulomatous ulcer with rolled edges Spread of granulomas into the groin results in edema or pseudobuboes Rare in the United States	Donovan bodies on biopsy	Doxycycline or trimethoprim-sulfamethoxazole Treat at least 3 wk
Lymphogranuloma venereum (LGV; Fig. 11-2)	*Chlamydia trachomatis* serovar L1, L2, or L3	**Painless** genital ulcer; painful inguinal lymphadenopathy (with groove sign); proctitis	Clinical syndrome; serology, complement fixation titers of at least 1:64; nucleic acid amplification tests	Doxycycline Treat for 3 wk

EIA, enzyme immunoassay; FDA, Food and Drug Administration; FTA-ABS, fluorescent treponemal antibody, absorbed; HSV-1, herpes simplex virus type 1; HSV-2, herpes simplex virus type 2; MHA-TP, microhemagglutination–*T. pallidum;* PCR, polymerase chain reaction; RPR, rapid plasma reagin; TP-PA, *T. pallidum* particle agglutination; VDRL, Venereal Disease Research Laboratory.

FIGURE 11-1 Chancroid presents as a painful ulcer and suppurative adenopathy. *(From www.cdc.gov.)*

- Quickly erodes and becomes indurated with a clean base and raised, firm borders
- Atypical lesions occur in 60% of cases
- Primary lesions may be accompanied by regional adenopathy that is classically rubbery, painless, and bilateral
- Secondary or disseminated syphilis (Fig. 11-5)
  - Begins 2 to 8 weeks after appearance of chancre
  - **May be associated with flu-like symptoms, generalized lymphadenopathy, and temporary patchy alopecia**
  - Characteristic rash may be macular, maculopapular, papular, or pustular and may involve the whole body or palms and soles
  - **Condylomata lata appear as raised, painless, gray-white lesions; are highly infectious; and develop in intertriginous areas and on mucous membranes**
- Latent syphilis
  - Defined by a lack of clinical manifestations with positive serology
  - Latent syphilis acquired within the preceding year is early latent syphilis
  - Late latent syphilis implies acquisition more than 1 year before diagnosis
- Tertiary syphilis
  - Slowly progressive, inflammatory disease
  - Gummatous syphilis results in skeletal, mucosal, ocular, and visceral lesions
  - Average time of onset is 4 to 12 years after infection

FIGURE 11-2 **A,** Early lymphogranuloma venereum (LGV) presents first as an ulcer and then as painful inguinal lymphadenopathy. **B,** Late complications of LGV include genital elephantiasis. *(From www.cdc.gov.)*

FIGURE 11-3 Primary genital herpes, along the shaft of the penis (**A**) and in the vulvar area (**B**). *(From www.cdc.gov.)*

- Cardiovascular syphilis causes endarteritis of the aortic vasovasorum
  - Average time of onset is 15 years
  - Presents as aortic aneurysm or aortic valve insufficiency
- Neurosyphilis
  - **Can occur at any syphilis stage**
  - Early neurosyphilis (meningovascular syphilis) usually presents during the first year after infection as a meningitis and/or ophthalmic symptoms—particularly among HIV-infected persons
  - Late neurosyphilis, occurring many years after primary infection, may be meningovascular (presenting as stroke) or parenchymatous, manifesting as tabes

dorsalis (electrical pains shooting down the legs) or general paresis (personality changes, hallucinations)
- Ocular manifestations may occur at any stage and include iritis, uveitis, neuroretinitis, and optic neuritis

Diagnosis

- Darkfield examination and direct fluorescent antibody tests of lesion exudates or tissue provide definitive evidence
- Two types of serologic tests are used for presumptive diagnosis:
  - Nontreponemal tests include rapid plasma reagin (RPR) and Venereal Disease Research Laboratory (VDRL) tests
    - Used as screening tests

FIGURE 11-4　The chancre of primary syphilis shown in a man (**A**) and in a woman (**B**). (*From www.cdc.gov.*)

FIGURE 11-5　The characteristic rash of secondary syphilis, commonly involving the palms and soles. (*From www.cdc.gov.*)

TABLE 11-2	Recommended Treatment Regimens for Syphilis	
Clinical Stage	**Treatment**
Primary and secondary syphilis	Benzathine penicillin G—2.4 million units IM in a single dose (If penicillin allergic—doxycycline 100 mg PO bid for 2 wk, except pregnant patients, who should be desensitized and treated with penicillin)
Early latent syphilis	Benzathine penicillin G—2.4 million units IM in a single dose
Late latent syphilis or latent syphilis of unknown duration	Benzathine penicillin G—7.2 million units, administered as 3 doses of 2.4 million units IM each at 1-wk intervals
Tertiary syphilis (gummatous and cardiovascular syphilis)	Benzathine penicillin G—7.2 million units, administered as 3 doses of 2.4 million units IM each at 1-wk intervals
Neurosyphilis	Aqueous crystalline penicillin G—18–24 million units per day, administered as 3–4 million units IV every 4 hr or continuous infusion, for 10–14 days *or* Procaine penicillin—2.4 million units IM qd, *plus* Probenecid—500 mg PO qid, both for 10–14 days

bid, twice daily; IM, intramuscularly; PO, orally; qd, daily; qid, four times daily.

- **Because of low specificity, must be confirmed by a treponemal test**
  - Treponemal tests include the fluorescent treponemal antibody, absorbed (FTA-ABS) and *T. pallidum* particle agglutination tests
  - Serologic tests may be negative in about 30% of primary syphilis cases; they are ~100% sensitive in secondary syphilis (a negative RPR essentially rules out the diagnosis of secondary syphilis)
- Neurosyphilis can occur at any stage of disease
  - Diagnosis is based on a combination of serologic tests, cerebrospinal fluid (CSF) abnormalities (>5 white blood cells [WBCs]/mm³ ± abnormal protein), or a reactive CSF VDRL
    - CSF VDRL is highly specific but insensitive (50%); negative study does not exclude the diagnosis
    - CSF FTA-ABS is less specific but very sensitive; negative study probably excludes neurosyphilis if the pretest probability is moderate to low
  - CSF examination indicated if neurologic or ophthalmologic abnormalities, evidence of active tertiary syphilis (aortitis, gumma, iritis), or treatment failure
  - HIV infection with CD4 ≤350 cells/mm³ or RPR ≥1:32 is associated with increased risk of asymptomatic neurosyphilis; CSF examination may be considered

Treatment

- **Parenteral penicillin G is the drug of choice (Table 11-2)**
  - Only accepted therapy with documented efficacy for neurosyphilis and syphilis during pregnancy is desensitization followed by penicillin therapy
  - **The Jarisch-Herxheimer reaction**
    - Acute febrile reaction associated with headache and myalgias; thought to be activation of inflammatory cascade associated with lysis of spirochetes

- Can occur within the first 24 hours after therapy (particularly in early syphilis)
  - Treatment is supportive with use of antipyretics and anti-inflammatory agents
- Response to therapy is monitored by change in titer of a nontreponemal test (e.g., RPR) 12 (for primary, secondary, and early latent stages of syphilis) to 24 (for late syphilis) months after therapy
  - A fourfold (or two-dilution) decrease in RPR or VDRL titer (e.g., from 1:64 to 1:16) indicates a cure
  - No change or increase in titer indicates failure of therapy
  - Documentation of a titer response followed by a fourfold increase indicates reinfection
  - Treponemal test (e.g., FTA-ABS) titers do not correlate with disease activity or therapy and will usually remain positive for life
- In neurosyphilis, quantitative nontreponemal serologic tests should be repeated at 6, 12, and 24 months and CSF examination should be repeated 6 months after therapy

Urethritis and Cervicitis

- Urethritis and cervicitis are characterized by discharge of mucopurulent or purulent material
- The principal etiologic agents are *Neisseria gonorrhoeae*, *Chlamydia trachomatis*, *Trichomonas vaginalis*; more recently, an association with *Mycoplasma genitalium* has been described

GONORRHEA

Basic Information

- Can involve the genital tract, rectum, or oropharynx, or become disseminated
- Incubation period is 3 to 7 days, and symptoms manifest within 10 to 14 days after exposure
- Disseminated gonococcal infection (DGI) occurs in 1% to 3% of cases

Clinical Presentation

- Disease presentations are variable and differ between men and women
  - In men, symptomatic disease occurs in ~70% with purulent urethral discharge or dysuria; causes 30% of epididymitis cases in young men
  - Women with cervicitis may have vaginal discharge or bleeding; 50% may be asymptomatic
  - Other syndromes in women include urethritis, Bartholin abscesses, or pelvic inflammatory disease (PID)
- DGI may present as triad of (1) dermatitis with petechial or pustular acral skin lesions, (2) tenosynovitis, and (3) asymmetrical migratory polyarthralgias, or as purulent arthritis without skin lesions
  - Perihepatitis, endocarditis, meningitis, and osteomyelitis occur less commonly

Diagnosis

- Stain of gram-negative intracellular diplococci; low sensitivity in asymptomatic persons and women

- Culture using modified Thayer-Martin medium; sensitivity ~85% to 90%
- Nucleic acid amplification (NAA) tests are the tests of choice for genital and extragenital sites; extragenital testing is not Food and Drug Administration (FDA) cleared but is routinely performed
- Sites for specimen collection for NAA tests include the vagina (preferred for women), cervix, urethra, urine (preferred for men), oropharynx, and rectum

Treatment

- A third-generation cephalosporin plus 1-g of oral azithromycin is first-line therapy; intramuscular ceftriaxone has excellent activity against genital and extragenital infections; oral cephalosporins are approved alternate agents but these may have lower activity against pharyngeal gonorrhea
- Fluoroquinolones are no longer recommended because of increased prevalence of drug resistance
- Azithromycin monotherapy at 2-g dosing is effective for both gonorrheal infections and chlamydial infections, but its use is limited by GI distress; this is the only available alternate agent if cephalosporins cannot be used to treat gonorrhea
- Patients with pharyngeal gonorrhea require a test-of-cure 2 to 3 weeks after therapy to verify response if treated with oral cephalosporins
- Sexual partners in the preceding 60 days or the last sexual partner should be referred for evaluation and treatment
- Patients with DGI are hospitalized and treated parenterally; 24 hours after clinical response, they may be discharged on oral cephalosporins to complete a 7-day course of therapy

CHLAMYDIA TRACHOMATIS

Basic Information

- *C. trachomatis* D through K serotypes are the most common bacterial STD in the United States [*C. trachomatis* L1–L3 serotypes cause LGV; see Table 11-1]
- Single biggest risk factor for D through K serotypes is young age

Clinical Presentation

- Infection in women may present as cervicitis or urethritis and may involve vaginal discharge, lower abdominal pain, or dysuria
- Men develop urethritis with dysuria and mucopurulent discharge
  - Epididymitis manifests as unilateral testicular pain and tenderness, edema, and hydrocele

Diagnosis

- Because asymptomatic infection is most common, yearly screening of all sexually active women ≤25 years old and older at-risk women is recommended to prevent sequelae
  - Untreated chlamydial infection in women is a major cause of PID, ectopic pregnancy, and infertility
  - In men, it may result in prostatitis

- Diagnostic methods include culture, antigen detection, gene probe hybridization, and NAA test (method of choice)

Treatment

- **The CDC recommends azithromycin or doxycycline as first-line agents**
- Alternatives include fluoroquinolones and erythromycin
- In pregnancy, doxycycline and fluoroquinolones are contraindicated. Test for cure is recommended after treatment with amoxicillin or erythromycin because these regimens may not be as efficacious and side effects may discourage compliance.
- Because reinfection following treatment is common and reinfection increases the risk for PID, repeat testing is warranted 3 months after therapy
- Sexual partners in the preceding 60 days or the last sexual partner should be referred for evaluation and treatment
- Other causes of urethritis include *Mycoplasma, Trichomonas,* and HSV

Pelvic Inflammatory Disease

Basic Information

- PID encompasses inflammatory conditions that produce one or more of the following: endometritis, salpingitis, tubo-ovarian abscess, and pelvic peritonitis
- Most commonly implicated organisms include *N. gonorrhoeae* and *C. trachomatis* as well as anaerobes, gram-negative bacilli, streptococci, and mycoplasmas

Clinical Presentation

- Fever and lower abdominal pain (usually bilateral) are the hallmarks of PID
- **Right upper quadrant tenderness from perihepatitis (Fitz-Hugh–Curtis syndrome) is seen in 10%**
- Pelvic examination may reveal cervical motion tenderness, adnexal tenderness, or purulent endocervical discharge
- A palpable adnexal mass suggests a tubo-ovarian abscess

Diagnosis

- **Clinical criteria for diagnosis are *one* of the following: uterine tenderness, adnexal tenderness, or cervical motion tenderness**
- Additional criteria include mucopurulent cervicitis, presence of WBCs in saline microscopy of vaginal secretions, documented *N. gonorrhoeae* or *C. trachomatis,* oral temperature above 38.3°C, and elevated erythrocyte sedimentation rate or C-reactive protein
- Definitive criteria are histopathologic evidence of endometritis, radiologic evidence on transvaginal ultrasound, and laparoscopic evidence of PID

Treatment

- **CDC first-line recommended treatment for PID is either cefotetan *or* cefoxitin *plus* doxycycline OR clindamycin *plus* gentamicin**
- Empirical therapy is broad spectrum to cover *N. gonorrhoeae, C. trachomatis,* anaerobes, gram-negative bacteria, and streptococci

- Inpatient therapy is provided when surgical emergencies cannot be excluded, the patient is pregnant, there is lack of response to or inability to take oral antibiotics, or the patient has a tubo-ovarian abscess

Epididymitis and Prostatitis

Basic Information

- *Epididymitis* is defined as inflammation of the epididymis caused by infection or trauma
- In men younger than 35 years, it is most often caused by *N. gonorrhoeae* (30%) or *C. trachomatis* (70%)
- **In men older than 35 years, non–sexually transmitted epididymitis is more commonly caused by gram-negative enteric organisms**
- Prostatitis, or inflammation of the prostate, is considered acute or chronic
  - Acute infection is caused by *Escherichia coli* and occasionally by *N. gonorrhoeae*
  - Chronic prostatitis is caused by gram-negative bacilli (*E. coli*) and enterococci

Clinical Presentation

- Epididymitis presents as unilateral testicular pain and tenderness, edema, and hydrocele
  - The major alternative diagnosis is testicular torsion, especially when onset of pain is sudden and pain is severe
  - Pyuria is generally seen in epididymitis, but not torsion
  - **Doppler ultrasound will show decreased or absent blood flow to the affected testicle in torsion but normal or increased blood flow with epididymitis**
- Acute prostatitis presents with fever, chills, perineal pain, back pain, dysuria
  - The prostate gland is tender on examination
- Chronic prostatitis is often indolent

Diagnosis

- For urethritis, perform Gram stain, culture, and/or NAA test of urethral exudates, intraurethral swab, or urine
- Diagnosis of prostatitis is usually clinical
  - "Milking" the prostate by digital examination before voiding may induce pyuria

Treatment

- In urethritis, CDC-recommended treatment is based on suspected etiology of infection
  - **For epididymitis most likely caused by gonococcal or chlamydial infection, treat to cover both organisms**
  - **For epididymitis in patients older than 35 years, treat with ofloxacin or levofloxacin**
- Treatment for acute prostatitis includes ceftriaxone, quinolones, or trimethoprim-sulfamethoxazole (TMP-SMX) for 14 days
- Treatment for chronic prostatitis includes 4 to 6 weeks of quinolone or 6 to 12 weeks of TMP-SMX

Vaginitis

Table 11-3 provides a summary of the types of organisms causing vaginitis and their specific diagnoses.

Treatment

Bacterial vaginosis is treated with a 7 day course of twice daily metronidazole (500 mg). Single dose (2 g) oral metronizadole is only recommended for the treatment of trichomoniasis and should not be used to treat bacterial vaginosis. Topical and oral antifungal agents may be used to treat vulvovaginal candidiasis.

Proctitis

- Defined as inflammation of the lining of the rectum
- Major causes of sexually transmitted proctitis
  - *Neisseria gonorrhoeae*
  - *Chlamydia trachomatis* serotypes D through K
  - *Chlamydia trachomatis* serotypes L1 through L3 (LGV) have made a resurgence in the United States and Western Europe in the last few years (see Table 11-1)
  - Syphilis
  - HSV-1 and 2
- All causes are indistinguishable based on symptoms. Testing for all these pathogens should be considered.
  - NAA tests have the highest sensitivity to detect *N. gonorrhoeae* and *C. trachomatis* (even though not FDA cleared for extragenital sites)
  - Culture for HSV
  - Serology is used to diagnose syphilis

Condylomata Acuminata or Anogenital Warts

Basic Information

- **Caused by human papillomavirus (HPV) infection**
- The most common viral STD in the United States; most infections asymptomatic and self-limited
- **Types 16, 18, 31, 33, and 35 have been strongly associated with cervical neoplasia**
- The same types are also associated with dysplastic and neoplastic anal lesions
- HPV types 6 and 11 are rarely associated with neoplasia but cause ~90% of warts

Clinical Presentation

- Exophytic verrucous white or pigmented lesions (Fig. 11-6)
- Symptoms vary according to site and size of the lesions
- Pain, bleeding, and pruritus may accompany lesions
- Large exophytic masses may result in obstruction or stricture

Diagnosis

- Diagnosis is based on visual inspection
- Evaluation should include anoscopy, sigmoidoscopy, colposcopy, and/or vulvovaginal examination
  - Acetic acid 5% can be applied to facilitate identification
- **Biopsy serves to evaluate for dysplasia**
- HPV DNA detection provides a definitive diagnosis but is not necessary for diagnosis

Treatment

- Treatment of external genital warts depends on size, location, and patient and provider preference
- **Treatments include surgical removal, cryotherapy, or topical therapy with podophyllin, imiquimod, or trichloroacetic acid**
- HPV quadrivalent vaccine for types 6, 11, 16, and 18 (Gardasil, by Merck) and bivalent vaccine for types 16 and 18 (Cervarix, by GSK) are licensed and recommended for all females ages 9 to 26 years; quadrivalent vaccine may be given to males ages 9 to 26 years
- Vaccination does not eliminate the need for cervical cancer screening because not all cancer-causing HPV types are included in the vaccine

Ectoparasite Infestations

Basic Information

- Includes pubic lice (pediculosis pubis) and scabies
- Scabies, caused by the mite *Sarcoptes scabiei*, is highly contagious
- **Pubic lice and scabies are transmitted by intimate personal contact and are associated with poverty, poor hygiene, and malnutrition**

Clinical Presentation

- Patients with pubic lice present with pruritus or notice nits or adult pubic lice attached to the base of pubic hair

TABLE 11-3	*Vaginitis*			
Diagnosis	**Organism**	**Type of Organism**	**Discharge**	**Specific Diagnosis**
Bacterial vaginosis	Replacement of normal *Lactobacillus* spp. with anaerobes	Bacteria	White, noninflammatory coating discharge	Clue cells seen on microscopy Vaginal pH >4.5 + whiff test (fishy odor on addition of 10% KOH)
Trichomoniasis	*Trichomonas vaginalis*	Protozoan	Foul-smelling, frothy, yellow-green discharge	Organism seen on microscopy of secretions (<70% sensitive); culture; PCR now FDA cleared
Vulvovaginal candidiasis	*Candida albicans*	Fungus (yeast)	White, "cottage cheese" discharge	Fungal elements seen on wet prep Vaginal pH 4–4.5

PCR, polymerase chain reaction.

FIGURE 11-6 Anal condylomata acuminata appear as exophytic verrucous lesions. *(From www.cdc.gov.)*

- Other affected areas may include eyelashes and coarse truncal and axillary hair
- Patients with scabies present with pruritic, erythematous papules and nodules and classic linear burrows, usually in web spaces between the fingers, around the nipples or periumbilical or extensor surfaces of extremities

Diagnosis

- Pubic lice are diagnosed by looking closely through pubic hair for nits, nymphs, or adults
- Scabies is confirmed by identifying the mite in skin scrapings

Treatment

- **Treatment of lice includes permethrin 1% cream or pyrethrins with piperonyl butoxide.** Malathion 0.5% lotion or ivermectin may be used in the setting of treatment failure due to drug resistance.
- **Recommended treatment of scabies is permethrin cream 5% or oral ivermectin**
  - Lindane 1% is no longer recommended because of systemic absorption and neurotoxicity

Urinary Tract Infections

Basic Information

- **Represent a broad spectrum of clinical illness from uncomplicated cystitis to pyelonephritis with bacteremia**
- Pregnancy increases the risk of UTI because of dilation of ureters, decreased ureteral peristalsis, and decreased bladder tone
  - About 20% to 40% of patients with untreated bacteriuria early in gestation progress to pyelonephritis later in pregnancy. Pyelonephritis has been associated with premature delivery.
  - Urine culture is therefore a routine part of prenatal screening
- Diabetic patients are predisposed to UTI and may progress to perinephric abscess, papillary necrosis, or emphysematous pyelonephritis

Clinical Presentation

- Uncomplicated acute bacterial cystitis
  - Characterized by dysuria, frequency, and urgency
  - Occurs in nonpregnant women with normal anatomy, no predisposing conditions, and no urologic instrumentation
  - Causative agents include primarily *E. coli* and *Staphylococcus saprophyticus*
- Complicated UTI is defined clinically by the presence of one of the following factors: pregnancy, diabetes, male sex, immunosuppression, catheter or urologic instrumentation, stone or abnormal structure of the genitourinary tract, or functional abnormality of the genitourinary tract
- **Acute pyelonephritis manifests with fever, flank pain, and urinary symptoms**
- Development of perinephric abscess is suggested by an acute pyelonephritis-like illness with persistent fever and symptoms despite medical therapy

Diagnosis

- Laboratory evaluation includes microscopic examination of the urine for pyuria and hematuria or urine dipstick test for leukocyte esterase and nitrites
- **Although a urine culture is not necessary for uncomplicated UTI, the microbiology of complicated UTI is less predictable and requires urine Gram stain and culture**
- Diagnosis of pyelonephritis is supported by significant bacteriuria or greater than 10^5 colony-forming units (CFUs)/mm^3 and pyuria of more than 10 WBCs/mm^3
  - Leukocyte casts are seen in 20% to 50% of cases
  - Blood cultures are positive in 20% of cases
- Diagnosis of a perinephric abscess should be confirmed by ultrasound or computed tomography scan

Treatment

- Treatment of uncomplicated UTI is empirical
  - **In areas where resistance to TMP-SMX is less than 20%, this drug can be used twice daily for 3 days**
  - Other agents include quinolone therapy for 3 days or nitrofurantoin for 5 days
  - **Amoxicillin or ampicillin should not be used for empirical treatment given the relatively poor efficacy**
- For complicated UTI, antibiotic selection is based on culture data and duration of therapy is generally 7 to 14 days depending on chosen antimicrobial agent
- For pyelonephritis, treatment is based on severity of illness and is guided by urine or blood culture results
  - In mild cases, treatment includes oral quinolones for 7 days or TMP-SMX for a 14-day course
  - Moderate to severe illness may initially require intravenous therapy with quinolones, aminoglycosides, extended-spectrum penicillins, third-generation cephalosporins, or carbapenems
- Catheter-associated bacteriuria should be treated in the setting of symptomatic infection, suspected sepsis, renal transplantation, or immunocompromise
  - **If possible, removal of catheter during treatment is advised**

- When chronic catheterization is required, intermittent catheterization rather than an indwelling catheter reduces the risk of infection
- For perinephric abscess, percutaneous drainage or surgery may be necessary
- Treat asymptomatic bacteriuria in pregnant women, prior to an invasive urologic procedure, in persons with renal transplant, or if neutropenia is present. Do NOT treat in diabetics and elderly persons.

Acknowledgment

This chapter was adapted from a chapter written by Lisa Spacek, MD, PhD for the third edition of *The Johns Hopkins Internal Medicine Board Review*.

REVIEW QUESTIONS

For review questions, please go to www.expertconsult.com.

SUGGESTED READINGS

Centers for Disease Control and Prevention: Sexually transmitted diseases treatment guidelines 2010, *MMWR Recomm Rep* 59(RR-12):1–110, 2010.

Gupta K, Hooton TM, Naber KG, et al: International clinical practice guidelines for the treatment of acute uncomplicated cystitis and pyelonephritis in women: a 2010 update by the Infectious Diseases Society of America and the European Society for Microbiology and Infectious Diseases, *Clin Infect Dis* 52(5):e103–e120, 2010.

11

Human Immunodeficiency Virus Infection

GAIL BERKENBLIT, MD, PhD

Today, more than 30 years since the first description of human immunodeficiency virus (HIV), over 1,100,000 people are infected nationwide, with more than 56,000 new cases per year. The use of chemoprophylaxis for opportunistic infections and the advent of more effective HIV therapy have led to a decline in overall mortality. Although guidelines regarding HIV therapy are continuously changing and are usually the purview of HIV specialists, the presentation of acute HIV, common opportunistic infections, and the complications of therapy should be recognized by the general internist.

Human Immunodeficiency Virus

Basic Information

- Biology of retroviruses
  - HIV-1 and HIV-2 are RNA retroviruses that cause acquired immunodeficiency syndrome (AIDS)
  - HIV entry into T cells is mediated via binding of the CD4 receptor and associated cofactors
  - Reverse transcriptase converts the RNA genome into double-stranded DNA, which then integrates into the host genome and co-opts cellular machinery for replication
  - HIV infection selectively depletes CD4 cells, resulting in immunodeficiency
- Epidemiology
  - HIV-1 is the dominant type in the United States and worldwide
  - HIV-2 is found mainly in West Africa and has a slower clinical course
  - Both are spread via blood-borne exposure (e.g., needle sharing, transfusions), sexual intercourse, and maternal-fetal transmission

Clinical Presentation

- Acute retroviral syndrome
  - Typical onset of symptoms 1 to 6 weeks after exposure to HIV (2 to 3 weeks most commonly), but it may manifest up to 6 months later
  - Symptoms often mimic infectious mononucleosis
  - **Most common presentation: fever, lymphadenopathy, pharyngitis, rash (Fig. 12-1), myalgias, and arthralgias**
  - Also reported: thrombocytopenia, leukopenia, diarrhea, headache, elevated transaminases, hepatosplenomegaly, aseptic meningitis, encephalopathy

- Symptoms resolve without treatment within 1 to 2 weeks
- Chronic HIV infection
  - May be clinically silent for years
  - Clinical manifestations depend on CD4 count (Table 12-1)
  - Opportunistic infections and associated conditions are discussed later in this chapter

Diagnosis and Evaluation

- HIV screening
  - Voluntary routine screening now recommended for all Americans ages 13 to 64 years by the Centers for Disease Control and Prevention and the American College of Physicians
  - Need for repeat testing determined by risk assessment
- Diagnostic testing
  - HIV antibody test (enzyme-linked immunosorbent assay [ELISA])
    - Positive 3 to 4 weeks after acute infection
    - **Test of choice in screening for chronic infection**
    - Western blot used to confirm diagnosis
  - CD4 count
    - Measure of severity of immunodeficiency
    - Decline in CD4 cells confers susceptibility to opportunistic infections
    - **CD4 count lower than 200/mm³ or the presence of an indicator condition defines AIDS**
  - HIV RNA viral polymerase chain reaction (PCR)
    - Positive 3 to 5 days after acute infection
    - **Test of choice in diagnosis of acute HIV infection, although count lower than 10,000 copies/ mm³ may be false positive**
    - Correlates with rate of disease progression
    - Used to follow response to antiretroviral therapy
  - HIV genotype
    - Detects mutations that confer resistance to antiretorival medications
    - Should be obtained as part of intial panel of tests for an individual with HIV
    - Nationwide, 10% to 20% of patients with new HIV infection have transmitted resistance to at least one class of antiretroviral medications

Antiretroviral Therapy

- Six main classes of antiretroviral agents have different potential adverse effects (Table 12-2)
- Initiation of therapy

95

FIGURE 12-1 Typical morbilliform rash associated with acute retroviral syndrome. *(From Forbes C, Jackson W: Color atlas and text of clinical medicine, ed 3, St. Louis, Mosby, 2003, Fig. 1-19.)*

- Current guidelines recommend initiation of antiretroviral therapy (ART) once the CD4 count declines to less than 500/mm³ or when symptoms are present
- Therapy may be considered on an individual basis when the CD4 count is greater than 500/mm³
- **Pregnant women, patients with HIV-associated nephropathy (HIVAN), and patients undergoing treatment for hepatitis B should all be treated regardless of CD4**
- **A combination of three antiretroviral agents from at least two different classes is recommended to prevent viral replication and inhibit the development of resistant HIV strains**
- The best choice of initial regimen remains controversial
  - Four regimens are currently recommended for initial therapy:
    - Efavirenz/tenofovir/emtricitabine
    - Ritonavir-boosted darunavir plus tenofovir/emtricitabine
    - Ritonavir-boosted atazanavir plus tenofovir/emtricitabine
    - Raltegravir plus tenofovir/emtricitabine
- Guidelines for monitoring and changing ART
  - Goal of therapy is viral suppression, which means that the viral load is undetectable or lower than 200 copies/mm³
  - CD4 count and viral load measured 2 to 8 weeks after initiation or change of therapy and every 12 to 24 weeks once viral load suppressed
  - **ART regimen should be changed if patient fails to achieve virologic suppression in 24 to 48 weeks or has an increase in viral load (>1000 copies/mm³)**
  - Generally, do not add a single drug to a failing regimen or switch single drugs in a regimen if there is ongoing viral replication
  - It is acceptable to switch single agents for side effect management if viral load is "undetectable"
- Prevention of HIV transmission: ART for postexposure prophylaxis (PEP)
  - PEP should be given for both percutaneous and mucocutaneous exposures with a combination of two drugs for lower-risk exposures and three drugs for higher-risk exposures
  - PEP should be given without delay (first dose within 1–2 hours) but is effective up to 72 hours after exposure

TABLE 12-1 Complications and Recommended Chemoprophylaxis for Opportunistic Infections by CD4 Cell Count

CD4 Cell Count*	Opportunistic Infections and Other HIV-Associated Conditions	Recommended Chemophylaxis Against Opportunistic Infections
>500/mm³	Acute retroviral syndrome HIV-associated nephropathy	None
200–500/mm³	Oral candidiasis Community-acquired pneumonia Pulmonary TB Kaposi sarcoma Herpes zoster CIN Lymphoma Anemia ITP	None
<200/mm³	*Pneumocystis jiroveci* pneumonia (PCP) Disseminated histoplasmosis Extrapulmonary TB Wasting HIV dementia	PCP prophylaxis with trimethoprim-sulfamethoxazole or dapsone or atovaquone or aerosolized pentamidine
<100/mm³	CNS toxoplasmosis Cryptococcosis CNS lymphoma	Toxoplasmosis prophylaxis (if patient is toxo IgG+) with trimethoprim-sulfamethoxazole *or* Dapsone/pyrimethamine/folinic acid or atovaquone
<50/mm³	Disseminated MAI Disseminated CMV Progressive multifocal leukoencephalopathy	MAI prophylaxis with azithromycin or clarithromycin

*At each stage of decline in CD4 cell count, patients become at risk for further opportunistic infections and other conditions and should receive appropriate chemoprophylaxis.
CIN, cervical intraepithelial neoplasia; CMV, cytomegalovirus; IgG, immunoglobulin G; ITP, idiopathic thrombocytopenia; MAI, *Mycobacterium avium-intracellulare*; TB, tuberculosis.

- High-risk factors for percutaneous transmission include hollow needle, visible blood, needle in vessel, and high viral load
- Recommended regimens vary, but exposed persons should be treated for 4 weeks
- Prevention of HIV transmission: ART for pre-exposure prophylaxis (PrEP)
  - **PrEP via administering daily tenofovir/emtricitabine to high-risk HIV-negative men who have sex with men (MSM) has been shown reduce risk of acquiring HIV by 44%**
  - However, regular condom use reduces risk by greater than 90%
  - Candidates for PrEP should be tested for HIV prior to initiation and at least every 3 months during use to avoid partial treatment of HIV infection

TABLE 12-2	Antiretroviral Medications and Commonly Associated Adverse Effects
Class of Antiretroviral Drug	**Adverse Effects**
Nucleoside Reverse Transcriptase Inhibitors	

Zidovudine (AZT)	Bone marrow suppression
	Lactic acidosis
	   Presents with fatigue, nausea, myalgias
	   Labs show anion gap acidosis and elevated lactic acid
	   Can occur any time during therapy

Stavudine (d4T)	Peripheral neuropathy Lipodystrophy Lactic acidosis
Didanosine (ddI)	Peripheral neuropathy Pancreatitis Lactic acidosis
Lamivudine (3TC)	
Emtricitabine (FTC)	

Abacavir	Fatal hypersensitivity reaction
	   Presents with fever, rash, flu-like symptoms
	   Usually in first 2–6 wk after starting
	   Can be fatal if drug not discontinued
	   Screen for susceptibility to hypersensitivity with an HLA-B*5701 test prior to initation

Tenofovir	Renal insufficiency Fanconi syndrome
Non-nucleoside Reverse Transcriptase Inhibitors	
Nevirapine	Rash Stevens-Johnson syndrome Hepatitis (especially at higher CD4 counts)
Efavirenz	CNS side effects (confusion, nightmares) Teratogenic
Etravirine	
Protease Inhibitors	**General side effects include diarrhea, lipodystrophy, central obesity with peripheral wasting, hyperlipidemia, and insulin resistance**
Atazanavir	Hyperbilirubinemia
Darunavir	
Fosamprenavir	
Indinavir	Nephrolithiasis
Lopinavir	
Nelfinavir	
Ritonavir	
Saquinavir	Q–T prolongation
Tipranivir	Intracranial hemorrhage
Membrane Fusion Inhibitors	
Enfuvirtide	Injection-site reactions
CCR5 Antagonist	
Maraviroc	Well tolerated, but only effective against CCR5 tropic virus
Integrase Inhibitor	
Raltegravir	Well tolerated, but twice daily

BOX 12-1	Immunization in HIV Patients

Indicated
Hepatitis A
Hepatitis B
Pneumococcus
Influenza
Tetanus-diphtheria

Contraindicated (Live Virus)
Varicella
Measles-mumps-rubella
Bacille Calmette-Guérin
Smallpox

- Candidates for PrEP should be tested for hepatitis B because this regimen is also active against hepatitis B, and patients may have a hepatitis flare when discontinued
- Other issues in the care of HIV-infected patients
  - Prophylaxis against certain opportunistic infections should be introduced once the CD4 count has declined to below predetermined levels (see Table 12-1)
  - Immunizations are an important component of HIV care, but live, attenuated virus vaccines should be avoided because of risk of disseminated infection (Box 12-1)
  - **Screening purified protein derivative (PPD) should be done at diagnosis and then annually if patent is at risk; PPD greater than 5 mm is considered positive**
  - Screening and vaccination for viral hepatitis should be performed
  - Cancer screening is as per usual guidelines with the exception of cervical cancer (8- to 10-fold elevated risk in HIV patients)
    - Perform a Papanicolaou (Pap) smear at the time of diagnosis and again in 6 months
    - If normal, can screen annually
  - Measures to increase adherence to medications are essential
    - Poor adherence is associated with resistance to ART
    - Factors associated with poor adherence include depression, poor social support, low self-efficacy ratings, active drug use, and complexity of regimen

Opportunistic Infections and Other HIV-Associated Conditions

CANDIDIASIS
Clinical Presentation
- At risk when CD4 count is lower than 250/mm^3
- **Most commonly seen as oropharyngeal creamy white plaques (thrush) that are removable by scraping (Fig. 12-2)**
- **Differential of white oral lesions includes oral hairy leukoplakia (Fig. 12-3)**
  - Characterized by painless, white, nonremovable plaques, usually on the lateral and dorsal tongue
  - Associated with Epstein-Barr virus infection
- Candidal esophagitis is the most common cause of odynophagia, followed by cytomegalovirus (CMV), herpes simplex virus (HSV), and aphthous ulcers

12

FIGURE 12-2 Oral candidiasis thrush. *(From Mandell GL, Bennett JE, Dolin R [eds]: Principles and practice of infectious diseases, ed 6, Philadelphia, Churchill Livingstone, 2005, Fig. 117-7.)*

FIGURE 12-3 Oral hairy leukoplakia. Note the predilection for the lateral tongue surface and the vertical ridges. *(From Cummings CW, Flint PW, Harker LA, et al [eds]: Cummings' otolaryngology: Head and neck surgery, ed 4, Philadelphia, Mosby, 2005, Fig. 64-8.)*

Diagnosis

- Oral candidiasis is usually diagnosed by appearance (see Fig. 12-2)
  - Swab or biopsy may be needed to differentiate from oral hairy leukoplakia
- Esophageal candidiasis is often diagnosed presumptively (odynophagia in HIV patient with low CD4 count)
  - Endoscopy is usually reserved for those for whom empirical therapy fails

Treatment

- Oral or vaginal candidal infection may be treated with topical azole therapy
- Candidal esophagitis is treated with a 2-week course of systemic fluconazole
- If azole resistance occurs, amphotericin B therapy may be necessary

PULMONARY INFECTIONS

See Table 12-3 and Figure 12-4 for common pulmonary conditions associated with HIV infection.

CNS MANIFESTATIONS

See Table 12-4 and Figure 12-5 for common CNS conditions associated with HIV infection.

DISSEMINATED *MYCOBACTERIUM AVIUM-INTRACELLULARE*

Clinical Presentation

- Presents when CD4 below $50/mm^3$
- **Symptoms include fevers, malaise, wasting, abdominal pain, lymphadenopathy**
- Often associated with anemia and leukopenia
- **Elevated alkaline phosphatase is often a clue to this infection**

TABLE 12-3		*Common Pulmonary Manifestations Associated with HIV Infection*			
	CD4 Count	**Clinical Presentation**	**Radiologic Appearance**	**Diagnostic Testing**	**Treatment**
Community-acquired pneumonia (CAP)	Any	Acute onset Fever Productive cough Pleuritic pain	Usually lobar infiltrate	Sputum Gram stain and culture	Antibiotic coverage for *Streptococcus pneumoniae* and typical CAP pathogens; cover gram-negative rods if CD4 low
Pneumocystis jiroveci pneumonia (PCP)	<200	Subacute onset Dry cough Hypoxia Fever Less likely if on prophylaxis	Usually "bat wing" perihilar infiltrate 20% have normal chest radiograph	Immunofluorescence, silver stain, or culture of induced sputum or bronchoalveolar lavage	Trimethoprim-sulfamethoxazole first-line agent Alternatives: dapsone/ trimethoprim; clindamycin/ primaquine; atovaquone; or IV pentamidine Add corticosteroids if PaO_2 <70 or A-a gradient >35
Pulmonary histoplasmosis	<200	Subacute onset Dry cough Oral ulcers common Geographic risk	Diffuse interstitial infiltrates	*Histoplasma* urine antigen; bronchoalveolar lavage culture	Itraconazole or amphotericin B
Pulmonary tuberculosis	Any	Gradual onset Extrapulmonary manifestations common if CD4 <200	Diffuse interstitial infiltrates Noncavitary in advanced HIV	AFB stain/culture PPD >5 mm considered positive in HIV-infected patients	Four-drug TB regimen for 2 mo, then two-drug maintenance for 6 mo total therapy

A-a, arterial-alveolar; AFB, acid-fast bacillus; Pao$_2$, arterial oxygen partial pressure; PPD, purified protein derivative; TB, tuberculosis.

FIGURE 12-4   Chest radiographs of common pulmonary conditions associated with HIV infection. **A,** Streptococcal pneumonia, presenting with focal lobar infiltrate. **B,** *Pneumocystis* pneumonia, typical presentation with "bat wing" infiltrates (*arrows*). **C,** Diffuse bilateral infiltrates in acute pulmonary histoplasmosis. **D,** Tuberculosis pneumonia, typically presents with noncavitary, lower-lobe infiltrates in advanced disease (key is an overlying artifact). *(A, B, and D, From Mason RJ: Murray and Nadel's textbook of respiratory medicine, ed 4, Philadelphia, Elsevier Saunders, 2005, Figs. 75-1, 75-5, and 75-2. C, From Mandell GL, Bennett JE, Dolin R [eds]: Principles and practice of infectious diseases, ed 6, Philadelphia, Churchill Livingstone, 2005, Fig. 262-5.)*

Diagnosis

- Most commonly diagnosed with mycobacterial blood cultures
  - Must hold cultures for weeks
- May suspect if acid-fast bacteria and granulomas are seen on biopsy of liver, lymph node, or bone marrow in a susceptible host

Treatment

- Treated with combination antimicrobial therapy (usually clarithromycin and ethambutol with or without rifabutin)

- **Azithromycin chemoprophylaxis is recommended when CD4 is lower than 50/mm³**

CYTOMEGALOVIRUS

Clinical Presentation

- Presents when CD4 count is lower than 50/mm³
- **Retinitis is most common end-organ complication of CMV (Fig. 12-6)**
- Symptoms include floaters and decreased visual acuity
- Retinal changes include fluffy white retinal infiltrates and hemorrhage

TABLE 12-4	*Common CNS Conditions Associated with HIV Infection*				
Disorder	**CD4 Count**	**Clinical Scenario**	**Appearance on MRI**	**Diagnosis**	**Treatment**
Toxoplasmosis	<100	Focal neurologic symptoms Seizures	Usually multiple ring-enhancing lesions Surrounding mass effect	Toxo IgG+ in 90% Presumptive diagnosis Follow response to therapy Clinical improvement MRI in 2 wk	Sulfadiazine + pyrimethamine Suppressive therapy until CD4 >200 for >3 mo
CNS lymphoma	<100	Focal neurologic symptoms Seizures	Usually single solid or ring-enhancing lesions Surrounding mass effect	First step is usually trial of toxoplasmosis therapy If no response, brain biopsy to diagnose lymphoma SPECT scan may be helpful if positive	Radiation therapy Begin antiretroviral therapy
Cryptococcal meningitis	<100	Severe headache High intracranial pressure Extra-CNS manifestations: skin lesions, pneumonia	Normal in 90% of patients Mass lesion in 10%	Classically, India ink test Now, usually serum and CSF cryptococcal antigen CSF culture Low CSF WBC count is poor prognosis sign	Amphotericin B + fluconazole for suppressive therapy until CD4 >100–200 for >6 mo
Progressive multifocal leukoence-phalopathy (PML)	<50	Rapidly progressive Focal neurologic symptoms Loss of speech, vision	Focal white matter changes No mass effect Definitive diagnosis requires brain biopsy	MRI appearance CSF for JC virus PCR	No specific therapy Antiretroviral therapy may be beneficial

CNS, central nervous system; CSF, cerebrospinal fluid; IgG, immunoglobulin G; MRI, magnetic resonance imaging; PCR, polymerase chain reaction; SPECT, single-photon emission computed tomography; WBC, white blood cell.

- Less common sites of involvement include GI tract (hemorrhagic ulcerations), lung (pneumonitis), and central nervous system (CNS) (encephalitis)

Diagnosis

- **Retina reveals characteristic "ketchup and cottage cheese" lesions on funduscopy, representing perivascular hemorrhage and exudates**
- Diagnosis at other sites is by CMV PCR, culture, or finding of viral inclusion bodies on histopathology

Treatment

- Systemic disease: Treat with either systemic ganciclovir or foscarnet
- CMV retinitis: Can use intraocular ganciclovir implants
  - Intraocular implants do not prevent nonophthalmologic manifestations of CMV

KAPOSI SARCOMA

Clinical Presentation

- Can be seen with a modestly depleted CD4 count (200–500/mm^3 range)
- **Indurated or nodular violaceous growths on the skin or in any visceral organ (Fig. 12-7)**
- Most common malignancy in HIV/AIDS
- Predominantly seen in men with same-sex contact as transmission risk

Diagnosis

- Biopsy shows proliferation of abnormal vascular structures on pathology

- Human herpesvirus 8 identified as causative agent but not used diagnostically

Treatment

- Cytotoxic chemotherapy
- Intralesional chemotherapy (if cutaneous)
- May regress with effective ART

NON-HODGKIN LYMPHOMA

Clinical Presentation

- Usually seen at CD4 count less than 200/mm^3
- Heterogeneous group of malignancies
- 70% are B-cell derived
- Intermediate or high-grade B-cell lymphomas are AIDS-defining events in individual with HIV infection
- **Extranodal presentation common (GI tract, visceral, bone marrow, body cavity)**

Diagnosis

- For accessible lesions, diagnosis made by biopsy
- For CNS lesions: **Thallium single-photon emission computed tomography (SPECT) scan is useful to differentiate lymphoma from similar-appearing lesions of toxoplasmosis; lymphoma lesions often enhance, whereas toxoplasmosis does not**
- **Biopsy warranted for lesions that do not respond to empirical therapy for toxoplasmosis**

Treatment

- Combination chemotherapy, brain radiation if CNS involvement, and ART

FIGURE 12-5   Imaging of common CNS conditions associated with HIV. **A,** CNS toxoplasmosis presents as multiple ring-enhancing lesions. **B,** CNS lymphoma usually presents as a solitary ring-enhancing lesion. **C** and **D,** Progressive multifocal leukoencephalopathy (PML) lesions are seen as areas of high signal intensity in the subcortical white matter (**C**) and do not enhance with gadolinium (**D**). *(A and B, From Haslett C, Chilvers ER, Boon NA, et al [eds]: Davidson's principles and practice of medicine, ed 19, New York, Churchill Livingstone, 2002, Figs. 1.88 and 1.89. C and D, From Mandell GL, Bennett JE, Dolin R [eds]: Principles and practice of infectious diseases, ed 6, Philadelphia, Churchill Livingstone, 2005, Fig. 120-4.)*

HIV-ASSOCIATED NEPHROPATHY

Clinical Presentation

- Can be seen at any CD4 level, but usually CD4 count is lower than 200/mm³
- Associated with high viral load
- **Presents with nephrotic syndrome**
- Progressive course; if untreated, leads to renal failure over 1 to 4 months

Diagnosis

- Large echogenic kidneys seen on ultrasound
- **Diagnosis made by biopsy that shows focal segmental glomerulosclerosis**

FIGURE 12-6 Cytomegalovirus (CMV) retinitis. **A**, Early disease with retinal involvement along blood vessels. **B**, Extensive retinal damage and retinal hemorrhages. **C**, CMV retinitis with papillitis. *(From Mandell GL, Bennett JE, Dolin R [eds]: Principles and practice of infectious diseases, ed 6, Philadelphia, Churchill Livingstone, 2005, Fig. 134-2.)*

FIGURE 12-7 Kaposi sarcoma can present cutaneously (**A**), in the oral mucosa (**B**), and internally in the lungs or GI tract (not shown). (*A, From Mandell GL, Bennett JE, Dolin R [eds]: Principles and practice of infectious diseases, ed 6, Philadelphia, Churchill Livingstone, 2005, Fig. 117-12. B, From Goldman L, Ausiello D: Cecil textbook of medicine, ed 23, Philadelphia, Elsevier Saunders, 2008, Fig. 414-12.)*

- Differential diagnosis includes: heroin nephropathy, drug toxicity (e.g., tenofovir, indinavir, trimethoprim-sulfamethoxazole), hepatitis-related nephropathy

Treatment

- ART
- Steroid therapy may slow progression until viral suppression is achieved

IMMUNE RECONSTITUTION SYNDROME (IRS)

Clinical Presentation

- Occurs 2 to 12 weeks after initiating ART
- Paradoxical clinical worsening owing to new ability to mount an inflammatory response against an underlying opportunistic infection or antigen (that was subclinical)
- Usually seen with low CD4 count (<100/mm³) and rapid decline in HIV viral load

Diagnosis

- Presentations of opportunistic infections may be atypical because of brisk inflammation; high clinical suspicion needed

Treatment

- Diagnose and treat the underlying opportunistic infection
- Anti-inflammatory treatment (corticosteroids or nonsteroidal anti-inflammatory drugs) may be effective, although not proven
- Continue ART

REVIEW QUESTIONS

For review questions, please go to www.expertconsult.com.

SUGGESTED READINGS

Bartlett JG, Gallant JE: *Pham Paul A: Medical management of HIV infection*, ed 15, Durham, NC, 2009–2010, Knowledge Source Solutions.

Sterling TR, Chaisson RE: General clinical manifestations of human immunodeficiency virus infection. In Mandell GL, Bennett JE, Dolin R, editors: *Principles and practice of infectious diseases*, ed 7, Philadelphia, 2010, Churchill Livingstone.

Mycobacterial Infections

SUSAN E. DORMAN, MD

Mycobacteria are aerobic bacteria that have the laboratory characteristic of retaining colorized stain when washed in an acid bath—hence they are "acid-fast" (Fig. 13-1). *Mycobacterium tuberculosis*, *Mycobacterium leprae*, and *Mycobacterium avium* complex are clinically among the most important mycobacteria. However, with the increasing prevalence of immunocompromised hosts, other mycobacterial species have become clinically relevant.

Tuberculosis

Basic Information

- Pathogenesis
  - Airborne transmission from patient with pulmonary tuberculosis (TB) disease (Fig. 13-2)
- Epidemiology
  - Global: Almost 9 million new cases and 2 million deaths per year
  - United States: 13,299 TB cases were reported in 2007 (4.4 cases per 100,000 population). African Americans and foreign-born persons are disproportionately affected.
- Impact of human immunodeficiency virus (HIV) on TB
  - **HIV increases risk of progression to active TB after *M. tuberculosis* infection**
  - **HIV increases risk of reactivation of latent *M. tuberculosis* infection**

FIGURE 13-1 Ziehl-Neelsen staining of a sputum sample of a patient with pulmonary tuberculosis demonstrating acid-fast bacilli. *(From Forbes C, Jackson W: Color atlas and text of clinical medicine, ed 3, St. Louis, Mosby, 2003, Fig. 4.14.)*

- HIV increases mortality from TB
- Highly active antiretroviral therapy decreases the risk of active TB in HIV-infected persons
- Multidrug-resistant TB (MDR-TB)
  - **Defined as resistance to at least isoniazid plus rifampin**
  - Clusters in geographic areas (Russia, Latvia, Estonia, China, Iran)
  - Other risk factors: prior TB treatment, noncompliance with TB treatment, adding one drug to a failing TB treatment regimen

Clinical Presentation

- **Primary infection: Usually asymptomatic**
  - Minority present with pleural effusion or pneumonia in mid- or lower lung fields with hilar or mediastinal lymphadenopathy
  - Most (>90%) immunocompetent people control initial infection and develop clinically silent latent infection (see Fig. 13-2)
  - **HIV-infected persons have high risk of progression to active TB after initial infection**
- Reactivation TB disease
  - Typically subacute illness over weeks or months with fever, sweats, weight loss, cough
  - **Pulmonary disease typically involves upper lobe(s) or upper segments of lower lobe(s).** Cavitation is classic, but infiltrates may be lobar, nodular, or interstitial
- Other comments
  - Nearly any organ system can be involved
  - HIV: Increased prevalence (compared with HIV-negative) of extrapulmonary TB, disseminated TB, miliary TB. Pulmonary TB (in HIV) can present with any chest radiographic pattern, including normal chest radiograph.
  - Miliary TB: Disease results from widespread hematogenous dissemination of bacilli. Classic chest radiographic appearance is innumerable tiny nodules (Fig. 13-3).

Diagnosis and Evaluation

- Detection of M. *tuberculosis* infection (either latent infection or active disease)
  - Tuberculin skin test (TST)
    - Intradermal inoculation of mycobacterial purified protein derivative. Readout is induration 48 to 72 hours after inoculation.
    - **False-positive result can be due to infection with nontuberculous mycobacteria (NTM) or prior bacille Calmette-Guérin (BCG) vaccination**

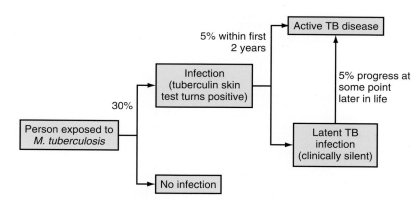

FIGURE 13-2 Pathogenesis of tuberculosis (TB) in immune-competent individuals exposed to *Mycobacterium tuberculosis*. HIV infection (not shown in this figure) substantially increases the proportion of patients who develop active TB disease after initial exposure and the proportion of patients who progress from latent infection to active TB.

FIGURE 13-3 Chest radiograph of a patient with miliary tuberculosis. *(From Swash M: Hutchinson's clinical methods, ed 21, Philadelphia, WB Saunders, 2002, Fig. 22.5.)*

- False-negative test can result from immunosuppression
- **Positive TST does not necessarily indicate active TB disease**
- Interferon-γ release assays (IGRAs)
  - **Whole-blood tests that can be used to diagnose *M. tuberculosis* infection**
  - **Currently, two IGRAs commercially available**
  - Measures a person's immune reactivity to *M. tuberculosis*
  - May be used in most instances in place of the TST
  - Cannot distinguish latent TB infection from active TB
  - Prior BCG vaccination will not cause a false-positive IGRA
- Detection of TB disease
  - Laboratory
    - Microscopic examination of sputum or other clinical specimen stained for acid-fast bacilli (AFB smear)

- **For diagnosis of pulmonary TB, obtain three morning sputum specimens (sent for AFB smear and mycobacterial culture)**
  - AFB smear not sensitive and not specific for *M. tuberculosis* (but positive smear is highly predictive of TB in TB-endemic settings)
- Culture
  - Sensitive and specific (in combination with other tests done on cultured material) for *M. tuberculosis*
  - Slow: Takes 3 to 6 weeks for *M. tuberculosis* to grow in culture
- Nucleic acid amplification (NAA) tests
  - Used to evaluate respiratory specimens from untreated patients
  - Highly specific for *M. tuberculosis*
  - Highly sensitive in AFB smear–positive patients; only 50% sensitive in AFB smear–negative patients
  - **If TB is suspected and NAA is negative, TB not excluded**
  - NAA test does not replace smear or culture

Treatment

- Treatment of latent TB infection (Fig. 13-4)
  - Decision to treat is based on individual's risk of recent *M. tuberculosis* infection and risk of progression to active TB disease if infected (Table 13-1)
  - Exclude active TB disease before starting treatment for latent TB
  - **Preferred regimen: Isoniazid daily for 9 months**
  - Alternative regimen: Rifampin daily for 4 months
  - **No age cutoff for treatment of latent TB infection**
- Treatment of drug-susceptible TB disease
  - Eight weeks of isoniazid plus rifampin plus pyrazinamide plus either ethambutol (commonly used) or streptomycin (not commonly used), followed by isoniazid plus rifampin "continuation phase" for an additional 4 months (total treatment duration, 6 months; Fig. 13-5)
  - Treatment extended to total of 9 months if delay (e.g., 2–3 months) in culture conversion
  - Treatment extended to 9 to 12 months for central nervous system TB
  - Streptomycin contraindicated in pregnant women; pyrazinamide not recommended for use in pregnant women
- Treatment of MDR-TB disease is 18 to 24 months, with complex regimens

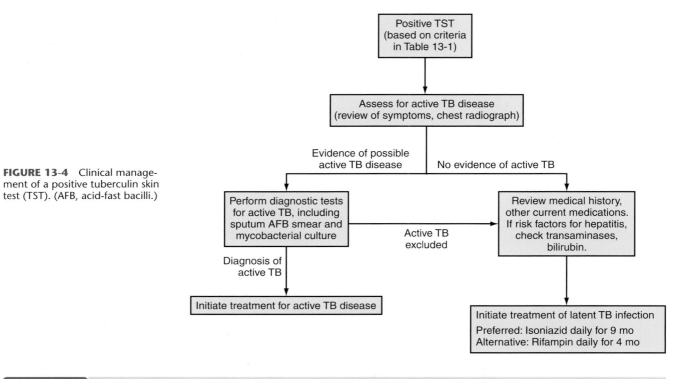

FIGURE 13-4 Clinical management of a positive tuberculin skin test (TST). (AFB, acid-fast bacilli.)

TABLE 13-1	*Risk Groups for Targeted Tuberculin Skin Testing (TST) and Treatment of Latent Tuberculosis (TB) Infection with Tuberculin Skin Test Cutpoints*
TST Induration Considered Positive	**Risk Group**
≥5 mm	HIV infection Recent contacts of active TB patients Fibrotic changes on chest radiograph Immunosuppression Use of anti–tumor necrosis factor-α drugs
≥10 mm	Recent immigrants Injection drug users Residents and employees of high-risk congregate settings (long-term care facilities, health care facilities, homeless shelters, prisons or jails) Mycobacteriology lab workers Persons with medical conditions that put them at risk (silicosis, diabetes mellitus, chronic renal failure, some malignancies, gastrectomy or jejunoileal bypass, underweight) Children <4 yr old Infants, children, or adolescents exposed to adults at high risk for TB ≥10 mm increase ≥10 mm increase within 2 yr is considered evidence of recent *Mycobacterium tuberculosis* infection (a positive TST reaction)
≥15 mm	Persons without any of above risk factors (TST not recommended in this group)

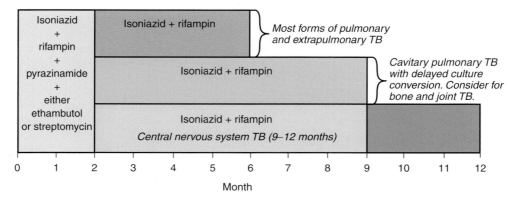

FIGURE 13-5 Recommended treatment for active tuberculosis disease, based on disease site.

TABLE 13-2	Toxicities of Commonly Used Antituberculosis Medications	
Drug	**Major Toxicities**	**Monitoring**
Isoniazid	Hepatotoxicity, peripheral neuropathy	Baseline liver chemistries. Repeat if baseline is abnormal or if other hepatitis risk factors or symptoms of hepatotoxicity are present.
Rifampin	Hepatotoxicity, fever, flu-like syndrome, thrombocytopenia, drug-drug interactions	Baseline liver chemistries and CBC. Repeat if baseline is abnormal or if other hepatitis risk factors or symptoms of adverse reaction are present.
Pyrazinamide	Hepatotoxicity, arthralgias, rash	Baseline liver chemistries, uric acid. Repeat if baseline is abnormal or if other hepatitis risk factors or symptoms of adverse reaction are present.
Ethambutol	Optic neuritis	Baseline and monthly tests of visual acuity and color vision.
Streptomycin	Ototoxicity, renal toxicity, teratogenic	Monthly audiometry, renal function, electrolytes. Contraindicated in pregnancy.

CBC, complete blood count.

13

- Treatment of TB disease in HIV-infected persons
  - TB treatment duration not affected by HIV
  - **Rifampin has drug-drug interactions with most protease inhibitors and non-nucleoside reverse transcriptase inhibitors**
  - **Worsening of TB signs or symptoms can be seen in first several weeks after starting HIV and/or TB treatment (paradoxical worsening)**
- Drug toxicities and monitoring for drug toxicity (Table 13-2)
  - Rifampin stimulates the cytochrome P450 system and enhances metabolism (thereby lowering blood levels and potentially decreasing effectiveness) of many drugs, including warfarin, oral contraceptives, methadone, most HIV protease inhibitors, most HIV non-nucleoside reverse transcriptase inhibitors

Prevention of Tuberculosis Transmission

- Respiratory isolation should be initiated for all persons suspected of having pulmonary TB disease who are hospitalized or in otherwise congregate settings (e.g., prison, nursing home)
- Care providers (for persons having or suspected of having infectious pulmonary TB disease) should use personal respiratory protection (e.g., N-95 mask)

Leprosy (Hansen Disease)

Basic Information

- Caused by M. leprae
- Prevalence highest in Africa, Asia

Clinical Presentation

- Broad spectrum of disease activity, including tuberculoid, borderline, and lepromatous forms
  - Tuberculoid: One or few asymmetrical anesthetic skin macules; nerve involvement (classically ulnar nerve at elbow) can be severe; biopsies of skin, nerves show few or no bacteria
  - Lepromatous: Symmetrical skin nodules and plaques on cool areas of body; affected tissues laden with mycobacteria; upper respiratory tract involvement

FIGURE 13-6 A patient with lepromatous leprosy demonstrating saddle-nose deformity. *(From Haslett C, Chilvers ER, Boon NA, et al: Davidson's principles and practice of medicine, ed 19, New York, Churchill Livingstone, 2002, Fig. 1.69.)*

common, manifest by nasal congestion, epistaxis, cartilage erosion/collapse (saddle-nose deformity; Fig. 13-6); peripheral neuropathy is common

Diagnosis and Evaluation

- Diagnosis based on clinical presentation plus biopsy (demonstration of AFB and histology)

Treatment

- Paucibacillary (skin smear negative, with five or fewer skin lesions): Dapsone daily plus rifampin monthly for 6 months
- Multibacillary (skin-smear positive, with more than five skin lesions): Dapsone daily plus rifampin monthly plus clofazimine for 1 year

TABLE 13-3	Clinical Features of Infections Caused by Nontuberculous Mycobacteria	
Species	**Reservoir**	**Common Clinical Manifestations**
Mycobacterium avium-intracellulare complex	Birds, cattle, swine, water, soil	Disseminated disease in AIDS (fevers, sweats, diarrhea, mesenteric adenopathy) Pulmonary disease (cavity, infiltrate, or bronchiectasis) in persons with underlying lung disease (COPD, cystic fibrosis) or older women
Mycobacterium kansasii	Water	Pulmonary disease resembling TB, or disseminated disease, especially in HIV-infected persons
Mycobacterium marinum	Water, marine organisms	"Fish-tank granuloma" Infection follows trauma, usually to extremities, occurring in water Presents as enlarging nodule(s) that ulcerate, drain
Mycobacterium fortuitum *Mycobacterium abscessus* *Mycobacterium chelonae* (rapid growers)	Water	Cutaneous disease, catheter-related infections, surgical wound infections, keratitis *M. abscessus* can cause pulmonary disease in cystic fibrosis

COPD, chronic obstructive pulmonary disease; TB, tuberculosis.

Nontuberculous Mycobacteria

Basic Information

- Rapid growers (visible growth within 7 days in culture): *Mycobacterium fortuitum*, *Mycobacterium chelonae*, *Mycobacterium abscessus*
- Slow growers (visible growth requires >7 days in culture): *Mycobacterium kansasii*, *Mycobacterium avium-intracellulare*, *Mycobacterium marinum*

Clinical Presentation

- Formerly known as mycobacteria other than tuberculosis
- Isolation of NTM from clinical specimen may result from contamination (e.g., from tap water), colonization in absence of NTM disease, or NTM disease
- **Immunosuppression is a risk factor for NTM disease**
- Common clinical syndromes listed in Table 13-3

Diagnosis and Evaluation

- Diagnosis is based on clinical presentation and positive culture of clinically relevant specimen (see Table 13-3)

Treatment

- Antimicrobial agents and treatment duration vary according to organism and site of disease

REVIEW QUESTIONS

For review questions, please go to www.expertconsult.com.

SUGGESTED READINGS

American Thoracic Society: Centers for Disease Control and Prevention: Treatment of tuberculosis, *Am J Respir Crit Care Med* 167:603–662, 2003.

Blumberg HM, Leonard MK Jr, Jasmer RM: Update on the treatment of tuberculosis and latent tuberculosis infection, *JAMA* 293:2776–2784, 2005.

Griffith DE, Aksamit T, Brown-Elliott BA, et al: An official ATS/IDSA statement: diagnosis, treatment, and prevention of nontuberculous mycobacterial diseases, *Am J Respir Crit Care Med* 175:367–416, 2007.

Horsburgh CR Jr, Rubin EJ: Clinical practice: latent tuberculosis infection in the United States, *N Engl J Med* 364:1441–1448, 2011.

Infectious Diarrhea

CYNTHIA L. SEARS, MD

Infectious diarrhea is the second leading cause of morbidity and mortality throughout the world, predominantly in developing countries. In the United States, at least 200 million episodes of acute diarrhea occur yearly, although a minority of those affected seek medical care. A systematic approach to the evaluation of the patient with diarrhea is useful in identifying the cause.

Approach to a Patient with Infectious Diarrhea

Clinical Presentation

- Acute diarrhea: Three or more episodes of liquid stool in a 24-hour period; symptoms typically last less than 14 days
- Chronic diarrhea: Duration exceeds 1 month
- Clinical classification of acute diarrhea (Table 14-1)
  - **Noninflammatory: Large-volume, watery stools containing no blood or pus. Some fecal inflammatory cells can be seen but frank pus is absent.**
  - **Inflammatory: Frequent, small-volume stools containing blood or pus. Fever and abdominal pain may be present.**
  - Frequent overlap occurs such that common causes of inflammatory diarrhea appear to be noninflammatory diarrhea clinically

Diagnosis and Evaluation

- History should focus on duration of symptoms, features of stool (hematochezia, tenesmus), associated symptoms (fever, abdominal pain), previous antibiotic use, immune status, travel history, exposure to children and risk for food-borne illness (see later discussion)
- Physical examination should include an evaluation of fever, hydration status, and abdominal tenderness
- Laboratory testing
  - Laboratory assessment is typically unnecessary unless inflammatory diarrhea is suspected or the patient is unstable or immunocompromised
  - Fecal leukocytes: Can help differentiate inflammatory from noninflammatory, but may be able to determine whether diarrhea is inflammatory by history alone
  - Stool culture: Indicated only if patient is clinically ill, immunocompromised, and/or presence of fecal leukocytes suggests an inflammatory process
  - Occult blood cards: A positive can serve as an indicator of inflammatory diarrhea

- **Ova and parasites: Reserve for persistent diarrhea (>14 days) or high-risk individuals (e.g., travel history or immunocompromised). Do not order routinely for acute diarrhea.**

Treatment

- Hydration: Cornerstone of therapy for all patients; oral usually sufficient
- Diet: No alteration other than avoidance of caffeine, dairy products, and sorbitol. Transient lactase deficiency may occur in diarrheal disease.
- Antidiarrheal medications
  - **Loperamide (Imodium): Delays passage through the intestine; safe in most situations; contraindicated in inflammatory diarrheas because of concern for decreased clearance of toxin or organism (particularly for Shiga toxin–producing *Escherichia coli* [STEC] and *Clostridium difficile*)**
  - Bismuth: Moderately effective but inconvenient and leaves a bad taste; can do harm when taken in excess; will darken stools
  - Diphenoxylate (Lomotil): Has central opiate effects, so try to avoid
- Antibiotics
  - Use is controversial; data are weak that they have impact on course of illness in all-comers
  - Rarely indicated in noninflammatory diarrhea unless the patient is unstable or at high risk (e.g., immunocompromised, recent travel, elderly)
  - **Most guidelines recommend empirical use of quinolones in inflammatory diarrhea; azithromycin is second choice**
  - Organisms such as *Vibrio cholerae*, *Shigella* organisms, and *Giardia* spp. should always be treated with antibiotics, but invasive *E. coli* and mild to moderate nontyphoidal *Salmonella* should not be treated with antibiotics

Food-borne Illness

Basic Information (Table 14-2)

- Can be caused by bacteria, viruses, and parasites or ingestion of bacterial toxins present in microbiologically contaminated foods
- **It is important for physicians to report cases caused by certain organisms (e.g., *Salmonella*) to their local or state health department.** Significant variations exist in state reporting guidelines.

TABLE 14-1	Clinical Classification of Acute Diarrhea
Classification	**Organisms**
Noninflammatory	Noroviruses, rotavirus, enterotoxigenic *Escherichia coli, Clostridium perfringens, Vibrio cholera, Giardia lamblia, Cryptosporidium*
Inflammatory	*Salmonella, Shigella, Campylobacter,* Shiga toxin–producing *E. coli* (O157 and non-O157), enteroinvasive *E. coli, Clostridium difficile, Yersinia, Vibrio parahaemolyticus, Entamoeba histolytica*

TABLE 14-2	Potential Reportable Food-borne Diseases
Category	**Illnesses or Organisms**
Bacteria	Botulism, brucellosis, cholera, *Escherichia coli* O157 (Shiga toxin–producing *E. coli*), salmonellosis, shigellosis, typhoid fever
Viruses	Hepatitis A
Parasites	Cryptosporidiosis, cyclosporiasis, trichinosis

Clinical Presentation

- Typically presents with GI symptoms (e.g., nausea, vomiting, diarrhea, abdominal pain)
- Neurologic symptoms such as paresthesias may be present in certain conditions (e.g., botulism)

Diagnosis and Evaluation

- Patients should be asked about ingestion of raw or poorly cooked food (e.g., fish, eggs, meats, shellfish); unpasteurized milk; home canned goods; or fresh produce (often imported)
- Source of food (if known) can be important in identifying a particular organism
  - Shellfish: *Vibrio cholerae, Vibrio parahaemolyticus*
  - Poultry and eggs: *Campylobacter, Salmonella* spp.
  - Meat: *Clostridium perfringens, Salmonella,* STEC
  - Dairy: *Salmonella,* STEC, *Yersinia*
  - Prepared protein-rich foods: *Staphylococcus* (ingestion of preformed toxin; Table 14-3)
  - Deli foods: *Listeria monocytogenes*
- Inquiries should be made about sick contacts, contact with day care centers, and travel
- Etiologies can be narrowed by determining whether the diarrhea is inflammatory or noninflammatory (see Table 14-1)
- **Timing of illness (incubation period) may be helpful**
  - 1 to 6 hours: *Staphylococcus aureus, Bacillus cereus*
  - 8 to 16 hours: *C. perfringens, B. cereus*
  - 16 to 72 hours: *Campylobacter jejuni, Salmonella, Shigella, E. coli* (including STEC), *Yersinia, Vibrio*

Common Pathogens

VIRAL PATHOGENS

- Account for at least 50% of all acute infectious diarrheal illnesses
- Usually the causative agent is never identified
- **Norovirus is the most commonly identified viral cause of endemic and epidemic diarrhea in adults**
  - Fecal-oral, food-borne, airborne, and fomite transmission common as a result of low inoculum required for disease
  - Incubation period is usually 24 to 48 hours
  - Noninflammatory diarrhea with or without vomiting; about 80% have both vomiting and diarrhea
  - Low-grade fever in about 50%
  - Treatment is supportive because symptoms usually are self-limited
- Rotavirus causes sporadic outbreaks in children; much less common in adults
  - Fecal-oral transmission usually seen
  - Vomiting, low-grade fever, transient lactase deficiency can be present
  - Episodes may last over 1 week
  - Treatment is supportive
- Hepatitis A (see Chapter 29)
  - Rare cause of food-borne disease
  - Long incubation period (15–50 days)
  - Transmitted by contaminated shellfish, raw produce, and foods contaminated after handling by infected people
  - Jaundice, abdominal pain, fever, elevated hepatic transaminases may be present
  - Diagnosis made by the presence of immunoglobulin M anti–hepatitis A antibodies
  - Treatment is supportive
  - Contacts should be given immune globulin

BACTERIAL PATHOGENS

See Table 14-3 for bacterial causes of diarrheal illness.

PARASITIC PATHOGENS

- *Giardia lamblia* (giardiasis)
  - Common cause of persistent or chronic diarrhea
  - Diarrhea usually watery but steatorrhea/malabsorption can arise
  - Bloating and mild nausea are common
  - **Major source is drinking water (usually well water); intrafamilial spread (person-to-person) occurs**
  - Usually responds to treatment with metronidazole
  - *Giardia* enzyme immunoassay (EIA) available for diagnosis
- *Cryptosporidium parvum* (cryptosporidiosis)
  - Regionally variable but can be similar in incidence to *Giardia*
  - **Source is often water but can be transmitted through person-to-person, fecal-oral routes**
  - Usually self-limited in normal host but can cause persistent (>14 days) or chronic diarrhea; in HIV-infected host (particularly with CD4 count <150–200 cells/mm³), often a chronic illness

TABLE 14-3	Bacterial Causes of Diarrheal Illness*		
Organism	**Usual Incubation Period**	**Associated Foods**	**Comments**
Bacillus cereus (preformed bacterial enterotoxin)	1–6 hr	Fried rice, other starchy foods	Usually presents as sudden nausea and vomiting Diarrhea may be present
Bacillus cereus (diarrhea toxin)	6–24 hr	Meats, vegetables	Diarrhea is the major manifestation
Campylobacter jejuni	1–3 days	Poultry, milk, water	Common bacterial pathogen Rarely, patients can develop Guillain-Barré syndrome or reactive arthritis after infection
Clostridium botulinum	3–30 days	Home-canned foods	Presents with vomiting, diarrhea, blurred vision, diplopia, and descending muscle weakness
Clostridium perfringens (diarrhea toxin)	6–24 hr	Meat, poultry, or gravy	Diarrhea is the major manifestation
Escherichia coli O157:H7/ other STEC	1–3 days	Beef, apple cider, water, unpasteurized milk	5–10% of infections lead to hemolytic uremic syndrome (HUS) Antibiotics not recommended because they may increase risk of HUS If infection suspected, enzyme immunoassay for Shiga-like toxin and stool culture for specific organism must be requested
Salmonella (nontyphoidal)	1–3 days	Poultry, eggs, milk, juice, fruits, vegetables (many foods possible)	Nontyphoidal *Salmonella* (many serotypes) are common causes of bacterial diarrhea In typhoid fever (*S. typhi*), diarrhea is uncommon; fever, fatigue, myalgias predominate
Shigella	1–3 days	Primarily person-to-person spread 20% of cases are food-borne	Variable presentation depending on infecting species Always treat with antibiotics (quinolones) for public health reasons
Staphylococcus aureus (preformed bacterial enterotoxin)	1–6 hr	Cream pastries, salads, poultry	Sudden onset of nausea and vomiting, followed later by diarrhea in some
Vibrio cholerae	1–3 days	Shellfish, contaminated water	Massive, noninflammatory diarrhea Antibiotics reduce length of illness
Vibrio parahaemolyticus	1–3 days	Raw fish, shellfish	Inflammatory diarrhea
Yersinia	1–3 days	Pork, milk	Inflammatory diarrhea Can cause right lower quadrant pain (pseudoappendicitis)

*Most causes of diarrhea can lead to postdiarrheal reactive arthritis and irritable bowel syndrome.
STEC, Shiga toxin–producing *E. coli*.

- Symptoms are variable but can cause large-volume losses or malabsorption
- Abdominal pain, fever, and vomiting can occur
- Symptoms may be relapsing
- Organisms appear on acid-fast stain as oocysts in stool (Fig. 14-1A)
- On pathology, life-cycle forms are detected in the brush border
- *Cryptosporidium* EIA available for diagnosis
- Nitazoxanide available for treatment of immunocompetent children and adults
- *Cyclospora cayetanensis*
  - Also increased in HIV but can infect immunocompetent host (e.g., outbreak associated with imported raspberries)
  - Symptoms similar to *Cryptosporidium*
  - Responds to sulfa antibiotics, including trimethoprim-sulfamethoxazole (TMP-SMX)
  - Organisms are also acid-fast positive in stool but twice the size of *Crytosporidium* (see Fig. 14-1B)

- **Entamoeba histolytica**
  - **Presents as an inflammatory process, often chronic, with bloody diarrhea and lower abdominal pain (similar to *Shigella*); can cause extraintestinal disease, especially liver abscess**
  - Diagnose by examining stool for trophozoites (Fig. 14-2), but morphologically indistinguishable from nonpathogenic *Entamoeba dispar*
  - Antigen detection methods for serum and stool to distinguish *E. histolytica* and *E. dispar* are available
  - Metronidazole is effective therapy; attention to elimination of tissue and cyst forms is important depending on the disease presentation
- *Trichinella spiralis*
  - Causes diarrhea, vomiting, abdominal pain, myalgias, fever, periorbital edema
  - Occurs days to weeks after ingestion of raw or undercooked meat (e.g., pork, bear, moose)

FIGURE 14-1 Acid-fast stain of intestinal pathogens. **A,** *Cryptosporidium* spp., 4 to 6 mm in diameter. **B,** *Cyclospora* spp., 8 to 10 mm in diameter. **C,** Elliptical-shaped *Isospora belli*. *(From Cohen J, Powderly W: Infectious diseases, ed 2, St. Louis, Mosby, 2004, Fig. 243-3.)*

FIGURE 14-2 Trophozoite of *Entamoeba histolytica*. Note the ingested red blood cells. *(From Cohen J, Powderly W: Infectious diseases, ed 2, St. Louis, Mosby, 2004, Fig. 242-1.)*

- Cardiovascular events may occur in up to 25% of patients
- Eosinophilia is usually present
- Treatment is supportive for mild cases. Mebendazole or albendazole is used in more severe cases. Prednisone is added if inflammation is severe.

TOXINS

- *Staphylococcus aureus* and *Bacillus cereus* are the most common toxin-mediated causes of food-borne disease. Consider botulism if neurologic symptoms are present.
- Ciguatera fish poisoning
  - Illness caused by toxins concentrated in the fish
  - **Causes diarrhea, nausea, and abdominal cramps followed by neurologic symptoms and signs such as tooth pain and paresthesias of the lips, tongue, and oropharynx**
  - Can lead to respiratory paralysis and bradycardia
  - Incubation is 1 to 6 hours; source is seafood; primarily seen in Florida and Hawaii
  - Duration of illness can be days to months
- Scombroid fish poisoning
  - Ingestion of histamine present in fish results in abdominal cramps, nausea, and diarrhea and, rarely, bronchospasm
  - Incubation is less than an hour; duration is a few hours
  - Treat with antihistamines in severe cases

FIGURE 14-3 Cytomegalovirus colitis. Biopsy specimen reveals the typical "owl's-eye" cell. *(From Kumar P, Clark M: Clinical medicine, ed 6, Philadelphia, Elsevier Saunders, 2005, Fig. 2.16.)*

Special Circumstances

HIV PATIENTS

- Approximately 50% of HIV patients develop diarrhea
- Many different causes
- Common infections include the following:
  - **Cryptosporidium (see preceding discussion): Most common protozoal cause of diarrhea in AIDS patients**
  - Cytomegalovirus (CMV)
    - Most common cause of viral colonic disease in HIV patients
    - Typically seen with CD4 counts below 50/mm^3
    - Presentation is variable and can range from mild diarrhea to an acute abdomen
    - Biopsy is required for diagnosis
    - See characteristic "owl's-eye" nucleus with basophilic intranuclear inclusion surrounded by clear halo (Fig. 14-3)
  - *Mycobacterium avium* complex (MAC)
    - Most infections seen when CD4 counts are less than 100/mm^3
    - Can involve large or small bowel; mucosa can appear normal on colonoscopy
    - Abdominal lymph nodes may be prominent
    - Diagnose by blood culture or tissue biopsy; stool culture is not diagnostic but is predictive of risk of disease over time
    - Combination therapy is important; can treat with clarithromycin/ethambutol
  - *Isospora belli*
    - Endemic to tropical areas; rare in the United States
    - Spread by fecal-oral route
    - Can cause chronic diarrhea
    - Diagnose by ova and parasite examination or biopsy (see Fig. 14-1C)
    - Can treat with TMP-SMX
  - Herpes simplex virus usually causes proctitis with anorectal pain and tenesmus
  - *Microsporidium*
    - Obligate intracellular pathogen seen on small bowel biopsies

- Seen almost exclusively in AIDS with CD4 count less than 100/mm^3
- Causes chronic diarrhea and malabsorption
- Giardiasis, strongyloidiasis, and *Cyclospora* also should be considered

TRAVELER'S DIARRHEA

- **Enterotoxigenic *E. coli* most common cause, but causative agent usually not identified**
- Up to 80% of cases are bacterial in origin
- Without treatment lasts 4 to 7 days; with antibiotics lasts 24 to 48 hours
- Patients should be advised to avoid tap water, ice, raw fruits and vegetables, and undercooked meats in underdeveloped countries
- Antibiotics of choice for treatment are quinolones. Due to increasing resistance, particularly in Southeast Asia with fluoroquinolone-resistant *C. jejuni*, azithromycin is an alternative therapy.
- Prophylaxis (with TMP-SMX or quinolones) considered only for high-risk patients

Antibiotic-Associated Diarrhea

Basic Information

- **Diarrhea can occur in up to 20% of patients receiving certain antibiotics (e.g., ampicillin, amoxicillin/clavulanate, cefixime, clindamycin)**
- Only 10% to 20% of cases of antibiotic-associated diarrhea are caused by *C. difficile* infection
- *C. difficile* does, however, account for most cases of colitis caused by antibiotics

Clinical Presentation

- *C. difficile* disease symptoms can range from mild, loose, or watery bowel movements to acute colitis with leukocytosis and abdominal pain. Fever occurs in only 10% to 15% of *C. difficile* patients; if present, it is a sign of severe disease.
- Symptoms of *C. difficile* can be delayed up to 4 to 8 weeks after antibiotic exposure
- **Community-associated *C. difficile* disease is increasing and occurring in some without antibiotic exposure**

Diagnosis and Evaluation

- Need to rule out *C. difficile* infection in most cases of diarrhea that are not mild and self-limited after antibiotic exposure
- Diagnosis is dependent on detection of *C. difficile* toxins in stool
- Most laboratories use EIAs for *C. difficile* that will have a false-negative rate of 10% to 30%. Polymerase chain reaction (PCR)–based tests offer high sensitivity and specificity.
- Most cases of *C. difficile* involve toxins A *and* B and, less frequently, toxin B alone.

Treatment

- Antibiotic-associated diarrhea not caused by *C. difficile* is self-limited after discontinuation of the antibiotic

14

- C. *difficile* infection should be treated and the inciting antibiotics discontinued if clinically feasible.
  - Oral metronidazole or vancomycin can be used
    - **In severe disease (e.g., fever, low albumin, white blood cell [WBC] count >15,0000/mm³, colon wall thickening on abdominal computed tomography; older patients are at increased risk), vancomycin is the drug of choice.** Vancomycin and metronidazole appear to be therapeutically similar in mild to moderate disease. Metronidazole is less expensive.
  - Avoid antiperistaltic agents
  - Usually treated for 10 to 14 days
- **There is a high relapse rate (20–25%) after initial treatment for C. difficile**
  - Initial relapses should be treated with another 10- to 14-day course of metronidazole or vancomycin
  - Method of treatment of patients with more than one relapse is controversial; prolonged, tapered treatment with vancomycin is most often used
  - Sequential therapy with vancomycin followed by rifaximin may be useful for recurrences

- Fidaxomicin may be useful in patients with relapsing C. *difficile* and in patients who cannot tolerate or do not respond to vancomycin
- For severe disease: IV metronidazole, vancomycin by nasogastric tube or enema, surgical consult, and consider IV immunoglobulin

REVIEW QUESTIONS

For review questions, please go to www.expertconsult.com.

SUGGESTED READINGS

Cohen SH, Gerding DN, Johnson S, et al: Clinical practice guidelines for Clostridium difficile infections in adults: 2010 update by the society for healthcare epidemiology of America (SHEA) and the infectious diseases society of America (IDSA), *Infect Control Hosp Epidemiol* 31:431–455, 2010.

Dupont HL: Clinical practice: bacterial diarrhea, *N Engl J Med* 361: 1560–1569, 2009.

Guerrant RL, Van Gilder T, Steiner TS, et al: IDSA practice guidelines for the management of infectious diarrhea, *Clin Infect Dis* 32:331–351, 2001.

Hessen MT: In the clinic: *Clostridium difficile* infection, *Ann Intern Med* 153:ITC4-1–ITC4-15, 2010.

Selected Topics in Infectious Disease I

ARUNA K. SUBRAMANIAN, MD

Patients seen by internists in both the inpatient and outpatient settings often present with a variety of infections. This chapter attempts to provide an overview of a number of infections, including meningitis, encephalitis, skin and soft tissue infections, infectious arthritis, and osteomyelitis. Additionally, an approach to the patient with fever of unknown origin (FUO) is presented.

Meningitis

Basic Information

- Defined as inflammation of the leptomeninges, the tissues surrounding the brain and spinal cord
- May be caused by bacteria, viruses, fungi, or other non-infectious etiologies
- Specific pathogens of acute bacterial meningitis: see Table 15-1
- Aseptic meningitis is strictly defined as meningeal inflammation with an absence of bacteria on cerebrospinal fluid (CSF) examination and culture
  - Mononuclear pleocytosis and normal glucose level are usually seen
  - Can result from a number of different causes (Table 15-2)
- Some pathogens may cause a subacute to chronic meningitis
  - Cryptococcal meningitis is more commonly seen in immunocompromised hosts, especially in advanced AIDS (see Chapter 12); however, it can cause a very indolent illness in healthy individuals
  - Tuberculous meningitis typically is quite protracted, with a CSF profile revealing a mononuclear pleocytosis and elevated protein and lowered glucose concentrations

Clinical Presentation

- Fever, headache, and nuchal rigidity (neck stiffness) are seen in most cases
- Mental status change and seizures can occur
- Diffuse maculopapular rash that becomes petechial is seen with meningococcemia (Fig. 15-1)
- Physical examination may reveal signs of meningeal irritation
  - Kernig's sign—pain in the back is elicited with passive extension of the knee while the hip is flexed
  - Brudzinski's sign—passive flexion of the neck results in spontaneous flexion of the hips and knees

Diagnosis

- Blood cultures should be obtained immediately
- Diagnosis relies on examination of the CSF (Table 15-3)
- **Neuroimaging with computed tomography (CT) or magnetic resonance imaging (MRI) is needed only in select** situations before performing a lumbar puncture (Table 15-4)
- **If neuroimaging is needed, empirical antibiotic therapy (and dexamethasone if indicated) must be started before scanning**

Treatment

- Bacterial meningitis
  - Empirical therapy
    - Age 1 month to 50 years: Vancomycin plus a third-generation cephalosporin (ceftriaxone or cefotaxime)
    - Older than 50 years: Ampicillin (to cover *Listeria* spp.), plus vancomycin, plus a third-generation cephalosporin
    - Penetrating head trauma, postneurosurgery, or CSF shunt: Vancomycin plus cefepime, ceftazidime, or meropenem
  - Role of adjunctive dexamethasone
    - **Recommended in adults with suspected or proven pneumococcal meningitis**
    - First dose 10 to 20 minutes before, or at least concomitant with, the first dose of antibiotics
    - Dosing: 0.15 mg/kg every 6 hours for 2 to 4 days
  - Organism-specific therapy (see Table 15-1)
- Aseptic meningitis
  - Treatment generally supportive
  - Acyclovir may be useful for herpesvirus infections

Encephalitis

Basic Information

- Inflammation of the brain parenchyma
- Frequently concurrent with meningitis (meningoencephalitis) or inflammation of the spinal cord (encephalomyelitis)
- Can be caused by a number of different viruses (Table 15-5)

Clinical Presentation

- Headache, fever, nuchal rigidity seen as in meningitis

TABLE 15-1	Common Etiologic Agents Causing Acute Bacterial Meningitis in Adults	
Pathogen	**Description**	**Treatment**
Streptococcus pneumoniae	Most common etiologic agent in United States Mortality 19–26% Sometimes associated with other foci of infection (e.g., pneumonia)	Vancomycin + 3rd-generation cephalosporin until antimicrobial susceptibility is known (some experts add rifampin if dexamethasone is given)
Neisseria meningitides	Affects mostly children and young adults Patients with terminal complement deficiency are predisposed Maculopapular rash progresses to petechiae on trunk, extremities, and mucous membranes	3rd-generation cephalosporin Switch to penicillin G or ampicillin once confirmed to be highly sensitive Chemoprophylaxis: Rifampin (or ciprofloxacin or ceftriaxone) recommended for household contacts, day care center members, those directly exposed to oral secretions
Haemophilus influenzae	Mostly occurs in children Disease in adults usually associated with sinusitis, otitis media, pneumonia, sickle cell disease, splenectomy, diabetes, immune deficiency, head trauma with CSF leak, or alcoholism	3rd-generation cephalosporin
Listeria monocytogenes	Disease of neonates, the elderly, and immunocompromised Outbreaks associated with contaminated coleslaw, milk, cheese Associated with hematologic malignancy, steroid use, iron overload	Ampicillin (or penicillin G) ± aminoglycoside
Staphylococcus aureus	Usually seen after head trauma	Nafcillin or oxacillin (if methicillin susceptible) Vancomycin ± rifampin (if methicillin resistant)

CSF, cerebrospinal fluid.

TABLE 15-2	Causes of Aseptic Meningitis
Category	**Examples**
Viral	Mumps, echovirus, poliovirus, coxsackievirus, herpes simplex virus
Bacterial	Tuberculosis, syphilis, partially treated bacterial
Miscellaneous infections	Toxoplasmosis, coccidioidomycosis, malaria, Whipple disease, leptospirosis
Noninfectious diseases	Brain tumors, sarcoidosis, meningeal carcinomatosis
Drugs	Trimethoprim-sulfamethoxazole, ibuprofen, carbamazepine

FIGURE 15-1 Typical rash of meningococcal sepsis. Fine erythematous macules and petechiae are present in some areas. *(From Cohen J, Powderly W: Infectious diseases, ed 2, St. Louis, Mosby, 2004, Fig. 227.9.)*

- Alterations in consciousness may clinically help distinguish from meningitis
  - Bizarre behavior, hallucinations, expressive aphasia can be seen with temporal lobe involvement with herpes simplex virus (HSV) infection (Fig. 15-2)
  - Focal neurologic signs and seizures can also develop
  - West Nile virus may be associated with flaccid weakness and reduced or absent reflexes

Diagnosis

- Basic CSF examination is similar to that seen in viral meningitis with lymphocytic pleocytosis, normal glucose level, and mildly elevated protein level
- CSF polymerase chain reaction (PCR) is useful for the detection of HSV, cytomegalovirus (CMV), Epstein-Barr virus (EBV), varicella-zoster virus (VZV), West Nile virus, and enteroviruses
- Serologic testing is useful for detection of arboviruses
- Brain biopsy only needed in patients who have negative CSF PCR and serology

Treatment

- Treatment is generally supportive (see Table 15-5)
- HSV encephalitis should be treated with IV acyclovir to lower morbidity and mortality
- Postexposure prophylaxis with antiserum is given for rabies exposure

TABLE 15-3 Typical Cerebrospinal Fluid Abnormalities in Acute Bacterial and Aseptic Meningitis

	Bacterial	Aseptic
Opening pressure	>20 cm H_2O	<25 cm H_2O
White blood cells	10–10,000/mm³	10–1000/mm³
Differential	Neutrophils predominate	Lymphocytes predominate*
Glucose	<40 mg/dL	>45 mg/dL
Protein	>100 mg/dL	<200 mg/dL
Gram stain	Positive in 60–90% of cases	Negative
Culture	Positive in 70–85% of cases	Negative
Latex agglutination (for antigens of *Streptococcus pneumoniae, Neisseria meningitides, Escherichia coli, Haemophilus influenzae,* and group B streptococcus)	Positive in 50–90% of cases	Negative
PCR of CMV, EBV, viral nucleic acid	Negative	Positive in some cases (i.e., HSV, CMV, EBV, VZV, enteroviruses)

*Neutrophils may predominate in very early viral meningitis.
CMV, cytomegalovirus; EBV, Epstein-Barr virus; HSV, herpes simplex virus; PCR, polymerase chain reaction; VZV, varicella-zoster virus.

Skin and Soft Tissue Infections

See Figure 15-3 and Table 15-6 for examples and summary of skin and soft tissue infections.

Basic Information
- Community-associated methicillin-resistant *Staphylococcus aureus* (CA-MRSA)
- Frequency: Varies by location, but incidence of infection is increasing; in Atlanta in 2003, 63% of community-onset skin and soft tissue infections due to *S. aureus* were CA-MRSA

Clinical Presentation
- Most present with skin or soft tissue infection; some develop necrotizing pneumonia, necrotizing fasciitis, endocarditis, osteomyelitis, or sepsis

Treatment
- Treatment options for MRSA
  - Vancomycin is the drug of choice
  - Many CA-MRSA strains may be sensitive to trimethoprim-sulfamethoxazole (TMP-SMX)
  - Clindamycin has been used with success in children; however, resistance can be inducible
  - Newer agents such as linezolid can be considered, if needed

TABLE 15-4 Indications for Head CT Before Lumbar Puncture When Acute Bacterial Meningitis Is Suspected

Category	Specific Indication
Immunocompromised host	HIV/AIDS, transplant patient, patient on immunosuppressive medications
History of CNS disease	Mass lesion, stroke, focal infection
New-onset seizure	Onset within 1 wk of presentation
Papilledema	Especially if no venous pulsations
Abnormal level of consciousness	Inability to follow 2 consecutive commands or answer 2 consecutive questions
Focal neurologic deficit	Dilated nonreactive pupil, ocular motility abnormalities, abnormal visual fields, gaze palsy, arm or leg drift

AIDS, acquired immunodeficiency syndrome; CNS, central nervous system; CT, computed tomography; HIV, human immunodeficiency virus.

- When to consider empirical treatment: One should base the need for treatment on the local antimicrobial susceptibility patterns in each community. **If the local rates are high, any patient presenting with a serious community-acquired skin or soft tissue infection should be empirically treated for CA-MRSA until a cause is confirmed.**

Acute Bacterial Arthritis

Basic Information
- Usually involves one joint (*monoarticular*)
- Route of infection is usually hematogenous
- Overall, *Neisseria gonorrhoeae* is the most common pathogen in healthy young adults (Fig. 15-4)
- *S. aureus*, groups A, B, C, and G streptococci, *Streptococcus pneumoniae*, and gram-negative bacilli account for most other infections
- Specific organisms should be suspected based on the underlying host (Table 15-7)

Clinical Presentation
- Pain, decreased range of motion, effusion, and erythema are typically seen
- Fever not always present
- Knee or hip most commonly affected

Diagnosis
- Aspiration of synovial fluid is essential to proper diagnosis
  - Ultrasonography, CT scan, or MRI may be helpful for detection and aspiration with involvement of certain joints (e.g., hip, sacroiliac joint)
  - **White blood cell (WBC) counts are usually greater than 50,000/mm³ with greater than 75% neutrophils**

TABLE 15-5	*Selected Viruses Causing Encephalitis*			
Virus	**Transmission**	**Diagnosis**	**Treatment**	**Comments**
Arboviruses California encephalitis (LaCrosse)	Mosquito	Serologic testing	Supportive	Mortality is low
St. Louis encephalitis	Mosquito	Serologic testing	Supportive	Mortality seen in up to 20% of patients
West Nile	Mosquito	PCR and/or IgM in CSF or serum	Supportive	Most infected patients present with febrile illness Advanced age is greatest risk factor for severe disease
Enteroviruses	Fecal-oral	CSF PCR	Supportive	Usually occurs in summer Rash, conjunctivitis, pleurodynia may occur
Herpes simplex virus (HSV)	Contact with mucosal surfaces	CSF PCR	Acyclovir	HSV-1 usually causes encephalitis/HSV-2 usually causes meningitis MRI frequently reveals abnormality in the temporal lobe
Rabies virus	Bite from a rabid animal (dog, cat, bat)	Viral antigen from a nape-of-neck biopsy	Supportive treatment Postexposure prophylaxis with antiserum and active immunization is important	Brainstem dysfunction causes diplopia, neuritis, excessive salivation, respiratory paralysis Consider diagnosis in spelunkers

CSF, cerebrospinal fluid; IgM, immunoglobulin M; MRI, magnetic resonance imaging; PCR, polymerase chain reaction.

FIGURE 15-2 Herpes simplex encephalitis. T2-weighted MRI views showing increased signal in left medial temporal lobe, inferior frontal lobe, and insular cortex. *(From Bradley WG, Daroff RB, Fenichel GM, Jankovic J: Neurology in clinical practice, ed 4, Burlington, MA, Butterworth-Heinemann, 2004, Fig. 59B.1.)*

- The presence of crystals does not rule out infection because crystal-induced arthritis and septic arthritis can occasionally occur together
- Gram stain is positive in one third of cases
- **Joint fluid cultures are positive in up to 90% of nongonococcal bacterial arthritis, but in less than 50% of gonococcal (GC) arthritis**
- Often need genital or pharyngeal culture to confirm GC
- Blood cultures are positive in up to 60% of cases of *S. aureus* but are less helpful with other pathogens

Treatment

- Empirical antimicrobial therapy after blood cultures and joint aspiration depends on Gram stain and patient's age and sexual activity
  - If GC arthritis is suspected, ceftriaxone should be started
  - If *S. aureus* is suspected, a penicillinase-resistant penicillin (e.g., oxacillin) should be used; if hospital acquired, consider vancomycin until sensitivity is known
  - If Gram stain is negative, a third-generation cephalosporin (e.g., ceftriaxone) is reasonable initial coverage
- Repeated aspirations may be necessary if effusions reaccumulate
- Indications for surgical drainage
  - Hip joint involvement (except in cases of GC)
  - Delay of therapy (>1 week after onset of symptoms)
  - Loculated infection or exudate too thick to aspirate
  - Poor response to therapy (e.g., failure to decrease synovial WBC)
  - Prosthetic joint infection (Box 15-1)

Chronic Monoarticular Arthritis

Basic Information

- Frequently caused by bacteria (and mycobacteria), fungi, and, rarely, parasites (Table 15-8)
- If joint culture is negative, synovial biopsy is necessary
- Treatment guided toward specific organism

FIGURE 15-3 **A,** Impetigo.
B, Erysipelas. **C,** Necrotizing fasciitis.
D, Extensive gas gangrene of the
arm. (**A, C,** and **D,** From Cohen J,
Powderly W: Infectious diseases, ed 2,
St. Louis, Mosby, 2004, Figs. 225.18,
225.20, and 10.19. **B,** From Habif TP:
Clinical dermatology, ed 4, St. Louis,
Mosby, 2004, Fig. 9-12.)

TABLE 15-6	**Skin and Soft Tissue Infections**			
	Description	**Pathogens**	**Treatment**	**Comments**
Impetigo (see Fig. 15-3A)	Superficial infection Vesicular with golden crusts	Group A streptococci *Staphylococcus aureus*	Topical and oral antibiotics	Can form bullae
Furuncle (boil)	Deep infection of hair follicle Usually on buttocks, face, neck Painful and tender	*S. aureus*	Moist heat Oral antibiotics Surgical drainage may be needed	Carbuncles are infections of contiguous follicles that extend into subcutaneous fat
Erysipelas (see Fig. 15-3B)	Superficial infection Involves cutaneous lymphatics Usually involves face or extremities Raised, violaceous, painful, spreading lesions with distinct border	Group A streptococci	Oral or IV penicillin	Bullae can develop Systemic toxicity can occur
Cellulitis	Spreading infection of skin and subcutaneous tissue Localized pain, swelling, and warmth No distinct border	Most common: Group A streptococci, *S. aureus* Diabetics: Mixed gram-positive and gram-negative aerobic/anaerobic bacteria Lymphedema: Groups A, B, C, G streptococci	Mild: Oral PRP or erythromycin Severe: PRP ± AG Diabetic: Broad coverage (e.g., cefoxitin + AG) Lymphedema: IV PRP. Can use oral penicillin to prevent recurrences	Tinea pedis may be a portal of entry in some patients Bullae may be present. In patients with cirrhosis and saltwater exposure, consider *Vibrio vulnificus*

Continued on following page

TABLE 15-6	Skin and Soft Tissue Infections *(Continued)*			
	Description	**Pathogens**	**Treatment**	**Comments**
Necrotizing fasciitis (see Fig. 15-3C)	Severe infection of the subcutaneous soft tissues Erythema and swelling progress rapidly to bullae and cutaneous gangrene Predilection for lower extremities, abdominal wall, and perineum (Fournier's gangrene)	Type I: Polymicrobial (anaerobes + streptococci + Enterobacteriaceae) Type II: Group A streptococci Recent cases now also associated with aggressive community-acquired MRSA	Surgical exploration and broad-spectrum antibiotics May need to include vancomycin if considering community-acquired MRSA	Risk factors include diabetes, peripheral vascular disease, surgery, trauma Systemic toxicity develops rapidly High mortality rate if surgical exploration not immediate
Gas gangrene (anaerobic cellulites; see Fig. 15-3D)	Begins as a localized infection in a superficial wound Rapidly spreads across fascial planes causing severe pain and swelling Crepitance may be palpable	*Clostridium perfringens* Other anaerobes	Surgical exploration Penicillin + clindamycin	Progresses from cellulitis to myositis to myonecrosis rapidly High mortality rate
Staphylococcal toxic shock syndrome	Fever, sunburn rash, hypotension progressing to multiorgan failure Desquamation occurs late	Associated with colonization of wound/vagina with toxin-producing *S. aureus* without invasive disease	IV fluid resuscitation Removal/drainage of the colonizing source Antibiotics: PRP or 1st-generation cephalosporins	Most commonly seen in the setting of menstruation Bacteremia or overt infection with *S. aureus* not usually seen
Streptococcal toxic shock syndrome	Fever and hypotension progressing to multiorgan failure Rash and desquamation usually not present	Usually associated with skin/soft tissue infection with toxin-producing group A streptococci	IV fluids Penicillin + clindamycin	Most patients are bacteremic

AG, aminoglycoside; IV, intravenous; MRSA, methicillin-resistant *S. aureus;* PRP, penicillinase-resistant penicillin.

FIGURE 15-4 Gonococcal septic arthritis with an associated papular skin lesion *(arrow)*. *(From Forbes C, Jackson W: Color atlas and text of clinical medicine, ed 3, St. Louis, Mosby, 2003, Fig. 3.8.)*

TABLE 15-7	Organisms Causing Acute Bacterial Arthritis
Organism	**Predisposing Factors and Conditions**
Neisseria gonorrhoeae	Age <30 yr
Staphylococcus aureus	Glucocorticoid therapy Rheumatoid arthritis Diabetes Post–surgical procedure
Streptococcus pneumoniae	HIV Alcoholism Sickle cell anemia Less than half have another focus of *S. pneumoniae* infection
Mycoplasma spp.	Primary immunoglobulin deficiency
Salmonella spp.	HIV Sickle cell disease
Pasteurella multocida	Cat bites or scratches
Other gram-negative bacilli	IV drug use Immunodeficiency Neonates Elderly

BOX 15-1	*Prosthetic Joint Infection*

Early infection: Acquired at surgery, usually low-grade pathogens (e.g., coagulase-negative staphylococci, diphtheroids)

    Late infection: Usually hematogenous seeding with *Staphylococcus aureus* or streptococci

    Wide spectrum of severity but usually have chronic, unremitting pain and may have loosening of the joint

    Definitive diagnosis made by culture of needle aspirate or surgical débridement

    Most successful therapy is removal of entire prosthesis and 6 weeks of antibiotic therapy

Viral Arthritis

Basic Information

- Caused by direct invasion of the synovium or by an immune reaction involving certain joints
- Usually a migratory polyarthritis
- Many viruses implicated
  - Rubella
    - Can occur following infection or immunization
    - Usually seen in women
    - Self-limited disease but, rarely, can persist for years
  - Mumps
    - More common in men
    - Develops within 2 weeks of parotitis
  - Parvovirus B19
    - Hands most frequently involved
    - Infection in adults can occur without fever or rash
    - Self-limited: Usually resolves within 8 to 10 weeks
  - Hepatitis B
    - Can manifest as arthralgias or symmetrical arthritis
    - Symptoms (arthralgias or arthritis) occur before jaundice and resolve when jaundice develops
- Most are self-limited: No specific treatment for the arthritis is available

Osteomyelitis

Basic Information

- Defined as an infection of bone
- Two basic types based on the route of infection
  - Hematogenous source
    - Caused by seeding of the bone during bacteremia
    - Primarily occurs in children and older adults
    - IV drug users
      - May have involvement of the vertebrae, sternoclavicular, sacroiliac, or symphysis pubis
      - *S. aureus, Pseudomonas, Serratia,* and *Eikenella* are the more common pathogens for this group
    - *S. aureus* is the organism most frequently isolated
    - Patients with sickle cell disease may be infected with *S. aureus* or *Salmonella*
    - Vertebral involvement caused by *S. aureus,* gram-negative bacilli, tuberculosis (TB; Pott disease), or *Candida*

TABLE 15-8	*Selected Pathogens Causing Chronic Monoarticular Arthritis*
Borrelia burgdorferi (Lyme disease)	50% of untreated patients develop monoarthritis or oligoarthritis of large joint(s) Serology is positive in almost all patients with arthritis See Chapter 16 for further information
Mycobacterium tuberculosis	Usually involves large joints (hips, knees, or ankles) Swelling and pain worsen over months to year; systemic signs and symptoms are frequently absent; synovial fluid examination reveals about 50% neutrophils; acid-fast stain is positive in less than half of cases; culture is frequently positive; synovial biopsy culture has higher yield Treat 6–9 mo with multiple agents (see Chapter 13)
Atypical mycobacteria	Usually involves smaller joints (wrists, hands) Infection occurs from inoculation from water or soil, so may see as a result of gardening or water-related activities Synovial biopsy necessary to make the diagnosis
Brucella spp.	Can cause acute or chronic monoarthritis or asymmetrical polyarthritis Febrile illness frequently coexists Transmission is through ingestion of unpasteurized milk or cheese, ingestion of raw meat, or inhalation during contact with animals (e.g., slaughterhouse workers) Treat with doxycycline + aminoglycoside
Sporothrix schenckii	Seen in gardeners or those who work with soil
Candida spp.	Results from surgical procedures or articular injections IV drug users may have involvement of spine or sacroiliac joint Treat with drainage and antifungal therapy

- Contiguous source
  - Accounts for most cases of osteomyelitis
  - Includes infections resulting from extension from adjacent soft tissue, injury, or surgery
  - Presentation is more indolent than with hematogenous spread
  - Diabetic foot ulcers and decubitus ulcers are common sources
  - **Most infections are polymicrobial,** although *S. aureus* is still frequently found
  - ***Pseudomonas aeruginosa* should be considered in the setting of a puncture wound of the foot**

Clinical Presentation

- Fever
- Bone pain over the affected site

Diagnosis

- Blood studies
  - Sedimentation rate and C-reactive protein elevated in most cases
  - Blood cultures more likely to be positive in cases of hematogenous spread

FIGURE 15-5 Diabetic abscess. **A,** Note discoloration proximal to abscess beneath first metatarsal head. **B,** Results of osteomyelitis of the first metatarsal with bony erosion (*arrow*) seen on radiograph. (*A, From Canale ST: Campbell's operative orthopaedics, ed 10, St. Louis, Mosby, 2003, Fig. 82-11A. B, From Forbes C, Jackson W: Color atlas and text of clinical medicine, ed 3, St. Louis, Mosby, 2003, Fig. 3.152.)*

- Radiologic and imaging studies
  - Plain radiographs
    - May show periosteal elevation, soft tissue swelling, or lytic changes (Fig. 15-5)
    - Findings not present during early infection
  - Technetium bone scan
    - Detects early lesions with high sensitivity
    - Best when bone was previously normal (false positives common with previously abnormal bone)
    - Cannot distinguish infection from tumor, fracture, or infarction
  - MRI
    - As sensitive as bone scan for acute osteomyelitis
    - **Test of choice for vertebral osteomyelitis because it better defines the surrounding soft tissue**
- Subperiosteal aspirate or bone biopsy cultures are needed to make a definitive diagnosis if blood cultures are negative
- **Swab cultures of sinus tract or ulcer base are unreliable for making a microbiologic diagnosis**

Treatment

- Early diagnosis and treatment are important to prevent bone necrosis
- Therapy for acute osteomyelitis usually consists of 6 weeks of IV antibiotics directed by the culture results
- Chronic osteomyelitis often requires therapy for more than 3 months (until erythrocyte sedimentation rate [ESR] normalizes)
- In patients with polymicrobial (aerobic and anaerobic) infections, amoxicillin/clavulanate or clindamycin plus ciprofloxacin can be used
- Surgery may be needed to remove devitalized bone or to restore vascular supply (if there is vascular insufficiency)

Fever of Unknown Origin

Basic Information

- Classified by a patient's condition and setting in which the fever manifests (Table 15-9)
- Most cases are caused by infections, noninfectious inflammatory diseases, or neoplasms
- Specific etiologies of classic FUO may be suggested by the patient's history (Table 15-10)

TABLE 15-9	Classification of Fever of Unknown Origin (FUO)	
Category	**Definition**	**Common Underlying Causes**
Classic FUO	Fever ≥38.3°C for ≥3 wk Blood cultures negative Lack of diagnosis with 3 outpatient visits or 3 inpatient days	Infection Cancer Collagen vascular diseases Granulomatous disease
Nosocomial FUO	Hospitalized patient with no fever on admission 3 days of investigation 2 days of negative incubating cultures	*Clostridium difficile* Phlebitis Sinusitis Drug fever
Neutropenic FUO	Absolute neutrophil count <500/µL 3 days of investigation 2 days of negative incubating cultures	Perianal infection *Aspergillus* spp. *Candida* spp.
HIV-associated FUO	HIV-positive patient Fever ≥3 wk in outpatients or >3 days for inpatients 3 days of investigation 2 days of negative incubating cultures	Mycobacteria Lymphoma Drug fever Cytomegalovirus *Pneumocystis jiroveci* (previously *P. carinii*) pneumonia

TABLE 15-10	Etiologic Considerations for Classic Fever of Unknown Origin
History	**Disease**
Foreign-born individuals	Extrapulmonary tuberculosis
Age >50 yr	Malignancy Giant cell arteritis
High fevers with arthralgias/arthritis	Still disease
Medical background with undocumented fevers	Factitious fever

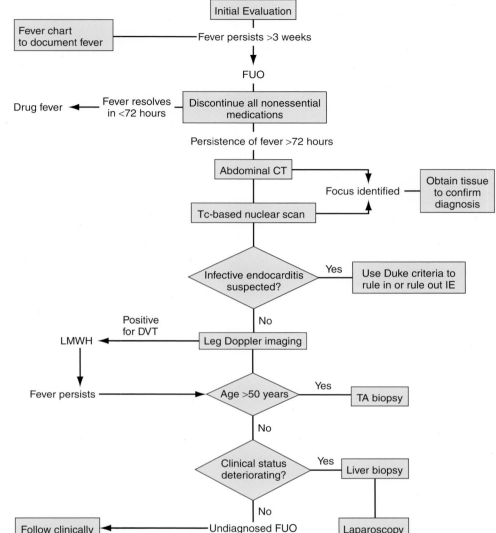

FIGURE 15-6 Diagnostic approach to fever of unknown origin (FUO). (CT, computed tomography; DVT, deep vein thrombosis; IE, infective endocarditis; LMWH, low-molecular-weight heparin; TA, temporal artery; Tc, technetium.) *(From Mourad O, Palda V, Detsky AS: A comprehensive evidence-based approach to fever of unknown origin. Arch Intern Med 163:549, 2003, Fig. 2.)*

Diagnosis

- A thorough history, including travel, hobbies, history of TB exposure, HIV risk factors, and medications, should be obtained to guide the evaluation
- Repeated physical examinations may be necessary to detect slowly progressing diseases
- Basic testing should include the following:
  - Complete blood count (CBC)
  - Comprehensive metabolic panel
  - Urinalysis
  - ESR and C-reactive protein
  - Blood cultures (>3 sets)
  - Chest radiograph
- Purified protein derivative should be placed and HIV testing considered
- CT scan of abdomen plus sinuses may be helpful in the absence of other localizing signs
- Further evaluation should be based on any findings from the history, physical, and basic laboratory tests

- Administration of naproxen may help distinguish between neoplasia and infection because the fever from neoplasms is thought to be more responsive to the medication
- Try to avoid empirical antibiotics because they may suppress, but not cure, an occult infection and may interfere with the ability to make a diagnosis
- Drug-induced fever should be considered a diagnosis of exclusion; it is confirmed by stopping the potentially offending agent
  - Usually patients do not appear as toxic as with other causes of FUO
  - **Rash and eosinophilia are sometimes present, but their absence does not rule out drug fever**
  - Some common causes are sulfonamides, β-lactam antibiotics, phenytoin, amiodarone, and nitrofurantoin
- Figure 15-6 shows an algorithm for diagnostic approach to FUO
- The cause of the FUO may not be found in approximately 30% of adults, but most of those without a diagnosis still have a good prognosis

REVIEW QUESTIONS

For review questions, please go to www.expertconsult.com.

SUGGESTED READINGS

Anaya DA, Dellinger EP: Necrotizing soft-tissue infection: diagnosis and management, *Clin Infect Dis* 44:705–710, 2007.

Cunha BA: Fever of unknown origin, *Infect Dis Clin North Am* 21:867–915, 2007.

Durack DT, Street AC: Fever of unknown origin reexamined and redefined, *Curr Clin Top Infect Dis* 11:35–51, 1991.

Mandell GL, Bennett JE, Dolin R, editors: *Principles and practice of infectious diseases*, ed 7, Philadelphia, 2010, Churchill Livingstone.

Smith JW, Chalupa P, Shabaz Hasan M: Infectious arthritis: clinical features, laboratory findings and treatment, *Clin Microbiol Infect* 12:309–314, 2006.

Tunkel AR, Hartman BJ, Kaplan SL, et al: Practice guidelines for the management of bacterial meningitis, *Clin Infect Dis* 39:1267–1284, 2004.

Tunkel AR, Glaser CA, Bloch KC, et al: The management of encephalitis: clinical practice guidelines by the Infectious Diseases Society of America, *Clin Infect Dis* 47:303–327, 2008.

Zimmerli W: Vertebral osteomyelitis, *N Engl J Med* 362:1022–1029, 2010.

Selected Topics in Infectious Disease II

JOHN N. AUCOTT, MD

This chapter is divided into three sections on selected topics in infectious disease encountered by the internist: (1) endocarditis, (2) tick-borne illnesses, and (3) infections from bite and scratch wounds.

Infective Endocarditis

Basic Information

- **Infective endocarditis may present as an acute infection with devastating consequences or with a slowly progressive course and subtle clinical findings.** The diagnosis may be straightforward or may require a combination of laboratory and clinical findings. Prolonged antibiotic treatment is required, with monitoring for progression despite therapy.
  - **Endocarditis most commonly refers to infection of one of the heart valves, but it may also occur on an atrial or ventricular septal defect or elsewhere in the endocardium**
  - Bacterial and fungal organisms may cause endocarditis
  - There are noninfectious inflammatory conditions of the endocardium and valves (e.g., Libman-Sacks endocarditis associated with systemic lupus erythematosus [SLE])
  - **In subacute bacterial endocarditis, the mitral valve is the most common valve infected, followed by the aortic valve.** Much less common is tricuspid valve involvement. Infection of the pulmonic valve is rare.
    - In acute bacterial endocarditis (usually caused by *Staphylococcus aureus*), infection of the aortic valve is most common (Fig. 16-1)
- Acute versus subacute endocarditis
  - Classically, acute endocarditis was caused by *S. aureus* and progressed to death if not treated in 6 weeks
  - Subacute endocarditis was most commonly caused by other organisms such as the viridans group of streptococci and even if not treated could persist for up to 1 year before death
  - However, the increasing prevalence of prosthetic heart valves, along with the evolving infectious etiologies of endocarditis, have made this distinction less clinically useful
  - **Etiologic agent, rather than acute versus subacute endocarditis, is now used to classify endocarditis since the etiologic agent determines treatment**

- Predisposing factors
  - Abnormal native heart valve is the most common predisposing factor
    - Mitral valve prolapse among most common (20–30% of cases), with murmur or thickened valve associated with highest risk
    - Rheumatic heart disease less common
    - Bicuspid aortic valves usually seen as predisposing factor for endocarditis in patients older than 60 years
  - Prosthetic valves
  - Congenital heart disease, including atrial and ventricular septal defects and patent ductus arteriosus
  - Prior endocarditis

Clinical Presentation

- Signs and symptoms
  - **Cardiac involvement: new regurgitant murmur, vegetations on echocardiography (absence of a visible vegetation does not exclude diagnosis), conduction abnormalities (especially with endocarditis of aortic valve), myocarditis, congestive heart failure**
  - Right-sided endocarditis: cough, chest pain, pleurisy, cavitating pulmonary infiltrates
  - Systemic inflammation: Fever, fatigue or failure to thrive, arthralgias; positive rheumatoid factor is seen in 50% of cases
  - Emboli: Seen in approximately one third of patients and may involve any organ; if central nervous system (CNS) is involved, middle cerebral artery is most commonly affected; large emboli are more common in fungal endocarditis
  - Mycotic aneurysms may be seen, usually in the cerebral arteries and aorta, but may also involve other major arteries
  - Immune complex disease: glomerulonephritis, Osler nodes (tender nodules on finger or toe pads), Janeway lesions (nodular hemorrhages on palms of hands or soles of feet), splinter hemorrhages (especially in proximal nail beds; Fig. 16-2)
  - Other: Roth spots (retinal hemorrhages; Fig. 16-3), petechiae, splenomegaly, digital clubbing
- Etiologic agents (Table 16-1)
  - Typical endocarditis organisms: Streptococci and staphylococci account for 80% to 90% of endocarditis

FIGURE 16-1 Infective endocarditis. Parasternal long-axis view echocardiogram of a patient with a large aortic valve vegetation (*arrow*). (Ao, aorta; LA, left atrium; LV, left ventricle.) *(From Zipes DP: Braunwald's heart disease: a textbook of cardiovascular medicine, ed 7, Philadelphia, Elsevier Saunders, 2005, Fig. 11-81.)*

FIGURE 16-2 Splinter hemorrhages and petechiae in a patient with infective endocarditis. *(From Zipes DP: Braunwald's heart disease: a textbook of cardiovascular medicine, ed 7, Philadelphia, Elsevier Saunders, 2005, Fig. 58-4.)*

- **Streptococci cause 60% to 80% of cases, with viridans streptococci the most common cause**
  - Pyogenic strep: Groups A, C rarely cause endocarditis
  - ***Streptococcus bovis:* Associated with GI neoplasms; should prompt evaluation of the colon for malignancy**
  - *Streptococcus mutans:* An oral pathogen; may cause endocarditis in the susceptible host with poor dentition

FIGURE 16-3 Roth spots in a patient with infective endocarditis. *(From Zipes DP: Braunwald's heart disease: a textbook of cardiovascular medicine, ed 7, Philadelphia, Elsevier Saunders, 2005, Fig. 58-5.)*

TABLE 16-1	*Causes of Bacterial Endocarditis*	
Endocarditis Subtype	**Most Common Organism**	**Other Common Organisms**
"Typical"	Viridans streptococci Many species highly associated such as *Streptococcus mutans*	*Staphylococcus aureus* Other streptococcal species *Staphylococcus epidermidis* (uncommon) Enterococci (uncommon)
Culture-negative	No dominant organism	*Haemophilus aphrophilus* *Haemophilus parainfluenzae* *Actinobacillus actinomycetemcomitans* *Cardiobacterium hominis* *Eikenella corrodens* *Kingella kingii*
Injection drug use	*S. aureus*	*Pseudomonas aeruginosa* *Candida* Enterococci *Streptococcus viridans* *S. epidermidis* Polymicrobial
Unusual causes	No dominant organism	Fungi: *Candida, Aspergillus* *Coxiella burnetii* *Bartonella* *Chlamydia* *Legionella* *Brucella* *Mycoplasma*
Early prosthetic valve	*S. epidermidis*	*S. aureus* Gram-negative bacilli Enterococci Diphtheroids Fungi
Late prosthetic valve	*S. epidermidis*	*S. viridans* *S. aureus* Gram-negative bacilli Enterococci

- Staphylococci cause 20% to 30% of cases, with *S. aureus* the most common cause
  - *S. aureus* infection, which may attack normal heart valves, results in rapid progression with valve destruction and is the most common cause of what is classically termed *acute endocarditis*
  - **Enterococci are an increasingly prevalent cause of endocarditis and are common in older men following genitourinary instrumentation or in women following obstetric procedures**
  - *Pseudomonas:* Typically in those with history of IV drug use; usually right-sided
- Culture-negative endocarditis: May present with endocardial vegetation or embolic events; blood culture should be held for 3 weeks if suspected
  - HACEK (*Haemophilus aphrophilus, Actinobacillus actinomycetemcomitans, Cardiobacterium hominis, Eikenella corrodens,* and *Kingella kingae*) group accounts for 3% to 5% of native valve infections (see Table 16-1)
- Unusual endocarditis organisms
  - *Coxiella burnetii* (Q fever): Diagnosed by serology; culture often negative
  - Fungi: *Candida* spp. most common, followed by *Aspergillus* spp.; susceptible hosts include those with history of injection drug use, prosthetic heart valve recipients, immunocompromised hosts
  - *Bartonella, Chlamydia, Legionella, Brucella, Mycoplasma* spp. are rare causes of endocarditis
- Prosthetic valves
  - Early prosthetic valve endocarditis is infection of a prosthetic valve within 60 days of valve insertion
  - Late prosthetic valve endocarditis occurs after 60 days of valve insertion
  - **Early infection makes up one third of prosthetic valve infections, whereas late infection makes up most cases of prosthetic valve endocarditis**
  - ***Staphylococcus epidermidis* is the most common cause of prosthetic valve endocarditis**
  - *Streptococcus viridans* is a rare cause of early prosthetic valve endocarditis but is a relatively common cause of late prosthetic valve endocarditis

Diagnosis and Evaluation

- Diagnosing endocarditis requires a high index of suspicion in the appropriate clinical setting, coupled with demonstration of microbial infection of the heart valves or endocardium
- Definite bacterial endocarditis is a pathologic diagnosis made by culture of a surgical specimen or at autopsy
  - Clinical criteria can be used to diagnose cases of definite endocarditis (Table 16-2), typically requiring demonstration of persistent bacteremia by blood culture, along with echocardiographic and clinical findings
    - Blood cultures: Standard initial drawing should be three separate sets of cultures drawn from three different sites over 1 hour
    - Echocardiography
      - Transthoracic echocardiography (TTE): First step with native valves; sensitivity is 44% to 63%

TABLE 16-2	*Diagnostic Criteria for Endocarditis**
Major Criteria	**Minor Criteria**
Positive blood culture Typical microorganism of endocarditis from two separate blood cultures Persistently positive blood cultures with a microorganism consistent with endocarditis, defined as blood cultures drawn more than 12 hr apart, or 3 of 3 positive sets of blood cultures drawn over the course of at least 1 hr Evidence of endocardial involvement Positive echocardiogram, demonstrating oscillating intracardiac mass or abscess, or dehiscent prosthetic valve New valvular regurgitation (excludes worsening of preexisting murmur)	Fever 38°C or higher Predisposing heart condition or injection drug use Vascular phenomena Arterial emboli Septic pulmonary infarcts Mycotic aneurysm Intracranial hemorrhage Conjunctival hemorrhage Janeway lesions Immunologic phenomena Glomerulonephritis Osler nodes Roth spots Rheumatoid factor Microbiologic evidence Positive blood cultures that do not meet major criteria Echocardiographic evidence Consistent with endocarditis but not meeting major criteria

*Endocarditis is diagnosed with two major criteria, one major plus three minor criteria, or five minor criteria.
Adapted from Durack DT, Lukes AS, Bright DK: New criteria for diagnosis of infective endocarditis: utilization of specific echocardiographic findings, *Am J Med* 96:200–209, 1994.

- Transesophageal echocardiography (TEE): Reserve for prosthetic valves or (−) TTE with abnormal valve (+) intermediate to high probability
- Possible endocarditis, in which diagnostic criteria are not met, should be treated as endocarditis until an alternate diagnosis is confirmed

Treatment

- Treatment principles in endocarditis
  - Parenteral antibiotics preferred to ensure consistent antibiotic levels
  - Extended therapy indicated because shorter courses associated with increased risk of relapse
  - Bactericidal antibiotics are superior to bacteriostatic antibiotics in achieving cure
    - **Antimicrobial choice should be guided by culture and sensitivity results (Table 16-3)**
- Surgical considerations
  - Failure of medical therapy
    - May be manifested by prolonged fever (often indicative of aortic valve ring abscess, which may be accompanied by evidence of atrioventricular conduction abnormalities)
    - New embolic events
    - Mycotic aneurysms
    - Persistent positive blood cultures may also be evidence of failure of medical therapy
  - Other indications for surgery
    - Major embolic events
    - Valvular dysfunction
    - Congestive heart failure
    - Fungal endocarditis

TABLE 16-3	Synopsis of Treatment of Bacterial Endocarditis	
Organism	**Standard Treatment**	**Comments**
Streptococcus viridans, with penicillin MIC <0.1	4 wk penicillin or ceftriaxone	2 wk penicillin or ceftriaxone, combined with gentamicin reasonable alternative
S. viridans, penicillin MIC >0.1	4 wk penicillin or ceftriaxone, combined with aminoglycoside for first 2 wk	
Staphylococcus aureus, left-sided	4 wk nafcillin combined with gentamicin for initial 3–5 days	MRSA treated with 4–6 wk daily vancomycin
S. aureus, right-sided	2 wk nafcillin combined with gentamicin	Treatment applies only to methicillin-sensitive staphylococci, with no embolic events
Prosthetic valve	6 wk therapy with penicillin derivative or vancomycin (depending on sensitivities) in combination with rifampin, plus aminoglycoside for initial 2 wk	Early surgical consultation advised Fungal infection of prosthetic valve requires surgery in most cases
Enterococcus	6 wk penicillin combined with gentamicin	If aminoglycoside resistance demonstrated, 8–12 wk penicillin indicated Other antimicrobial resistance common and should prompt consultation with infectious disease team
Fungal	Early surgery usually required	

MIC, minimum infective concentration; MRSA, methicillin-resistant *Staphylococcus aureus.*

Prevention of Endocarditis
- Endocarditis prophylaxis
  - Endocarditis prophylaxis recommendations were recently revised because the risk of endocarditis from dental procedures is thought to be less than previous estimates
  - Prophylaxis should be done in patients with high-risk cardiac conditions, defined as:
    - Prosthetic cardiac valve or prosthetic material used for cardiac valve repair
    - Previous infective endocarditis
    - Congenital heart disease (CHD), specifically:
      - Unrepaired cyanotic CHD, including palliative shunts and conduits

- Completely repaired congenital heart defect with prosthetic material or device, whether placed by surgery or by catheter intervention, during the first 6 months after the procedure
- Repaired CHD with residual defects at the site or adjacent to the site of a prosthetic patch or prosthetic device
- Cardiac transplant recipients who develop cardiac valvulopathy
- Dental or respiratory procedure (prophylaxis not recommended for bronchoscopy): Single-dose amoxicillin (2 g) 1 hour before procedure (clindamycin, clarithromycin, or azithromycin if penicillin allergic)
- Bowel or genitourinary procedures: Ampicillin (vancomycin if penicillin allergic) plus gentamicin 1 hour before procedure, ampicillin 6 hours later
- Low-risk patients for whom antibiotic prophylaxis is not recommended
  - Mitral valve prolapse
  - Bicuspid aortic valve
  - Acquired aortic or mitral valve disease
  - Pacemakers
  - Defibrillators
- Low-risk procedures for which antibiotic prophylaxis is not recommended
  - GI endoscopy (except sclerosis or dilatation/endoscopic retrograde cholangiopancreatography [ERCP])
  - Restorative dentistry
  - Gynecologic procedures: vaginal hysterectomy, vaginal delivery, cesarean section
  - Cardiac procedures: cardiac catheterization, balloon angioplasty

Tick-Borne Illnesses

Basic Information
- Tick-borne illnesses are best understood by understanding not only their clinical manifestations but also their vectors, reservoirs, geographic distribution, and seasonal variations (Table 16-4)
- Most people with tick-borne infections do not remember a recent tick bite, and most tick bites do not result in a tick-borne infection
- **In most cases, early manifestations of tick-borne disease are nonspecific flu-like symptoms of fever, fatigue, generalized achiness with or without a rash**
- Lyme disease may present with later symptoms of arthritis or neurologic manifestions of VIIth nerve palsy, symptoms of CNS infection, or peripheral neuropathy

Clinical Presentation
Table 16-5 compares the clinical features of tick-borne illnesses
- Rocky Mountain spotted fever (RMSF)
  - After incubation period of 2 to 14 days, flu-like symptoms of fever, myalgias, and GI upset develop
  - Characteristic rash develops 3 to 5 days after onset of fever (Fig. 16-4)

TABLE 16-4	*Comparison of Tick-Borne Illnesses*			
Illness	**Etiologic Agent**	**Vector**	**Reservoir**	**Geographic Distribution**
Rocky Mountain spotted fever	*Rickettsia rickettsii*	Eastern United States: Dog tick (*Dermacentor variabilis*) Western United States: Rocky Mountain wood tick (*Dermacentor andersoni*)	Vector tick is also reservoir	South-central and mid-Atlantic states (uncommon in western United States and Rocky Mountains)
Human monocytic ehrlichiosis	*Ehrlichia chaffeensis*	Lone-star tick (*Amblyomma americanum*)	Deer	Midwest; south-central and southeastern United States
Human granulocytic anaplasmosis	*Anaplasma phagocytophilum*	Deer tick (*Ixodes scapularis*)	Unknown	Scattered east and west coast states; northern states; Florida
Babesiosis	United States: *Babesia microti* Europe: *Babesia divergens, Babesia bovis*	Ticks (*I. scapularis*)	Rodents (especially white-footed mouse); cattle	Northeast coastal states
Lyme disease	*Borrelia burgdorferi*	Deer tick (*I. scapularis*)	Mouse	Northeast; Wisconsin and Minnesota; Pacific Northwest

TABLE 16-5	*Comparison of Clinical Features of Tick-Borne Illnesses*		
	Rash	**Laboratory**	**Diagnostic Test of Choice**
Rocky Mountain spotted fever	Begins distally (palms or soles) Spreads to involve arms, legs, then trunk Begins as maculopapular eruption, evolving to petechial or purpuric appearance Seen in 90%	Laboratory findings nonspecific WBC typically normal Renal insufficiency and acute tubular necrosis common CSF may show elevated protein if neurologic involvement	Early clinical diagnosis required to prevent death; occasionally rickettsiae may be demonstrated in biopsy of rash; diagnosis may be confirmed by acute and convalescent serology.
Human monocytic ehrlichiosis (HME)	Rash seen in ⅓ Maculopapular eruption; rarely petechial	Leukopenia and thrombocytopenia, neutropenia common Transaminitis and renal insufficiency common	Clinical diagnosis but fourfold increase in antibody titer to *Ehrlichia chaffeensis*; monocytic inclusions may be seen.
Hemolytic granulocytic anaplasmosis (HGA)	Same as HME	Same as HME	Clinical diagnosis, but fourfold increase in antibody titer to *Anaplasma phacocytophilum* granulocytic inclusions may be seen. PCR available for acute diagnosis.
Babesiosis	Rash from babesiosis unusual, but coinfection with Lyme disease is common and should be investigated in all patients with babesiosis	Hemolytic anemia (pronounced) Mild transaminitis	Thick or thin blood smear demonstrates intraerythrocytic parasites PCR of blood.
Lyme disease	Erythema migrans rash 80% Not always "bull's-eye" rash	WBC typically normal without leukocytosis Mild transaminitis rarely	ELISA; negative in 70–80% in weeks 1–2; positive when repeated weeks 4–6.

CSF, cerebrospinal fluid; ELISA, enzyme-linked immunosorbent assay; PCR, polymerase chain reaction; WBC, white blood cell.

- **Disease may be fatal, especially if not diagnosed and treated early in illness (case fatality rate approaches 20%)**
- Ehrlichiosis and anaplasmosis (human monocytic ehrlichiosis [HME] and human granulocytic anaplasmosis [HGA])
  - After an incubation period of 1 week, flu-like symptoms of high fever (>103°F), headache, myalgias, and malaise develop; often accompanied by thrombocytopenia and mild elevation of aspartate aminotransferase (AST) and alanine aminotransferase (ALT)
- **Presenting symptoms may be mild; rash is uncommon, and its absence helps distinguish these disorders from RMSF and Lyme disease**
- HGA may occur as coinfection with Lyme disease
- Most patients have mild illness. Severe illness, with renal failure and respiratory insufficiency is uncommon but has been described.

FIGURE 16-4 Florid petechial rash on the arm of a patient with Rocky Mountain spotted fever. *(From Mandell GL, Bennett JE, Dolin R [eds]: Principles and practice of infectious diseases, ed 6, Philadelphia, Churchill Livingstone, 2005, Fig. 184-4.)*

FIGURE 16-5 Erythema migrans rash of Lyme disease with classic "bull's-eye" appearance.

- Babesiosis
  - **Mild symptoms are the rule in North America, except in patients with asplenia, who may experience overwhelming infection with hypotension, acute respiratory distress syndrome**
  - After incubation of 1 to 3 weeks, flu-like symptoms of fever, headache, myalgias, and arthralgias occur, often accompanied by dark urine (resulting from hemolysis)
  - Coinfection with *Borrelia burgdorferi* (Lyme disease) common and should be considered in all patients with babesiosis
- Lyme disease
  - Occurs as both acute localized cutaneous rash and as disseminated early and late manifestations; as previously discussed, always consider coinfection with babesiosis or HGA when diagnosing Lyme disease
    - **Localized erythema migrans is most common acute presentation** (spreading erythematous rash; minority of rashes have central clearing or classic "bull's-eye" appearance; Figs. 16-5 and 16-6)
      - The rash is noted in at least 80% of cases
  - Malaise, headache, migratory myalgias, and arthralgias are common and may occur with or without rash
    - Disseminated infection may occur within days to weeks of infection (Fig. 16-7)
      - Cutaneous dissemination with multiple areas of distant skin involvement with pleomorphic-appearing rash
      - Neurologic symptoms may include cranial neuritis (most commonly VIIth nerve), meningitis, radicular pain syndromes
      - Cardiac symptoms may include atrioventricular block and myocarditis
    - Late infection results from persistent infection at systemic sites seeded during primary infection
      - Persistent infection occurs months to years after infection, manifested primarily with musculoskeletal disease
      - **Classic manifestation is monoarthritis of the knee, with effusion occurring months after infection**
      - Radiculopathy or symmetrical sensory neuropathy can occur

FIGURE 16-6 Erythema migrans rash of Lyme disease with uniform erythema.

FIGURE 16-7 Cutaneous dissemination of Lyme disease presenting with pleomorphic rash.

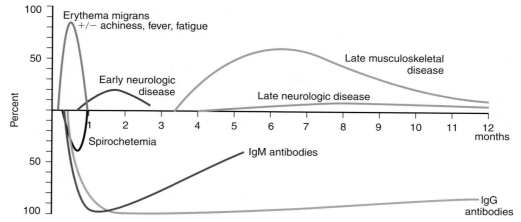

FIGURE 16-8 Natural history of untreated Lyme disease showing both acute and chronic phases of illness. (IgG, immunoglobulin G; IgM, immunoglobulin M.)

Diagnosis

Figure 16-8 provides an algorithm of the history of untreated Lyme disease (see also Table 16-5)

- Early features of most tick-borne illnesses are similar; high index of suspicion coupled with geographic distribution contribute to diagnosis
- Clinical presentation of many of these disorders should prompt initiation of treatment before definitive test results available
- Rash may assist in diagnosis of patients, particularly with RMSF and Lyme disease (see Table 16-5)
- **Other laboratory features may support diagnosis, such as thrombocytopenia (which suggests anaplasmosis), but many findings, such as mild elevation of AST and ALT, are shared across disorders**

Treatment

- **RMSF, ehrlichiosis, anaplasmosis, and Lyme disease all respond to doxycycline**
  - RMSF: Doxycycline 100 mg twice daily for 1 week
  - Anaplasmosis and ehrlichiosis: Doxycycline 100 mg twice daily for 10 days
  - Lyme disease: Doxycycline 100 mg twice daily for 14 days, which will treat possibility of coinfection with HGA
    - Amoxicillin used for children where doxycycline contraindicated
  - Lyme arthritis: 30 days oral doxycycline or amoxicillin; re-treatment for recurrent arthritis with 28 days of oral therapy or IV ceftriaxone
  - Neuroborreliosis (i.e., meningitis or radiculopathy due to Lyme disease) or cardiac involvement: Ceftriaxone IV for 14 to 28 days
  - Lyme disease prophylaxis
    - A 200-mg single dose of doxycycline may be effective as postexposure prophylaxis; the Infectious Disease Society of America recommends its use only when all of the following criteria are met:
      1. Attached tick identified as an adult or nymphal *Ixodes scapularis* tick (deer tick)
      2. Tick is estimated to have been attached for ≥36 hours (by degree of engorgement or time of exposure)
      3. Prophylaxis is begun within 72 hours of tick removal
      4. Local rate of infection of ticks with *B. burgdorferi* is ≥20% (these rates of infection have been shown to occur in parts of New England, parts of the mid-Atlantic states, and parts of Minnesota and Wisconsin)
    - Vaccine for Lyme disease discontinued; long-term protection unclear, especially without availability of boosters
- Babesiosis may be asymptomatic and may not require treatment. Symptomatic patients and those with asplenia should be treated with atovaquone and azithromycin. Exchange transfusion may be necessary in cases with high-grade parasitemia greater than 10%. Relapses of symptomatic disease have been observed in patients with asplenia or underlying malignancy.

Infection from Bite and Scratch Wounds

Basic Information

- Humans, dogs, and cats harbor bacterial pathogens in the oral cavity that can cause significant infection in humans when bitten. In addition, a well-described illness may follow scratch wounds from cats.
  - **Treatment of infection before symptoms develop is the standard of care with bite wounds, although dog bites become infected in a minority of cases**
  - Immunization for tetanus should be current (or updated, if not), and consideration should be given to the possibility of rabies

Clinical Presentation

- Most bite wounds occur on the upper extremities but are also commonly seen on the face and lower extremities
- **Superficial abrasions should be cleaned and otherwise need no treatment**
  - Deep bite wounds and wounds inflicted on a closed fist may need extensive débridement and surgical evaluation

- Human bites may introduce infection with *S. viridans*, *S. epidermidis*, *S. aureus*, *Eikenella*, and other species
- Dog bites may introduce infection with *Pasteurella multocida*, *S. aureus*, and, less commonly, *Bacteroides*, *Fusobacterium*, and *Capnocytophagia*
- **Cat bites may introduce infection with *P. multocida* or *S. aureus*; deep bites risk the development of osteomyelitis**
- The major risk from cat scratches (almost always from kittens) is infection with *Bartonella henselae* (i.e., cat-scratch disease)
    - Regional adenopathy developing 2 weeks after a cat scratch (by which time the injury is likely to have healed) is the most common presentation and may be accompanied by malaise and fever
    - Adenopathy may progress to lymphadenitis and rarely to suppuration
    - More serious manifestations include seizures and coma and are more common in children

Diagnosis

- Bite wounds present with an obvious history and present little in the way of clinical dilemmas
    - Cat-scratch disease may be missed in a patient presenting with adenopathy unless an inciting injury is specifically queried
    - Antibody titers for *B. henselae* are available but unlikely to be of use in the acute setting
- *Pasteurella* infection typically becomes symptomatic in 24 hours
- Treatment for bite wounds is empirical and not based on culture results
- If the patient with a history of cat bite presents late (i.e., days or weeks after injury), consideration should be given to osteomyelitis

Treatment

- **The major consideration for pathogens in animal bites, particularly in cat bites, is treatment to cover infection with *P. multocida***
    - *P. multocida* is resistant to typical agents used to cover cellulitis (i.e., dicloxacillin, cephalexin, erythromycin)

- **Treatment is typically with amoxicillin/clavulanate or clindamycin plus a fluoroquinolone (in penicillin-allergic patients)**
- Dog bites may introduce *P. multocida* and rarely cause infection with *Capnocytophagia*, which in asplenic patients may result in sepsis
    - *Capnocytophagia* infection responds to amoxicillin/clavulanate or clindamycin
- If rabies is a consideration, treatment should be rabies immune globulin and rabies vaccine
- Human bites are more commonly associated with cellulitis from *Staphylococcus* or *Streptococcus* spp. and should be treated with amoxicillin/clavulanate or clindamycin
    - *Eikenella* spp. may be resistant to both and often require a fluoroquinolone for treatment
- Cat-scratch disease is treated with macrolides (clarithromycin, azithromycin) or fluoroquinolones

REVIEW QUESTIONS

For review questions, please go to www.expertconsult.com.

SUGGESTED READINGS

Dumler JS, Bakken JS: Ehrlichial diseases of humans: emerging tick-borne infections, *Clin Infect Dis* 20:1102–1110, 1995.

Durack DT, Lukes AS, Bright DK: New criteria for diagnosis of infective endocarditis: utilization of specific echocardiographic findings. Duke Endocarditis Service, *Am J Med* 96:200–209, 1994.

Wilson W, Taubert KA, Gewitz M, et al: Prevention of infective endocarditis: guidelines from the American Heart Association. A guideline from the American Heart Association Rheumatic Fever, Endocarditis, and Kawasaki Disease Committee, Council on Cardiovascular Disease in the Young, and the Council on Clinical Cardiology, Council on Cardiovascular Surgery and Anesthesia, and the Quality of Care and Outcomes Research Interdisciplinary Working Group, *Circulation* 116:1736–1754, 2007.

Wilson WR, Karchmer AW, Dajani AS, et al: Antibiotic treatment of adults with infective endocarditis caused by streptococci, enterococci, staphylococci, and HACEK microorganisms. American Heart Association, *JAMA* 274:1706–1713, 1995.

Wormser GP, Dattwyler RJ, Shapiro ED, et al: The clinical assessment, treatment, and prevention of Lyme disease, human granulocytic anaplasmosis, and babesiosis: clinical practice guidelines by the Infectious Diseases Society of America, *Clin Infect Dis* 43:1089–1134, 2006.

SECTION THREE

BOARD REVIEW

Pulmonary and Critical Care Medicine

Obstructive Lung Disease

ROBERT A. WISE, MD; and M. BRADLEY DRUMMOND, MD, MHS

Obstructive lung disease encompasses a wide range of processes all involving obstruction to airflow. Roughly 50% of patients die within 10 years of initial diagnosis of smoking-related chronic obstructive pulmonary disease (COPD). The most common chronic obstructive lung diseases include those that are smoking-related (chronic bronchitis and emphysema) and those that are not smoking-related (asthma, bronchiectasis, cystic fibrosis [CF], and bronchiolitis obliterans).

Asthma

Basic Information

- **Asthma is a chronic inflammatory disease of the airways that is characterized by episodes of cough, wheezing, and dyspnea**
- **It is characterized by increased sensitivity of the airways to constrict in response to nonspecific stimulation (i.e., bronchial hyper-reactivity)**
- **Approximately 80% of patients with asthma have an allergic tendency (atopy) characterized by positive immediate hypersensitivity skin tests (Fig. 17-1)**

Clinical Presentation

- Asthma may manifest with different syndromes, often overlapping
- Extrinsic asthma
  - Usual onset in **childhood**
  - Attacks **triggered by exposure to inhaled allergen**
    - Dust mites
    - Cockroaches
    - Cat antigen
    - Molds, particularly *Alternaria*
    - Pollens (e.g., ragweed, trees, grasses)
- Intrinsic asthma
  - Usual onset in **early adulthood**
  - Attacks **triggered by viral infections, nonspecific irritants**
  - May lead to chronic asthmatic bronchitis
  - Obesity is a risk factor, particularly for women
- Exercise-induced asthma
  - Characterized by **bronchospasm 10 to 20 minutes after exhausting exercise** (Fig. 17-2)
  - Occurs in majority of asthmatics, but may occur as sole manifestation of asthma
  - **Triggered by drying or cooling (or both) of airways** with hyperventilation, particularly cold, dry air
  - **Can be prevented with inhaled bronchodilators (e.g., albuterol), or leukotriene antagonists (e.g., montelukast)**

- Triad asthma (Samter syndrome)
  - **Asthma,** often requiring systemic corticosteroids for control
  - **Nasal polyps (Fig. 17-3)**
  - **Aspirin (or other NSAID) sensitivity**
  - May require leukotriene antagonist for control of symptoms
- Cough-variant asthma
  - May manifest as **cough in the absence of wheezing**
  - Responds to treatment for asthma
  - Airways hyper-reactivity present
  - One of the **three most common causes of chronic cough** (along with gastroesophageal reflux disease and chronic sinusitis/postnasal drip syndrome)
- Occupational asthma
  - Presents as **"Monday morning" symptoms** that abate during weekends
  - Symptoms usually **worse in the evening,** better in the morning
  - Prolonged exposures may lead to irreversible airflow obstruction
  - Common causes
    - Pigeons, chickens
    - Epoxy resins
    - Laboratory animals
    - Metals (nickel, chromium)
    - Plastics and rubber
- Refractory asthma
  - **Chronic unremitting wheezing** requiring long-term systemic corticosteroids
  - Often leads to chronic airway remodeling with chronic airflow obstruction
  - Possible causes for refractory asthma: see Box 17-1
- Disorders that may **mimic asthma**
  - **Congestive heart failure**
  - **Mitral stenosis**
  - **Upper airway obstructions** (e.g., laryngeal tumors, subglottic stenosis, Wegener granulomatosis)
  - Paradoxical **vocal cord dysfunction** (more common in women and health-care workers)

Evaluation and Diagnosis

- **Consider diagnosis of asthma in patients with history of wheezing or variable dyspnea with specific triggers**
- **Diagnosis confirmed by presence of obstructive lung disease on pulmonary function tests at the time of symptoms that normalize when asymptomatic**
- Diffusing capacity of the lungs for carbon monoxide ($D_{L_{CO}}$) normal between episodes

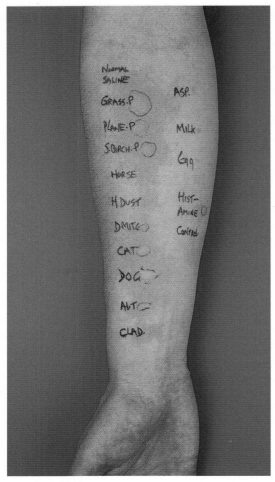

FIGURE 17-1 Multiple positive skin test results in a patient with extrinsic asthma. *(From Forbes CD, Jackson WF: Color atlas and text of clinical medicine, ed 3, St. Louis, Mosby, 2003, Fig. 4.18.)*

FIGURE 17-2 Forced expiratory volume in 1 second (FEV_1) in a patient with exercise-induced asthma. Note the sudden fall of FEV_1, followed by gradual recovery. *(From Haslett C, Chilvers ER, Boon NA, et al: Davidson's principles and practice of medicine, ed 19, New York, Churchill Livingstone, 2003, Fig. 13.25.)*

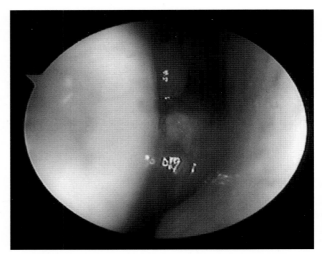

FIGURE 17-3 Endoscopic view of nasal polyps protruding from middle meatus. *(From Adkinson NF Jr, Yunginger J, Busse W, et al: Middleton's allergy: principles and practice, ed 6, St. Louis, Mosby, 2003, Fig. 78-1.)*

BOX 17-1	*Causes of Refractory Asthma*

Chronic exposure to an allergen (e.g., molds), irritant (e.g., air pollution), or sensitizing agent (e.g., toluene di-isocyanate)

Use of β-blockers (e.g., timolol eye drops for glaucoma)

Use of aspirin-containing drugs

Mucocutaneous fungal infections

Allergic bronchopulmonary aspergillosis

Churg-Strauss vasculitis

- Home monitoring with peak flowmeter may be helpful for diagnosing or monitoring disease
- **Negative methacholine challenge test makes active asthma unlikely**

Treatment

Figure 17-4 shows a stepwise approach to asthma treatment.

- **The goal of asthma treatment is to avoid symptoms, minimize use of short-acting bronchodilators for relief of symptoms, prevent nocturnal awakening from asthma, and minimize systemic side effects of treatment**
- Four components of asthma treatment
  - **Monitor symptoms and pulmonary function**
  - **Control environmental exposures**
  - **Educate patient regarding avoidance of triggers and proper treatment**
  - **Drug treatment (Box 17-2)**
- Stepwise drug treatment of chronic asthma (see Fig. 17-4)
  - **For intermittent symptoms (up to two episodes per week), occasional inhaled short-acting bronchodilators**
  - **For persistent symptoms (e.g., use of short-acting bronchodilator more than twice per week),**

17

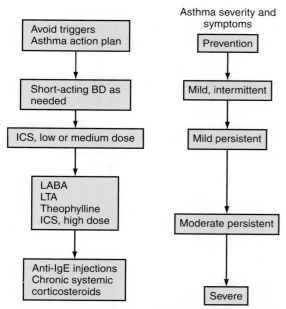

FIGURE 17-4 Stepwise approach to asthma treatment. Severity of asthma is defined by the abnormality of lung function, frequency of symptomatic use of bronchodilators, and frequency of nocturnal awakenings. For patients who use their short-acting bronchodilator more than twice weekly, drugs are prescribed to control or prevent symptoms. Usually treatment is initiated with inhaled corticosteroids, and then additional controller drugs are added. Patients with recalcitrant asthma may require long-term corticosteroids or anti–immunoglobulin E (anti-IgE) therapy. (BD, bronchodilator; ICS, inhaled corticosteroids; LABA, long-acting β-agonist; LTA, leukotriene antagonist.)

BOX 17-2 *Drug Therapy for Asthma*

β_2-Agonists
  Short-acting (albuterol)
  Long-acting (salmeterol, formoterol, arformoterol)
    (in combination with inhaled corticosteroids)
Antimuscarinics
  Tiotropium
  Theophylline, aminophylline
Corticosteroids
  Systemic
  Inhaled
Antileukotrienes
  Leukotriene receptor antagonist
  Lipoxygenase inhibitors

- **Systemic bronchodilators** (e.g., subcutaneous terbutaline or IV aminophylline) may be used in selected cases
- Indications for **hospitalization**
- **Peak flow less than 40% of baseline** after 4 to 6 hours of treatment
- **Persistent hypoxemia**
- **Hypercapnia**—blood gas pH may normalize if severe attack and patient is becoming fatigued
- **Altered sensorium**
- History of **previous near-fatal asthma** attacks

Smoking-Related Chronic Obstructive Pulmonary Disease

Basic Information

- Chronic bronchitis (chronic mucus hypersecretion syndrome)
  - Occurs in about **one out of three smokers**
  - Can occur with **occupational exposures to dust**
  - **Often remits when exposure to dust or tobacco ceases**
  - Definition
    - **Daily production of sputum for 3 or more months per year for 2 consecutive years**
    - With obstructive ventilatory defect, may be called chronic obstructive bronchitis
  - Morbid anatomy
    - **Hyperplasia of the airway mucous glands and goblet cells**
    - Mucus plugging, thickening, tortuosity, and **fibrosis** of the peripheral airways (Fig. 17-5)
  - Pathophysiology
    - Not always associated with obstructive ventilatory defect
    - Airway resistance may be increased
  - Chest radiograph
    - **Hyperinflation**
    - **Increased peribronchial markings at lung bases**
    - Thickening of **airway walls**
- Emphysema
  - **Definition** based on anatomic demonstration of **airspace enlargement**

controller therapy with inhaled corticosteroids or leukotriene antagonists, supplemented by bronchodilators as needed
- For persistent symptoms that do not respond to moderate doses of inhaled corticosteroids, **leukotriene antagonists, theophylline, or long-acting β-agonists (e.g., salmeterol, formoterol) may be added to inhaled corticosteroids.** Long-acting antimuscarinics (e.g., tiotropium) are also effective for asthma if other agents are not tolerated.
- For persistently low lung function, frequent exacerbations, or severe attack, **systemic corticosteroids** may be needed to gain control of disease
- Review treatment at 1- to 6-month intervals. Consider step-down of therapy if asthma has been well controlled for at least 3 months.
- Treatment of the acute asthmatic attack
  - Inhaled **short-acting bronchodilators** (e.g., albuterol) every 20 minutes for three doses
  - Inhaled **ipratropium** for individuals with severe airflow obstruction failing to improve after repeated short-acting β-agonist treatment
  - **Supplemental oxygen** if hypoxemia is present
  - Intravenous magnesium sulfate (2 gm infused over 20 minutes) can be helpful in individuals with severe attacks
  - If no relief, **systemic corticosteroids** (e.g., prednisone 60–120 mg PO or IV and repeat every 6 hours as needed)

- **Progressive destruction of alveolar septa** and capillaries
- **Airspace enlargement** and the development of macroscopic bullae
- Smoking-related disease usually involves respiratory bronchiole in the center of the pulmonary lobule (centrilobular or centriacinar emphysema; see Fig. 17-5)
- α_1-Antitrypsin deficiency usually involves the entire pulmonary lobule (panlobular or panacinar) emphysema (see later discussion)
- **Centrilobular emphysema mostly affects the upper lung zones**
- **Panacinar emphysema mostly affects the lower lung zones**
- Pathophysiology
  - Reduced elastic recoil of the lung (increased compliance)
  - Slowing of maximum expiratory airflow (decreased forced expiratory volume in 1 second/forced vital capacity [FEV_1/FVC] ratio)

| Narrowing of small airways in chronic bronchitis | Centriacinar emphysema | Panacinar emphysema |

Narrowing; mucus plugging

FIGURE 17-5 Pathologic features of chronic bronchitis and emphysema. *(From Kumar P, Clark M: Clinical medicine, ed 5, Philadelphia, Elsevier Saunders, 2005, Fig. 14.23.)*

FIGURE 17-6 Chest radiograph of patient with severe COPD, showing arterial deficiency pattern of emphysema. Lungs are hyperinflated, diaphragms are low and flat, and there is paucity of vascular markings. *(From Weinberger SE: Principles of pulmonary medicine, ed 4, Philadelphia, Saunders, 2004, Fig. 6-8.)*

- Hyperinflation (increased static lung volumes)
- Decreased alveolar surface area for gas exchange (reduction in $D_{L_{CO}}$); ventilation-perfusion mismatch (hypoxemia)
- Chest radiograph
  - **Flattening of the diaphragm** (Fig. 17-6)
  - Attenuation of vascular markings
  - Enlargement of the central pulmonary arteries
  - **Hyperinflation**
  - Enlargement of the anterior airspace
  - Increase of the sternophrenic angle
- Computed tomography (CT) of chest
  - **Bullae** (avascular regions)
  - Regions of decreased lung density (less than −910/−950 Hounsfield units)
- Natural history of COPD (Fig. 17-7)
  - One in seven patients who smoke develops COPD
  - COPD develops over many years of smoking
  - Those who develop COPD have **increased rate of FEV₁ decline**
  - **Smoking cessation stops accelerated loss of lung function and prolongs survival**
  - Patients are usually **asymptomatic until FEV₁ is 30% to 50% predicted**
  - Risk factors for development of COPD in smokers: see Box 17-3
  - Survival is lower in patients with higher **BODE** index based on
    - Low **b**ody mass index
    - Severe **o**bstructive ventilatory defect

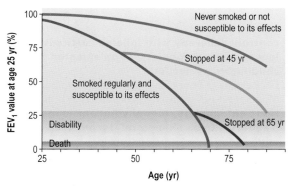

FIGURE 17-7 Natural history of COPD. Nonsmokers and smokers who are not susceptible to develop COPD lose about 25% of the early adulthood FEV₁ as a consequence of aging. Susceptible smokers lose lung function at a rate two to three times faster. By middle age, they develop symptomatic obstructive lung disease. If they continue to smoke, the disease progresses and eventually leads to disability and death. At any degree of impairment of lung function, smoking cessation leads to slowing of disease progression and extends the period of relative health.

| **BOX 17-3** | *Risk Factors for Development of Chronic Obstructive Pulmonary Disease in Smokers* |

Airways reactivity
Family history of COPD
Childhood lung disease
Occupational dust exposures (e.g., silica, cotton dust, grain dust)

COPD, chronic obstructive pulmonary disease.

- Severe **d**yspnea
- Poor **e**xercise tolerance on 6-minute walk test

Clinical Presentation

- Spectrum of COPD (Table 17-1)
  - COPD includes patients with chronic obstructive bronchitis, emphysema, or both
- Physical findings in COPD (Figs. 17-8 and 17-9; Box 17-4)
  - **Physical examination not helpful in detecting mild COPD**
  - **Physical examination not helpful in ruling out COPD**

TABLE 17-1	Clinical Spectrum of Chronic Obstructive Pulmonary Disease	
Characteristic	**Type A**	**Type B**
Underlying lung disease	Emphysema	Chronic bronchitis disease
Lung volumes	Hyperinflated	May be normal
Physique	Slender	Obese
Dyspnea	Very dyspneic	Not dyspneic
$Paco_2$	Low until end stage	Elevated
Oxygenation with exercise	Worsens	May improve
Oxygenation at rest	Satisfactory	Low

$Paco_2$, arterial partial pressure of carbon dioxide.

FIGURE 17-8 Respiratory failure. The patient is breathless at rest and exhibits central cyanosis with blueness of the lips and face. The lips are pursed during expiration, a characteristic feature of COPD. This facial appearance is often accompanied by heart failure with peripheral edema (cor pulmonale). The term *blue bloater* derives from this combination of cyanosis and edema. *(From Swash M, Glynn M: Hutchison's clinical methods, ed 22, Philadelphia, Elsevier Saunders, 2007, Fig. 6.1.)*

- An abnormal physical examination is about 90% specific for a diagnosis of COPD

Diagnosis

- Spirometry in COPD
  - **Most sensitive measure** of disease presence and progression
  - Earliest abnormalities are decreased maximal flow at low lung volumes (seen on flow-volume loops)
  - **FEV_1/FVC less than 70%** is reasonable threshold for diagnosing obstructive lung disease, but this may be within normal range in elderly patients and may underdiagnose younger patients
  - **FEV_1 determines the severity** (<30% predicted is very severe)

Treatment

- Treatment of stable COPD (Fig. 17-10)
  - **Smoking cessation**
    - Strong personalized message
    - Nicotine replacement (e.g., gum, patch, inhaler, lozenge, nasal spray)

FIGURE 17-9 A "pink puffer" with emphysema. Pao_2 is maintained, but breathlessness is common, combined in the term *pink puffer*. *(From Forbes CD, Jackson WF: Color atlas and text of clinical medicine, ed 3, St. Louis, Mosby, 2003, Fig. 4.91.)*

BOX 17-4	Physical Findings in Moderate Chronic Pulmonary Disorder

Diaphragm moves <2 cm
Hyper-resonant percussion
Decreased cardiac dullness
Decreased breath sounds
Forced expiration time >10 seconds
Abdominal point of maximum cardiac impulse

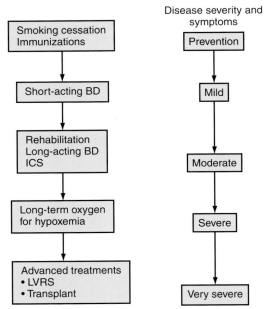

FIGURE 17-10 The stepwise approach to treatment of COPD. The severity of disease is judged by the impairment of FEV_1 as a percent predicted: greater than 80%, mild; 50% to 80%, moderate; 30% to 50%, severe; and less than 30%, very severe. (BD, bronchodilator, either β-agonist or anticholinergic or combined; ICS, inhaled corticosteroids; LVRS, lung volume reduction surgery.)

- Bupropion
- Varenicline
- Set quit date
- Group support
- Follow-up
- See Chapter 71 regarding discontinuation of addictive substances
- **Bronchodilators** for maintenance bronchodilation
  - Anticholinergic (e.g., ipratropium, tiotropium)
  - β-Agonists (e.g., salmeterol, formoterol, arformoterol, indacaterol)
  - Short-acting for symptom relief (e.g., albuterol)
  - Oral theophylline or phosphodiesterase type 4 inhibitors (roflumilast)
- Inhaled corticosteroids (ICS) to reduce exacerbation frequency
  - Not useful to prevent disease progression
  - Reduce frequency of exacerbations
  - Associated with an increased risk of pneumonia
- **Exercise training/rehabilitation** to improve exercise tolerance
  - Improves efficiency of exercise
  - No effect on lung function
- **Chronic low-flow oxygen therapy** (e.g., 2 L/min by nasal cannula)
  - **Improves survival** in patients with hypoxemia
  - Indications
    - **Partial pressure of oxygen (Pao_2) less than 55 mm Hg (O_2 saturation less than 89%)** in usual health
    - **Pao_2 less than 60 mm Hg (O_2 saturation less than 90%) with evidence of cor pulmonale or neurocognitive impairment**

- Lung transplantation candidates
  - **FEV_1 less than 20% predicted**
  - **Age under 60 to 65 years**
  - Sufficient social support
  - **Lung volume reduction surgery (LVRS)**
    - Procedure removes 20% to 30% of lung volume
    - Best results in patients with upper lung zone emphysema and poor exercise capacity after rehabilitation
  - **Bullectomy**
    - For single bulla occupying one third of a hemithorax
    - Best results with normal compressed lung and normal $D_{L_{CO}}$
- Treatment of COPD exacerbation
  - **About 50% are associated with lower airway bacterial infection**
    - **Antibiotics if change in sputum volume, color, associated dyspnea**
  - **Bronchodilators** by metered-dose inhaler as effective as by nebulizer in compliant patients
  - **Systemic corticosteroids** shorten duration of exacerbation
    - **No benefit of more than 2 weeks of corticosteroids**

Other Forms of Obstructive Lung Disease

α₁-ANTITRYPSIN DEFICIENCY

Basic Information

- Autosomal recessive trait
  - Also referred to as α₁-antiprotease deficiency
- Alleles of antiprotease activity (3 most common of more than 75 identified)
  - M: Normal
  - S: Intermediate
  - Z: Marked decrease
  - Null: Absent (rare)
- Phenotypes
  - **M, MS, MZ: No increased risk**
  - **SZ: Mild increased risk**
  - **ZZ: Increased risk for emphysema; 10% also develop chronic liver disease**
- **Panacinar emphysema** is the typical manifestation of ZZ disease
  - Affects entire respiratory lobule uniformly
  - Predominates at **lung bases**

Clinical Presentation

- Found in about **1% of patients with emphysema**
- **Premature lung disease** (age 30–40 years in smokers, age 50–60 years in nonsmokers)
- Absence of the antiprotease enzymes thought to allow proteases from inflammatory cells to damage alveolar septae
- **Bronchiectasis and chronic bronchitis may occur in deficient states along with mucous gland hyperplasia**
- **About 10% of patients have concomitant liver disease**

- Many patients have COPD that is not distinguishable from other smoking-related presentations

Diagnosis

- **Low α₁ fraction** on serum protein electrophoresis
- Plasma levels of α₁-**antitrypsin reduced**
- Direct **genotyping**

Treatment

- Smoking cessation
- Genetic counseling
- **Augmentation therapy with human α₁-protease inhibitor is most useful in those with moderate disease severity**

BRONCHIOLITIS OBLITERANS

Basic Information

- Causes of bronchiolitis obliterans (BO)
  - Inhalation of **toxic fumes**
    - Methane
    - Hydrochloric acid
    - Chlorine
    - Ammonia
    - Sulfuric acid
    - Nitric acid (silo filler's disease)
  - **Viral infections** (e.g., respiratory syncytial virus, adenovirus, and influenza)
  - Connective tissue diseases—**rheumatoid arthritis**
  - **Organ transplantation:** lung, heart, and bone marrow
  - **Neuroendocrine cell hyperplasia**
  - Idiopathic

Clinical Presentation

- Cough
- Dyspnea
- Airflow obstruction
- Air trapping
- Physical findings
  - **Inspiratory squeaks and diffuse crackles**
  - Chest may be quiet

Diagnosis

- Chest CT
  - May appear **normal**
  - Diffuse **centriacinar nodules**
  - Diffuse **ground-glass** infiltrates
  - Mosaic pattern with segmental hyperinflation on expiratory views
- Histology
  - Often requires lung biopsy for diagnosis
  - Inflammation, thickening, occlusion, and disappearance of bronchioles

Treatment

- Immunosuppressive drugs, but often there is little response
- Macrolide antibiotics useful in some cases, particularly post–lung transplantation
- **BO should not be confused with bronchiolitis obliterans with organizing pneumonia (BOOP,** also called

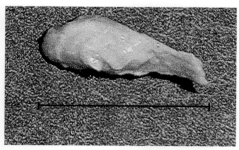

FIGURE 17-11 Typical sputum plug of allergic bronchopulmonary aspergillosis. *(From Forbes CD, Jackson WF: Color atlas and text of clinical medicine, ed 3, St. Louis, Mosby, 2003, Fig. 4.12.)*

cryptogenic organizing pneumonia, or COP), which is a different entity involving plugging of airways with granulation tissue and postobstructive chronic pneumonia. **BOOP is often responsive to corticosteroids, whereas BO is not** (see Chapter 20).

ALLERGIC BRONCHOPULMONARY ASPERGILLOSIS

Basic Information

- **Hypersensitivity reaction to *Aspergillus* manifesting as worsening asthma**
- Patients with CF are also susceptible to allergic bronchopulmonary aspergillosis (ABPA), and this may be an important factor in rapid clinical deterioration

Clinical Presentation

- **Chronic steroid-dependent asthma or rapidly progressive CF**
- Recurrent **pulmonary infiltrates**
- **Brown, black, or green sputum plugs and airway casts expectorated** (Fig. 17-11)
- Culture of *Aspergillus* species from sputum
- Perihilar evanescent oval shadows on chest radiograph from mucoid impactions
- **Marked eosinophilia**
- **Elevated serum immunoglobulin E (IgE)**
- Positive *Aspergillus* skin test and serum precipitins
- Dilation of central airways, "gloved finger" bronchiectasis

Pathophysiology

- Immune arthus-type reaction to *Aspergillus* colonizing airways

Diagnosis

- Major criteria
  - **Asthma**
  - Blood **eosinophilia**
  - Immediate skin reactivity (IgE-dependent reaction) to *Aspergillus* antigens
  - Immunoglobulin G (IgG) antibodies (type III reaction) to *Aspergillus* antigens
  - **Transient or fixed pulmonary infiltrates**
  - Central bronchiectasis
  - **High serum IgE titer (normal level in symptomatic patient excludes ABPA)**

FIGURE 17-12 Characteristic CT scan from patient with lymphangioleiomyomatosis. The bullae within the left lung appear as typical punched-out "Swiss cheese" lesions. The interlobular septae are thickened, giving the remaining lung parenchyma a more opaque appearance.

- Minor criteria
  - Presence of *Aspergillus* in sputum
  - Expectoration of brown mucous plugs
  - Late-phase skin test reactivity to *Aspergillus* antigen

Treatment

- **Corticosteroids** with dose adjusted by IgE levels
- Oral antifungal agents may help in some cases
- Check for CF genotype in affected patients

LYMPHANGIOLEIOMYOMATOSIS

See Figure 17-12 for a characteristic CT scan showing lymphangioleiomyomatosis.

Basic Information

- This is a rare disorder; etiology is unknown
- Affects **only fertile women**
- Excess proliferation of lymphatic smooth muscle
- Cystic lung disease with increased interstitial markings
- Associated in some cases with polymorphisms of tuberous sclerosis gene complex

Clinical Presentation

- Presents with progressive **dyspnea**
- Repeated **hemoptysis** may occur
- **Interstitial infiltrates** and airflow obstruction
- May present with pneumothorax or chylothorax

Diagnosis

- Obstructive pattern on pulmonary function tests; low $D_{L_{CO}}$
- **Characteristic "Swiss cheese" appearance on chest CT from multiple cystic spaces**
- Diffuse **proliferation of smooth muscle** within the airway walls, interstitium, and lymphatics

Treatment

- **Sirolimus (rapamycin) prevents disease progression**
- **Lung transplantation for severe disease**

CYSTIC FIBROSIS

Basic Information

- Most common lethal **autosomal recessive** disease in whites in the United States
- **Obstruction of exocrine glands** by viscous secretion
- Forty percent may not be diagnosed until adolescence
- ABPA and asthma are seen more frequently in patients with CF

Clinical Presentation

- COPD
- Bronchiectasis
- **Nasal polyps**
- **Pancreatic insufficiency**
- **Hemoptysis**
- Chronic mucoid *Pseudomonas* infection

Diagnosis

- Abnormal sweat chloride test (**elevated** chloride)
- Genotyping

Treatment

- Management of obstructive lung disease
- Chest physiotherapy with manual percussion, flutter valves, pneumatic vest
- Long-term antibiotics, including inhaled antibiotics
- Nutritional support and replacement of pancreatic enzymes

UNUSUAL CAUSES OF OBSTRUCTIVE LUNG DISEASE

- Immunoglobulin deficiency with bronchiectasis
  - Immunoglobulin A (IgA), IgG subclasses 2 and 4
- Immotile cilia syndromes
  - Kartagener syndrome with situs inversus
  - Absence of dynein arms of cilia on electron microscopy
- Yellow nails syndrome with bronchiectasis
  - Pleural effusions, lymphedema, yellow nails
- Sarcoidosis with upper or lower airway involvement (see Chapter 20)
- Eosinophilic granuloma
- Sjögren syndrome
- HIV with premature emphysema

REVIEW QUESTIONS

For review questions, please go to www.expertconsult.com.

SUGGESTED READINGS

Celli BR, MacNee W: ATS/ERS Task Force: Standards for the diagnosis and treatment of patients with COPD: a summary of the ATS/ERS position paper, *Eur Respir J* 23:932–946, 2004.
Global Initiative for Asthma (GINA): *Global strategy for asthma management and prevention (updated 2010)* Available at, www.ginasthma.com.
Global Initiative for Chronic Obstructive Lung Disease (GOLD): *Global strategy for the diagnosis, management, and prevention of chronic obstructive pulmonary disease (updated 2010)* Available at, www.goldcopd.org.
National Asthma Education and Prevention Program Expert Panel Report III: *Guidelines for the diagnosis and management of asthma: update of selected topics*, August 2008, Available atwww.nhlbi.nih.gov/guidelines/asthma/.

Pulmonary Function Testing

ROBERT A. WISE, MD; and MEREDITH C. McCORMACK, MD, MHS

Pulmonary function tests (PFTs) are used in the evaluation of lung diseases. The quality of the tests may vary depending on the patient's effort. The tests most commonly employed are spirometry, flow-volume loops, broncho-provocation testing, carbon monoxide diffusing capacity, lung volume measurements, and measures of respiratory muscle strength. The 6-minute walk test, a simple measure of functional exercise capacity, is also performed in many pulmonary laboratories.

Pulmonary Function Tests

Spirometry

- Widely available and the most useful pulmonary function test
  - Can be performed in office or clinic, as well as laboratory setting
  - Measured using flow sensors (pneumotachometers) or volume sensors (spirometers)
- **Helpful in evaluation of obstructive lung disease (e.g., chronic obstructive pulmonary disease [COPD]/asthma)**
- Performed as a forced expiration following maximum inspiration
- Recorded as volume expired per unit of time
- **Forced expiratory volume is the volume expired in 1 second (FEV$_1$) (Fig. 18-1)**
  - Correlated with maximum ventilation and with exercise
  - **Reduced in both obstructive and restrictive disorders**
  - **Predictive of mortality** in general population, lung cancer risk, disability
- **Forced vital capacity (FVC)** is the maximum volume expired from the lung (see Fig. 18-1)
  - **May be reduced due to low total lung capacity (TLC) in restrictive ventilatory defect or due to elevated residual volume (RV) from air trapping in obstructive disease**
- **FEV$_1$/FVC is an index of the rate of emptying of the lung**
  - **Ratio less than 0.7 usually indicates obstructive ventilatory defect (Box 18-1)**
- Maximum midexpiratory flow rate (MMFR) or forced expiratory flow (FEF) 25% to 75% (forced expiratory flow at 25–75% of vital capacity) measures the mean flow during the middle 50% of expiration
  - Often considered a measure of small airways function, the test is variable and nonspecific

Flow-Volume Loops

Figure 18-2 illustrates flow-volume loops.
- Displays forced expiratory and inspiratory maneuvers as flow (i.e., slope of spirogram) versus volume
- **Useful for diagnosis of upper airway obstruction**
  - Abnormality in both inspiration and expiration (fixed)
  - Abnormality in inspiration only (variable extrathoracic obstruction)
  - Abnormality in expiration only (variable intrathoracic obstruction)
- Fixed upper airway obstructions
  - Cause greater reduction in peak expiratory flow rates, but inspiratory flow rate also decreased
  - Common causes
    - **Bilateral vocal cord paralysis**
    - **Tracheal stenosis** (e.g., following prolonged endotracheal intubation or in relapsing polychondritis)
    - **Laryngeal or tracheal tumors**
    - **Granulomatous diseases** (e.g., sarcoid, Wegener granulomatosis)
- Variable extrathoracic obstruction
  - Flow during inspiration is normally greater than expiratory flow
  - In variable extrathoracic obstruction, **inspiratory flow is less than expiratory flow at middle lung volumes**
  - Common with **vocal cord dysfunction** or **unilateral vocal cord paralysis**
  - Found in obese individuals and those with **sleep apnea** syndrome
- Variable intrathoracic obstruction
  - **Expiratory flow is decreased,** whereas inspiratory flow is not altered
  - **Tracheal tumors, subglottic stenosis** may present this way
- Chronic obstructive pulmonary disease (COPD)
  - **Curvilinear flow volume curve caused by slowly emptying lung units**
  - Peak flow is relatively preserved, making it poor measure of COPD severity
  - Flow rates at low lung volumes are more impaired
  - Asthma produces similar curve shape but with reduced flow rates at all lung volumes, including peak flow
- Vocal cord dysfunction (VCD)
  - **VCD presents as "asthma," but without hyperinflation on chest radiograph, and is unresponsive to steroids**
  - More common in women than men

■ Definitive diagnosis is made by visualizing vocal cord abnormalities with laryngoscopy during an attack

■ Diagnosis may be suggested by abnormal inspiratory flow patterns on flow-volume loops (presents as variable extrathoracic obstruction)

Bronchoprovocation Testing

See Figure 18-3 for a methacholine challenge test.

■ Performed by inhaling increasing concentrations of methacholine, followed by spirometry after each concentration

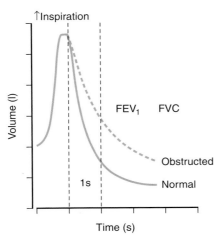

FIGURE 18-1 A spirometer tracing. The patient breathes out as fast as possible after maximum inhalation. Volume expelled is related to lung capacity. The forced expiratory volume in 1 second (FEV_1) is compared with the forced vital capacity (FVC). In the normal person, this ratio is greater than 80%; abnormal (i.e., obstructive defect) is a ratio less than 70%. *(From Davies A, Blakeley A, Kidd C: Human physiology, New York, Churchill Livingstone, 2001, Fig. 7.1.9.)*

BOX 18-1	*Potential Indications for Spirometry*

Diagnosis of obstructive lung disease

Evaluation of severity of lung disease

Screen high-risk individuals (e.g., smokers)

Preoperative assessment (see Chapter 72)

Evaluation of disability/impairment

Monitoring of treatment

Assess toxic effects of exposure or drug toxicity

■ **A positive test is defined by achieving a 20% or greater fall in FEV_1 with a dose of 16 to 25 mg/mL methacholine or less**

■ The concentration required to achieve a 20% fall in FEV_1 is called the PC_{20}

■ Half of COPD patients have positive methacholine challenge testing

■ **Positive test is nonspecific**

■ **Negative methacholine challenge makes active asthma unlikely**

■ **Useful in the case of chronic cough to rule out cough-variant asthma**

Carbon Monoxide Diffusing Capacity (DL_{CO})

■ Tests the integrity of the alveolar-capillary surface area for gas exchange

■ Carbon monoxide diffusing capacity (DL_{CO}) less than 80% predicted is abnormal

■ DL_{CO} less than 50% predicted predicts oxygen desaturation with exercise

■ DL_{CO} is **decreased in disorders that decrease pulmonary capillary blood volume**

■ **Interstitial lung diseases**

■ **Emphysema**

■ **Pulmonary vascular disease**

■ **Normal DL_{CO} makes clinically important interstitial disease unlikely**

■ DL_{CO} changes in disease states: see Table 18-1

■ Utility

■ **Distinguishing emphysema from asthma (low in emphysema, normal or high in asthma)**

■ Evaluation of dyspnea

■ Monitoring occupational/toxic exposures (e.g., bleomycin, amiodarone)

Lung Volume Measurements

■ **Useful for distinguishing restrictive lung diseases from obstructive lung diseases (Figs. 18-4 and 18-5)**

■ Resident gas methods (helium dilution and nitrogen washout) may underestimate lung volumes with obstructive defects

■ Body plethysmography is more accurate in obstructive diseases

■ **Restrictive ventilatory defects have a reduction in all subdivisions of lung volume, including TLC, vital capacity (VC), and RV**

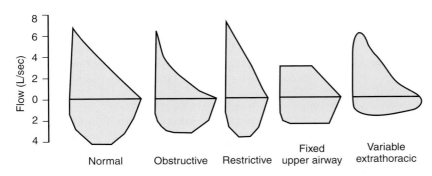

FIGURE 18-2 Flow-volume loops. Curve begins at left axis and, with forced expiration, follows a clockwise pattern. The normal pattern appears as a triangle over a half circle. With development of chronic obstructive pulmonary disease, the expiratory limb becomes curvilinear. In restrictive lung diseases, the flows are relatively preserved and the width of the curve is narrowed. With a fixed upper airway obstruction, the inspiratory and expiratory limbs are flattened.

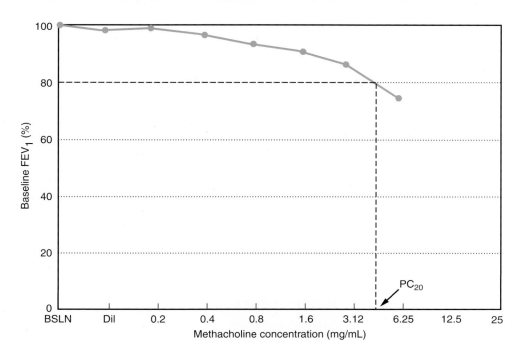

FIGURE 18-3 Methacholine challenge test. Progressively greater concentrations of inhaled methacholine are given with a nebulizer. After each concentration, spirometry is performed. In patients with airways reactivity, the forced expiratory volume in 1 second (FEV_1) will decline by more than 20% before the maximum concentration is reached (usually 25 mg/mL). The provocative concentration (PC_{20}) is determined by interpolation between concentrations. Patients with active asthma will usually show a drop in FEV_1 at less than 10 mg/mL. A positive test for airways reactivity is not diagnostic, however, as many normal individuals and patients with chronic obstructive pulmonary disease have a positive test.

TABLE 18-1	$D_{L_{CO}}$ Changes in Disease States	
$D_{L_{CO}}$ Normal or Increased	**$D_{L_{CO}}$ Decreased**
Asthma	Emphysema
Polycythemia	Anemia
Obesity	Interstitial lung disease
Left-to-right shunt	Pneumonectomy
Supine position	Pulmonary hypertension
Postexercise	Pulmonary embolism
Pulmonary hemorrhage	

$D_{L_{CO}}$, diffusing capacity of the lungs for carbon monoxide.

- **Obstructive ventilatory defects typically cause elevation of TLC (hyperinflation) and RV (gas trapping) with reduction in VC**
- Obesity typically causes a disproportionate reduction in functional residual capacity (FRC) with small reductions in TLC and VC

Respiratory Muscle Strength

- **Definitive test for respiratory muscle weakness is transdiaphragmatic pressure (Pdi)**
- Measured with balloon-tipped catheter to determine the pressure difference between esophagus (pleural pressure) and stomach (abdominal pressure)
- Maximum inspiratory pressure (MIP) is useful for screening for respiratory muscle weakness (i.e., diaphragmatic weakness/paralysis)

  - Normal values between −100 and −140 cm H_2O
- Bilateral diaphragm paralysis usually causes hypercapnia at moderate levels of restriction
- Clues to diaphragm paralysis
  - Orthopnea
  - Paradoxical abdominal motion with inspiration

Six-Minute Walk Test

- Simple assessment of functional exercise capacity
- Used to assess functional status (e.g., lung transplantation evaluation) and response to treatment
- Predicts morbidity and mortality (e.g., in COPD, pulmonary hypertension, heart failure)
- Test is performed under standard conditions
  - Patient walks as far as possible in 6 minutes
  - Patient can stop and rest during the 6 minutes as needed (clock continues)
  - Patients can use oxygen and necessary walking aids, such as canes
  - Scripted language at each minute interval without coaching
  - Dyspnea and leg pain are recorded pre- and post-test (Borg scale)
- Results reported as absolute and percent predicted

REVIEW QUESTIONS

For review questions, please go to www.expertconsult.com.

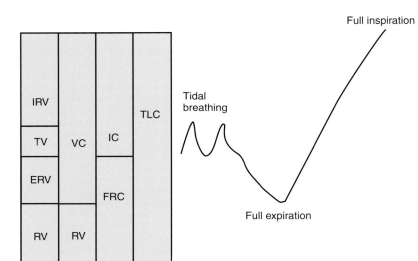

FIGURE 18-4 Lung volume subdivisions. Lung volumes are determined by measurement of FRC using a resident gas method (nitrogen washout or helium dilution) or Boyle's law method (body plethysmography). The remaining lung volumes are calculated from a period of tidal breathing followed by a slow vital capacity maneuver as shown in the right panel. (ERV, expiratory reserve volume; FRC, functional residual capacity; IC, inspiratory capacity; IRV, inspiratory reserve volume; RV, residual volume; TLC, total lung capacity; TV, tidal volume; VC, vital capacity.)

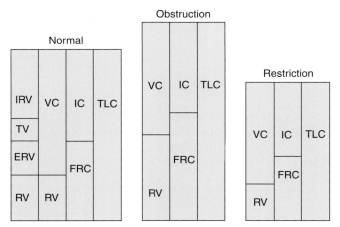

FIGURE 18-5 Abnormalities of lung volumes. Obstructive lung diseases cause elevation of TLC (hyperinflation) and RV (air trapping) with a net increase in the ratio of RV/TLC and a reduction in VC. Restrictive lung diseases cause proportionate reduction in all of the lung volumes. In obesity, however, a mild reduction in TLC is accompanied by a more marked reduction in FRC. (ERV, expiratory reserve volume; FRC, functional residual capacity; IC, inspiratory capacity; IRV, inspiratory reserve volume; RV, residual volume; TLC, total lung capacity; TV, tidal volume; VC, vital capacity.)

SUGGESTED READINGS

American Thoracic Society: ATS Statement: guidelines for the six-minute walk test, *Am J Respir Crit Care Med* 166:111–117, 2002.

Macintyre N, Crapo RO, Viegi G, et al: Standardisation of the single-breath determination of carbon monoxide uptake in the lung, *Eur Respir J* 26:720–735, 2005.

Miller MR, Hankinson J, Brusasco V, et al: Standardisation of spirometry, *Eur Respir J* 26:319–338, 2005.

Pellegrino R, Viegi G, Brusasco RO, et al: Interpretative strategies for lung function tests, *Eur Respir J* 26:948–968, 2005.

Wanger J, Clausen JL, Coates A, et al: Standardisation of the measurement of lung volumes, *Eur Respir J* 26:511–522, 2005.

West JB: *Respiratory physiology: the essentials*, Philadelphia, Lippincott, 2004, Williams & Wilkins.

Chest Radiograph Review

CHRISTIAN A. MERLO, MD, MPH; and PETER B. TERRY, MD, MA

Pattern reading is the approach used by most radiologists to narrow the differential diagnosis when interpreting chest radiographs. This entails evaluation of both the character (e.g., nodule, mass, or infiltrate) and distribution (e.g., upper vs. lower lung field, and unilateral vs. bilateral) of pulmonary parenchymal abnormalities.

Nodules and Masses

Basic Information

- A nodule (Fig. 19-1) is defined as a lesion that measures less than 4 cm in diameter, and a mass (Figs. 19-2 to 19-5) is one that is greater than 4 cm in diameter. Lesions greater than 3 cm in diameter have a greater than 75% probability of being malignant.

Clinical Presentation

- **Smaller lesions are usually benign** because to be visible on a chest radiograph, they must be of high density, a property usually associated with calcification. Certain patterns of calcification suggest that the nodule is benign. **Eccentric calcification, although usually benign, may be associated with a malignant cause.** More benign patterns of calcification include
  - Diffuse complete calcification
  - Laminated calcification
  - Eggshell calcification
  - Central/"bull's-eye" calcification
  - Popcorn calcification
  - Onion skin calcification

Diagnosis and Evaluation

- The **differential diagnosis of nodules** includes
  - Infections
    - Bacterial (including abscesses)
    - Mycobacterial
    - Fungal
    - Parasitic (e.g., human infection with *Dirofilaria immitis* [dog heartworm])
  - Granulomata
  - Rheumatoid nodules
  - Wegener granulomatosis
  - Vascular malformations
  - Bronchogenic cysts
  - Hamartoma
  - Primary or secondary lung neoplasms
- **The differential diagnosis of masses includes the preceding possibilities and is expanded to include sarcomas, fibromas, and progressive massive fibrosis (PMF)**

- The differential diagnosis for anterior mediastinal masses ("terrible Ts") deserves particular attention and includes
  - **T**eratoma
  - **T**hymoma
  - **T**hymolipoma
  - **T**hymic carcinoma/carcinoid
  - **T**hymic cyst
  - **T**horacic thyroid
  - **T**errible lymphoma

Infiltrates

Basic Information

- The radiographic pattern and constituents of infiltrates provide clues to their etiology

Clinical Presentation

- **Alveolar infiltrates (Figs. 19-6 to 19-8) are marked by their homogeneity, their irregular and often fluffy appearance, and the presence of air bronchograms (Fig. 19-9);** they may consist of
  - Water
    - Cardiogenic pulmonary edema
    - Noncardiogenic pulmonary edema
  - Blood
    - Goodpasture syndrome
    - Idiopathic pulmonary hemosiderosis
    - Systemic lupus erythematosus (SLE)
  - Cells
    - Malignant
      - Bronchoalveolar cell carcinoma
    - Benign
      - Eosinophilic pneumonia
      - Desquamative interstitial pneumonitis
  - Pus
    - Bacterial pneumonia
  - Protein
    - Alveolar proteinosis
    - *Pneumocystis jiroveci* pneumonia (PCP)–associated protein in alveoli
  - Calcium
    - Alveolar microlithiasis (very rare)
- **Interstitial infiltrates (Figs. 19-10 and 19-11) have a broad differential diagnosis, although the pattern helps to narrow the diagnostic possibilities:**
  - Reticular
  - Nodular
  - Combined—a very common pattern with a broad differential diagnosis

FIGURE 19-1 Nodule.

FIGURE 19-2 Mass.

FIGURE 19-3 Mass.

FIGURE 19-4 Mass.

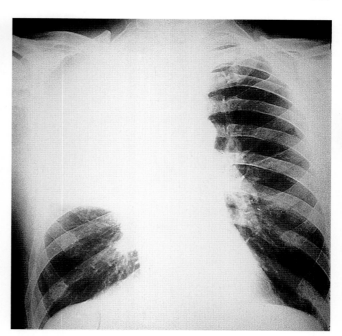

FIGURE 19-6 Alveolar infiltrate.

FIGURE 19-5 Mass.

FIGURE 19-7 Alveolar infiltrate.

FIGURE 19-8 Alveolar infiltrate.

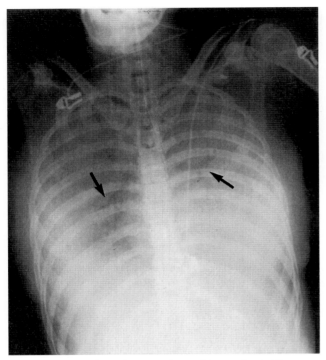

FIGURE 19-9 Air bronchograms (*arrows*) in a patient with alveolar infiltrates due to *Pneumocystis jiroveci* pneumonia. *(From Souhami R: Textbook of medicine, New York, Churchill Livingstone, 2002, Fig. 13.12.)*

FIGURE 19-11 Interstitial infiltrate.

- Linear
- **Honeycomb—implies scarring and end-stage disease and is usually seen with idiopathic pulmonary fibrosis (IPF)**
- Ground glass
  - Bronchiolitis obliterans with organizing pneumonia
  - Sarcoidosis
  - Viral pneumonitis

Diagnosis and Evaluation

- **The pattern of distribution of interstitial infiltrates may provide clues to the specific diagnosis**
- The **differential diagnosis of upper lobe infiltrates is generally small** and depends on the clinical history and whether the abnormality is unilateral or bilateral
  - Diffuse **bilateral** upper lobe infiltrates (Figs. 19-12 and 19-13)
    - Sarcoidosis
    - Eosinophilic granuloma
    - Ankylosing spondylitis
    - Cystic fibrosis
    - Hypersensitivity pneumonitis
    - Old tuberculosis or histoplasmosis
    - Pneumoconiosis (e.g., silicosis)
  - **Unilateral** upper lobe infiltrates (Figs. 19-14 to 19-16)
    - Infections
      - Tuberculosis
      - Histoplasmosis
      - Coccidioidomycosis
      - *Klebsiella* pneumonia
    - Primary lung neoplasms
- **The differential diagnosis of lower lobe infiltrates (Fig. 19-17) is generally much broader, but 80% of the time the differential is found within the following list:**
  - **Bronchiectasis (look for "tram tracks")**
  - **Aspiration (usually found in the superior or posterior basilar segments)**
  - Dermatomyositis/polymyositis
  - **Asbestosis (always associated with crackles on examination)**
  - Scleroderma, SLE, Sjögren syndrome

FIGURE 19-10 Interstitial infiltrate.

FIGURE 19-12 Bilateral upper lobe infiltrate.

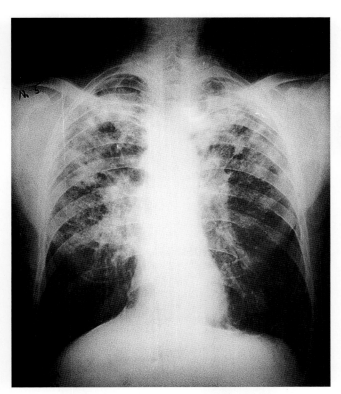

FIGURE 19-13 Bilateral upper lobe infiltrate.

FIGURE 19-14 Unilateral upper lobe infiltrate.

FIGURE 19-15 Unilateral upper lobe infiltrate.

FIGURE 19-16 Unilateral upper lobe infiltrate.

FIGURE 19-18 Pleural effusion.

FIGURE 19-17 Lower lobe infiltrate.

- Sarcoidosis (pleural thickening and effusions are seldom seen)
- Early Hamman-Rich syndrome/IPF (pleural disease is uncommon)
- Rheumatoid arthritis

Pleural Effusions

Basic Information

- **Both the size and side of a pleural effusion provide clues to its etiology**
  - **A pleural effusion filling more than half (Fig. 19-18) of the hemithorax is likely caused by**
    - Trauma
    - Tumor

- Tuberculosis
- Hepatic hydrothorax (in patients with cirrhosis and ascites)
- Chylothorax (caused by thoracic duct obstruction or disruption)
- **An effusion that is bilateral and with a normal heart** is generally caused by
  - Tumor
  - Connective tissue disease
  - Viral infection
  - Congestive heart failure (less often)
- **An effusion that is bilateral and with an enlarged heart is generally caused by congestive heart failure**
- **Right-sided effusions** suggest
  - Congestive heart failure
  - Hepatic hydrothorax
  - Meigs syndrome (in patients with benign ovarian tumors or fibroids)
- **Left-sided effusions** suggest
  - Aortic aneurysm dissection
  - Boerhaave syndrome (esophageal rupture)
  - Pancreatitis
  - Splenic rupture or infarction

REVIEW QUESTIONS

For review questions, please go to www.expertconsult.com.

SUGGESTED READINGS

Fraser RG, Pare JAP, Pare PD, et al: *Diagnosis of diseases of the chest*, Philadelphia, 1991, WB Saunders.
Sherman CB: Inflammatory disease of the lung. In Barondess JA, Carpenter CJ, editors: *Differential diagnosis*, Philadelphia, 1994, Lea & Febiger.
Teeter JG, Terry PB: Pulmonary nodules, masses and mediastinal disease. In Barondess JA, Carpenter CJ, editors: *Differential diagnosis*, Philadelphia, 1994, Lea & Febiger.

Interstitial Lung Disease

MAUREEN R. HORTON, MD; and ROBERT W. HALLOWELL, MD

This chapter covers a group of diseases that produce diffuse involvement of the lung parenchyma with distinct pathophysiology. Some are primary pulmonary diseases; others are seen in association with systemic disorders. The pace of symptom onset, the presence or absence of extrapulmonary signs and symptoms, and the radiographic pattern of the process often provide clues to the etiology.

Idiopathic Pulmonary Fibrosis

Basic Information

- Two thirds of patients have disease onset **when older than 60 years of age**
- Slight male predominance
- Most common idiopathic interstitial pneumonia; over 60% of cases
  - Majority of patients have a history of smoking; environmental exposures may play a role
  - Familial forms, while reported, are rare
- No known cause, cure, or effective treatment

Clinical Presentation

- Insidious onset over years; symptoms are usually present for 3 to 5 years prior to diagnosis
- Acute exacerbations portend a worse prognosis
- **Exertional dyspnea; nonproductive cough; rare constitutional symptoms**
- Physical examination
  - Dry, "Velcro-like" crackles
  - Clubbing
  - Signs of elevated right-sided pressure on cardiac examination late in disease (e.g., elevated jugular venous pressure, edema, and right ventricular heave)

Diagnosis, Evaluation, and Treatment

- Imaging
  - Subpleural, reticular and nodular infiltrates with basilar predominance and areas of honeycombing on high-resolution computed tomography (HRCT) (Figs. 20-1 and 20-2)
  - Minimal ground-glass infiltrates that may be asymmetrical
  - Decreasing lung volumes on serial chest radiographs
  - Honeycombing on CT scan correlates with fibrosis on biopsy
- Labs are nonspecific

- Pulmonary function tests (PFTs)
  - **Restrictive disease with decreased forced vital capacity (FVC), total lung capacity (TLC), and diffusing capacity for carbon monoxide (D_{LCO})**
- Diagnosis
  - Made from the constellation of clinical history, classic HRCT findings, and the **absence of other identifiable causes for fibrosis** (e.g., environmental exposures, connective tissue disease, drug toxicity)
  - Surgical lung biopsy demonstrating usual interstitial pneumonitis (UIP) is the gold standard for diagnosing idiopathic pulmonary fibrosis (IPF), **although UIP on biopsy alone is not adequate to make a diagnosis of IPF**
  - Not all patients require surgical lung biopsy if the clinical picture is overwhelmingly suggestive in the setting of a UIP pattern on HRCT
  - Table 20-1 lists diagnostic categories of alternative idiopathic interstitial pneumonias
- Therapy/natural history
  - Lung transplantation remains the only effective treatment
  - *N*-acetylcysteine 600 mg three times daily has been demonstrated in one study to slow the progression of IPF compared with placebo
  - While often used in acute exacerbations, steroids have not proven effective, with historic response rates less than 5% to 10%
  - Cytotoxic agents (azathioprine, cyclophosphamide) are also ineffective

Desquamative Interstitial Pneumonia

Basic Information

- Desquamative interstitial pneumonia (DIP) is a misnomer; histologic finding is a pigmented macrophage infiltrate, not desquamated cells
- Rare
- Ninety percent of patients are smokers
  - Presents as the insidious onset of cough and dyspnea over several weeks
- The relationship between respiratory bronchiolitis-associated interstitial lung disease (RBILD) and DIP is controversial, although both may fall within a spectrum of the same disease

FIGURE 20-1 Reticular infiltrates in a patient with idiopathic pulmonary fibrosis. Note the subpleural, peripheral distribution of infiltrates.

FIGURE 20-2 Lungs of a patient with end-stage idiopathic pulmonary fibrosis.

- RBILD is less severe and also smoking-related. It involves an infiltration of pigmented macrophages into the bronchioles and alveolar ducts.

Imaging
- Linear opacities on chest radiograph. HRCT shows ground glass (50% basilar predominant); reticular, consolidative, and honeycomb patterns uncommon

Diagnosis
- Histology shows diffuse accumulation of intra-alveolar macrophages

Treatment
- Resolution of symptoms may be seen in some patients following smoking cessation. Steroids may have some benefit. Up to 25% of patients progress despite therapy (see Table 20-1).

TABLE 20-1	Idiopathic Interstitial Pneumonias			
	UIP	**DIP**	**AIP**	**NSIP**
Onset	Insidious	Insidious	Acute	Subacute
Steroid response	Poor	Good	Poor	Good
Complete recovery possible?	No	Yes	Yes	Yes

AIP, acute interstitial pneumonitis; DIP, desquamative interstitial pneumonitis; NSIP, nonspecific interstitial pneumonitis; UIP, usual interstitial pneumonitis.

Connective Tissue Diseases

SYSTEMIC LUPUS ERYTHEMATOSIS

Basic Information
- Systemic lupus erythematosus (SLE) is a systemic, autoimmune disease that may involve the lung or pleura
- Rarely causes chronic interstitial lung disease (ILD)
- More than one manifestation may be present in a single patient

Clinical Presentation
Table 20-2 summarizes the clinical presentations of pulmonary SLE.
- Other clinical presentations may include:
  - **Alveolar hemorrhage**
    - Acute fever, dyspnea, cough, with or without hemoptysis
    - **Falling hematocrit with new infiltrates suggests alveolar hemorrhage**
    - Can be diagnosed with bronchoscopy
    - May be seen in the presence or absence of the antiphospholipid antibody syndrome
  - **Diaphragm dysfunction**
    - "Shrinking lung syndrome": **Smaller lung volumes resulting from diaphragm weakness**

RHEUMATOID ARTHRITIS

Basic Information
- Although rheumatoid arthritis (RA) is more common in females, **RA lung disease is more common in males (3:1)**
- **RA lung disease precedes joint symptoms in 20% of cases**
- Multiple pulmonary manifestations of RA

Clinical Presentation
See Table 20-2 for a summary of the clinical presentation of RA.
- Other clinical presentations may include:
  - Rheumatoid (necrobiotic) nodules
    - **May be single or multiple; may cavitate**
    - Pathology of nodules reveals histiocytic palisades specific for RA
    - Caplan syndrome: Rheumatoid nodules in coal miners

TABLE 20-2	*Pulmonary Manifestations of Connective Tissue Diseases*			
	SLE	**RA**	**Scleroderma**	**PM**
Acute pneumonitis	May be initial manifestation of SLE Acute-onset fever, pneumonic symptoms Diffuse or patchy infiltrates in chest film Pleuritis, pericarditis are common	None	Aspiration pneumonia is common consequence of esophageal dysmotility	None
Interstitial disease	Progression from acute pneumonitis is gradual; dyspnea, ± pleuritis, ± productive cough Lower lobe infiltrates on chest film, with increasing restriction of PFTs	Similar to IPF Dyspnea and cough are common Clubbing is common Lower lobe infiltrates, with or without honeycombing Variable response to corticosteroids	Can be seen in patients with CREST or diffuse disease Usually after skin disease Infiltrates are predominantly lower lobe Clubbing is rare Recurrent aspiration may present as interstitial disease	Progressive DOE ± Muscle symptoms Lower lobe infiltrates
Pleural disease	Pain, dyspnea, fever, and effusion are common Pleural fluid is exudative, with normal glucose and normal pH Pleural fluid ANA may be increased LE cells diagnostic	Symptoms related to pleural disease are present in 20% of patients Pleural fluid: Low pH, glucose <30 mg/dL in 70–80% of patients Pleural fluid RF may be increased and greater than serum RF	Thickening or effusions in 10–25%, but rarely symptomatic	None
Pulmonary hypertension	Rare without parenchymal disease May be primary arteriolar disease or secondary to interstitial lung disease	Secondary to hypoxia with severe ILD Idiopathic secondary to RA	Seen in 10% of patients with CREST Pulmonary hypertension in patients with scleroderma is a primary vascular disease, and occurs independent of parenchymal disease	Usually secondary to parenchymal disease

ANA, antinuclear antibody; CREST, calcinosis, Raynaud syndrome, esophageal dysmotility, sclerodactyly, telangiectasia; DOE, dyspnea on exertion; ILD, interstitial lung disease; IPF, idiopathic pulmonary fibrosis; LE, lupus erythematosus; PFTs, pulmonary function tests; PM, polymyositis; RA, rheumatoid arthritis; RF, rheumatoid factor; SLE, systemic lupus erythematosus.

- Bronchiolitis obliterans
  - **Dyspnea, dry cough; chest radiograph is clear or hyperinflated**
  - Obstruction on PFTs
  - Pathology reveals lymphoplasmacytic infiltration of airway wall
  - Poor response to therapy
- Cricoarytenoid arthritis
  - **Pain, hoarseness, dyspnea, stridor, obstruction**
  - Symptoms in 25% of patients with RA

SCLERODERMA

Basic Information

- **60% to 100% of patients with scleroderma have ILD at autopsy**
- There are several manifestations of lung disease in scleroderma
  - Pulmonary hypertension occurs in 5% to 37% of patients and is more common with CREST syndrome. It can be secondary to ILD or as a result of primary vascular involvement.

Clinical Presentation

See Table 20-2.

POLYMYOSITIS/DERMATOMYOSITIS

Basic Information

- More common in females
- 10% present with ILD prior to myositis
- Associated with anti-Jo, anti-PL-12, or other antisynthetase antibodies
  - Biopsy can show UIP or nonspecific interstitial pneumonitis (NSIP) pattern
- The antisynthetase syndrome is characterized by ILD with minimal or subclinical muscle symptoms
- Patients may be steroid responsive

Clinical Presentation

- Dyspnea on exertion, proximal muscle weakness, skin rash, "heliotrope" rash around eyes, "mechanic's hands." While often present, elevated creatine kinase and aldolase are not needed for the diagnosis.

| TABLE 20-3 | Comparison of Pulmonary-Renal Disorders |

	Wegener Granulomatosis	Microscopic Polyangiitis	Goodpasture Syndrome
Presentation	Ears, nose, and throat are involved in 85% of patients Kidney is ultimately involved in 85% of cases Cough and dyspnea Pleural effusion, subglottic/bronchial stenoses or endobronchial lesions seen Can involve skin, joints, eyes, and neurologic system	Upper respiratory tract is involved in only 35% Kidneys are most common organ affected (90%) Cough and dyspnea Pleural effusion, subglottic/bronchial stenoses or endobronchial lesions Can involve skin, joints, eyes, and neurologic system	Hemoptysis, dyspnea, cough, and fatigue are the primary symptoms Fever, chills, and weight loss occur in <25% of patients
Radiographic findings	Infiltrates, nodules, or cavitation may be seen Infiltrates or nodules may be unilateral or bilateral	Similar to WG	Bilateral infiltrates are the most common chest radiographic finding
Diagnostic studies	ESR commonly increased Abnormal urinalysis 80% PR3-ANCA most strongly correlated with WG, but sensitivity and specificity variable MPO-ANCA can be positive in up to 20% of cases Lung or kidney biopsy demonstrates **granulomatous** inflammation	Elevated ESR Abnormal urinalysis MPO-ANCA is most strongly correlated with MPA, but PR3-ANCA can also be positive No granulomas on biopsy; most common lung finding is pulmonary capillaritis	Anemia is common Hematuria and proteinuria are seen in 90% of patients Anti-GBM antibodies are seen in 90% of patients Suspect when patient has the constellation of alveolar infiltrates, anemia, and renal disease Linear IgG in biopsy, or anti-GBM antibodies are diagnostic
Treatment	Limited disease: Methotrexate plus prednisone Life- or organ-threatening disease: Oral daily cytoxan plus prednisone If patient is severely ill, give solumedrol 1 g/day for 3 days followed by oral prednisone Cyclophosphamide for 3–6 mo; taper steroids over 6 mo 75–90% complete remission Plasmapharesis is only indicated for severe pulmonary hemorrhage or cases with positive anti-GBM	Treatment is the same as for WG MPA is less likely to relapse than WG	Corticosteroids, cyclophosphamide, **plasmapheresis**

ANCA, antineutrophil cytoplasmic antibody; ESR, erythrocyte sedimentation rate; GBM, glomerular basement membrane; IgG, immunoglobulin; MPA, microscopic polyangiitis; MPO, myeloperoxidase; PR3, proteinase 3; WG, Wegener granulomatosis.

Anti-neutrophil Cytoplasmic Antibody (ANCA)–Associated Vasculitides

WEGENER GRANULOMATOSIS

Basic Information
- Also known as "ANCA-positive granulomatous vasculitis"
  - 90% of cases have ANCA antibodies
- Two forms described
  - **Classic disease: Involving the upper and lower respiratory tracts and kidney**
  - **Limited disease: Isolated respiratory tract involvement. Up to 40% may be negative for ANCA antibodies.**
- Characteristic pathology reveals necrotizing granulomatous inflammation and small-vessel vasculitis of the upper and lower respiratory tracts and necrotizing glomerulonephritis in the kidney
- Majority of cases demonstrate positive proteinase 3 (PR3)-ANCA

Clinical Presentation
See Table 20-3.

MICROSCOPIC POLYANGIITIS

Basic Information
- Most common ANCA-associated small-vessel vasculitis
- Similar to Wegener granulomatosis, only without the presence of granulomas on biopsy
- Upper respiratory tract involvement is much less common
- Majority of cases demonstrate positive myeloperoxidase (MPO)-ANCA
- Less likely to relapse than Wegener granulomatosis

FIGURE 20-3 Immunofluorescence study demonstrating linear staining (immunoglobulin G) of alveolar walls in a patient with Goodpasture syndrome. (Original magnification ×10.) *(From Mason RJ: Murray and Nadel's textbook of respiratory medicine, ed 4, Philadelphia, Elsevier Saunders, 2005, Fig. 56.8.)*

CHURG-STRAUSS SYNDROME

Basic Information

- 50% are ANCA positive; MPO-ANCA is most common
- Discussed further below (see Eosinophilic Lung Diseases)

GOODPASTURE SYNDROME

Basic Information

- Disease affecting the lung and kidney associated with **circulating anti–glomerular basement membrane antibodies** that may be the cause of the process (Fig. 20-3)
- MPO-ANCA can be positive in 10% to 40% of cases
- The **lung and kidney are both involved in 60% to 80% of cases;** in the remainder the kidney is involved alone

Clinical Presentation

See Table 20-3.

Eosinophilic Lung Diseases

Basic Information

- Comprise a diverse group of diseases, all of which exhibit blood or tissue eosinophilia

Clinical Presentation and Treatment

- *Acute eosinophilic pneumonia*
  - Acute presentation with infiltrates and hypoxemia with or without peripheral eosinophilia
  - **Diagnosis requires eosinophilia in bronchoalveolar lavage (BAL) fluid or lung tissue**
  - Very steroid-responsive
- *Chronic eosinophilic pneumonia*
  - Subacute presentation with constitutional symptoms, cough, dyspnea, and **peripheral eosinophilia**
  - Chest radiograph with peripheral infiltrates ("**reverse pulmonary edema**"; Fig. 20-4)

FIGURE 20-4 Chest radiograph of a patient with idiopathic chronic eosinophilic pneumonia showing bilateral alveolar opacities predominating in the upper lobes ("reverse pulmonary edema"). *(From Mason RJ: Murray and Nadel's textbook of respiratory medicine, ed 4, Philadelphia, Elsevier Saunders, 2005, Fig. 57-3.)*

  - Diagnosis requires BAL eosinophilia (>40% diagnostic) or lung tissue eosinophilia
  - Very steroid-responsive
  - May develop severe asthma and require chronic steroid use
- *Hypereosinophilic syndrome*
  - Defined as more than **1500 eosinophils/mm³ in peripheral blood for 6 months**
  - Primary targets include the **heart, central nervous system, peripheral nervous system, and skin. The lung is less commonly involved.**
  - Treat with corticosteroids or cytotoxic agents (or both)
- *Allergic bronchopulmonary aspergillosis (ABPA)*
  - Clinical constellation of **asthma, eosinophilia, infiltrates, and mucus plugs**
  - Bronchiectasis may result (Fig. 20-5)
  - Diagnosis is made by demonstrating eosinophilia, a positive skin test or antibodies to *Aspergillus*, an increased total and specific immunoglobulin E, and recurrent infiltrates on chest film
  - Very responsive to corticosteroids and itraconazole
- *Allergic angiitis and granulomatosis (Churg-Strauss syndrome)*
  - Clinical constellation of **asthma, eosinophilia, and systemic vasculitis**
  - Lung biopsy reveals eosinophilia and extravascular granulomas
  - **Asthma is present in more than 80% of patients** and radiographic infiltrates are present in more than 90% of patients; 30% have pleural effusions
  - Disease may be unmasked after tapering systemic steroids in an asthmatic

FIGURE 20-5 Axial computed tomography scan of a patient with allergic bronchopulmonary aspergillosis showing central bronchiectasis with mucoid impaction. A diffuse bilateral inhomogeneous lung opacity is present, with areas of low attenuation throughout the pulmonary parenchyma representing mosaic perfusion resulting from a combination of large and small airway inflammation. *(From Mason RJ: Murray and Nadel's textbook of respiratory medicine, ed 4, Philadelphia, Elsevier Saunders, 2005, Fig. 57-7.)*

- **This is a systemic illness, with skin (75% of patients) and peripheral nervous system (mononeuritis multiplex in 60% of cases) involvement**
  - **The heart and GI tract may also be involved**
  - The kidney is *rarely* involved
  - Usually responsive to corticosteroids
- *Eosinophilic granuloma (pulmonary Langerhans cell histiocytosis, pulmonary histiocytosis X)*
  - Non-neoplastic collection of Langerhans cells (differentiated cells of the monocyte-macrophage lineage)
  - Despite name, not actually an eosinophilic lung disease, since eosinophils may or may not be present in lesions. Rather, it is a variant of histiocytosis X seen in smoking adults (Box 20-1).
  - Mid-upper lung zone predominance
  - Lesions extend from bronchovascular structures into the surrounding parenchyma to form **stellate lesions**
  - Almost all are smokers
  - 10% to 20% develop spontaneous pneumothorax, often with recurrence
    - Treatment includes smoking cessation with lung transplantation in severe cases. Steroids are generally ineffective.

Bronchiolitis Obliterans with Organizing Pneumonia/ Cryptogenic Organizing Pneumonia

Basic Information

- Pathologic diagnosis of fibroblast and inflammatory cell plugs filling bronchioles, alveolar ducts, and alveoli
- This is a nonspecific histologic reaction that can be **seen in response to infections, connective tissue diseases, or drugs. May also be idiopathic.**

BOX 20-1 | *Eosinophilic Granuloma*

Pulmonary Langerhans cell histiocytosis
Cough and dyspnea in two thirds of patients
Smoking history in 90% of patients
Radiographic manifestations: Progression from diffuse nodules to reticulonodular pattern to diffuse cystic changes in severe disease
Spares costophrenic angles
Pneumothorax common
May have associated central diabetes insipidus and bone cysts
Biopsies reveal CD1a(+), s100+ Langerhans cells on light microscopy with Birbeck granules on electron microscopy
Prognosis usually good with smoking cessation

- A diagnosis of bronchiolitis obliterans with organizing pneumonia (BOOP) typically means the idiopathic form
- This is a different entity from bronchiolitis obliterans (Box 20-2)

Clinical Presentation

- Idiopathic BOOP commonly presents as a subacute illness with an infectious-like onset
  - Cough, dyspnea, and fever are the most common symptoms
  - Crackles or squeaks are present on lung examination in 75% of patients

Evaluation and Diagnosis

- **Patchy infiltrates,** which may migrate, are the most common radiographic finding
- **PFTs reveal restriction and hypoxemia, in contrast to bronchiolitis obliterans, which is characterized by an obstructive PFT pattern**
- Obstruction is seen in only 20% of patients with BOOP; nearly all are smokers

Treatment

- Idiopathic **BOOP is steroid responsive**, with typical doses 0.75 to 1.5 mg/kg prednisone/day
- Relapse is common if the duration of therapy is less than 6 months
- The response to therapy in drug- and connective tissue disease–associated BOOP is much less predictable

Asbestos-Related Lung Disease

Basic Information

- Disease results from chronic exposure over prolonged periods, usually years
- Sources of exposure include the auto industry (brakes), construction, demolition, shipbuilding and renovation, the cement industry, and mining

Clinical Presentation

- Asbestosis
  - Manifests as progressive dyspnea, usually 10+ years after exposure

| BOX 20-2 | *Bronchiolitis Obliterans (Obliterative Bronchiolitis)* |

Basic Information

A variety of associations, including postinfection (viral primarily); post-transplantation; toxin/fumes exposure; drugs (e.g., penicillamine, gold); and connective tissue diseases

There is also an idiopathic form

Clinical Presentation

The primary clinical manifestation is dyspnea

Evaluation and Diagnosis

Pulmonary function tests reveal obstruction or air trapping with high residual volumes

Chest radiographs may reveal hyperinflation or may be normal

Lung biopsies demonstrate a constrictive bronchiolitis

Treatment

The response to corticosteroid therapy is generally poor

FIGURE 20-6 Mesothelioma. Axial thoracic computed tomography scan shows diffuse right pleural thickening (*arrows*) associated with marked volume loss in the right thorax. Note the presence of mediastinal pleural involvement (*arrowhead*). (*From Mason RJ: Murray and Nadel's textbook of respiratory medicine, ed 4, Philadelphia, Elsevier Saunders, 2005, Fig. 70.2.*)

- Intensity of asbestos exposure affects expression and latency
- Interstitial fibrosis, primarily in the lower lobes, similar to IPF
- Pleural disease
  - Benign pleural disease is typically the first manifestation; includes pleural plaques, thickening, and benign effusions
  - **Mesothelioma is a malignant tumor of the pleura,** presenting with chest pain (often pleuritic), dyspnea, weight loss, and cough, after a latency of 20 to 40 years (Fig. 20-6)
  - **Mesothelioma is not affected by smoking**
  - There is no effective therapy
- Lung cancer and asbestos
  - The risk of lung cancer in an asbestos-exposed individual is increased 4- to 5-fold in a nonsmoker and by 50-fold in smokers, compared with non–asbestos-exposed nonsmokers

Sarcoidosis

Basic Information

- Sarcoidosis is a systemic disease of unknown origin
- Pathologic **hallmark is the noncaseating granuloma**
- Presentation
  - Most instances (70–80%) occur between the ages of 20 and 50 years
  - More common in blacks and females in the United States
  - 30% to 60% of cases are asymptomatic

Clinical Presentation

- Constitutional symptoms including weight loss, fatigue, fever, and malaise may occur
- Respiratory tract
  - The lung is involved in more than 90% of cases

- Cough, dyspnea, sputum production, and hemoptysis can be seen
- Endobronchial disease may produce obstructive symptoms
- The upper respiratory tract can be involved, producing nasal and upper airway obstruction or hoarseness
- Mycetomas can be seen in fibrocystic sarcoid lesions
- Eye
  - Uveitis and keratoconjunctivitis
  - Sicca syndrome (dry eyes and mouth)
  - Uveoparotid fever in sarcoidosis (Heerfordt-Waldenström syndrome) is the constellation of bilateral lacrimal and parotid gland enlargement, fever, and anterior uveitis
- Heart
  - Myocardial granulomatous inflammation can produce conduction abnormalities, tachyarrhythmias, cardiomyopathy, and sudden death
  - Cor pulmonale can be seen in patients with chronic severe pulmonary disease
- Neurologic
  - Up to 5% of patients with sarcoidosis have neurologic manifestations
  - Central nervous system findings may precede other findings, but peripheral nerves are typically involved late
  - Cranial nerves (II, VII, VIII, IX, X), meninges, and pituitary gland most often involved
  - Lumbar puncture may reveal increased cells (typically monocyte predominant), protein, or opening pressure, in addition to decreased glucose. Cerebrospinal fluid is normal in up to 30% of patients with neurosarcoid.
- Skin
  - Erythema nodosum most common skin finding (Fig. 20-7)
  - **Löfgren syndrome: Erythema nodosum with hilar adenopathy, arthralgias, and fever—spontaneous resolution common**

FIGURE 20-7 Erythema nodosum. *(From Habif TP: Clinical dermatology: a color guide to diagnostic therapy, ed 4, St. Louis, Mosby, 2004, Fig. 18-9.)*

TABLE 20-4	*Chest Radiographic Staging in Sarcoidosis*	
Type	Distribution	Frequency (%)
0	Normal	5–10
I	Hilar nodes	45–65
II	Hilar nodes + reticular opacities	25–30
III	Reticular opacities alone	15
IV	Pulmonary fibrosis	5–10

FIGURE 20-8 Posteroanterior chest radiograph of stage I sarcoidosis. Important features include prominent hilar lymphanopathy and normal lung fields. *(From Mason RJ: Murray and Nadel's textbook of respiratory medicine, ed 4, Philadelphia, Elsevier Saunders, 2005, Fig. 55-1.)*

- Lupus pernio: Purplish nodules or plaques on cheeks, nose, and ears
- Treatment of skin disease may be with chloroquine or pentoxifylline, rather than corticosteroids
- Liver
  - Hepatic granulomas in 75% of patients
  - Only 35% have elevated liver function tests; alkaline phosphatase is the best clinical predictor
  - Symptomatic liver disease uncommon

Evaluation and Diagnosis

- Chest radiographs in patients with sarcoidosis have been typed (or staged) based on the pattern of abnormalities (Table 20-4 and Fig. 20-8)
- Disease progression is not necessarily from one stage to next
- **Tissue biopsy revealing noncaseating granulomas is required for the diagnosis**
- Serum angiotensin-converting enzyme level may be elevated in patients with sarcoidosis and may track with disease activity. However, it is nonspecific and nondiagnostic, so its role in management is undefined.

Treatment

- Treatment should be limited to symptomatic or progressive pulmonary disease or any involvement of heart, eye, or nervous system
- Corticosteroids (usually low to moderate doses) are the mainstay of therapy; alternative regimens including methotrexate or azathioprine may be used in refractory cases or as steroid-sparing agents

REVIEW QUESTIONS

For review questions, please go to www.expertconsult.com.

SUGGESTED READINGS

Browne K: Asbestos-related disorders. In Parkes WR, editor: *Occupational lung disorders*, Boston, 1994, Butterworth Heinemann.

Delaney P: Neurologic manifestations of sarcoidosis, *Ann Intern Med* 87:336–345, 1977.

Epler GR, editor: *Diseases of the bronchioles*, New York, 1994, Raven Press.

Johns CJ, Scott PP, Schonfeld SA: Sarcoidosis, *Annu Rev Med* 40:353–371, 1989.

Katzenstein A- L: *Katzenstein and Askin's surgical pathology of non-neoplastic lung disease*, Philadelphia, 1997, WB Saunders.

Katzenstein A-L, Myers JL: Idiopathic pulmonary fibrosis, *Am J Respir Crit Care Med* 157:1301–1315, 1998.

Ragu GA, et al: An Official ATS/ERS/JRS/ALAT Statement. Idiopathic pulmonary fibrosis: evidence-based guidelines for diagnosis and management, *Am J Respir Crit Care Med* 181:788–824, 2011.

Schwarz MI, King TE, Cherniak RM: Principles of and approach to the patient with interstitial lung disease. In Murray JF, Nadel JA, editors: *Textbook of respiratory medicine*, ed 3, Philadelphia, 2000, WB Saunders.

20

Venous Thromboembolic Disease

DAVID B. PEARSE, MD

Venous thromboembolism, which includes deep venous thrombosis (DVT) and pulmonary thromboembolism (PE), occurs for the first time in approximately 100 persons per 100,000 in the United States each year. **More than 80% of clinically significant pulmonary emboli occur from DVTs in the lower extremities;** the remaining emboli originate from pelvic and upper extremity veins. The estimated short-term mortality rate from untreated PE (30%) is markedly reduced (<5%) by successful diagnosis and appropriate therapy. Unfortunately, the diagnoses of DVT and PE are frequently missed, and effective prophylactic treatment is underused.

Deep Venous Thrombosis

Basic Information

- Virchow's triad
  - **Venous stasis**
    - Immobility
    - Elevated venous pressure
    - Elevated blood viscosity
  - **Vessel wall damage**
  - **Increased blood coagulability**
    - Activation of clotting
    - Inhibition of fibrinolytic system
    - Deficiencies of coagulation factors
- Mechanisms
  - **Most important clinical risk is venous stasis from immobility**

Clinical Risk Factors

- Lower extremity DVT
  - Recent surgery
  - Major trauma **(>50% develop DVT if prophylaxis not implemented)**
  - Previous DVT **(25% recurrence over 5 years after first DVT)**
  - Increasing age (exponential increase after age 50 years)
  - Pregnancy/puerperium (PE is second leading cause of death; 75% occur postpartum)
  - Oral contraception
  - Medical conditions with immobility/hypercoagulability
    - Common: cancer, heart failure, myocardial infarction, obesity, myeloproliferative disorder, nephrotic syndrome

- Uncommon: systemic lupus erythematosus, antiphospholipid antibody, sickle cell anemia, homocystinuria, Behçet syndrome
- Upper extremity DVT
  - Central venous catheter
  - Cancer

Familial Thrombophilic Disorders

- Common
  - Activated protein C resistance (factor V Leiden)
    - Autosomal dominant defect of factor V (incomplete penetrance): Prevents inactivation by protein C
    - **5% of normal white population is heterozygous;** rare in those of African or Asian descent
    - 20% of unselected DVT patients; 60% of idiopathic, recurrent DVTs are heterozygous
    - DVT recurrence risk significant in homozygotes; insignificant in heterozygotes
  - Prothrombin 20210A
    - Gene defect causing increased prothrombin and thrombin
    - **2% of normal white population;** rare in those of African or Asian descent
    - 5% of unselected DVTs, problematic when coexisting with other defects
- Rare
  - Deficiencies of antithrombin III, protein C, protein S
    - Autosomal dominant
    - **Protein C or S deficiency associated with warfarin-induced skin necrosis**

Clinical Presentation

- **Symptoms and signs neither sensitive nor specific**
  - Only 35% of symptomatic patients have leg DVT
  - Leg pain or swelling may be present
  - Homans' sign (pain and tenderness with dorsiflexion of ankle) present in less than 40%
- Starts in calf (except leg trauma, orthopedic surgery); most self-limited
- 25% of calf DVTs extend to thigh
- **Thigh DVTs strongly associated with PE**
  - Untreated symptomatic proximal DVT: 20% mortality from acute PE
  - 40% to 50% of patients with symptomatic thigh DVT have silent PE
- DVT recurs in 25% by 5 years; **50% of recurrences in contralateral leg**

Diagnosis and Evaluation

- Noninvasive
  - B-mode compression ultrasonography (US)
    - Visualizes noncompressible clot in proximal veins; **poor for calf DVT**
    - 97% sensitive and specific for **symptomatic** proximal leg DVT
    - 30% to 60% sensitive, 98% specific for **asymptomatic** proximal leg DVT
    - **Initial test of choice for upper extremity DVT evaluation** but sensitivity and specificity 80%
    - Addition of Doppler flow or color adds little to sensitivity
  - Computed tomographic (CT) venography
    - Performed with CT angiography (CTA); able to visualize clot in thigh, pelvic veins, inferior vena cava (IVC)
    - Contrast dye load
    - **Sensitivity and specificity comparable to compression US so not routinely recommended**
    - **Useful with injured or casted leg** as US cannot be performed in this scenario
  - Magnetic resonance imaging (MRI)
    - Able to visualize clot in calf, thigh, pelvic veins, IVC, upper extremities
    - Performed with injured or casted leg as US cannot be performed in this scenario
    - Requires administration of high-dose gadolinium
      - Can cause nephrogenic systemic fibrosis
    - Sensitivity and specificity greater than 90%
- D-Dimer
  - Degradation product of cross-linked fibrin
  - Elevated in DVT/PE but also in
    - Surgery, trauma, malignancy, disseminated intravascular coagulopathy, pregnancy, infection, normal elderly
  - Assay
    - Enzyme-linked immunosorbent assay (ELISA) more sensitive than latex agglutination
    - **Positive D-dimer not helpful;** negative (i.e., normal) D-dimer more clinically useful as follows
      - Normal D-dimer with low pretest probability for DVT or PE excludes thromboembolism
      - Normal highly sensitive D-dimer with nondiagnostic ventilation-perfusion $(\dot{V}/\dot{Q})$ scan excludes PE
  - **Usefulness limited in inpatients and the elderly**
- Invasive: Venography
  - **Gold standard,** detects thigh, calf, and upper extremity DVT regardless of symptoms
  - **Can distinguish between acute and recurrent clot**
  - Risks of contrast dye
  - Painful, can cause thrombosis
  - Decreasing availability
- DVT diagnosis in the symptomatic lower extremity
  - Determine pretest clinical risk using Well's prediction rule (Table 21-1)
  - Low clinical suspicion and normal D-dimer
    - Further testing unnecessary, low incidence of DVT/PE if no therapy given
  - Low clinical suspicion and negative US (if D-dimer not available)

TABLE 21-1	*Assessment of Pretest Probability of Deep Venous Thrombosis (DVT)*	
Variables		**Points**
Active cancer		1
Paralysis, paresis, or recent plaster immobilization of lower extremities		1
Bedridden >3 days or major surgery within 12 wk		1
Localized tenderness along deep veins		1
Swelling of entire leg		1
Calf swelling >3 cm larger than other side		1
Pitting edema of symptomatic leg		1
Collateral superficial veins		1
Alternative diagnosis at least as likely as DVT		−2

Clinical pretest probability for PE: low, <1; intermediate, 1–2; high, >2. Data from Wells PS, Hirsh J, Anderson DR, et al: Accuracy of clinical assessment of deep-vein thrombosis, *Lancet* 345:1326–1330, 1995.

- Further testing unnecessary, low incidence of DVT/PE if no therapy given
- Moderate or high clinical suspicion: US necessary
- **Negative initial US:** 15% of these patients have calf DVT; 20% to 30% of these will extend to thigh
  - US should be repeated at 1 week
- Negative serial US: Acceptable 1% to 2% risk of thromboembolism if untreated
- Immediate venogram is alternative to serial US

DVT Treatment/Prophylaxis

- Treatment of DVT—see Treatment section under Pulmonary Embolism
- Prophylaxis choice depends on the risk of thrombosis for an individual (Table 21-2)

Pulmonary Embolism

Basic Information

- Effects of pulmonary emboli on gas exchange
  - Dead space increased but **arterial partial pressure of carbon dioxide ($Paco_2$) normal or low** (from hyperventilation)
  - **Hypoxemia variable** because it is epiphenomenon of thrombus (e.g., atelectasis, edema, interatrial shunting, low mixed venous oxygen tension)
- Effects of pulmonary emboli on pulmonary and systemic hemodynamics
  - In previously healthy patients
    - Peripheral vascular resistance (PVR) increase proportional to obstruction
    - Pulmonary artery pressure (P_{PA}) increases after 30% to 50% of bed occluded
    - Normal right ventricle (RV): **Maximal mean P_{PA} of 40 mm Hg**
  - In patients with preexisting heart/lung disease
    - No correlation of clot burden with PVR or P_{PA}
  - Shock
    - Increased right atrial pressure decreases venous return

TABLE 21-2	*DVT Prophylaxis*	
	Clinical Risks	**Prophylaxis**
Low risk (<10% DVT*)	Minor surgery in mobile patients Medical patients who are fully mobile	Early ambulation Compression stockings
Moderate risk (10–40% DVT)	Most general, open gynecologic or urogenital surgery Medical patients, bed rest or sick Moderate risk plus high bleeding risk	LMWH (e.g., enoxaparin 40 mg SQ qd) LDUH (5000 U SQ bid or tid), fondaparinux Mechanical thromboprophylaxis†

High risk (40–80% DVT)	Hip or knee arthroplasty
	Hip fracture surgery
	Extensive trauma
	Stroke, spinal cord injury
	Major cancer surgery or major surgery
	  with history of DVT
		LMWH (e.g., enoxaparin 40 mg qd or
		  30 mg bid), fondaparinux (hip surgery
		  or fracture), or moderate-dose warfarin
		  (INR 2–3)
		Continue LMWH after hospital discharge for
		  up to 28 days

*Rates based on objective diagnostic screening for DVT in patients not receiving thromboprophylaxis.
†Mechanical thromboprophylaxis includes intermittent pneumatic compression and/or graduated compression stockings.
DVT, deep venous thromboembolism; INR, international normalized rate; LDUH, low-dose unfractionated heparin; LMWH, low-molecular-weight
  heparin.
From Geerts WH, Bergqvist D, Pineo GH, et al: Prevention of venous thromboembolism, *Chest* 133:381S–453S, 2008.

FIGURE 21-1 Proposed diagnostic algorithm for pulmonary embolism (PE) in patients with low or intermediate pretest probability using either V̇/Q̇ scan or computed tomographic angiography (CTA) as initial test. (MD-CTA, multidetector CT angiogram; V̇/Q̇, ventilation-perfusion scan; VUS, venous ultrasound; *dashed line* indicates optional choice; *using a highly sensitive assay.) (Modified from Torbicki A, Perrier A, Konstantinides S, et al: Guidelines on the diagnosis and management of acute pulmonary embolism. Eur Heart J 29:2276–2315, 2008.)*

- RV distention leads to shift of interventricular septum, causing impaired left ventricular function

Clinical Presentation

- **PE presents as**
  - **Infarction-like syndrome: chest pain, cough, hemoptysis (65%)**
  - **Dyspnea syndrome (22%)**
  - **Circulatory collapse (8%)**
- **Major symptoms: dyspnea, chest pain, cough**
- **Major signs: tachypnea, crackles, tachycardia**

- Dyspnea, tachypnea, or pleuritic chest pain present in 97% of PE cases

Diagnosis and Evaluation

See Figures 21-1 and 21-2.
- Chest radiograph and electrocardiogram (ECG)
  - Abnormal in 70% to 90%, but nonspecific
    - Atelectasis, consolidation, diaphragm elevation on chest film
    - Nonspecific ST-segment changes on ECG
- Arterial blood gases

- **Wide alveolar-to-arterial O₂ gradient**
- **Respiratory alkalosis**
- **Hypoxemia** with the following caveats
  - 12% to 25% of patients have an arterial partial pressure of oxygen (PaO_2) greater than 80 mm Hg
  - 20% have normal age-defined alveolar-to-arterial O_2 gradient
- PE diagnosis in the symptomatic patient
  - Determine pretest clinical risk using Well's prediction rule (Table 21-3)
  - Low or intermediate clinical risk and normal D-dimer
    - Further testing unnecessary, low incidence of DVT/PE if no therapy given
  - Low/intermediate clinical risk and elevated D-dimer or high clinical risk
    - Further testing necessary
    - Lung imaging with $\dot{V}/\dot{Q}$ scan (Fig. 21-3 and Table 21-4) or CTA
  - Normal $\dot{V}/\dot{Q}$ scan rules out PE regardless of clinical suspicion or ventilation scan findings
  - High-probability $\dot{V}/\dot{Q}$ scan and moderate/high clinical probability: 88% to 96% positive predictive value
  - High-probability $\dot{V}/\dot{Q}$ scan and low clinical probability: 50% positive predictive value
  - All other abnormal $\dot{V}/\dot{Q}$ scan/clinical probability combinations: PE risk unpredictable but substantial (20–40%)
  - Specificity of high-probability $\dot{V}/\dot{Q}$ scan not altered by underlying lung disease such as chronic obstructive pulmonary disease

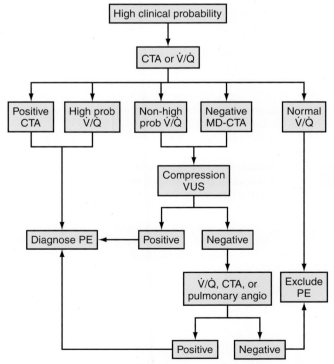

FIGURE 21-2 Proposed diagnostic algorithm for pulmonary embolism (PE) in patients with high pretest probability using either $\dot{V}/\dot{Q}$ scan or computed tomographic angiography (CTA) as initial test. (MD-CTA, multidetector CT angiogram; $\dot{V}/\dot{Q}$, ventilation-perfusion scan; VUS, venous ultrasound.) *(Modified from Torbicki A, Perrier A, Konstantinides S, et al: Guidelines on the diagnosis and management of acute pulmonary embolism. Eur Heart J 29:2276–2315, 2008.)*

- Proximal filling defects on CTA diagnostic (Fig. 21-4); **single distal filling defects can be false positive,** so further testing may be justified
- Negative multidetector CTA adequate stopping point only if low or intermediate pretest risk
- If additional testing needed, can perform $\dot{V}/\dot{Q}$ scan, CTA, pulmonary angiography, or lower extremity US as secondary test depending on initial test choice
- Role for serial leg studies following $\dot{V}/\dot{Q}$ testing
  - Low/intermediate clinical probability, intermediate- or low-probability $\dot{V}/\dot{Q}$ scan, negative leg US, and good cardiopulmonary reserve (no shock, syncope, RV dysfunction, or respiratory failure)
    - Two additional leg studies at 7 and 14 days off anticoagulant; if negative, no treatment
    - If cardiopulmonary reserve poor: proceed with lung imaging with spiral CT or angiography
  - This strategy results in
    - Less than 10% overall need for pulmonary angiography in PE work-up
    - Less than 3% subsequent thromboembolism at 3 months if anticoagulant withheld

Treatment

- Acceptable forms of therapy
  - Low-molecular-weight heparin (LMWH) 100 units/kg every 12 hours or 200 units/kg once per day (no monitoring, contraindicated if renal failure), *or*
  - Unfractionated heparin (UH) 80 units/kg IV bolus, then 18 units/kg/hr, activated partial thromboplastin time (aPTT) 1.5 to 2.5 continuous *or*
  - UH 17,500 units subQ every 12 hours, aPTT 1.5 to 2.5 continuous, *then*
  - Warfarin 5 mg/day started day 1, overlapped with heparin 2 days, target international normalized ratio (INR) 2 to 3
    - Proteins C and S decline when warfarin is started during an active thrombotic state. This decline causes an increase in thrombogenic potential. Heparin can counteract this temporary procoagulant effect.

TABLE 21-3	Assessment of Pretest Probability of Pulmonary Embolism	
Variables		**Points**
Clinical signs and symptoms of DVT		3.0
Alternative diagnosis less likely than PE		3.0
Heart rate >100/min		1.5
Immobilization or surgery in preceding 4 weeks		1.5
Previous DVT or PE		1.5
Hemoptysis		1.0
Cancer		1.0

Clinical pretest probability for PE: low, <2; intermediate, 2–6; high, >6.
DVT, deep venous thromboembolism; PE, pulmonary thromboembolism.
From Wells PS, Ginsberg JS, Anderson DR, et al: Use of a clinical model for safe management of patients with suspected pulmonary embolism, *Ann Intern Med* 129:997–1005, 1998.

A Posterior perfusion

B Equilibrium

FIGURE 21-3 Lung ventilation and perfusion scintigraphy. **A,** Multiple perfusion defects in left upper lobe and right midzone on perfusion scan. **B,** Normal ventilation scan. This combination is consistent with high probability of pulmonary embolism. *(From Haslett C, Chilvers ER, Boon NA, et al: Davidson's principles and practice of medicine, ed 19, New York, Churchill Livingstone, 2002, Fig. 13.6.)*

- PE/DVT: Duration of therapy
  - **Three months with reversible major risk factors**
  - **Six months with reversible minor risk factors** (estrogen therapy, partial immobilization)
  - **Six months to indefinite for idiopathic DVT/PE**
    - Indefinite if low bleeding risk and patient agrees
    - Six months if significant bleeding risk or patient refuses indefinite treatment
  - **Twelve months to indefinite for**
    - First DVT/PE with cancer, antiphospholipid antibody, deficiency of antithrombin III, *or*
    - Second DVT/PE, which is idiopathic or associated with thrombophilic disorder
    - Indefinite if low bleeding risk and patient agrees
    - Twelve months if significant bleeding risk or patient refuses indefinite treatment
- Thrombolytic therapy (TT)
  - TT indicated for
    - **PE with severe hemodynamic/oxygenation compromise**
      - In PE, TT accelerates resolution of physiologic abnormalities and scan defects
      - **However, no difference at 7 days compared with heparin**
    - Extensive iliofemoral DVT
      - Decreases postphlebitic syndrome
    - Use of TT in submassive PE (normal blood pressure but RV dysfunction) controversial
    - Submassive PE associated with increased mortality on heparin therapy
    - TT not shown to decrease mortality in this subgroup
  - Risk of TT
    - Serious bleeding 6% to 45% (threefold > heparin)
    - Fatal bleeding 2% (10-fold > heparin)
  - Approved drugs
    - Recombinant tissue-type plasminogen activator (rt-PA) infusion over 2 hours
    - Streptokinase infusion over 24 hours
    - Urokinase infusion over 12 to 24 hours
  - Contraindications to TT
    - Absolute
      - **Intracranial or intraspinal disorders, surgery, trauma in preceding 2 months**
      - **Active bleeding**

TABLE 21-4	*Ventilation-Perfusion Lung Scanning: The PIOPED Study Criteria*	
Scan Pattern (Prevalence)	**Original Definition**	**Revised Definition**
High probability (13%)	Segmental mismatches: ≥2 large 1 large + 2 moderate ≥4 moderate	≥2 moderate/large segmental mismatch
Intermediate (39%)	Not high or low	1 moderate/large segmental mismatch or match Not high or low
Low (34%)	1 moderate/large segmental mismatch ≥4 moderate/large segmental matches	>3 small subsegmental defects Nonsegmental perfusion defects
Very low/normal (14%)	Normal perfusion ≤3 small subsegmental perfusion defects	Normal perfusion ≤3 small subsegmental perfusion defects

PIOPED, Prospective Investigation of Pulmonary Embolism Diagnosis.

FIGURE 21-4 CT scan demonstrating filling defect in proximal left pulmonary artery (*arrow*) from thrombus. Distal branches of artery are occluded. *(From Souhami R: Textbook of medicine, New York, Churchill Livingstone, 2002, Fig. 13.6.2A.)*

- Relative
  - Surgery, organ biopsy, large-vessel puncture, cardiopulmonary resuscitation, within 10 days postpartum
- Surgical or catheter embolectomy
  - Alternative to TT when TT contraindications present
  - Effective in small case series; morbidity and mortality poorly defined
- IVC filters
  - Indications
    - Contraindication to anticoagulation
    - Recurrence of DVT/PE on therapeutic anticoagulation
  - Effects
    - Decrease early recurrent PE after anticoagulation without mortality effect
    - Increase incidence of later DVT

REVIEW QUESTIONS

For review questions, please go to www.expertconsult.com.

SUGGESTED READINGS

Baarslag HJ, van Beek EJ, Koopman MM, et al: Prospective study of color duplex ultrasonography compared with contrast venography in patients suspected of having deep venous thrombosis of the upper extremities, *Ann Intern Med* 136:865–872, 2002.

Bounameaux H, Perrier A, Righini M: Diagnosis of venous thromboembolism: an update, *Vasc Med* 15:399–406, 2010.

Carrier M, Righini M, Djurabi RK: VIDAS d-dimer in combination with clinical pre-test probability to rule out pulmonary embolism, *Thromb Haemost* 101:886–892, 2009.

Decousus H, Leizorovicz A, Parent F, et al: A clinical trial of vena caval filters in the prevention of pulmonary embolism in patients with proximal deep-vein thrombosis, *N Engl J Med* 338:409–415, 1998.

Elliott CG, Lovelace TD, Brown LM, et al: Diagnosis: imaging techniques, *Clin Chest Med* 31:641–657, 2010.

Geerts WH, Bergqvist D, Pineo GH, et al: Prevention of venous thromboembolism, *Chest* 133:S381–S453, 2008.

Haas S: Venous thromboembolism in medical patients: the scope of the problem, *Semin Thromb Hemost* 29:17–21, 2003.

Kearon C: Duration of therapy for acute venous thromboembolism, *Clin Chest Med* 24:63–72, 2003.

Kearon C, Crowther M, Hirsh J, et al: Management of patients with hereditary hypercoagulable disorders, *Annu Rev Med* 51:169–185, 2000.

Kyrle PA, Rosendaal FR, Eichinger S: Risk assessment for recurrent venous thrombosis, *Lancet* 376:2032–2039, 2010.

Musset D, Parent F, Meyer G, et al: Diagnostic strategy for patients with suspected pulmonary embolism: a prospective multicentre outcome study, *Lancet* 360:1914–1920, 2002.

Qaseem A, Snow V, Barry P, et al: Current diagnosis of venous thromboembolism in primary care: a clinical practice guideline from AAFP and ACP, *Ann Family Med* 5:57–62, 2007.

Stein PD, Fowler SE, Goodman LR, et al: for PIOPED II: Multidetector computed tomography for acute pulmonary embolism, *N Engl J Med* 354:2317–2327, 2006.

Stein PD, Terrin ML, Hales CA, et al: Clinical, laboratory, x-ray, and EKG findings in patients with acute PE and no preexisting cardiac or pulmonary disease, *Chest* 100:598–603, 1991.

Tamariz LJ, Eng J, Segal EB, et al: Usefulness of clinical prediction rules for the diagnosis of venous thromboembolism: a systematic review, *Am J Med* 117:676–684, 2004.

Tapson VF: Acute pulmonary embolism, *N Engl J Med* 358:1037–1052, 2008.

Todd JL, Tapson VF: Thrombolytic therapy for acute pulmonary embolism, *Chest* 135:1321–1329, 2009.

Torbicki A, Perrier A, Konstantinides S, et al: Guidelines on the diagnosis and management of acute pulmonary embolism, *Eur Heart J* 29:2276–2315, 2008.

21

Selected Topics in Pulmonary Medicine

ALBERT J. POLITO, MD

Pulmonary medicine encompasses a variety of disorders that fall outside such traditionally broad topics as chronic obstructive pulmonary disease (COPD), asthma, interstitial lung disease, and thromboembolic disease. This chapter addresses four important smaller topics: (1) sleep disorders, (2) the solitary pulmonary nodule, (3) hemoptysis, and (4) pulmonary hypertension.

Sleep Disorders and Obstructive Sleep Apnea

Basic Information

- Apnea: Cessation of airflow for more than 10 seconds
- **Obstructive apnea: Patient continues to make respiratory efforts against an obstruction (typically a narrowing or closure in the upper airway)**
  - Occurs in 3% to 4% of women and 6% to 9% of men (Box 22-1 lists risk factors)
  - Recurrent decrements in airflow (i.e., apneas or hypopneas) most commonly occur during sleep (obstructive sleep apnea, OSA)
  - Events usually more prominent during rapid-eye-movement sleep, caused by associated hypotonia of upper airway musculature
- **Central apnea: Patient makes no respiratory effort during the apnea** (Box 22-2 lists diseases associated with central apnea)
  - Occurs most commonly during sleep (central sleep apnea, CSA)
  - During sleep, transient abnormalities of central drive to the respiratory muscles occur in affected individuals
  - Much less common than OSA
- Mixed apnea: Apnea with features of both OSA and CSA
- Hypopnea: A 50% or greater decrease in airflow or a less than 50% decrease in airflow associated with at least a 4% drop in oxygen saturation or an arousal
- Apnea-hypopnea index (AHI) = total number of apneas and hypopneas per hour of sleep; normal is five or fewer events per hour
- Respiratory disturbance index (RDI) is frequently larger than the AHI, as it includes not only apneas and hypopneas, but other respiratory disturbances that can disrupt sleep (e.g., respiratory effort–related arousals; RERAs)

- Upper airway resistance syndrome (UARS)
  - Repeated arousals secondary to increased upper airway resistance ("crescendo snoring")
  - AHI is normal; RDI is elevated
  - No significant oxygen desaturation episodes
- Obesity-hypoventilation syndrome ("Pickwickian syndrome")
  - Syndrome of morbid obesity and chronic hypoventilation with daytime hypercapnia (arterial partial pressure of carbon dioxide [$PaCO_2$] >45 mm Hg)
  - OSA present in majority of patients
- Cheyne-Stokes respirations
  - Cyclic rise and fall in respiratory pattern with recurrent periods of apnea
  - Apneas are typically central
  - Most commonly seen with congestive heart failure, central neurologic disease, or administration of sedative agents, but may occur in normal patients

Clinical Presentation

- OSA
  - History obtained from the patient alone may be unreliable
    - Input of bed partner or housemate often helpful
    - Symptoms of OSA include loud, disruptive snoring (patient "wakes the dead"); daytime sleepiness; witnessed apneas (most sensitive medical history question: "Have you ever been told that you stop breathing while you are sleeping?")
    - Patients also describe sleep as nonrefreshing, complain of morning headaches, and experience irritability/personality change/depression, cognitive impairment, and decreased libido
    - Nocturia/enuresis may also be seen
  - **Physical examination findings in OSA include obesity, increased neck circumference, large tonsils and adenoids, large uvula, low soft palate, systemic hypertension, and lower extremity edema**
    - Retrognathia, micrognathia, and other craniofacial abnormalities also described
    - Medical consequences of OSA are listed in Table 22-1
- CSA
  - History findings include daytime sleepiness and witnessed apneas
    - Snoring not a prominent finding
  - Physical examination findings in CSA

BOX 22-1 *Risk Factors for Obstructive Sleep Apnea*

Gender
　Male:female ratio, 2:1
　Risk increases for postmenopausal women
Age
　Predominantly 40–70 years old
Body habitus
　Obese (BMI >30 kg/m²)
Alcohol use
Medications
　Sedatives
　Hypnotics
Endocrine disease
　Acromegaly
　Hypothyroidism

BMI, body mass index.

BOX 22-2 *Clinical Conditions and Diseases Associated with Central Sleep Apnea*

Stroke
Stable methadone maintenance treatment
Multiple system atrophy (Shy-Drager syndrome)
Autonomic dysfunction
Myasthenia gravis
Neuromuscular disease
Bulbar poliomyelitis
Encephalitis

TABLE 22-1 *Medical Consequences of Obstructive Sleep Apnea*

Cardiovascular Effects	Noncardiovascular Effects
Systemic hypertension	Cognitive impairment
Pulmonary hypertension	Motor vehicle accidents
Congestive heart failure	Work-related accidents
Coronary artery disease	Sexual dysfunction
Nocturnal arrhythmias	Impaired quality of life
Stroke	

FIGURE 22-1 Polysomnogram in obstructive sleep apnea. The study shows a period when ventilation is obstructed and there is no airflow (V). At this time, the diaphragm continues to contract (EMG$_{di}$), esophageal (P$_{es}$) and gastric (P$_{ga}$) pressure swings occur, and there is ribcage and abdominal movement (RC and AB). As obstruction continues, arterial oxygen saturation (So$_2$) falls. Eventually the activity of the upper airway muscles, including the genioglossus muscle (EMG$_{ge}$), increases, the upper airway becomes patent, and airflow is restored. Patients can have hundreds of similar episodes during the night. *(From Onal E, Lopata M, O'Connor T: Pathogenesis of apneas in hypersomnia-sleep syndrome, Am Rev Respir Dis 125:167, 1982; and Souhami R: Textbook of medicine, New York, Churchill Livingstone, 2002, Fig. 13.42.)*

- Patients may have any body habitus
- Underlying neurologic disease, if present, determines many of the physical findings

Diagnosis and Evaluation

- Diagnosis of a suggested apnea syndrome is obtained with an overnight polysomnogram ("sleep study"; Fig. 22-1)
- Physiologic parameters measured include airflow, chest/abdominal wall effort, oxygen saturation, electroencephalogram (EEG), electrocardiogram (ECG), electrooculogram (EOG), and body position
- Recording time should be 6 to 8 hours

- **If AHI is more than five events per hour, sleep study is positive for sleep apnea**
  - **OSA versus CSA is determined by presence versus absence of chest/abdominal wall efforts, respectively**
    - Mild: 6 to 15 events per hour
    - Moderate: 16 to 30 events per hour
    - Severe: More than 30 events per hour

Treatment

- OSA
  - Three components to treatment: Behavioral, medical, and surgical (Table 22-2 and Fig. 22-2)
  - **Behavioral treatment is commonly the only intervention recommended for patients with mild OSA**
  - Compliance a major problem with nasal continuous positive airway pressure (CPAP); discomfort of apparatus, claustrophobia, aerophagia, and difficulty with exhalation are common side effects

- CSA
  - Nasal CPAP usually not effective
  - Treatment of choice: Nocturnal nasal noninvasive ventilation with a backup respiratory rate and bilevel (inspiratory and expiratory) positive airway pressure (BiPAP) settings
  - Ventilatory stimulants (e.g., acetazolamide) have not proven useful

Solitary Pulmonary Nodule

Basic Information

- Pulmonary nodule: A single, well-defined lesion, usually rounded or slightly ovoid, surrounded by normal lung tissue
  - **Diameter must be 3 cm or less**
    - **If diameter greater than 3 cm, process is called a mass, of which 90% are malignant**
- Solitary pulmonary nodules are found in 1 of every 500 chest radiographs

- Nodular mimics: nipple shadows, skin moles, prominent costochondral junction
- Etiologies (Table 22-3)
  - **60% benign (most common: healed granulomas secondary to tuberculosis or fungal infection)**
  - **40% malignant (most common: bronchogenic carcinoma)**

Clinical Presentation

- The solitary pulmonary nodule is usually an unexpected finding on routine chest film
  - Most patients are asymptomatic; some have cough

Diagnosis and Evaluation

- Key features of the history include
  - Age (malignancy uncommon in patients younger than 35 years)
  - Smoking (increases likelihood of malignancy)
  - Occupational exposure (asbestos, silica)
  - Prior history of cancer
  - Travel or history of living in endemic area

TABLE 22-2   Treatment of Obstructive Sleep Apnea (OSA)

Modality	Options	Comments
Behavioral	Weight loss Avoidance of alcohol, sedatives, and hypnotics Position therapy	Small amounts of weight loss can significantly improve symptoms Lateral decubitus sleeping position helps alleviate symptoms in many
Medical	Nasal continuous positive airway pressure (CPAP) Oral appliances Protriptyline Medroxyprogesterone acetate Oxygen	Nasal CPAP is treatment of choice for moderate to severe OSA; apnea, snoring, daytime somnolence, and hypertension all may improve Oral appliances most useful in retrognathia and micrognathia; not effective in severe OSA No medication has been shown to be successful in treating OSA Medroxyprogesterone increases respiratory drive and improves daytime arterial blood gases but has no effect on OSA
Surgical	Nasal surgery (e.g., septoplasty, sinus surgery) Tonsillectomy/adenoidectomy Uvulopalatopharyngoplasty (UPPP) Laser-assisted uvuloplasty Maxillofacial surgery Tracheostomy	Nasal surgery rarely effective in directly treating OSA Tonsillectomy/adenoidectomy most effective in children with OSA UPPP most common surgical procedure for OSA; at least 50% will not improve despite surgery Tracheostomy 100% effective but should be reserved for patients with severe/incapacitating disease that has failed standard aggressive therapy

Untreated obstructive sleep apnea

Obstructive sleep apnea treated with continuous positive airway pressure

FIGURE 22-2 Effect of continuous positive airway pressure (CPAP) on obstructive sleep apnea (OSA). The chief mechanism of CPAP in the treatment of OSA is airway splinting and dilation of obstructed pharyngeal segments. *(From Albert RK, Spiro SG, Jett JR: Clinical respiratory medicine, ed 2, St. Louis, Mosby, 2004, Fig. 71-9.)*

- **Mississippi and Ohio River valleys: Suggests histoplasmosis (most common); blastomycosis**
- **Southwestern United States: Suggests coccidioidomycosis**
- Physical examination
  - Most patients have normal lung examinations
  - Occasionally, with a proximally located nodule, a localized wheeze (from airway impingement) may be present
  - Clubbing may be present with a malignant pulmonary nodule
- Further imaging (Fig. 22-3)
  - The initial step is always to locate older chest radiographs to evaluate stability or change in size of the nodule; allows approximate calculation of doubling time
  - **Doubling time of 25 to 450 days suggests a malignant process**
  - **Doubling time of less than 25 days or more than 450 days suggests a benign process**
  - Doubling time refers to the volume of the nodule (i.e., an increase of 28% in nodule diameter indicates doubling)
- Chest computed tomography (CT): Important for defining the characteristics of the nodule (Table 22-4)
- The pattern of calcification may be useful in diagnosis (Figs. 22-4 and 22-5)
  - Hamartomas show a "popcorn" calcification pattern or areas of low-attenuation fat deposits (or both) (Fig. 22-6)
  - Pulmonary arteriovenous malformations (AVMs) fill with contrast material
- Positron emission tomography (PET): Used to define metabolic activity of pulmonary nodule
  - In general, malignant lesions have an increased rate of label uptake compared with benign lesions or normal tissue; however, active infections, granulomatous diseases, and other inflammatory conditions also can have increased uptake (false positives)
  - False negatives can occur with small tumors (<1 cm), tumors with low metabolic activity (e.g., bronchial carcinoid), and hyperglycemia
  - For diagnosis of malignant solitary pulmonary nodules, sensitivity is 97% and specificity is 82%
- Role in evaluating solitary pulmonary nodules is still being determined; most useful in borderline cases, with biopsy recommended if PET scan positive

Treatment

- General principles
  - If a nodule has grown with a doubling time of 25 to 450 days and the patient's cardiopulmonary status permits surgery, thoracotomy with resection is indicated
  - If no previous films are available, the patient's risk of cancer must be assessed to determine whether the approach should be observation or biopsy (see Fig. 22-3)

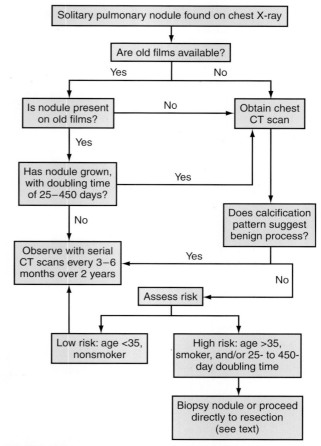

FIGURE 22-3 Management of the solitary pulmonary nodule. (CT, computed tomography.)

TABLE 22-3	Causes of the Solitary Pulmonary Nodule	

Benign Causes	Malignant Causes
Infectious granuloma (tuberculosis, histoplasmosis, coccidioidomycosis)	Bronchogenic carcinoma
	Bronchial carcinoid
Hamartoma	Pulmonary lymphoma
"Round" pneumonia	Pulmonary sarcoma
Bronchogenic cyst	Solitary metastasis from extrapulmonary site
Pulmonary infarction	
Arteriovenous malformation	
Rheumatoid nodule	
Wegener granulomatosis	
Amyloidosis	
Parasitic infection (Ascaris, Echinococcus)	

TABLE 22-4	Characteristics Suggestive of Benign and Malignant Pulmonary Nodules	

Characteristic	Benign	Malignant
Size	<2 cm	>2 cm
Edge	Smooth, sharp	Spiculated, ragged
Cavitation	No	Yes
Satellite lesions	Yes	No
Doubling time	<25 days or >450 days	25–450 days

- Patient preferences must always be taken into account; some patients fear the uncertainty of observation and want to "do something" right away to make a diagnosis (this may not be possible or appropriate)
- Biopsy techniques
  - Fiberoptic bronchoscopy: Limited usefulness in evaluation of the solitary pulmonary nodule
    - Most useful if the nodule is greater than 2 cm in diameter, is located proximally, or has a bronchus leading into it on chest CT
    - Diagnostic yield: 10% to 20% if less than 2 cm, 55% if greater than 2 cm
  - Percutaneous transthoracic needle aspiration: Usually performed with CT guidance
    - Most useful for peripheral lesions in the outer one third of the lung
    - **Higher diagnostic yield than bronchoscopic biopsy: 80% to 95% (even in lesions <2 cm)**
    - Major limitation: 10% to 30% rate of pneumothorax
  - Once diagnosis is confirmed, treat the underlying disease

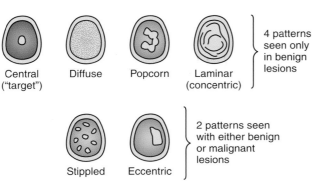

FIGURE 22-4 Calcification patterns in solitary pulmonary nodules. *(Adapted from Lillington GA: Management of solitary pulmonary nodules, Dis Mon 37:271, 1991.)*

Hemoptysis

Basic Information

- Hemoptysis: Expectoration of blood from the airways
- Pathophysiology: **In the majority of cases, hemoptysis originates from bronchial arterial circulation**
  - Bronchial arteries increase in size and number in the setting of chronic inflammation (e.g., bronchiectasis) or malignancy and are susceptible to rupture
  - Bleeding may be profuse because of the high pressure of the systemic circulation
  - **Clinically significant bleeding from pulmonary arterial circulation is rare because it is a low-pressure system and hypoxic pulmonary vasoconstriction diverts blood flow away from diseased portions of the lung**
- Causes are listed in Box 22-3
  - Bronchitis and bronchogenic carcinoma, the two most common causes, account for 40% and 25% of cases, respectively

Clinical Presentation

- Amount of blood may be small or large; massive hemoptysis is defined most commonly as loss of more than 600 mL of blood in 24 hours
- Hemoptysis may be accompanied by mucopurulent sputum and fever (bacterial pneumonia), hematuria (pulmonary-renal syndromes, including Goodpasture syndrome), or prominent sinusitis (i.e., Wegener granulomatosis), the presence of which may offer clues to etiology

Diagnosis and Evaluation

- Key features of the history start with a careful questioning of the patient's symptoms to help determine source of blood; many patients confuse hemoptysis with hematemesis or epistaxis

FIGURE 22-5 The use of CT to characterize a solitary pulmonary nodule. **A,** Chest radiograph shows a peripheral nodule *(arrow)* that does not appear to be calcified. **B,** CT scan through the nodule demonstrates dense, diffuse calcification, consistent with a benign lesion. The other gray densities on the scan are pulmonary vessels rather than nodules. *(From Mason RJ: Murray and Nadel's textbook of respiratory medicine, ed 4, Philadelphia, Elsevier Saunders, 2005, Fig. 20-36.)*

FIGURE 22-6 Hamartoma. CT scan shows low attenuation within the solitary pulmonary nodule, consistent with fat. *(From Mason RJ: Murray and Nadel's textbook of respiratory medicine, ed 4, Philadelphia, Elsevier Saunders, 2005, Fig. 20-37.)*

- Other features include estimation of the quantity of blood and the duration of bleeding
- Physical examination
  - Crackles or rhonchi may be present in the area of the bleeding and can help localize site of bleeding
- Radiographic studies
  - Chest radiograph should be obtained in every patient and may suggest the diagnosis
    - Nodule or mass suggests neoplasm
    - Lobar atelectasis suggests obstructing endobronchial lesion
    - **Mass within a cavity ("air crescent sign") suggests aspergilloma** (fungus ball; Fig. 22-7)
    - Thickened bronchial walls ("tram tracking") suggest bronchiectasis
  - 30% of patients have normal or nonlocalizing chest films
  - Chest CT is generally not an important tool for evaluation of hemoptysis, except in those patients with normal or nonlocalizing chest radiographs
- Fiberoptic bronchoscopy: The invasive procedure of choice for nonmassive hemoptysis
  - Helpful for localizing the bleeding side or the specific site of bleeding
  - Not useful for massive hemoptysis (field of vision through bronchoscope is obscured by large amounts of blood)

Treatment

- Therapy should be directed at the underlying cause of the hemoptysis (e.g., antibiotics for bronchitis or pneumonia; diuresis for congestive heart failure; resection and chemotherapy/radiotherapy for bronchogenic carcinoma)
- Massive hemoptysis requires special attention
  - **Airway protection: Position patient with the bleeding lung in the dependent position (prevents spillage of blood into the nonbleeding lung)**

BOX 22-3 *Causes of Hemoptysis*

Infectious
Bronchitis
Bronchiectasis
Pneumonia
Tuberculosis

Neoplastic
Bronchogenic carcinoma
Bronchial carcinoid
Pulmonary metastasis from other site

Cardiovascular
Congestive heart failure
Mitral stenosis
Pulmonary embolism/infarction
Pulmonary arteriovenous malformation

Miscellaneous
Idiopathic (as much as 20–30% of cases)
Lung contusion
Goodpasture syndrome
Wegener granulomatosis
Smoking freebase cocaine ("crack")
Pseudohemoptysis (from *Serratia marcescens* pneumonia)

FIGURE 22-7 Chest radiograph showing an aspergilloma in the left lower lung zone of an asymptomatic patient. A dark rim of air is readily seen around the upper edge of the fungus ball ("air crescent sign"). *(From Mason RJ: Murray and Nadel's textbook of respiratory medicine, ed 4, Philadelphia, Elsevier Saunders, 2005, Fig. 34-15.)*

- Intubation may be needed to isolate the lungs from each other, using a double-lumen endotracheal tube
  - Fluid resuscitation to support volume
    - Initial management: crystalloid intravenous fluids
    - Blood products in patients who are anemic, coagulopathic, and/or bleeding rapidly
  - Gentle cough suppression to prevent the airway trauma of vigorous coughing
    - Avoid excessive cough suppression because airway compromise can result
  - Correction of coagulopathy, if present
  - Bronchial artery embolization is effective at immediately halting bleeding in 80% to 95% of patients
    - 30% will rebleed within 3 months
  - Surgery: Indicated for massive, unilateral hemoptysis unresponsive to other measures, provided that the patient has adequate pulmonary reserve
    - High mortality rate (35%) for patients actively bleeding at the time of surgery

Pulmonary Hypertension

Basic Information

- Normal pulmonary artery (PA) pressures are 18 to 30 mm Hg systolic and 4 to 12 mm Hg diastolic
- **Pulmonary hypertension is defined as mean PA pressure greater than 25 mm Hg at rest**
  - Severe pulmonary hypertension is defined as mean PA pressure ≥40 mm Hg at rest
- **Traditionally classified as either primary or secondary (Box 22-4 lists causes of secondary pulmonary hypertension)**

Clinical Presentation

- Demographics
  - **Primary pulmonary hypertension, now usually called idiopathic pulmonary arterial hypertension (IPAH), is three times more common in women than in men and generally occurs in younger patients (typical age of onset is 20–40 years)**
- Symptoms
  - Similar for both primary and secondary etiologies, though for the latter, other symptoms of the underlying disorder may be present (e.g., snoring and hypersomnolence in OSA, skin changes in scleroderma)
  - Patients with mild pulmonary hypertension are usually asymptomatic
  - Exertional dyspnea is most common presenting complaint
  - May also have chest pain or dizziness; syncope portends a poor prognosis

Diagnosis and Evaluation

- Physical examination
  - **Prominent pulmonic component (P$_2$) of the second heart sound is a reliable indicator of elevated PA pressure**
  - May also see elevated jugular venous pressure with large a-wave, left parasternal heave (from right ventricular hypertrophy), right-sided S$_3$, or tricuspid regurgitation murmur
  - Pedal edema common

BOX 22-4	*Causes of Secondary Pulmonary Hypertension*

Cardiac Disease
Congenital
Eisenmenger syndrome
Left-sided heart failure

Parenchymal Lung Disease
Chronic obstructive pulmonary disease
Interstitial lung disease

Vascular Impairment
Chronic thromboembolic disease
Pulmonary veno-occlusive disease
Sickle cell disease

Infections
HIV
Schistosomiasis

Drugs/Toxins
Anorexigens

Miscellaneous
Obstructive sleep apnea
Collagen vascular diseases (through either direct vascular effect or interstitial changes in the parenchyma)

- Chest radiography
  - Shows enlarged pulmonary arteries with rapid tapering of vessels toward the periphery of the lungs (a "pruned tree" appearance; Fig. 22-8)
  - May also see right-heart enlargement
  - For secondary pulmonary hypertension caused by parenchymal lung disease, look for hyperinflation and bullous disease (suggestive of COPD) or increased interstitial markings (suggestive of interstitial lung disease)
- Other studies
  - Echocardiography:
    - Permits evaluation for signs of right ventricular pressure overload, including paradoxic bulging of septum into left ventricle during systole and hypertrophy of the right ventricular free wall
    - Doppler estimates of PA pressure based on velocity of tricuspid regurgitation can be suggestive of pulmonary hypertension but are also very prone to inaccuracy
  - Pulmonary function tests: Typically show decreased diffusing capacity
  - Ventilation-perfusion scan: Helps identify patients with secondary pulmonary hypertension because of chronic thromboembolic disease, but IPAH can also produce abnormal scans
  - Right-heart catheterization: Permits direct measurement of PA pressure and, with angiography, definitive diagnosis of chronic thromboembolic disease

FIGURE 22-8 Progressive pulmonary arterial hypertension. **A,** The patient initially had a normal chest radiograph. **B,** Several years later, however, increasing heart size and marked dilation of the main pulmonary artery (MPA) and right pulmonary artery (RPA) are noted. Pulmonary artery enlargement can be recognized by a bulging along the left cardiac border just below the aortic arch. *(From Mettler FA: Essentials of radiology, ed 2, Philadelphia, Elsevier Saunders, 2005, Fig. 5-12.)*

Treatment

- IPAH
  - Right-heart catheterization should be performed in all patients to determine if there is a positive response to acute administration of a vasodilator (typically nitric oxide)
    - **5% to 10% of patients are "responders" (PA pressure declines by at least 10 mm Hg to a value <40 mm Hg) and should be treated with oral calcium channel blockers**
    - **"Nonresponders" have an increased risk of death with calcium channel blockers and should receive other therapy (prostacyclin, endothelin receptor antagonist, or phosphodiesterase 5 inhibitor)**
  - Continuous infusion of epoprostenol (prostacyclin), a direct pulmonary vasodilator, is indicated in patients with New York Heart Association class III or IV symptoms
    - Adverse effects of epoprostenol include flushing and diarrhea
    - Prostacyclin analogues: trepostinil, iloprost
  - Other treatment options
    - Endothelin receptor antagonists (bosentan, ambrisentan) directly oppose the vasoconstricting effects of endothelin-1
    - Phosphodiesterase 5 inhibitors (sildenafil, tadalafil) enhance nitric oxide–mediated vasodilation
  - Clinical studies are evaluating combination therapy with more than one of the various classes of drugs
  - **Chronic anticoagulation is indicated in all patients to prevent intravascular thrombosis in the pulmonary circulation as well as deep venous thrombosis**
  - Many patients require chronic diuretic therapy
  - Supplemental oxygen
- Secondary pulmonary hypertension
  - Treat underlying disease
  - Epoprostenol and bosentan are used frequently for secondary pulmonary hypertension caused by scleroderma
  - Sildenafil is used increasingly in a variety of secondary settings
  - Chronic anticoagulation should be instituted for all patients with severe pulmonary hypertension, provided there is no contraindication
  - Supplemental oxygen helps reduce hypoxic pulmonary vasoconstriction
  - For severe chronic thromboembolic pulmonary hypertension, consider pulmonary thromboendarterectomy

REVIEW QUESTIONS

For review questions, please go to www.expertconsult.com.

SUGGESTED READINGS

Badesch DB, Champion HC, Sanchez MA, et al: Diagnosis and assessment of pulmonary arterial hypertension, *J Am Coll Cardiol* 54:S55–S66, 2009.

Corder R: Hemoptysis, *Emerg Med Clin North Am* 21:421–435, 2003.

Epstein LJ, Kristo D, Strollo PJ Jr, et al: for the Adult Obstructive Sleep Apnea Task Force of the American Academy of Sleep Medicine: Clinical guideline for the evaluation, management and long-term care of obstructive sleep apnea in adults, *J Clin Sleep Med* 5:263–276, 2009.

Farber HW, Loscalzo J: Pulmonary arterial hypertension, *N Engl J Med* 351:1655–1665, 2004.

Flemons WW: Clinical practice: obstructive sleep apnea, *N Engl J Med* 347:498–504, 2002.

Jean-Baptiste E: Clinical assessment and management of massive hemoptysis, *Crit Care Med* 28:1642–1647, 2000.

Lillington GA: Management of solitary pulmonary nodules, *Dis Mon* 37:271–318, 1991.

Malhotra A, White DP: Obstructive sleep apnoea, *Lancet* 360:237–245, 2002.

Ost D, Fein AM, Feinsilver SH: Clinical practice: the solitary pulmonary nodule, *N Engl J Med* 348:2535–2542, 2003.

Runo JR, Loyd JE: Primary pulmonary hypertension, *Lancet* 361:1533–1544, 2003.

Wahidi MM, Govert JA, Goudar RK, et al: for the American College of Chest Physicians: Evidence for the treatment of patients with pulmonary nodules: when is it lung cancer? ACCP evidence-based clinical practice guidelines (ed 2), *Chest* 132:94S–107S, 2007.

Critical Care Medicine

GEOFFREY R. CONNORS, MD; and JONATHAN SEVRANSKY, MD, MHS

Critical care medicine focuses on the management of acute organ failure and other life-threatening illnesses. Treatment of acute respiratory failure and its common causes, including pneumonia, chronic obstructive pulmonary disease (COPD), and the acute respiratory distress syndrome (ARDS), is an important component of critical care management. The timely diagnosis and rapid treatment of septic, cardiogenic, and hypovolemic shock are crucial to the survival of patients with these life-threatening conditions. Recent emphasis on minimizing and preventing the complications of critical care therapies is also highlighted here. Because toxin exposures often require acute management in a critical care setting, a review of the major types of toxin exposures is included.

Acute Respiratory Failure

Basic Information

- Two pathophysiologic causes of acute respiratory failure
  - **Failure of oxygenation**
    - Defined as an **inadequate arterial partial pressure of oxygen (Pao$_2$)** despite high levels of supplemental inspired O$_2$
    - Five major etiologic classes
      - Right-to-left shunt via pathologic vascular communications (e.g., pulmonary arteriovenous malformations [AVMs], intracardiac right-to-left shunts), or space-filling pulmonary parenchymal lesions (e.g., atelectasis or pneumonia). These patients will not correct with supplemental oxygen.
      - Ventilation-perfusion ($\dot{V}/\dot{Q}$) mismatch: Regional imbalances between blood flow and ventilation (e.g., pulmonary embolism or lung parenchymal disease); corrects, partially or completely, with the addition of supplemental oxygen
      - Reduced diffusion capacity (e.g., interstitial lung disease, emphysema); may be minimal at rest; more pronounced with exercise
      - Alveolar hypoventilation (e.g., from central nervous system [CNS] depression, neuromuscular disease, or chest wall abnormality); the only type of hypoxic failure with a normal alveolar-arterial (A-a) gradient
      - Low fraction of inspired oxygen (Fio$_2$) (e.g., high altitude)
  - **Failure of ventilation**
    - Defined as elevated arterial partial pressure of carbon dioxide (Paco$_2$) with decreased pH

- Caused by either
  - Increased CO$_2$ production (e.g., sepsis, overfeeding, thyrotoxicosis)
  - Decreased CO$_2$ elimination
- Decreased minute ventilation (e.g., CNS depression)
- Decreased alveolar ventilation (e.g., COPD, acute increase in dead space from pneumonia or large pulmonary embolus)

Clinical Presentation

- Depends on underlying cause
- Agitation or altered mental status commonly seen in hypoxia and hypercarbia
- **Cyanosis occurs only once deoxyhemoglobin level is greater than 5 g/dL, which corresponds to an arterial oxygen saturation (Sao$_2$) around 67%**

Diagnosis and Evaluation

- **Pulse oximeter may be unreliable in the following situations:**
  - On the steep portion of the oxyhemoglobin dissociation curve (i.e., at saturation levels <90%; Fig. 23-1)
  - Patients with carboxyhemoglobin or methemoglobin
  - Patients with decreased peripheral perfusion (e.g., shock)
  - Patients with pigmented skin or nail polish
- Arterial blood gas measurement is the gold standard
  - Most oxygen is delivered to tissues bound to hemoglobin, which is reflected in measured saturation obtained with arterial blood gas rather than dissolved in the plasma (i.e., measured by Pao$_2$)
  - **Consider mechanical ventilation, in conjunction with a tight-fitting mask (noninvasive) or endotracheal intubation when Pao$_2$ is less than 60 to 70 mm Hg with Fio$_2$ greater than 80% or Paco$_2$ ≥45 mm Hg with pH <7.35**
  - **Work of breathing (high respiratory rate with use of accessory muscles) and ability to protect airway are additional important considerations**

Treatment

- Supplemental oxygen to **maintain O$_2$ saturation greater than 88% or Pao$_2$ greater than 55 mm Hg**
- Do not deliver inadequate amounts of oxygen out of concern about suppressing central respiratory drive; this is a rare complication
- Mechanical ventilation (Box 23-1)
  - Consider whether patient is noninvasive ventilation candidate (Table 23-1)

FIGURE 23-1 Oxyhemoglobin dissociation curve. *(From Goldman L, Bennett JC, Ausiello D: Cecil textbook of medicine, ed 22, Philadelphia, Saunders, 2004, Fig. 100.5.)*

BOX 23-1 *Mechanical Ventilation*

Types

Volume cycled: Ventilator delivers a set volume, using whatever pressure is required to overcome airway resistance and lung compliance. Examples include assist control and synchronized intermittent mandatory ventilation.

  Assist control: Patient receives a set tidal volume for every initiated breath. A preset number of breaths per minute prevents hypoventilation.

  Synchronized intermittent mandatory ventilation (SIMV): Patient receives a set tidal volume for only a designated number of breaths per minute. Additional patient-initiated breaths have no support.

Pressure cycled: Ventilator maintains a set pressure; tidal volume delivered depends on lung mechanics. Examples include pressure-regulated volume control and pressure support.

  Pressure-regulated volume control (PRVC): Patient receives set tidal volume for every initiated breath as long as the pressure required to deliver remains below a preset value.

  Pressure support: Ventilator provides a constant preset pressure for each patient-initiated breath; primarily used in awake patients or as a weaning mode. Should not be used in patients without intact respiratory drive.

Complications

Auto–positive end-expiratory pressure (PEEP) (dynamic hyperinflation): Caused by air trapping because of inadequate emptying during expiration in patient with airflow obstruction (e.g., asthma or chronic obstructive pulmonary disease)

The increased intrathoracic pressure causes increased work of breathing and may decrease venous return to the heart, producing hypotension

Treatment includes disconnecting the patient from the ventilator as a temporary measure if decompensating; changing the ventilator parameters to allow increased expiratory time by increasing inspiratory flow rate; decreasing tidal volume and respiratory rate; and increasing sedation

Volutrauma or barotrauma: Can cause pneumothorax, pneumomediastinum, and diffuse alveolar damage

Increased infection rate: Ventilator-associated pneumonia

Endotracheal tube complications: Subglottal stenosis, vocal cord dysfunction, tracheoesophageal fistula, sinusitis

Noninvasive Ventilation

Definition: Mechanical ventilation without endotracheal intubation

Does not protect airway; avoid using in patients with depressed level of consciousness

Continuous positive airway pressure (CPAP): Constant pressure provided throughout respiratory cycle

Bilevel positive airway pressure (BiPAP): Different pressures provided upon inspiration and expiration

---

TABLE 23-1 *Criteria for Use of Noninvasive Ventilation*

Disease	Patient Characteristics	Contraindications
COPD exacerbation	Hypercapneic respiratory failure (pH 7.25–7.35, RR, 20–25) Able to manage secretions	Shock Not able to tolerate mask GCS score <8
Respiratory failure in immunosuppressed patients with bilateral infiltrates	Immunosuppression (e.g., s/p bone marrow transplantation, HIV, or post-chemotherapy neutropenia)	Shock Not able to tolerate mask GCS score <8

COPD, chronic obstructive pulmonary disease; GCS, Glasgow Coma Scale; HIV, human immunodeficiency virus; RR, respiratory rate; s/p, status post.

- Noninvasive ventilation decreases complications such as ventilator-associated pneumonia, decreases length of intensive care unit (ICU) stay, and improves mortality rates for selected patients with hypercarbic respiratory failure in setting of COPD and immunosuppressed patients with bilateral infiltrates and hypoxemic respiratory failure
- Treat underlying cause (e.g., antibiotics for pneumonia, bronchodilators and corticosteroids for status asthmaticus)
- The use of a protocol to assure daily interruption of sedation in combination with daily spontaneous breathing trials for ventilated patients decreases the time on the ventilator, time in the ICU, as well as overall 1-year mortality
- Benzodiazepines, a historical mainstay of sedation for mechanically ventilated patients, should be limited as they contribute to agitation, delirium, and time spent on the ventilator, especially when used as a continuous infusion

FIGURE 23-2 Chest radiograph of a patient with acute respiratory distress syndrome. Note diffuse bilateral infiltrates. *(From Mason RJ: Murray and Nadel's textbook of respiratory medicine, ed 4, Philadelphia, Elsevier Saunders, 2005, Fig. 51.2.)*

Acute Respiratory Distress Syndrome

Basic Information

- Divided into pulmonary and nonpulmonary causes (although no clear difference in outcomes)
  - **Sepsis and pneumonia are most common causes**
  - Other causes: aspiration, irritant gases and smoke inhalation, medications, blood transfusions, burns, pancreatitis, and trauma
- Incidence increases with increasing age
  - Estimated 15 to 78 cases per 100,000 population
  - At-risk patients who develop ARDS generally do so within 48 to 72 hours of acquiring risk factor, although some may take as long as a week to meet criteria
  - Some suggestion that African Americans may have higher risk than whites
- **Overall mortality related to number of organ system failures**
  - Single-organ system failure mortality rate 25% to 40%
  - Three-organ system failure has up to 90% mortality rate
  - Mortality rates increase with age
- **Sepsis and multiorgan system failure most common causes of death**
  - Rare for patients to die solely from intractable hypoxemia
  - May be difficult to diagnose ventilator-associated pneumonia in patients with ARDS
- Survivors of acute illness may have long-term sequelae
  - Two thirds of survivors have minimal to moderate respiratory impairment 1 year after event
  - Recent studies have reported muscle wasting, weakness, and post-traumatic stress disorder as late as 1 year after illness in survivors of ARDS. Only half of the survivors return to work 1 year after discharge. Some neuromuscular and psychiatric sequelae persist 5 years after hospital discharge.

Clinical Presentation, Diagnosis, and Epidemiology of ARDS

- Syndrome definition from the European-American Consensus Statement requires
  - **Acute onset of symptoms**
  - **Diffuse bilateral infiltrates on chest radiograph** (Fig. 23-2)
  - **Pao_2/Fio_2 ratio less than 200** (Pao_2/Fio_2 ratio <300 defines acute lung injury [ALI])
  - **No evidence of left-heart failure (pulmonary capillary wedge pressure <18 mm Hg)**

Prevention

- Early antibiotics and resuscitation for severe sepsis, use of lower tidal volumes in at-risk patients, and **higher thresholds to transfuse blood and plasma products may reduce the incidence of ALI and ARDS**
- The early administration of continuous positive airway pressure (CPAP) ventilation in heme malignancy patients with signs of respiratory failure decreases incidence of ARDS

Treatment

- **Use lung-protective ventilatory strategy**
  - **Small tidal volumes (6 mL/kg) coupled with low plateau pressures (<30 cm H_2O) help to minimize ventilator-induced lung injury**
  - This approach decreases mortality from ARDS, reduces incidence of multi–organ system failure, and decreases measures of local and systemic inflammation
  - Higher levels of positive end-expiratory pressure (PEEP) coupled with lung-protective ventilation do not change mortality rates in patients with ALI, but may decrease duration of ventilation. More severely ill patients may have a mortality benefit when higher levels of PEEP are used.

- Use of a conservative fluid management strategy (limiting fluid balance after initial resuscitation has been accomplished) improves lung function and decreases the need for mechanical ventilation without worsening cardiac or renal failure rates
- Supportive care: Mechanical ventilation, treatment of underlying cause, hemodynamic and renal support, and nutritional support if necessary; when to start nutrition, and what formulation to use, remain controversial
- **Routine modulation of proinflammatory mediators is of no proven value**
- **Corticosteroids' role uncertain** in treatment of late-phase ARDS, with conflicting results from studies
- Prone positioning and inhaled nitric oxide improve oxygenation in many patients but have no effect on length of ventilation or survival
- Alternate modes of mechanical ventilation, such as high-frequency oscillatory ventilation and airway pressure release ventilation (APRV), may be considered in patients who fail conventional therapy. It is reasonable to consider transfer of such patients to high-volume centers with expertise in rescue modes, including extracorporeal membrane oxygenation (ECMO).
- Early, short-term use of neuromuscular blockers, specifically cis-atracurium, in sicker ARDS patients may have clinical benefit without causing prolonged neuromuscular weakness

Sepsis

Basic Information

- Etiology
  - Bacterial products (e.g., endotoxin, peptidoglycans, teichoic acid) stimulate host defense cells (monocyte or macrophage)
  - Host defense cells respond by **producing proinflammatory mediators** (e.g., tumor necrosis factor-α [TNF-α], interleukin-1 [IL-1], arachidonic acid metabolites, platelet-activating factor, complement components, and nitric oxide)
  - Proinflammatory mediators cause **dysregulation of the coagulation cascade**
- Epidemiology
  - Incidence: 80 cases per 100,000 population
    - More common at the extremes of age (i.e., very young or very old)
    - Incidence may be increased in African Americans
  - May occur in the setting of a wide number of infections (i.e., gram-positive, gram-negative, viral, or fungal organisms)
  - Infections may occur in community, facility, or hospitalized person; both immunocompetent and immunosuppressed patients may develop sepsis
  - The lungs, central venous catheters, and bladder catheters are the most common sites of nosocomial infections in ICU patients

- **Gram-positive organisms now most common cause of sepsis, followed closely by gram-negative organisms**
- Mortality related to number of organs that fail (may also be affected by underlying disease)

Clinical Presentation and Diagnosis

- Bacteremia is defined as the **presence of bacteria in the bloodstream**
- Sepsis syndrome is defined as the presence of the following four components:
  - Temperature (>38°C or <36°C)
  - Pulse (>90 beats/min)
  - Respiration rate (>24 breaths/min, $PaCO_2$ <32 mm Hg), or need for mechanical ventilation
  - White blood cell (WBC) count (>12,000/mm^3 or <4000/mm^3)
    - Evidence of infection (i.e., positive blood, urine, or sputum cultures; positive Gram stain; or presence of pus)
      - Microbiologic proof not required since patients sometimes are on antibiotics when sepsis develops
  - Note definition of syndrome is not specific, as there are many causes of elevated pulse, temperature, respiration rate in hospitalized patients
- **Severe sepsis defined as sepsis plus organ failure (e.g., renal, hematologic, respiratory, cardiovascular, neurologic)**
- **Septic shock is defined by hypotension unresponsive to fluid resuscitation and the presence of end-organ damage**
  - Mortality rates 15% to 20% for sepsis; 50% to 60% for septic shock

Treatment

- Timely antibiotics, fluids, and hemodynamic support; renal support if necessary
  - Appropriate antibiotics should be infused within 1 hour in patients with hypotension caused by sepsis (door-to-infusion time <1 hour); selection of antibiotics should be driven by patient characteristics and place that patient developed infection (i.e., home versus hospital)
- **Early antibiotic administration in conjuction with early goal-directed therapy (e.g., protocol-based strategy using fluids, vasopressors, and, if necessary, packed red blood cell transfusions, inotropes, and endotracheal intubation/mechanical ventilation). Appropriate treatment goals include mean arterial pressure greater than 65 mm Hg, central venous pressure greater than 8 mm Hg, and urine output greater than 0.5 mL/kg/hr; may also include either mixed venous O_2 saturation greater than 70% or decreasing lactate levels.**
  - Similar goal-directed therapy late in management (i.e., after 24 hours) does not improve outcomes
- **Corticosteroids may reduce the incidence of hypotension in sepsis but have no effect on mortality, regardless of the results of a corticotropin stimulation test. There may, however, be a role for steroids in patients with sepsis who remain hypotensive despite adequate fluid resuscitation and vasopressor use.**

- No role for high-dose (pulsed) corticosteroids
- Laboratory analysis of hypothalamic-pituitary-adrenocortical axis (random cortisol levels, corticotrophin stimulation testing) are of limited value in selecting whether to use stress-dose steroids in septic shock
- No benefit seen with attempts to modulate proinflammatory cytokines (e.g., anti-TNF monoclonal antibody, soluble TNF receptor, IL-1 receptor antagonist)
- Routine use of **dopamine to prevent renal failure is of no proven value**

Shock

Basic Information
- Shock is defined as **inadequate end-organ perfusion** (not synonymous with hypotension)
- Results from any combination of malfunction of
  - Arterial perfusion
  - Cardiac performance
  - Vascular performance
  - Cellular function

Clinical Presentation
- Decreased urine output
- Decreased peripheral perfusion (e.g., cool extremities, cyanosis)
- Altered mental status
- Tissue hypoxia (elevated lactic acid)

Diagnosis
See Figure 23-3 for a diagnostic algorithm for treating shock.
- Four types of shock are distinguished (Table 23-2)
- Pulmonary artery (Swan-Ganz) catheter
  - May be useful as diagnostic tool to measure cardiac output and filling pressures (noninvasive methods less accurate)
  - Limitations on usefulness
    - Varied levels of interpretation skills
    - Pulmonary artery occlusion pressure is not always a good surrogate for left ventricular end-diastolic volume
  - Routine placement of a pulmonary artery catheter does not improve clinical outcomes

Treatment for Septic Shock
- Volume resuscitation
  - Crystalloids (e.g., saline, lactated Ringer's solution) are the initial fluid of choice
    - Inexpensive, readily available
    - No proven benefit to use of colloids (e.g., albumin) in critically ill patients requiring fluid resuscitation in randomized trials; some forms of volume-expanding starches may worsen clinical outcomes
- In patients with critical illness **without coronary artery disease or active bleeding,** a transfusion threshold of hemoglobin of 7 g/dL was as effective as, and possibly superior to, using a transfusion threshold of hemoglobin of 10 g/dL

- Vasopressor support to maintain organ perfusion
  - Septic shock patients treated with dopamine or norepinephrine have similar mortality rates. Dopamine may increase mortality in patients with cardiogenic shock.
  - Dopamine is more likely to cause tachyarrhythmias
  - Norepinephrine is more potent vasopressor
    - No proven benefit (or harm) to adding vasopressin to norepinephine as opposed to using norepinephrine alone
- Supplemental oxygen to increase oxygen delivery
- Antibiotics directed at likely pathogens (site of infection and location of infection important determinants)

Preventing Complications
- Most life-sustaining therapies used in the ICU have potential mechanical or infectious complications (e.g., ventilator-induced lung injury, ventilator-associated pneumonia, central line–associated bloodstream infections, medication-induced delirium, critical illness weakness)
- Important to use these therapies only when necessary and to discontinue when risk-benefit ratio no longer favors use
  - Use ventilator protocols, especially daily spontaneous breathing trials, to wean patients off ventilators
  - Use sterile technique to place catheters; full-body as opposed to local sterile field preferred, chlorhexidine should be used, povidone-iodine (Betadyne) solution no longer considered adequate
    - Subclavian or internal jugular site less likely to have mechanical or infectious complications than femoral site
    - Central venous catheters should be placed under bedside ultrasound guidance when available
    - Remove catheters when no longer essential
  - Use deep venous thromboembolism prophylaxis for all ICU patients without a strong contraindication
  - Stress ulcer prophylaxis for at-risk patients (mechanical ventilation >48 hours or coagulopathy)
  - Tight glucose control is no longer indicated given the risks of hypoglycemia, though hyperglycemia should be avoided as well; glucose values should be maintained between 110 and 150 mg/dL
  - Sedation protocols to minimize dose of sedatives
    - Daily interruption or nurse-driven protocols both are acceptable
    - Both decrease length of intubation and ICU stay
  - Limiting the use of benzodiazepines, using a daily delirium assessment tool, and attempting to regulate day/night cycles in the ICU to decrease the incidence and duration of delirium
  - Elevation of head of bed 30° to 45° to reduce risk of ventilator-associated pneumonia in intubated patients
  - The use of checklists (e.g., when placing a central line, performing a thoracentesis, daily rounding checklists) decreases complications, nosocomial infections, and length of stay in critically ill patients in the ICU
  - Early mobility, ideally through a nurse-directed protocol to identify eligible patients, should be used in most ICU patients, including many who are still orally intubated

FIGURE 23-3 Diagnosis of shock. (BUN, blood urea nitrogen; CT, computed tomography; ECG, electrocardiogram; ICU, intensive care unit; LV, left ventricular; MAP, mean arterial pressure; MRI, magnetic resonance imaging; PA, pulmonary artery; PCWP, pulmonary capillary wedge pressure; PT, prothrombin time; PTT, partial thromboplastin time; RV, right ventricular; WBC, white blood cells.) *(From Goldman L, Bennett JC, Ausiello D: Cecil textbook of medicine, ed 22, Philadelphia, 2004, Saunders, Fig. 102.3.)*

Toxin Exposures

MANAGEMENT PRINCIPLES FOR TOXIN EXPOSURES

- Obtain history: time since ingestion, number and type of pills taken, formulation (e.g., extended release), concomitant ingestions (alcohol, illicit drugs)
- Obtain IV access, nasogastric intubation

TABLE 23-2	Differentiation of the Four Different Types of Shock*			
Type of Shock	**Cardiac Output**	**Filling Pressure**	**SVR**	
Distributive 　Septic 　Anaphylactic 　Neurogenic	↑	↓ or normal	↓	
Hypovolemic	↓	↓	↑	
Cardiogenic (pump failure)	↓	↑	↑	
Extracardiac obstructive 　Pericardial tamponade 　Acute PE 　Air embolus	↓	↓ or ↑	↑	

PE, pulmonary embolism; SVR, systemic vascular resistance.
*Can be made based on pulmonary artery catheter parameters.

- Activated charcoal blocks absorption of most drugs
  - **Exceptions include alkalis, lithium, iron, and insecticides**
  - **Ipecac is no longer routinely recommended to induce emesis**
    - May be used in the alert, awake patient
  - **Gastric lavage is of unproven efficacy but often used, and may be useful if recent ingestion (<1 hour)**
  - **Endotracheal intubation should be considered in patients who are obtunded or have a poor gag reflex**

TOXIN-SPECIFIC MANAGEMENT

Analgesics and Sedatives

See Table 23-3 for a summary of analgesic and sedative toxin exposures.

Cardioactive Medications

- Tricyclic antidepressants
  - Basic information
    - Possess anticholinergic, α-adrenergic blocking, and adrenergic uptake–inhibiting properties
    - Ingestion of 10 to 20 mg/kg may cause moderate to severe toxicity, and 30 to 40 mg/kg may be life-threatening
    - Best predictor of toxicity is **QRS interval greater than 100 ms**
  - Clinical presentation
    - Arrhythmias, hypotension, and anticholinergic effects (e.g., hyperthermia, flushing, dilated pupils, intestinal ileus, urinary retention, and sinus tachycardia) (Fig. 23-4)

TABLE 23-3	Toxin Exposures: Analgesics and Sedatives			
Toxin Exposure	**Basic Information**	**Clinical Picture**	**Diagnosis**	**Treatment**
Acetaminophen	Toxicity caused by reactive metabolite Metabolite detoxified by glutathione	Hepatotoxicity: 　If ingestion >7.5 g 　Less in alcoholics	Acetaminophen level Nomogram helpful in determining potential for toxicity over time	N-Acetylcysteine Best results within 8 hr of exposure May be beneficial up to 24 hr
Salicylate	Uncouples oxidative phosphorylation	Acute toxicity: 　Respiratory alkalosis 　Anion gap acidosis 　Hyperthermia 　Coagulopathy 　Pulmonary edema 　Hyper- or hypoglycemia 　Seizures	Salicylate level: 　>40 mg/dL in acute ingestion 　>30 mg/dL in chronic ingestion Potential toxicity by dose: 　<150 mg/kg low risk 　>300 mg/kg severe toxicity 　>500 mg/kg may be lethal	Hydration Alkalinization of urine Gastric lavage, activated charcoal Hemodialysis (for seizures, refractory acidosis, or levels >90–100 mg/dL)
Opiates	Bind opiate receptors	Hypotension Respiratory depression CNS depression	Urine testing for opiate metabolites	Naloxone 　Opiate antagonist 　Short acting
Benzodiazepines	Bind the GABA receptor	Hypotension Respiratory depression CNS depression Synergistic effect with opiates	Urine testing for metabolites	Flumazenil 　Benzodiazepine receptor antagonist 　Short acting. Use with caution. May precipitate seizures in patients with chronic benzodiazepine use or concomitant TCA overdose.

GABA, γ-aminobutyric acid; TCA, tricyclic antidepressant.

FIGURE 23-4 Electrocardiogram (ECG) in tricyclic antidepressant overdose. **A,** Sinus tachycardia, QRS widening, and Q–T prolongation in a patient with tricyclic antidepressant overdose. **B,** Normal ECG in the same individual 4 days later. *(From Goldberger AL: Clinical electrocardiography: a simplified approach, ed 6, St. Louis, Mosby, 1999, Fig. 10-4.)*

- CNS effects are common, with initial agitation followed by seizures and depressed consciousness
  - Treatment
    - **Alkalinization** to serum pH of 7.4 to 7.5 with IV sodium bicarbonate is indicated to reduce occurrence of arrhythmias
    - If patient is on a ventilator, may also hyperventilate
    - Carefully monitor pH during therapy (pH >7.55 increases risk of seizures)
- β-Blockers
  - Basic information
    - Negative inotropic and chronotropic effects
    - Non–β_1-selective agents may have respiratory effects, and lipophilic agents (e.g., propranolol) can cross blood-brain barrier, causing CNS depression
  - Clinical presentation
    - Hypotension, bradycardia, and varying degrees of heart block
  - Treatment
    - Glucagon
    - IV fluids if hypotensive
    - If needed, pacing and vasopressor or inotrope with β_1 activity
- Calcium channel blockers
  - Basic information
    - Negative inotropic and chronotropic effects
  - Clinical presentation
    - Hypotension, bradycardia, and low cardiac output
  - Treatment
    - 10% calcium chloride
    - If needed, pacing and vasopressor with β and α activity
- Digitalis
  - Basic information
    - Therapeutic inotropic agent/antiarrhythmic with a narrow therapeutic window

- Clinical presentation
  - Nausea, malaise, weakness, bradycardia, heart block, hyperkalemia, visual complaints of seeing yellow halos around lights
- Treatment
  - **Digoxin-specific antibody**
    - Indicated for **hemodynamically compromising conduction disturbances or for hyperkalemia**
  - Calcium is relatively contraindicated in this setting because hypercalcemia may potentiate digitalis toxicity
  - Cardiac monitor for at least 6 hours after ingestion
- Theophylline
  - Basic information
    - Methylxanthine bronchodilator with a narrow therapeutic window
  - Clinical presentation
    - Nausea and vomiting, agitation, seizures and arrhythmias, especially supraventricular
  - Treatment
    - **Hemodialysis or charcoal hemoperfusion may be initiated for markedly elevated levels (>60–100 mg/mL), seizures, or persistently unstable hemodynamics**
    - Supraventricular arrhythmias may be treated with β-blockers

Toxins That Alter Hemoglobin/Oxygen-Binding Properties

- Carbon monoxide poisoning
  - Basic information
    - Colorless, odorless gas emitted by faulty heaters
    - Seen primarily in winter months

TABLE 23-4	*Alcohol-Induced Toxicity*				
Alcohol	**Example**	**Clinical Presentation**	**Anion Gap***	**Osmolar Gap†**	**Treatment**
Methanol	Antifreeze Bootleg whiskey	Abdominal pain Nausea/vomiting Loss of vision	+	+	Fomepizole (alcohol dehydrogenase inhibitor)
Ethylene glycol	Antifreeze Windshield deicer	Ataxia Seizures Abdominal pain Nausea/vomiting	+	+	Fomepizole
Isopropanol	Rubbing alcohol	Abdominal pain Nausea/vomiting Headache Ataxia Coma	−	+	Fomepizole

*Anion gap = $[Na^+] - ([Cl^-] + [HCO_3^-])$.
†Osmolar gap = measured osmolality − $\{2[Na^+] + (BUN/2.8) + ([glucose]/18)\}$.

- Clinical presentation
  - Dizziness, headache, weakness, confusion, dyspnea, chest pain
  - In severe cases: loss of consciousness, focal CNS symptoms, cardiac ischemia
  - Lips and skin may appear cherry red, but this is an insensitive sign
  - Diagnosis is made by measurement of carboxyhemoglobin
- Treatment
  - Remove patient from the source
  - **Deliver 100% Fio_2 by non-rebreathing mask**
  - **Hyperbaric oxygen** appears to prevent delayed neurologic sequelae in high-risk patients (loss of consciousness, confusion, lactic acidosis)
- Methemoglobinemia
  - Basic information
    - Occurs when the ferrous ions (Fe^{2+}) of heme are oxidized to the ferric (Fe^{3+}) state that has a lower affinity for oxygen
    - Methemoglobin formation may be caused by exogenous agents, including sulfonamides, nitrates, topical anesthetics, antimalarials, and occupational exposures
    - Higher levels of methemoglobin occur in individuals with deficiency of the cytochrome b_5 reductase enzyme, which reduces Fe^{3+} to the Fe^{2+} state
  - Clinical presentation
    - Hypoxia, cyanosis, and chocolate color of arterial blood
    - Suggested in a patient with **a low pulse oximetry reading, but a normal arterial blood gas Pao_2**
  - Diagnosis
    - Measurement of methemoglobin level
  - Treatment
    - Discontinuation of the offending agent
    - Administration of **methylene blue** to reduce the methemoglobin to hemoglobin

Alcohols

See Table 23-4 for a summary of alcohol-induced toxicity.

REVIEW QUESTIONS

For review questions, please go to www.expertconsult.com.

SUGGESTED READINGS

The Acute Respiratory Distress Syndrome Network: Ventilation with lower tidal volumes as compared with traditional tidal volumes for acute lung injury and the acute respiratory distress syndrome, *N Engl J Med* 342:1301–1308, 2000.

Dellinger RP, Levy MM, Carlet JM, et al: Surviving Sepsis Campaign: international guidelines for management of severe sepsis and septic shock, *Crit Care Med* 36:296–327, 2008.

Finfer S, Bellamo R, Boyce N, et al: A comparison of albumin and saline for fluid resuscitation in the intensive care unit, *N Engl J Med* 350:2247–2256, 2004.

Girard TD, Kress JP, Fuchs BD, et al: Efficacy and safety of a paired sedation and ventilator weaning protocol for mechanically ventilated patients in intensive care (Awakening and Breathing Controlled trial): a randomised controlled trial, *Lancet* 371:126–134, 2008.

Harvey S, Harrison DA, Singer M, et al: Assessment of the clinical effectiveness of pulmonary artery catheters in management of patients in intensive care (PAC-Man): a randomised controlled trial, *Lancet* 366:472–477, 2005.

Hebert PC, Wells G, Blajchman MA, et al: A multicenter, randomized, controlled clinical trial of transfusion requirements in critical care. Transfusion Requirements in Critical Care Investigators, Canadian Critical Care Trials Group, *N Engl J Med* 340:409–417, 1999.

Knaus WA, Zimmerman JE, Wagner DP, et al: APACHE—Acute Physiology and Chronic Health Evaluation: physiologically based classification system, *Crit Care Med* 9:591–597, 1981.

National Heart, Lung, and Blood Institute: Acute Respiratory Distress Syndrome (ARDS) Clinical Trials Network: Comparison of two fluid-management strategies in acute lung injury, *N Engl J Med* 354:2564–2575, 2006.

Tobin MJ: Advances in mechanical ventilation, *N Engl J Med* 344:1986–1996, 2001.

23

Pleural Disease

ALBERT J. POLITO, MD

Pleural diseases are among the most frequently encountered problems in chest medicine. Two of the most common such diseases are pleural effusions and pneumothoraces. The former reflect an excessive accumulation of fluid in the pleural space, whereas the latter occur when air enters the pleural space.

Pleural Effusions

Basic Information

- The most common causes of pleural effusion in the United States are congestive heart failure, pneumonia, malignancy, and pulmonary embolism
- Pathophysiology of pleural effusions
  - Pleural fluid originates from capillaries in parietal pleura and is drained by lymphatics in parietal pleura
  - Pleural effusion forms when more fluid is formed than can be reabsorbed
  - Effusion can also originate from interstitial spaces of lung, intrathoracic lymphatics, or the peritoneal cavity
    - Mechanisms of pleural fluid accumulation are shown in Table 24-1
  - Subpulmonic effusions develop when fluid becomes loculated between the lower aspect of the lung and the diaphragm
  - Parapneumonic effusions and empyema are pleural effusions associated with bacterial pneumonia or lung abscess; they are associated with a higher mortality rate than pneumonia and abscess without effusions

Clinical Presentation

- Symptoms of pleural effusion differ markedly according to cause and rapidity of onset
  - Pleural effusions are often asymptomatic, but small to moderate effusions may be symptomatic if they develop rapidly
  - Dyspnea; pleuritic chest pain (although pain may be dull and aching); and dry, nonproductive cough are typical symptoms of pleural effusion
    - Patients with infectious causes (e.g., pneumonia, tuberculosis) present with acute febrile illness and chest pain
    - **Patients with malignant pleural effusions typically present with dyspnea**
      - **Malignancy is the most common cause of massive pleural effusions that cause complete opacification of one hemithorax**

- Patients with a pulmonary embolus present with pleuritic chest pain and dyspnea
  - Effusions (seen in 30–50% of cases) are usually small to moderate in size and unilateral
- Rheumatoid pleurisy may be asymptomatic and occur in the absence of joint disease activity
  - Classic presentation is an elderly man with subcutaneous rheumatoid nodules and a unilateral pleural effusion
  - **Frequently mimics a complicated parapneumonic effusion, with high lactate dehydrogenase (>1000 U/L), low glucose (<40 mg/dL), and low pH (<7.2)**
- Lupus pleuritis is typically painful and occurs in 15% to 40% of patients with lupus at some point in the disease
  - Small, bilateral effusions commonly seen
  - It is the presenting feature of lupus in 5% of cases
  - **Lupus pleuritis may be seen in drug-induced lupus because of procainamide, hydralazine, or isoniazid, among others**
- Chylothorax manifests with (typically) unilateral pleural effusion (Fig. 24-1)
  - Thoracic duct course (Fig. 24-2): Originates in abdomen as cisterna chyli, enters the thorax with the aorta, runs along the right anterolateral surface of the vertebrae, crosses the midline at the fourth thoracic vertebra, continues up along the left anterolateral vertebral surface, and empties into the junction of the left internal jugular and subclavian veins
  - **Site of interruption of thoracic duct determines side of pleural effusion (right-sided if below the fourth thoracic vertebra; left-sided if above it)**
  - **Lymphoma is cause in 75% of cases**
  - Thoracic duct trauma from injury or surgery makes up the majority of the remainder of cases
  - Occasionally idiopathic; rarely seen with tuberculosis or sarcoid
- Patients with asbestos exposure may present with benign asbestos pleural effusion (BAPE) 5 to 15 years after exposure to asbestos
  - Effusions are typically unilateral, persist for a mean of 4 months, and resolve spontaneously
  - Patients may go on to develop pleural plaques (20 years after exposure) or mesothelioma (20–30 years after exposure)

TABLE 24-1	*Mechanisms of Pleural Fluid Accumulation*
Mechanism	**Representative Disease State**
Increased hydrostatic pressure of vasculature	Congestive heart failure
Decreased oncotic pressure of vasculature	Nephrotic syndrome
Decreased pleural pressure	Atelectasis
Obstruction of lymphatic drainage	Malignancy
Increased capillary permeability	Parapneumonic effusion
Rupture of thoracic duct	Chylothorax
Increased fluid in peritoneal cavity	Hepatic hydrothorax
Iatrogenic	Placement of central line into pleural space

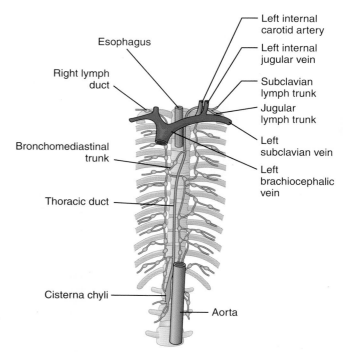

FIGURE 24-2 Lymphatics of the thorax. *(From Jacob S: Atlas of human anatomy, New York, Churchill Livingstone, 2002, Fig. 3.4h.)*

FIGURE 24-1 Chylothorax. The classic milky-appearing pleural fluid of a chylothorax. *(From Forbes CD, Jackson WF: Color atlas and text of clinical medicine, ed 3, St. Louis, Mosby, 2003, Fig. 4.53.)*

- **Physical examination findings over the site of the effusion include dullness to percussion, with decreased or absent breath sounds and the absence of tactile fremitus**
  - Pleural rub (creaky, leathery sound) not common; suggests pleural inflammation alone or with small effusion
  - Other physical findings vary depending on cause of effusion

Diagnosis and Evaluation

- Evaluation of pleural effusions is done by imaging of the effusion and sampling of the effusion with thoracentesis
- Imaging
  - As pleural effusion develops, small amounts of fluid obscure posterior costophrenic angle on lateral imaging, followed by blunting of lateral costophrenic angle on posteroanterior imaging (Fig. 24-3)
    - Sensitivity of posteroanterior and lateral films is 200 mL
    - Lateral decubitus film extremely helpful in detecting effusion; can detect as little as 15 mL of fluid

FIGURE 24-3 Large left pleural effusion. This patient had a previous mastectomy on the right, and the pleural effusion is malignant. The mediastinal shift to the right results from the space-occupying effects of the fluid. *(From Albert RK, Spiro SG, Jett JR: Clinical respiratory medicine, ed 2, St. Louis, Mosby, 2004, Fig. 1.83.)*

- **If lateral decubitus film shows fluid is free-flowing and depth of pleural fluid is greater than 10 mm, diagnostic thoracentesis can be performed**
  - Consider subpulmonic effusion if one hemidiaphragm appears elevated and apex of diaphragm is laterally displaced
    - On left side, consider if top of hemidiaphragm is separated from gastric air bubble

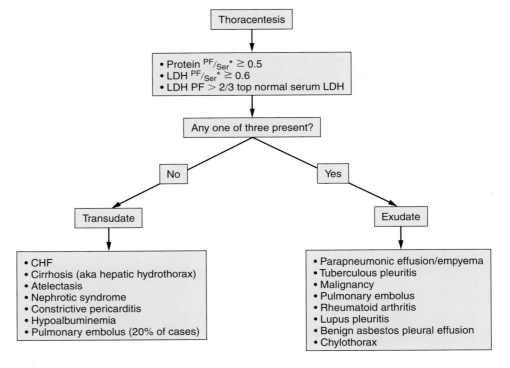

FIGURE 24-4 Transudates and exudates. (CHF, congestive heart failure; LDH, lactate dehydrogenase.) *Pleural fluid value (PF) divided by serum value (Ser).

- Ultrasound is useful for identifying loculated areas of pleural fluid or for localizing placement of thoracentesis needle and distinguishing pleural fluid from pleural thickening
- Computed tomography (CT) scanning helps distinguish between pleural and parenchymal disease and can differentiate between empyema and lung abscess
- Thoracentesis
  - For undiagnosed pleural effusions, thoracentesis is indicated
  - Differential diagnosis of pleural effusion is narrowed by determining whether pleural fluid is transudate or exudate (Fig. 24-4)
    - Note that pulmonary embolus usually (80%) results in an exudative effusion but manifests with a transudate in 20% of cases
  - **If any one of the three criteria shown in Figure 24-4 (known as Light's criteria) is met, the effusion is classified as an exudate**
    - **Application of Light's criteria occasionally leads to misclassification of a transudate as an exudate, but does not lead to misclassifying exudates**
- Cytopathology: Important for diagnosing malignant effusions
  - Most common causes of malignant pleural effusions include lung cancer (33%, usually adenocarcinoma), breast cancer (25%), and lymphoma/leukemia (15%)
  - **Sensitivity of single thoracentesis sample for diagnosing malignancy is 60%; three sequential thoracenteses increase sensitivity to 80%**
  - Cytology more likely to be positive with pleural metastases or with mediastinal lymph node involvement

- Culture
  - Most common organisms in parapneumonic effusion are *Staphylococcus aureus*, anaerobes such as *Bacteroides* and *Peptostreptococcus*, *Streptococcus pneumoniae*, and gram-negative organisms such as *Escherichia coli* and *Klebsiella*
  - **Yield for mycobacterial cultures is only 35%; pleural biopsy typically performed if tuberculosis suggested**
    - **With pleural biopsy, granulomas seen in 80% of cases; acid-fast bacteria (AFB) stain positive in 25% of cases; and AFB culture positive in 55% of cases**
    - **Tuberculin skin test (purified protein derivative [PPD]) positive in only two thirds of patients with a tuberculous pleural effusion**
- Other tests used in evaluation of pleural fluid are shown in Table 24-2
- In patients with pneumonia, characteristics used to distinguish parapneumonic effusion from empyema are shown in Table 24-3

Treatment

- Treatment of pleural effusions determined by size of effusion, presence of symptoms, and cause of effusion
- Treatment of underlying etiology of effusion is most important, but definitive mechanical removal of fluid may also be needed
  - Options include therapeutic thoracentesis, chest tube drainage, thoracotomy with decortication, and pleurodesis (fusion of visceral and parietal pleura to prevent recurrence of symptomatic effusion; particularly useful with empyemas and malignant effusions)
    - Chemical pleurodesis: Sclerosant agent is introduced through chest tube after fluid is drained and lung has reexpanded

TABLE 24-2	Tests Used in the Evaluation of Pleural Fluid
Test	**Result**

Cell counts	RBC count >100,000/μL suggests
	  Trauma
	  Malignancy
	  Pulmonary embolism with infarction
	WBC count
	  <1000/μL suggests transudate
	  >1000/μL suggests exudate
	WBC differential
	  >10,000 neutrophils/μL suggests
	    parapneumonic effusion or empyema;
	    occasionally seen with pulmonary
	    embolus, pancreatitis, or early tuberculosis
	  >50% lymphocytes suggests tuberculosis
	    or malignancy; also seen after coronary
	    artery bypass graft surgery
	  Eosinophilia nonspecific, but may suggest
	    parasitic infection, drug reaction,
	    malignant effusion, or Churg-Strauss
	    syndrome

pH	pH <7.2 suggests
	  Complicated parapneumonic effusion
	  Empyema
	  Esophageal rupture
	  Rheumatoid pleurisy
	  Malignant effusion
	pH >7.8 suggests *Proteus* infection

Glucose	Glucose <60 mg/dL suggests
	  Parapneumonic effusion
	  Empyema
	  Rheumatoid pleurisy
	  Malignant effusion
	  Tuberculous pleuritis

Amylase	If elevated, suggests
	  Pancreatic disease
	  Esophageal rupture (salivary isoenzymes
	    elevated); typically results in left-sided
	    effusion
	  Malignant effusion (salivary isoenzymes
	    not elevated)

Triglycerides (TG)	TG >110 mg/dL indicates chylothorax
	If TG 50–110 mg/dL, send fluid for
	  chylomicrons
	  Presence of chylomicrons indicates
	    chylothorax
	TG <50 mg/dL indicates no chylothorax

Cholesterol	Causes a "pseudochylothorax" (milky fluid
	  but not a true chylothorax)
	Usually seen in long-standing effusions
	  Old tuberculous effusion
	  Rheumatoid pleurisy
	  Nephrotic syndrome

Antinuclear antibody (ANA)	Pleural fluid ANA titer commonly elevated to
	  >1:160 in lupus, but is not specific for the
	  disease

Adenosine deaminase	Typically >50 units/L in tuberculous pleurisy

Interferon-γ	Elevated in tuberculous pleurisy but cutoff
	  value not well established
	Note that interferon-γ release assays
	  (IGRA), such as commercially available
	  QuantiFERON-TB Gold and T-SPOT.TB,
	  are not useful for diagnosing tuberculous
	  pleuritis

RBC, red blood cell; WBC, white blood cell.

TABLE 24-3	Parapneumonic Effusions and Empyema	
Effusion Type	**Definition**	**Treatment***

Simple parapneumonic effusion	pH >7.2
	Glucose >40 mg/dL
	LDH <3 times top
	  normal serum LDH
		Antibiotics alone
		  often sufficient

Complicated parapneumonic effusion	Gross appearance
	  does not resemble
	  pus
	pH <7.0
	Glucose <40 mg/dL
	"Borderline"
	  complicated pH
	  7.0–7.2, with
	  glucose >40 mg/
	  dL and/or LDH
	  <3 times normal
		Antibiotics
		Chest tube
		Serial thoracentesis
		  acceptable in
		  borderline cases

Empyema	Appearance of frank
	  pus
	pH <7.0
	Glucose <40 mg/dL
	WBC count typically
	  >15,000/μL
	Bacterial culture
	  commonly
	  positive
		Antibiotics
		Chest tube
		Decortication
		  may be required
		Fibrinolytics or
		  thoracoscopy
		  occasionally
		  used if
		  loculations
		  present

LDH, lactate dehydrogenase; WBC, white blood cell.

*Treatment of each disorder will be determined in part by volume of fluid and presence of loculations.

- **Talc, administered in a slurry, is the most effective agent but does carry a small risk of respiratory failure**
- Doxycycline also is commonly used—slightly less effective than talc but not associated with respiratory failure
- Surgical pleurodesis via thoracotomy using one of two techniques
  - Mechanical abrasion of pleura
  - Insufflation of talc (equally effective as talc slurry, and with same risk of respiratory failure)
- Specific treatment
  - Parapneumonic effusion (see Table 24-3)
  - **Chylothorax: Treatment includes chest tube, bed rest, enteral feeding with medium-chain triglycerides (absorbed to circulation via portal vein, avoiding thoracic duct)**
    - Occasionally thoracic duct ligation or placement of pleuroperitoneal shunt needed
    - Lack of treatment results in loss of protein, fat, and lymphocytes, risking malnutrition and infection

Pneumothorax

Basic Information

- Pneumothorax results from the introduction of air into the pleural space
  - May occur spontaneously or result from trauma or iatrogenic causes (e.g., surgery, central venous access placement, thoracentesis)

- Primary spontaneous pneumothorax occurs when no clinically apparent lung disease is present
  - **Incidence in men compared with women is 6 to 1**
  - **Typical patient is a tall, thin male younger than age 40 years who smokes**
  - Most patients have radiographically inapparent subpleural bullae
- Secondary spontaneous pneumothorax occurs as a result of underlying lung disease
  - Obstructive lung diseases associated with secondary spontaneous pneumothorax include asthma, chronic obstructive pulmonary disease, and cystic fibrosis
  - Associated interstitial lung diseases include idiopathic pulmonary fibrosis, eosinophilic granuloma, and lymphangioleiomyomatosis
  - *Pneumocystis jiroveci* (formerly *carinii*) pneumonia and Marfan syndrome also are associated with secondary spontaneous pneumothorax

Clinical Presentation

- Typical symptoms include ipsilateral pleuritic chest pain and dyspnea
- Physical findings normal with small pneumothorax (<15%)
  - **Tachycardia is the most common finding in pneumothorax**
  - **Hyperresonance to percussion, decreased chest wall movement, decreased fremitus, and decreased or absent breath sounds common with large pneumothorax**
  - Hypotension, cyanosis, and shift of the trachea to the contralateral side seen with tension pneumothorax

Diagnosis and Evaluation

- Radiographic imaging used to confirm diagnosis
  - Visceral pleural edge separated from chest wall on chest radiograph (Fig. 24-5)
  - May be difficult to diagnose with underlying lung disease (e.g., bullous emphysema)
  - Chest CT may be needed if suggested but not apparent on chest film

Treatment

- Treatment is similar for primary and secondary spontaneous pneumothorax, although the threshold for placing a chest tube is lower (i.e., done sooner) for secondary spontaneous pneumothorax
  - **Administer 100% oxygen and observe patient if pneumothorax is small (<15%)**
    - **Increases rate of reabsorption of air from pleural space fourfold**
  - Larger (>15%) pneumothoraces require removal of air, either with catheter (works best with young patients) or with chest tube (required for most patients)

FIGURE 24-5 Anteroposterior chest radiograph of simple pneumothorax. Note absence of lung marking on the affected side and deviation of the trachea contralaterally. *(From Roberts JR: Clinical procedures in emergency medicine, ed 4, Philadelphia, WB Saunders, 2004, Fig. 10-1.)*

- Recurrence rate
  - Similar for primary and secondary forms
  - **30% after first episode; more than 50% after second episode**
  - Usually occurs within 2 years after initial pneumothorax
  - Advise patients to avoid scuba diving
  - **After second pneumothorax, recommend intervention to prevent recurrence**
    - Chemical pleurodesis through chest tube
    - If present, blebs/bullae should be surgically resected, with concomitant surgical pleurodesis
    - Pleurodesis agents and techniques are same as those used for persistent pleural effusions (see above)

REVIEW QUESTIONS

For review questions, please go to www.expertconsult.com.

SUGGESTED READINGS

Haynes D, Baumann MH: Management of pneumothorax, *Semin Respir Crit Care Med* 31:769–780, 2010.

Heffner JE, Klein JS: Recent advances in the diagnosis and management of malignant pleural effusions, *Mayo Clin Proc* 83:235–250, 2008.

Light RW: *Pleural diseases*, ed 5, Philadelphia, Lippincott, 2007, Williams & Wilkins.

Light RW: Update on tuberculous pleural effusion, *Respirology* 15:451–458, 2010.

Schiza S, Siafakas SM: Clinical presentation and management of empyema, lung abscess, and pleural effusion, *Curr Opin Pulm Med* 12:205–211, 2006.

Wrightson JM, Davies RJ: The approach to the patient with a parapneumonic effusion, *Semin Respir Crit Care Med* 31:706–715, 2010.

SECTION FOUR

BOARD REVIEW

Gastroenterology

Peptic Ulcer Disease and Gastrointestinal Bleeding

JOHN O. CLARKE, MD; and LINDA A. LEE, MD

Causes of gastrointestinal (GI) blood loss have been divided into two basic categories based on the anatomic location of the bleeding source in relation to the ligament of Treitz. *Upper GI bleeding* refers to blood loss originating above this area, whereas *lower GI bleeding* stems from sources below. This chapter focuses on the approach to patients with suspected upper or lower GI bleeding and describes the most common specific causes within each category.

Background

Stomach Anatomy

Figure 25-1 illustrates the anatomy of the stomach.
- Antrum
  - Pyloric glands
    - G cells: Secrete gastrin, which stimulates acid production
    - D cells: Secrete somatostatin, which inhibits gastrin secretion
    - Goblet cells: Secrete mucus to coat and protect the stomach from corrosive injury
- Fundus/body
  - Oxyntic glands
    - Parietal cells: Secrete acid (HCl)
    - Chief cells: Secrete pepsinogen, which is converted to pepsin by HCl. Pepsin can damage the gastric epithelium.

Gastric Acid Secretion

- Three pathways by which acid production/secretion occurs
  - Vagus innervation leads to release of acetylcholine, which leads to stimulation of H^+/K^+–adenosine triphosphatase (ATPase) and acid production/secretion
  - Gastrin release leads to direct stimulation of H^+/K^+-ATPase, which leads to acid production/secretion
  - Histamine release leads to stimulation of adenylate cyclase, which leads to cyclic adenosine monophosphate (cAMP), which leads to stimulation of H^+/K^+-ATPase and leads to acid production/secretion
- Regulation of acid secretion
  - Basal acid secretion: Mediated by vagal tone; highest levels at nighttime
  - Food-stimulated secretion

- Cephalic phase: Sight, smell, and taste stimulate the vagus nerve
- Gastric phase: Triggered by gastric distention and protein digestion caused by food entering the stomach; gastrin is then released
- Intestinal phase: Triggered by protein in small bowel

Peptic Ulcer Disease

Causes

- Direct mucosal injury (e.g., toxins, ethanol, nonsteroidal anti-inflammatory drugs [NSAIDs], *Helicobacter pylori*, bile)
- Inhibition of prostaglandin synthesis (NSAIDs)
- Disruption of the protective mucus layer (NSAIDs, *H. pylori*)
- Increased gastric acid secretion (*H. pylori*, gastrinoma, hypercalcemia, sepsis, central nervous system, burns)
- Mucosal ischemia (anastomotic ulcers)

Epidemiology

- **Most patients have normal acid secretion**
- Gastric ulcers may represent an underlying malignancy (~3%)
- Duodenal ulcers rarely represent an underlying malignancy
- Lifetime prevalence of peptic ulcer disease (PUD) is 5% to 10%

Clinical Presentation

- Epigastric abdominal pain is the most common symptom
- Nausea and vomiting may occur
- Gastrointestinal bleeding (see later discussion): 20% of patients will bleed and can present with hematemesis, coffee-grounds emesis, hematochezia, or melena
- Perforation
  - Seen in 5% of patients
  - Abdominal examination reveals rigid abdomen with rebound tenderness
  - Duodenal ulcers may penetrate posterior to the pancreas, resulting in elevations in amylase and lipase
- Gastric outlet obstruction
  - Usually caused by peripyloric scar formation

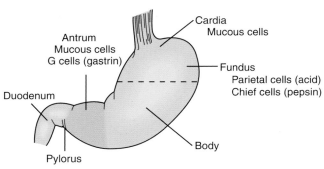

FIGURE 25-1 Anatomy of the stomach. *(From Kumar V, Fausto N, Abbas A: Robbins & Cotran's pathologic basis of disease, ed 7, Philadelphia, WB Saunders, 2004, Fig. 17-12A.)*

- Presents with abdominal bloating, nausea, vomiting, weight loss

Diagnosis

- Endoscopy has been shown to be far superior to barium studies for the detection of gastric and duodenal ulcers

Therapy

- Antacids
  - Neutralize acid
  - Magnesium and aluminum compounds can be toxic in patients with renal failure
  - Calcium carbonate antacids can cause milk-alkali syndrome (hypercalcemia, hyperphosphatemia) with prolonged use
- Histamine$_2$ (H$_2$) blockers (e.g., cimetidine, ranitidine, famotidine, nizatidine)
  - Block H$_2$ receptor on parietal cells
  - Work relatively quickly (approximately 30 minutes)
  - Effective for both duodenal and gastric ulcers
  - Associated with tachyphylaxis and may not provide long-term benefit (but effective in acute treatment or intermittent use)
  - Inhibit cytochrome P-450 drug metabolism (more common with cimetidine); need to monitor levels of some drugs (e.g., warfarin, phenytoin, theophylline)
- Proton pump (H$^+$/K$^+$-ATPase) inhibitors (e.g., omeprazole, lansoprazole, rabeprazole, pantoprazole, esomeprazole, dexlansoprazole)
  - **Irreversibly block H$^+$/K$^+$-ATPase; take 3 days to block 90% of pumps**
  - Increase gastrin levels
  - Most effective when given prior to meals (typically prior to breakfast if once daily and prior to breakfast/dinner if twice daily)
  - Effective for both duodenal and gastric ulcers
  - Can interfere with the absorption of other drugs (e.g., ketoconazole, ampicillin, iron, digoxin)
  - Emerging data suggest long-term use may be associated with decreased bone mineral density and increased community-acquired infection
  - Emerging data suggest that they may decrease efficacy of clopidogrel and protease inhibitors
  - Have not been shown to increase the risk of gastric cancers

- Can be associated with rebound acid hypersecretion upon cessation
- Sucralfate
  - Stimulates endogenous prostaglandins and enhances mucosal defenses and repair
  - Effective for duodenal ulcer
  - Avoid in patients with renal insufficiency because of the potential for aluminum toxicity

Duration of Therapy

- Duodenal ulcers: 4 to 6 weeks
- **Gastric ulcers: 6 to 8 weeks; repeat endoscopy with biopsies to rule out gastric cancer in 8 weeks**

NSAID-Associated GI Toxicity

Epidemiology

- Dyspepsia occurs in 10% to 20% of patients taking NSAIDs
- 1.3% of those taking NSAIDs for arthritis have a serious GI complication
- Mortality rate for those hospitalized with NSAID-related bleeding is 5% to 10%
- **An increased risk of GI bleeding is associated with even low-dose aspirin use (<75 mg/day)**
- Enteric-coated aspirin has a rate of complication similar to non–enteric-coated preparations

Risk Factors

- Prior history of ulcer
- Concomitant use of corticosteroids
- Concomitant use of other anticoagulants
- High doses of NSAIDs
- Advanced age (>70 years)
- *H. pylori*—controversial

Mechanisms

- Topical: NSAIDs are acidic and can migrate through the protective layer of mucus to the gastric epithelium, where they dissociate into the ionized form. The disruption in the layer of mucus also permits further injury by gastric acid and pepsin.
- Inhibition of prostaglandin synthesis: most important cause of gastroduodenal NSAID injury

Therapy

- Withdraw NSAIDs
- Treat *H. pylori* (see later discussion) if ulcer is present
- Proton pump inhibitor

Prophylaxis

- Not indicated in the absence of prior PUD or symptoms
- Misoprostol
  - Prostaglandin E derivative shown to decrease the incidence of NSAID-induced ulceration
  - Diarrhea is a common side effect
  - Contraindicated in pregnancy (or in women considering pregnancy as it acts as an abortifacient)
- Proton pump inhibitor is also effective
- H$_2$ blockers found to be inferior to proton pump inhibitors and misoprostol

- **Eradicate *H. pylori* before initiating NSAID therapy if patient is *H. pylori* positive and has a history of PUD**

Alternative to Prophylaxis

- Cyclooxygenase-2 (COX-2)–selective inhibitors
- Based on the fact that cyclooxygenase-1 (COX-1) is constitutively expressed and maintains GI mucosal integrity and COX-2 expression is induced by inflammation
- Studies show that COX-2–selective inhibitors are less likely to cause PUD than are nonselective NSAIDs
- Lack cardiovascular protective effects (COX-1 participates in platelet aggregation)
- There are increasing data to show that all drugs in this class appear to have potential cardiovascular risk that may be dose dependent. Should be used with caution in patients with cardiac risk factors.
- **Protective effect of COX-2–selective inhibitor is lost if the patient uses regular or baby acetylsalicylic acid concomitantly**

Helicobacter pylori Infection

Features

- Gram-negative, spiral-shaped, flagellated rod
- Accounts for most cases of PUD in the United States
- Found in mucus layer; produces a urease that splits urea into ammonia and bicarbonate
- Humans are the principal reservoir
- Mode of transmission thought to be fecal-oral and/or oral-oral routes
- Infection thought to occur in childhood
- In the United States, 40% to 50% of those older than 60 years are infected
- More prevalent in developing countries
- Risk factors for infection include low socioeconomic status, domestic crowding, exposure to unclean food or water
- Over half the world is infected with *H. pylori*; however, only approximately 15% of people with *H. pylori* report GI symptoms

Diagnosis

- Noninvasive tests
  - Serum immunoglobulin G (IgG): About 90% sensitivity
    - Serum qualitative antibody test
    - Whole-blood qualitative antibody test
    - Quantitative antibody test: A 30% decrease in titer can be used to document post-treatment eradication (rarely done). A qualitative test is not useful to document post-treatment eradication because IgG remains positive after treatment.
  - Urea breath test (95% sensitivity, >95% specificity)
    - Urea labeled with C-13 or C-14 cleaved by urease into ammonia and CO_2
    - Stop proton pump inhibitor 1 week and antibiotics 4 weeks before test; should also stop bismuth and high doses of H_2-receptor antagonists
  - Stool *H. pylori* antigen test
    - Sensitivity 93.2%, specificity 93.2%

  - Useful for initial diagnosis and also documentation of post-therapy eradication
  - More widely available than breath test
- Invasive tests
  - Rapid urease test (~90% sensitivity, >95% specificity)
    - Biopsy is placed on a card that is spotted with urea; when urease is present, it cleaves the urea, inducing a pH and color change on the card
  - Histology
  - Presence of active chronic gastritis suggests the presence of *H. pylori* even in the absence of visible organisms
  - Organisms can be detected by Giemsa, hematoxylin and eosin, and silver stains
  - Culture
    - Useful only for detecting antibiotic resistance and not often obtained in clinical practice
- Use of *H. pylori* testing
  - Antibody tests are useful in those who have not been previously treated
  - **Stool antigen test or urea breath test is useful to detect active infections or monitor response to therapy**
  - Endoscopy is useful to detect *H. pylori*–associated ulcers or cancers; of note, while endoscopy with histology is specific for *H. pylori*, sensitivity is less than either the stool antigen test or urea breath test

Therapy

- Overview
  - **Triple-drug therapy superior to dual-drug therapy**
  - Reinfection is rare
  - Metronidazole resistance is 43%
  - Clarithromycin resistance is 8%
- Food and Drug Administration–approved regimens
  - 14 days: Bismuth subsalicylate 2 tablets four times a day, metronidazole 250 mg four times a day, tetracycline 500 mg four times a day, H_2 blocker (H_2 blocker should be continued for 4 weeks)
  - 10 days: Lansoprazole 30 mg twice a day, amoxicillin 1 g twice a day, clarithromycin 500 mg twice a day (LAC)
  - 10 days: Omeprazole 20 mg twice a day, amoxicillin 1 g twice a day, clarithromycin 500 mg twice a day (OAC)
  - 10 days: Esomeprazole 40 mg once per day, amoxicillin 1 g twice per day, clarithromycin 500 mg twice per day
  - 7 days: Rabeprazole 20 mg twice per day, amoxicillin 1 g twice per day, clarithromycin 500 mg twice per day

Diseases Associated with *H. pylori*

- Peptic ulcer disease
  - ***H. pylori* is present in 70% of patients with gastric ulcers and in nearly 100% of patients with duodenal ulcers**
- Active chronic gastritis
- Gastric adenocarcinoma

- **Gastric mucosa-associated lymphoid tissue (MALT) lymphoma: Treatment of infection causes tumor regression in most patients with this disease**

Zollinger-Ellison Syndrome

Basic Information

- Hypersecretion of gastrin from tumors arising from the pancreas or wall of the duodenum (*gastrinoma*)
- Presents with peptic ulceration, which may be refractory to treatment
- Ulceration may be single or multiple and involve the stomach, duodenum, or jejunum (classic location is postbulbar duodenum)
- Diarrhea results from the high volumes of gastric acid produced. Steatorrhea may result from inactivation of pancreatic enzymes as a result of the high volume of gastric acid in the duodenum.
- Two thirds of gastrinomas are malignant and may metastasize to the lymph nodes or liver
- About one third of gastrinomas are associated with multiple endocrine neoplasia type 1, so adenomas of the parathyroid (causing hypercalcemia) and pituitary may also be seen

Diagnosis

- Elevated basal acid output levels (not sensitive)
- **Increased serum gastrin levels (value >1000 pg/mL) with a gastric pH less than 2 mEq/mL is virtually diagnostic**
- Patients with gastrin levels less than 1000 pg/mL and with a pH less than 2 mEq/mL need provocation testing
  - Secretin test: IV infusion of secretin results in a paradoxical rise in serum gastrin in patients with Zollinger-Ellison syndrome but not in other conditions. A secretin stimulation test has a sensitivity of approximately 85%.
    - Calcium infusion test has a much lower sensitivity and specificity and should be used only if the secretin test does not confirm the diagnosis and suspicion is high
- Tumor localization
  - Radiologic imaging: Abdominal computed tomography (CT)—**90% of gastrinomas are located within the "gastrinoma triangle,"** bordered by the head of the pancreas, the second portion of the duodenum, and the cystic and common bile ducts
  - Octreotide scintigraphy scan: ^{111}In-DTPA-D-Phe1 octreotide binds to the somatostatin type 2 receptors on gastrinomas. Using whole-body scintigraphy, gastrinomas can be localized with a sensitivity of 71% to 75% and a specificity of 86% to 100%.

Dyspepsia

- Definition: Chronic or recurrent epigastric pain in the absence of reflux symptoms, acute severe pain, abdominal wall pain, or dysphagia
- Differential diagnosis of dyspepsia
  - Functional dyspepsia: 60% of cases

- Disordered motility
  - Visceral hypersensitivity
  - Altered intestinogastric reflexes
  - Psychological stress
- Peptic ulcer disease: 15% to 25% of cases
- Gastroesophageal reflux disease: 5% to 15% of cases
- Malignancy: Less than 2% of cases
- Clinical evaluation and therapy
  - 2005 American Gastroenterology Association Guidelines
    - If age younger than 55 years and no warning symptoms (e.g., weight loss, dysphagia, anemia), check for *H. pylori* (breath test or stool antigen test preferred), and treat if positive; trial of antisecretory therapy if serology negative; if no response, then endoscopy
    - If age older than 55 years or warning symptoms are present, proceed directly to endoscopy

Gastrointestinal Bleeding

Approach to the Patient with Gastrointestinal Bleeding

- Evaluation
  - Determine heart rate, blood pressure, the presence of orthostatic hypotension
  - Check hematocrit—may initially be misleadingly normal in patients with severe bleeding
- **Volume resuscitation with IV fluids or blood**
- Differentiate between upper (UGIB) and lower GI bleeding (LGIB)
  - Hematemesis: Indicates an upper source (above the ligament of Treitz)
  - Melena: Indicates that blood has been present in the GI tract for a number of hours; can be seen in upper GI as well as proximal lower (i.e., right colon) GI bleeding
  - Hematochezia: Usually suggests a lower GI source but can be from a massive upper GI bleed
  - Nasogastric aspirate: Look for fresh blood or "coffee grounds"; can occasionally see a nonbloody aspirate in patients with UGIB
- Diagnosis (Fig. 25-2)
  - Suspected UGIB: Proceed with upper endoscopy
  - Suspected LGIB: Controversial; many sources recommend performing sigmoidoscopy or colonoscopy first and then proceeding with angiography or technetium-99m (^{99m}Tc)–labeled red cell scan if bleeding persists; however, because of issues of preparation and timing, if the bleed is significant, in practice the order is often reversed and a tagged red blood cell scan or angiography is obtained first to evaluate for bleeding activity and offer potential therapy
  - Hematochezia with hemodynamic instability: **Initially perform upper endoscopy to rule out an upper GI source**
  - Occult GI bleed: Refers to hemoccult-positive stool without a clear source; work-up usually consists of an upper endoscopy and lower endoscopy (yield, ~50%); if negative, the small bowel should be evaluated (push enteroscopy, video capsule endoscopy, single/double balloon enteroscopy or small bowel series; yield of additional studies ~70%)

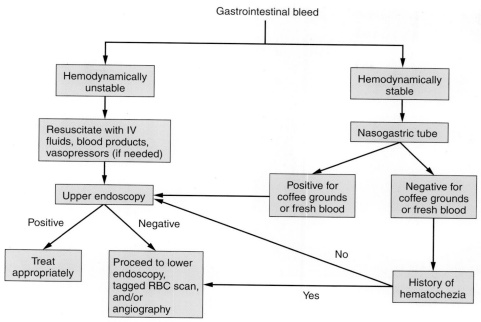

FIGURE 25-2 Evaluation of patient with gastrointestinal bleeding. (IV, intravenous; RBC, red blood cell.)

TABLE 25-1	Causes of Gastrointestinal (GI) Bleeding	
	Upper GI	**Lower GI**
Acute GI bleeding	Peptic ulcer disease Gastric erosions Esophagitis Mallory-Weiss tear (5–15%) Portal hypertension–related Dieulafoy lesion	Diverticulosis Vascular ectasia Colitis Neoplasms
Chronic GI bleeding	Esophagitis Gastric ulcer Gastritis Duodenal ulcer Vascular ectasia	Adenomas >1 cm Carcinoma Colitis Vascular ectasia

- Treatment: Based on the cause of the bleed; H_2 blockers and proton pump inhibitors do not reduce the risk of rebleeding in the absence of endoscopic stigmata of recent bleeding; if UGIB is suspected, may wish to start IV proton pump inhibitor empirically as multiple studies have now shown the IV proton pump inhibitors reduce the rate of rebleeding and need for surgery in patients with bleeding ulcers

Etiology

See Table 25-1 for a summary of the causes of GI bleeding.
- Upper GI source
  - Consider in a patient who presents with melena, hematemesis, or brisk hematochezia associated with orthostatic hypotension
- Lower GI source
  - Accounts for only 20% of all episodes of acute GI bleeding
  - Consider in a patient who presents with hematochezia, occasionally with melena

- In more than half the cases of acute LGIB, diverticular bleed is the cause

Specific Etiologies

- Gastric/duodenal ulcers
  - Bleeding ulcers tend to be located on the lesser curve or in the posterior duodenal bulb, where erosion into large vessels may occur
  - H. pylori does not appear to be a risk factor for ulcer bleeding, unlike age and NSAID use
  - Endoscopic therapy is warranted in patients with a visible vessel observed in an ulcer crater, even if there is no active bleeding; chance of rebleeding is 50% to 70% without therapy, 20% with therapy
  - IV omeprazole administered after endoscopic therapy decreased the rate of recurrent bleeding from 22.5% to 6.7%
  - Refer patients for surgery if endoscopic therapy is unsuccessful
  - Consider long-term prophylactic therapy in those who have bled; 33% PUD recurrence rate in 3 years without prophylaxis
- Mallory-Weiss tear
  - Laceration of the mucosa at the gastroesophageal junction
  - **Often associated with a history of vomiting or dry heaves before the bleeding episode**
  - May also be associated with heavy alcohol use
  - Bleeding usually stops spontaneously, although rebleeding may occur in 5% of patients
  - Angiography with embolization can be performed. Surgery is rarely required.
  - **Distinguished from Boerhaave syndrome, which is esophageal perforation caused by retching**
- Vascular malformations
  - Angiodysplasia

FIGURE 25-3 Endoscopic view of watermelon stomach. *(From Feldman M: Sleisenger and Fordtran's gastrointestinal and liver disease, ed 7, Philadelphia, WB Saunders, 2002, Fig. 120-9.)*

A

B

FIGURE 25-4 Diverticulosis of the colon. **A,** Double-contrast barium enema showing outpouchings *(arrows)* that represent diverticula. **B,** CT scan showing outpouchings *(arrows)* and a focal mass (M), a developing abscess. *(From Mettler FA: Essentials of radiology, ed 2, Philadelphia, Elsevier Saunders, 2005, Fig. 6-73.)*

- Flat, red lesions; can be found anywhere in the small intestine and colon
- Diagnosed by endoscopy
- Associated with chronic renal failure, valvular heart disease
- Treat with iron supplements or with estrogens
- Brisk bleeds can be evaluated by bleeding scan or arteriography and treated by embolization, surgical resection
- Watermelon stomach (Fig. 25-3)
  - Vascular ectasia of the gastric antrum
  - Seen predominantly in elderly women
  - Association with chronic liver disease and scleroderma
  - Usually manifests as iron deficiency anemia
  - Treat with iron supplementation, but sometimes cautery or rarely surgery is necessary
- Dieulafoy lesion
  - Ectatic artery that erodes into the stomach, causing brisk bleeding
  - Endoscopy may fail to identify the lesion if the bleeding has ceased
  - Treat endoscopically with cautery; embolization or surgery may be necessary
  - Uncommon (1% of upper GI bleeds) but can be catastrophic
- Diverticulosis—"outpouchings" of colonic mucosa and submucosa (Fig. 25-4)
  - Most common cause of acute LGIB
  - Usually affects the left colon, but bleeding is often from the right colon
  - Low recurrence rate of bleeding
  - In only 20% of cases will the bleeding diverticulum be identified
  - **Most patients do well, and bleeding stops spontaneously**
  - Resection in those with refractory bleeding or recurrent bleeding

- Diverticulitis
  - Inflammation around the diverticular sac
  - Usually occurs in the left colon
  - Typically presents with abdominal pain, fever, and leukocytosis
  - Microscopic bleeding can occur commonly, but gross bleeding is rare
  - **CT scan can aid in the diagnosis, but barium enema and colonoscopy should be avoided with acute infection**
  - Complications include perforation, peritonitis, abscess, and fistula formation
  - Treat with broad-spectrum antibiotics (e.g., oral ciprofloxacin plus metronidazole or IV pipercillin/tazobactam) to cover gram-negative aerobes and anaerobes

- Bleeding associated with portal hypertension
  - Bleeding can occur if portal pressure is greater than 12 mm Hg
  - Prevent bleeding with β-blockers, which also reduce mortality associated with bleeding
  - Esophageal/gastric varices
    - Likelihood of varices in cirrhotic patients is 35% to 80%, with 30% experiencing bleeding
    - Mortality rate for each bleeding episode is 35% to 50%
    - **Poor prognostic indicator: Only one third of patients with a history of variceal bleeding are alive at 1 year**
    - Acute therapy
      - Volume replacement/blood products
    - Sengstaken-Blakemore tube is only a temporizing measure for another therapy
    - Octreotide (minimal impact on systemic hemodynamics, in contrast to vasopressin)
    - Endoscopic sclerotherapy or band ligation
    - Transjugular intrahepatic portosystemic shunt (TIPS)
      - No mortality advantage over endoscopic therapy
      - High incidence of hepatic encephalopathy
      - Useful as a bridge to transplantation
    - Surgical shunting
    - Orthotopic liver transplantation
  - Portal hypertensive gastropathy
    - Vascular congestion of the gastric mucosa, imparts a "mosaic appearance" endoscopically
    - Treat with somatostatin to lower splanchnic blood flow
    - Consider TIPS
  - Secondary prevention of recurrent bleeding associated with portal hypertension
    - Nonselective β-adrenergic blocker drugs (e.g., propranolol)
    - Variceal banding: Useful for esophageal varices only; not gastropathy or gastric varices
    - TIPS
- Colitis
  - Infectious (see Chapter 14)
  - Inflammatory: Crohn disease, ulcerative colitis (see Chapter 28)
  - Ischemic
    - Patients usually over age 60 years
    - Arises from low flow rate, not occlusion
    - **Watershed areas affected—right colon, splenic flexure, and rectum**
    - Symptoms include mild abdominal pain, cramping, bloody diarrhea
    - Diagnose by clinical presentation, colonoscopy
    - Can be associated with estrogen use, hypercoagulable states, vasculitis
- Chronic GI bleeding
  - Can present as iron deficiency anemia from causes such as PUD, colon cancer, vascular malformations
    - Can also present with heme-positive stool in the absence of iron deficiency
  - UGIB causes include esophagitis, gastritis, PUD
  - LGIB causes include colon cancer, colonic adenomas larger than 1 cm, colitis, vascular ectasia
  - Presence of upper GI symptoms is usually associated with detection of an upper GI lesion
  - In patients with or without symptoms, upper GI lesion is more common than lower GI lesion
    - Work-up: Upper endoscopy, colonoscopy, push enteroscopy, capsule enteroscopy, single/double balloon enteroscopy, dedicated small bowel series; bleeding scan and angiography are only useful if there is acute bleeding at a fairly brisk rate (0.1 mL/min for scan, 0.5 mL/min for angiography); diagnostic yield of capsule enteroscopy is greater than for push enteroscopy; single/double balloon enteroscopy allows both diagnosis and treatment, but it is time-consuming and not widely available

REVIEW QUESTIONS

For review questions, please go to www.expertconsult.com.

SUGGESTED READINGS

Barkun AN, Bardou M, Kuipers EJ, et al: International consensus recommendations on the management of patients with nonvariceal upper gastrointestinal bleeding, *Ann Intern Med* 152:101–113, 2010.

Gralnek IM, Barkun AN, Bardou M: Management of acute bleeding from a peptic ulcer, *N Engl J Med* 359:928–937, 2008.

Green BT, Rockey DC: Lower gastrointestinal bleeding—management, *Gastroenterol Clin North Am* 34:665–678, 2005.

Lanza FL, Chan FK, Quigley EM: Guidelines for prevention of NSAID related ulcer complications, *Am J Gastroenterol* 104:728–738, 2009.

Rockey DC, Cello JP: Evaluation of the gastrointestinal tract in patients with iron-deficiency anemia, *N Engl J Med* 329:1691–1695, 1993.

Rockey DC, Koch J, Cello JP, et al: Relative frequency of upper gastrointestinal and colonic lesions in patients with positive fecal occult-blood tests, *N Engl J Med* 339:153–159, 1998.

25

Esophageal Disease

JOHN O. CLARKE, MD; and LINDA A. LEE, MD

Diseases of the esophagus include a number of conditions caused by abnormalities in anatomic structure or function. This chapter reviews many of those conditions, including gastroesophageal reflux disease (GERD) and esophagitis, esophageal cancer, and dysmotility syndromes. Before describing specific disease processes, basic esophageal anatomy is reviewed.

Normal Esophageal Structure and Function

Figure 26-1 shows the anatomy of the esophagus.
- Upper esophageal sphincter
  - Striated muscle
  - Relaxes in response to a swallow
  - Functions to prevent aspiration
- Esophageal body
  - Upper one third striated muscle, lower two thirds smooth muscle
  - Innervated by the vagus nerve
  - Swallowing initiates contractions in the upper esophagus, and enteric nervous system perpetuates them through the body
- Lower esophageal sphincter (LES)
  - High-pressure zone in distal esophagus
  - Relaxes in response to a swallow (vagally mediated)
  - Prevents GERD
  - Relaxation regulated by a variety of neuropeptides and hormones

Gastroesophageal Reflux Disease

Basic Information
- Protective mechanisms against reflux include the LES, peristalsis, saliva, and gravity
- **Caused by increased frequency of transient relaxations of the LES and decreased LES tone**
- There are numerous potential complications of GERD (Box 26-1)

Clinical Presentation
- Heartburn, indigestion
- Acid regurgitation
- Water brash: Vagal-mediated saliva production that occurs in response to esophagitis; distinguished from regurgitation
- Dyspnea: Vagal-mediated bronchoconstriction, microaspiration

- Dysphagia: Triggered by esophageal spasm
- Chronic cough
- Hoarseness
- Chest pain

Diagnosis and Evaluation
- In patients who present "typically" (heartburn and/or acid regurgitation), testing might not be necessary; a therapeutic trial (see following) may be sufficient
- Testing is indicated when atypical presentations, refractory symptoms, weight loss, or dysphagia is present
- Endoscopy with biopsies is often the first-line diagnostic study and is very specific for reflux (>95%) if esophagitis or Barrett esophagus is identified; however, it is relatively insensitive (~20% in most studies)
- A 24-hour catheter-based pH probe has been the traditional gold standard when symptoms are persistent and endoscopy is unrevealing. However, two new modalities have now entered the clinical arena: (1) a wireless pH capsule that can be attached temporarily to the esophageal wall and records the pH telemetrically; and (2) combined 24-hour pH/impedance, which combines standard pH monitoring with impedance flow, thereby allowing detection of flow (allowing detection of nonacid reflux). Wireless pH testing allows pH testing without the need for a nasal tube, increased patient comfort, and a longer duration of testing. The addition of impedance improves sensitivity as nonacid reflux can be detected.
- Barium swallow: Used primarily to evaluate dysphagia; insensitive for nonerosive esophagitis
- Bernstein test (acid infusion): A provocative test to evaluate atypical chest pain; symptoms are reproduced with the infusion of 0.1 N HCl but not with the infusion of saline; not used clinically in most centers and of limited diagnostic utility

Treatment
- Greater amount of acid suppression is needed to control GERD than to control peptic ulcer disease
- Lifestyle changes
  - Smoking cessation
  - Avoidance of alcohol
  - Low-fat diet
  - Elevate the head of the bed (6 inches)
  - Eat several hours before going to bed
  - Avoid medications that lower LES tone (e.g., anticholinergics, sedatives, nitrates, calcium channel blockers, theophylline)
  - Avoid foods known to lower LES tone (e.g., tomatoes, citrus, garlic, onions, peppermint, chocolate)

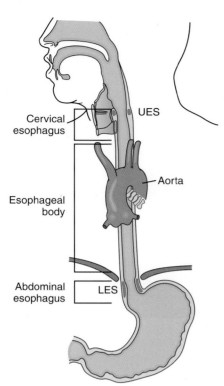

FIGURE 26-1 Anatomy of the esophagus showing the upper esophageal sphincter (UES), lower esophageal sphincter (LES), and esophageal body.

Labels in figure: Cervical esophagus, UES, Aorta, Esophageal body, Abdominal esophagus, LES

26

BOX 26-1	*Potential Complications of GERD*

Esophagitis

Esophageal ulceration

Esophageal stricture

Pulmonary aspiration

Barrett esophagus

  Occurs in up to 14% of patients with reflux symptoms undergoing endoscopy

  Replacement of the squamous epithelium with columnar epithelium

  Increased cancer risk associated only with specialized columnar epithelium (i.e., goblet cells present)

  Increased rate of adenocarcinoma estimated to be 10%

  Surveillance endoscopy every 3 years with biopsies from multiple levels is recommended but has not yet been shown to reduce mortality

  Treatment is antireflux therapy, although this may not cause regression of Barrett esophagus or reduce the risk of progression to high-grade dysplasia or cancer

  Presence of high-grade dysplasia is an indication for endoscopic ablative therapy or potentially esophagectomy, particularly for those patients who are not good surgical candidates

---

- Antacids: Treat symptoms, not esophagitis
- Histamine$_2$ (H$_2$) blockers (cimetidine, ranitidine, famotidine, nizatidine) are useful for cases of moderate severity
- Proton pump inhibitors (omeprazole, pantoprazole, rabeprazole, lansoprazole, esomeprazole)

- **Superior to H$_2$ blockers in controlling symptoms and healing esophagitis**
  - Duration of therapy should be at least 2 weeks
  - Prolonged use is necessary for severe cases
  - No increased risk of tumors (carcinoid or gastrinoma) with long-term use
  - Emerging data to suggest long-term use may be associated with decreased bone mineral density and increase in community-acquired infections
  - May interfere with the antiplatelet activity of clopidogrel
- Prokinetic agents (e.g., metoclopramide) increase LES pressure and/or gastric emptying
- γ-Aminobutyric acid (GABA) agonists (e.g., baclofen) decrease the frequency of transient LES relaxation and subsequently the number of reflux episodes; limited utility because of dose-related side effects
- Endoscopic antireflux devices: Of limited utility as most devices either have been withdrawn from the market or have had limited efficacy in clinical trials. At present, this option should be reserved only for carefully selected patients in clinic trials.
- Antireflux surgery (fundoplication) is indicated in patients with refractory symptoms. Laparoscopic Nissen fundoplication is a proven effective alternative to proton pump inhibitor (PPI) use and may be effective in up to 90% of cases.
- **In cases of refractory GERD, consider alternative diagnoses, such as gastroparesis, gastrinoma (rare), gallbladder dysfunction, eosinophilic esophagitis or cardiac etiology**

Esophagitis: Causes

- GERD (see preceding)
- Pill-induced
  - Common offenders include KCl, nonsteroidal anti-inflammatory drugs (NSAIDs), tetracycline, alendronate, quinidine, FeSO$_4$, and ascorbic acid
- Occurs more often in elderly patients
- Caustic ingestion
  - **Ingestion of alkali worse than acid**
    - Induction of vomiting is not recommended for lye ingestion
    - Increased risk of squamous cell carcinoma with lye strictures
  - Stricture formation is common
  - Can also cause perforation, bleeding, and death
- Eosinophilic esophagitis
  - Deposition of eosinophils in esophagus leads to a ringed esophagus
  - Results in solid-food dysphagia
  - Believed to be related to either food or airborne allergies but mechanism uncertain
  - Clusters with asthma and atopic disorders
  - Diagnosed with endoscopic biopsy
  - Increasing markedly in incidence and prevalence
  - Treated in most cases with dietary modification or topical steroids
- Infectious
  - Presence or absence of oral lesions does not correlate with esophagitis

- Diagnosis best made by endoscopy
- Viral esophagitis
  - Cytomegalovirus (CMV)
    - Typically seen in immunocompromised patients
    - Endoscopy shows serpiginous ulcers within normal mucosa
    - Histology shows intranuclear and intracytoplasmic inclusions
    - Treat with ganciclovir or foscarnet (if resistance occurs)
  - Herpesvirus
    - Type 1 rarely causes esophagitis in immunocompetent patients
    - Type 1 or 2 can cause esophagitis in immunosuppressed patients
    - Endoscopy shows vesicles and small ulcers
    - Histology can show eosinophilic intranuclear inclusions and giant cell formation
    - Treat with acyclovir or foscarnet (if acyclovir resistance occurs)
  - Varicella-zoster virus (VZV)
    - Can cause esophagitis in immunocompetent and immunosuppressed patients
    - Similar presentation to herpes simplex virus (HSV)
    - Acyclovir can reduce symptom duration
  - HIV (see Chapter 12)
    - Self-limited ulceration can accompany seroconversion
    - Persistent ulceration can exist in patients with more advanced disease; glucocorticoids or thalidomide may be used to treat
  - Candidal esophagitis
    - Endoscopy shows whitish-yellow plaques (Fig. 26-2)
    - Diagnose by demonstrating yeast or hyphal forms on KOH preparation
    - Fluconazole is the preferred treatment
    - Ketoconazole and amphotericin are acceptable alternatives
  - Bacterial esophagitis (rare): In immunocompromised hosts, *Lactobacillus* and β-hemolytic streptococci can be the cause

Structural Disorders

- Zenker diverticulum
  - Outpouching of the wall above the upper esophageal sphincter
  - Symptoms include halitosis and regurgitation of saliva and food
  - Commonly associated with underlying dysmotility
  - Treatment with surgery (cricopharyngeal myotomy/diverticulectomy), if needed
- Esophageal webs and rings
  - Schatzki ring
    - Causes intermittent dysphagia to solids ("steak-house syndrome")
    - Congenital ring at distal esophagus just above or at the LES
    - Endoscopic dilation usually effective in treating
  - Plummer-Vinson syndrome

FIGURE 26-2 Endoscopic appearance of candidal esophagitis. *(From Cohen J, Powderly W: Infectious diseases, ed 2, St. Louis, Mosby, 2004, Fig. 237-2.)*

  - Web(s) in cervical esophagus
  - Presents as intermittent dysphagia
  - Associated with iron deficiency anemia
  - Associated with squamous cell esophageal cancer
- Hiatal hernia: Movement of part of the stomach into the thoracic cavity
  - Sliding type
    - Very common with increasing age
    - Gastroesophageal junction (GEJ) and fundus slide upward
    - Can contribute to reflux esophagitis
  - Paraesophageal type
    - GEJ remains fixed
    - Pouch of stomach herniates through the esophageal hiatus next to the GEJ
    - Can cause bleeding and strangulation
    - **Surgery is often necessary for symptomatic or large hernias of this type**

Esophageal Dysmotility Syndromes

- Oropharyngeal dysmotility
  - Diminished ability to move food to esophagus
  - Characterized by dysphagia, nasal regurgitation, coughing, and aspiration
  - Most often caused by neurologic disorders (e.g., myasthenia gravis, multiple sclerosis, amyotrophic lateral sclerosis)
  - Collagen vascular diseases that affect striated muscle (polymyositis, dermatomyositis) can also cause oropharyngeal dysmotility
- Achalasia
  - Most cases in the United States are idiopathic
  - Presentation: dysphagia, regurgitation, chest pain, weight loss

FIGURE 26-3 Barium swallow showing an air-fluid level in the esophagus and a "bird's-beak" deformity consistent with achalasia.

- Diagnosis: Barium swallow can be highly suggestive, but manometry is the most sensitive study
- Radiologic studies
  - Barium swallow—dilated esophagus that tapers to a "bird's beak" and air-fluid level in the esophagus (Fig. 26-3)
  - Chest radiograph—absent gastric bubble
  - Esophageal manometry—absence of peristalsis and failure of the LES to relax in response to a swallow
- Esophagogastroduodenoscopy (EGD) is necessary to rule out pseudoachalasia/secondary cause
- Therapy
  - Medications (smooth muscle relaxants)—rarely effective
  - Endoscopic dilation of LES (success rates of 60–90%)
  - Myotomy—surgical or laparoscopic; reflux esophagitis and stricture may be a complication of surgery (success rates of up to 90%)
  - Botulinum toxin produces short-term results only but can be diagnostically helpful in atypical presentations
- Secondary causes
  - Gastric cancer involving the GEJ (pseudoachalasia)
  - Neurologic disorders (e.g., myasthenia gravis, amyotrophic lateral sclerosis)
  - Chagas disease (American trypanosomiasis)
    - Transmission: Through reduviid bugs carrying the parasite *Trypanosoma cruzi*; transmission also occurs through blood transfusions

FIGURE 26-4 Diffuse esophageal spasm leading to "corkscrew" esophagus. *(From Feldman M: Sleisenger and Fordtran's gastrointestinal and liver disease, ed 7, Philadelphia, WB Saunders, 2002, Fig. 32-14.)*

- Epidemiology: Found mainly in Central and South America, although cases have been reported in the southern United States
- Presentation
  - Acute disease (usually self-limited): Skin induration (chagoma), fever, lymphadenopathy; myocarditis and heart failure can occur
  - Chronic disease (years or decades after primary infection): cardiomyopathy, arrhythmias, megaesophagus, megacolon, aspiration pneumonia
- Diagnosis: Examination of blood smear for parasites in acute disease; serologic tests for antibodies to *T. cruzi* for chronic disease
- Treatment: Nifurtimox or benznidazole recommended; referral for cardiac transplantation may be needed for severe cardiomyopathy
- Scleroderma (see Chapter 45)
  - Presentation: Severe GERD, dysphagia
  - More than 90% have esophageal involvement
  - More than 90% have Raynaud's phenomenon
  - Peptic stricture in distal esophagus may occur
  - Diagnosis: Esophageal manometry shows absent peristalsis and low LES tone; barium swallow shows dilation and loss of peristaltic contractions

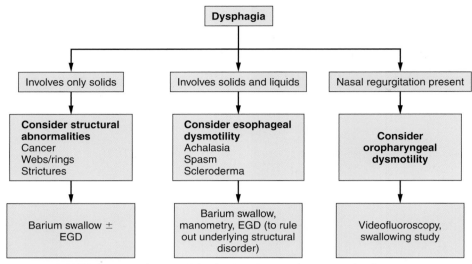

FIGURE 26-5 Evaluation of dysphagia. EGD, esophagogastroduodenoscopy.

- Therapy
  - PPIs
  - Esophageal dilation for peptic stricture
- Diffuse esophageal spasm
  - Presentation: Dysphagia, chest pain that can be aggravated by stress
  - Commonly associated with GERD (70%)
  - Diagnosis
    - Esophageal manometry test may be normal if patient is asymptomatic at the time
    - Barium swallow can show "corkscrew" esophagus, uncoordinated contractions along the esophageal wall (Fig. 26-4)
  - Treatment
    - Treat GERD
    - Smooth muscle relaxants (isosorbide dinitrate, dicyclomine, calcium channel blockers) if GERD is not present
    - Antidepressants (selective serotonin reuptake inhibitors, trazodone)
    - Benzodiazepines

Esophageal Cancer

- Can present with solid-food dysphagia, odynophagia, weight loss, and/or pneumonia from tracheoesophageal fistulas
- Squamous cell carcinoma
  - Incidence decreasing
  - More common in men and African Americans
  - Usually occurs in mid- to lower esophagus
  - Risk factors include alcohol, smoking, achalasia, nitrate consumption, lye ingestion, Plummer-Vinson syndrome
- Adenocarcinoma
  - Incidence increasing
  - More common in men and in whites
  - Usually occurs in the distal esophagus
  - Major risk factor is GERD and Barrett esophagus (see Box 26-1)

- Diagnosis: Endoscopic biopsy and tumor brushings; computed tomography scan and endoscopic ultrasound to assess regional spread
- Therapy
  - Prognosis is generally poor (5-year survival is 5%)
  - Surgical resection appropriate for less than half of all patients; 5-year survival rate after esophagectomy is about 20%
  - Palliative measures include radiation, chemotherapy, photodynamic therapy, stenting, and endoscopic fulguration with lasers

Approach to the Patient with Dysphagia/Odynophagia

- Age, gender, immunosuppression, duration of symptoms, and associated symptoms (e.g., weight loss, chest pain) may suggest a particular cause
- Barium swallow is almost always the first test to obtain
- Symptom-based evaluation is often helpful (Fig. 26-5)

REVIEW QUESTIONS

For review questions, please go to www.expertconsult.com.

SUGGESTED READINGS

American Gastroenterological Association Institute technical review on the management of gastroesophageal reflux disease, *Gastroenterology* 135:1392–1413, 2008.

American Gastroenterological Association medical position statement on treatment of patients with dysphagia caused by benign disorders of the distal esophagus, *Gastroenterology* 117:229–233, 1999.

DeVault KR, Castell DO: Updated guidelines for the diagnosis and treatment of gastroesophageal reflux disease, *Am J Gastroenterol* 100:190–200, 2005.

Kahrilas PJ: Clinical practice: gastroesophageal reflux disease, *N Engl J Med* 359:1700–1707, 2008.

Shaheen NJ, Richter JE: Barrett's oesophagus, *Lancet* 373:850–861, 2009.

Pancreatic and Biliary Disease

KERRY B. DUNBAR, MD

The pancreas is a lobular structure responsible for secretion of digestive enzymes, bicarbonate, and certain hormones. The gallbladder and biliary tree serve to excrete cholesterol, assist in the absorption of fats, and influence water and electrolyte transport. Diseases of the pancreas and biliary system include a number of acute and chronic conditions responsible for visits to both internists and gastroenterologists.

Pancreatic Disease

OVERVIEW OF PANCREATIC STRUCTURE AND FUNCTION

- Anatomy and physiology (Fig. 27-1A)
  - Pancreas: Soft, elongated gland that lies behind the peritoneum of the posterior abdominal wall
  - Anatomic parts of the pancreas are the head with the uncinate process, the neck, the body, and the tail
  - Main pancreatic duct (duct of Wirsung) opens in the major duodenal papilla
  - The accessory pancreatic duct (duct of Santorini) drains via the minor duodenal papilla
  - The pancreas has a lobular structure and consists of an exocrine portion, which secretes digestive enzymes and bicarbonate, and an endocrine portion, which secretes hormones into the blood
  - The exocrine portion is composed of ductal, acinar, and centroacinar cells
  - **More than 95% of pancreatic masses arise from acinar cells**
  - The endocrine pancreas consists of islet cells (1–2%) that produce insulin, glucagon, somatostatin, and pancreatic polypeptide
  - Exocrine pancreatic secretion occurs via acinar cell secretion into pancreatic ductules; islet cells secrete hormones directly into the blood
- Developmental abnormalities
  - Pancreas divisum (see Fig. 27-1B)
    - Incomplete fusion of the ducts results in the duct of Wirsung draining only the ventral pancreas and the duct of Santorini draining the entire dorsal pancreas
    - Present in 5% to 10% of the general population
    - Can be associated with pancreatitis, but most patients are asymptomatic
  - A long common channel between the bile duct and pancreatic duct may facilitate reflux of bile into the pancreatic duct. This can increase the risk of acute pancreatitis.

- Annular pancreas
  - Congenital anomaly in which a concentric band of pancreatic tissue forms around the duodenum
  - Typically presents in infancy as duodenal obstruction but can also present in adulthood
  - Can be seen with other congenital abnormalities, such as intestinal malrotation, Meckel diverticulum, Down syndrome, and tracheoesophageal fistulas

ACUTE PANCREATITIS

Basic Information

- Epidemiology
  - Acute pancreatitis is a common disorder that results in thousands of hospitalizations
  - The incidence of acute pancreatitis ranges from 5 to 35 per 100,000 per year
- Etiology (Table 27-1)
  - **Gallstones and ethanol are the two most common causes of acute pancreatitis**
  - Drug-induced pancreatitis usually occurs within the first month of drug administration
  - The incidence of post–endoscopic retrograde cholangiopancreatography (ERCP) pancreatitis is 1% to 10%, and may be as high as 30% following sphincter of Oddi manometry
  - Autoimmune pancreatitis causes recurrent episodes of acute pancreatitis and chronic pancreatitis
    - Characterized by pancreatic and biliary strictures
    - Computed tomography (CT) shows diffuse enlargement of the pancreas or a focal inflammatory mass
    - Serum immunoglobulin G, subclass 4 (IgG4), is often elevated
    - Responds to corticosteroids
  - About 10% to 30% of acute pancreatitis is idiopathic
  - Biliary sludge, or microlithiasis, can cause recurrent acute pancreatitis
- Pathophysiology
  - Poorly understood, but the triggering event is thought to vary according to the cause
  - The initiating event includes intra-acinar activation of pancreatic enzymes. Trypsinogen is converted to trypsin with damage to the microcirculation and autodigestion of the pancreas.
  - Activation and release of phospholipase, elastase, kallikrein, complement, and coagulation factors further damage the pancreas. Release of cytokines can lead to systemic inflammatory response syndrome (SIRS) in severe cases of pancreatitis.

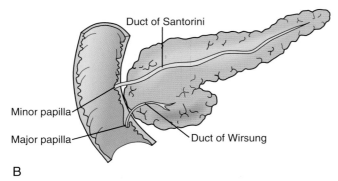

FIGURE 27-1 **A,** Normal anatomy of the pancreatic ductal system. **B,** Pancreas divisum.

Clinical Presentation

- Symptoms
  - Epigastric abdominal pain radiating to the back
  - Nausea, vomiting, abdominal distention
- Physical examination
  - Fever, tachycardia, hypotension
  - Abdominal tenderness
  - Diminished bowel sounds
  - **Discoloration around umbilicus (Cullen's sign) or flanks (Grey-Turner sign) suggests hemoperitoneum and hemorrhagic pancreatitis**
- Clinical course and complications
  - Most patients with acute pancreatitis have mild, self-limited disease
  - In those with recurrent attacks, the first attack is usually the most severe and has the highest associated risk of death
  - Early complications are those that develop less than 14 days from admission (Box 27-1)
  - Late complications are those that develop after 14 days
    - Pseudocyst formation with or without infection (Fig. 27-2)
      - Most pseudocysts resolve spontaneously within 6 weeks
      - Those that persist, enlarge, become infected, or become symptomatic need endoscopic, percutaneous, or surgical drainage
    - Infected pancreatic necrosis leading to phlegmon
  - Pancreatic sepsis is the most common cause of death in patients with severe acute pancreatitis

TABLE 27-1	Etiologic Association of Acute Pancreatitis
Category	**Examples**
Obstruction	Choledocholithiasis, biliary microlithiasis, ampullary or pancreatic tumor, pancreas divisum, mucinous ductal ectasia or intraductal papillary mucinous neoplasm, choledochocele, parasites, periampullary duodenal diverticula, hypertensive sphincter of Oddi, duodenal loop obstruction
Toxins	Ethanol, methanol, scorpion venom, organophosphorus insecticides, cigarette smoking
Drugs	Azathioprine, 6-mercaptopurine, valproic acid, estrogens, tetracycline, metronidazole, pentamidine, furosemide, sulfonamides, methyldopa, cimetidine, ranitidine, sulindac, dideoxyinosine, nitrofurantoin
Metabolic	Hypertriglyceridemia (types I, IV, V), hypercalcemia
Trauma	Blunt trauma to abdomen, postoperative, post-ERCP/endoscopic sphincterotomy/sphincter of Oddi manometry
Infections	Parasites (ascariasis, chlonorchiasis), viral (mumps; rubella; hepatitis: A, B, non-A, non-B; coxsackievirus; echovirus; adenovirus; cytomegalovirus; varicella; Epstein-Barr virus; HIV)
Vascular	Ischemia (post–cardiac surgery), atherosclerotic emboli, malignant hypertension, vasculitis (SLE, PAN)
Miscellaneous	Penetrating peptic ulcer, Crohn disease of the duodenum, autoimmune pancreatitis, pregnancy-associated, Reye syndrome, idiopathic
Hereditary	Mutations of *PRSS1, SPINK1,* and *CFTR;* can develop into chronic pancreatitis
Idiopathic	

ERCP, endoscopic retrograde cholangiopancreatography; HIV, human immunodeficiency virus; PAN, polyarteritis nodosa; SLE, systemic lupus erythematosus.

BOX 27-1	*Early Complications of Pancreatitis*

Vascular instability and SIRS
Pulmonary complications: ARDS, effusions, atelectasis
Renal: acute renal failure, acute tubular necrosis
Endocrine and metabolic derangements: hyperglycemia, acidosis, hypocalcemia
Infected pancreatic necrosis
Pancreatic or retroperitoneal hemorrhage
Hemosuccus pancreaticus: massive GI bleeding caused by pseudoaneurysm of the splenic artery
Disseminated intravascular coagulation
Splenic vein thrombosis

ARDS, acute respiratory distress syndrome; GI, gastrointestinal; SIRS, systemic inflammatory response syndrome.

FIGURE 27-2 CT scan: Pancreatic pseudocyst in the tail of the pancreas (*arrow*).

FIGURE 27-3 CT scan: Acute pancreatitis (*arrow*).

Diagnosis and Evaluation

- Blood tests
  - Serum amylase and lipase: Most often used to diagnose pancreatitis
    - Amylase is the most commonly used test, but it is less sensitive and specific than serum lipase
    - Pancreatitis is more likely when the amylase and lipase are elevated to at least three times the upper limit of normal
    - **If the amylase is elevated but lipase is not, consider a nonpancreatic process**
  - Both amylase and lipase can be elevated in other intra-abdominal processes (e.g., bowel infarction, perforation, or obstruction) that may also present with an acute abdomen
  - **The levels of pancreatic enzymes do not correlate with the severity of disease**
  - Renal failure alone and diabetic ketoacidosis (without pancreatitis) may be associated with elevated amylase and lipase
- Serum liver function tests
  - Serum alanine aminotransferase (ALT) is a useful predictor of biliary origin of pancreatitis. An ALT more than three times the upper limit of normal is suggestive of gallstone pancreatitis. However, a normal ALT does not rule out gallstone pancreatitis as sensitivity is low.
  - Elevations of serum bilirubin and alkaline phosphatase are not specific for the diagnosis of gallstone pancreatitis
- Radiologic tests
  - Plain radiographs
    - Useful for detecting free air, which suggests bowel perforation
    - Abnormal gas signs in pancreatitis include local "sentinel loop" and general small bowel ileus
    - Chest radiograph may show pleural effusions (left greater than right), atelectasis, or acute respiratory distress syndrome–like pattern

- Transabdominal ultrasonography
  - Useful for diagnosis of gallstone disease and bile duct dilation in gallstone pancreatitis
  - Not usually helpful in visualizing the pancreas itself because of overlying bowel gas
- **CT is the most informative radiologic test**
  - Mild pancreatitis may be associated with a normal CT scan
  - Severe pancreatitis can result in pancreatic enlargement, peripancreatic fluid or debris, abdominal fluid collections, hemorrhage, and necrosis. IV contrast can help identify pancreatic necrosis (Fig. 27-3).
  - Serial CT scans can be helpful in detecting pancreatic abscesses; gas in fluid collections may suggest a pancreatic abscess caused by gas-forming organisms
- Magnetic resonance cholangiopancreatography (MRCP) can be used to identify the cause of acute pancreatitis and stage severity
  - Provides a better view of pancreatic and bile ducts than CT
  - Can detect choledocholithiasis, fluid collections, necrosis, and pseudocysts
- ERCP helps to diagnose the cause of acute recurrent pancreatitis, such as choledocholithiasis (gallstone pancreatitis), papillary stenosis, complete or incomplete pancreas divisum, tumor, stones, and sphincter of Oddi dysfunction
- Endoscopic ultrasonography (EUS) may be helpful for diagnosing tumors not evident by CT scan that may present with acute pancreatitis
- Clinical measurements of severity
  - Ranson's criteria (Table 27-2)
    - Traditionally used for predicting mortality
    - Fulfillment of three or more criteria indicates severe disease and poor prognosis. Those with three or four risk factors have a 15% mortality rate; those with seven or more risk factors have a 100% mortality rate.

TABLE 27-2	Ranson's Criteria for Acute Pancreatitis	
On Admission	**Within 48 Hours**
Age >55 yr	Hematocrit decrease = 10%
WBC >16,000/mm^3	BUN increase = 5 mg/dL
Glucose >200 mg/dL	Calcium <8 mg/dL
Lactate dehydrogenase >350 units/L	Po$_2$ <60 mm Hg
Aspartate aminotransferase >250 units/L	Base deficit >4 mEq/L
	Fluid deficit >6 L

BUN, blood urea nitrogen; Po$_2$, partial pressure of oxygen; WBC, white blood cell count.

- More recent studies have suggested that the Ranson score is not an adequate predictor of severity
- Acute Physiology and Chronic Health Evaluation II (APACHE II) score
  - Also used to assess illness severity. Uses vital signs, selected laboratory studies (white blood cell count, hematocrit, arterial pH, creatinine), age, comorbid illnesses to predict mortality
  - CT scan: The presence of pancreatic necrosis, abscess, or pseudocyst usually predicts severe disease

Treatment

- Supportive care: bowel rest, IV fluids, analgesic and antiemetic medications
- Enteral nutrition: Jejunal feeding in acute pancreatitis reduces the incidence of infection and shortens length of stay in the hospital
- Parenteral nutrition: May be required for moderate and severe pancreatitis
- Antibiotics: Use of antibiotics in pancreatitis is a source of controversy. Studies show conflicting results. Patients with severe necrotizing pancreatitis are most likely to benefit from antibiotics. Imipenem and meropenem achieve high pancreatic tissue levels and may be effective for reducing the incidence of pancreatic sepsis in patients with severe necrotizing pancreatitis; **empirical antibiotic therapy is currently recommended only for such severe cases.**
- A CT scan should be obtained if there is no clinical improvement within 72 hours. If necrosis is found and infection is suspected, endoscopic or CT-guided fine-needle aspiration (FNA) should be considered.
- Surgery is indicated for drainage of pancreatic abscess and debridement of infected pancreatic phlegmon
- ERCP
  - Urgent ERCP is indicated for gallstone pancreatitis, especially with coexisting cholangitis, jaundice, dilated common bile duct, or in patients with clinical deterioration (Fig. 27-4)
  - ERCP with sphincterotomy and stenting of the minor papilla is also useful for treatment of acute recurrent pancreatitis in patients with pancreas divisum
- Cholecystectomy is recommended for patients with gallstone pancreatitis after recovery

FIGURE 27-4 Endoscopic retrograde cholangiopancreatography: Gallstone pancreatitis caused by stone impacted in major duodenal papilla.

- Nasogastric tube suction, histamine$_2$ (H$_2$) receptor antagonists, fresh-frozen plasma, and peritoneal lavage have no proven efficacy for treatment of acute pancreatitis. Pancreatic duct stents have been shown to reduce the risk of post-ERCP pancreatitis.

CHRONIC PANCREATITIS

Basic Information

- Definition and cause
  - Chronic pancreatitis is manifested by abdominal pain and abnormal secretory function of the exocrine pancreas associated with histologic findings of atrophy and fibrosis of exocrine parenchyma
  - If alcoholism is excluded, most patients in the United States with chronic pancreatitis have no identifiable cause
  - Idiopathic chronic pancreatitis presents at any age
  - Hereditary pancreatitis—several mutations lead to hereditary pancreatitis
    - PRSS1—Autosomal dominant mutation in the serine protease 1 gene. Can present as acute or chronic pancreatitis with prominent pancreatolithiasis.
    - SPINK1—Acute or chronic pancreatitis caused by mutations in the serine protease inhibitor Kazal type 1 gene. Inheritance is complex.
    - CFTR—Autosomal recessive mutation of the cystic fibrosis transmembrane conductance regulator gene
  - Autoimmune pancreatitis can also cause chronic pancreatitis
  - Cigarette smoking increases the risk of chronic pancreatitis
- Pathophysiology
  - Pancreatic duct obstruction occurs from hypersecretion of pancreatic fluid, rich in protein and calcium carbonate, which can precipitate in branches of the pancreatic duct

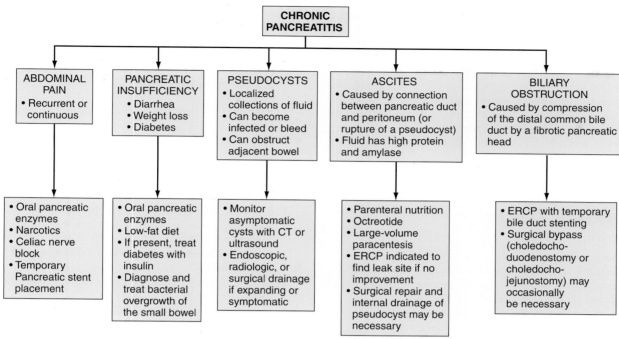

FIGURE 27-5 Sequelae and treatment of chronic pancreatitis. (CT, computed tomography; ERCP, endoscopic retrograde cholangiopancreatography.)

- Patchy mononuclear cell parenchymal infiltration, atrophy, and fibrosis of the exocrine tissue may be seen on pathology

Clinical Presentation

- Signs and symptoms
  - Abdominal pain: Recurrent episodes or continuous pain
  - Pancreatic insufficiency: Diarrhea (steatorrhea) and weight loss caused by malabsorption
  - Diabetes: Occurs in advanced chronic pancreatitis
  - Occasionally, patients may have no pain but may have malabsorption with or without diabetes
  - May be completely asymptomatic
- **Painful attacks tend to diminish over time (5–10 years) as the exocrine and endocrine insufficiency progresses**
- Cessation of alcohol intake may decrease the frequency of painful attacks, but pancreatic insufficiency may still develop despite abstinence
- Complications include pseudocysts, ascites, and biliary obstruction (Fig. 27-5)

Diagnosis and Evaluation

- Blood tests
  - Amylase and lipase levels are typically normal
- Pancreatic function tests
  - Bentiromide test
    - Bentiromide is *N*-benzoyl-L-tyrosyl-*para*-aminobenzoic acid (NBT-PABA), which is cleaved by pancreatic chymotrypsin in the duodenum
    - PABA is absorbed by the small intestine, conjugated by the liver, and excreted in the urine if pancreatic exocrine function is normal

- Assuming small bowel function is normal, decreased urinary excretion or serum levels suggest pancreatic exocrine insufficiency
- Mainly of historical interest, not commonly used clinically
- Pancreatic intubation function tests: Bicarbonate and enzyme concentrations measured from direct samples obtained from an ERCP
- Stool tests
  - **72-hour fecal fat collection: Still the most definitive test for diagnosing steatorrhea, which may be pancreatic or nonpancreatic**
    - Greater than 7 g/24 hours of fecal fat while consuming a high-fat diet is considered abnormal
    - Pancreatic steatorrhea does not occur until the pancreatic lipase output decreases to less than 5% to 10% of normal
  - Fecal chymotrypsin and fecal elastase are simpler tests of pancreatic exocrine function. Low fecal levels of chymotrypsin or fecal elastase suggest pancreatic dysfunction, but may not be sensitive for mild cases of chronic pancreatitis.
- Radiology and imaging studies
  - Plain radiographs: Useful for detecting pancreatic calcifications, which are suggestive of chronic pancreatitis
  - Ultrasound: Can occasionally see portions of the pancreas, but often the tail and body are obscured by bowel gas. Not the test of choice.
  - CT scan: Can detect atrophy, pancreatic calcifications, pseudocysts, tumors, focal fibrotic masses, and associated bile duct and/or pancreatic duct dilation
  - MRCP: Best for visualizing the pancreatic duct and cysts and in diagnosing pancreas divisum. Can detect calcifications, pseudocysts, tumors.

- ERCP: Useful for evaluating pancreatic ductal changes, but can be normal in mild cases. Due to the risk of post-ERCP pancreatitis, ERCP is performed infrequently for diagnosis. MRCP is often used instead and ERCP reserved for therapy of strictures due to pancreatitis.
- EUS: High-resolution images of the pancreas identify irregularities in the pancreatic ducts, cysts, parenchymal atrophy and lobularity, calcifications, and masses. Can help in diagnosing early chronic pancreatitis, even when ERCP and/or other imaging is normal.

Treatment
See Figure 27-5 for treatment options.

PANCREATIC CANCER
Basic Information
- Epidemiology
  - Pancreatic cancer is the second most common GI malignancy (after colorectal cancer) in the United States
  - Types of pancreatic cancer
    - Adenocarcinoma is the most common type of malignancy and has the worst prognosis
    - Cystadenocarcinoma, papillary cystic carcinoma, ampullary carcinoma, neuroendocrine tumors, and lymphoma are rarely seen
  - Intraductal papillary mucinous neoplasms (IPMNs) are cystic lesions of the pancreas
    - Associated with acute and chronic pancreatitis
    - Risk of pancreatic adenocarcinoma depends on IPMN type, size and features
    - Many are detected incidentally on imaging studies (CT, magnetic resonance imaging of the abdomen) in patients with no history of pancreatitis
    - Evaluation with CT, MRCP, and EUS-guided FNA can be used to assess
    - Large cysts, cysts with a solid component, dilation of the pancreatic duct, symptomatic cysts have a higher risk of malignancy and should be considered for surgical resection
- Etiology
  - Risk factors for pancreatic cancer include cigarette smoking, obesity, age, male sex, African American race, chronic pancreatitis
  - Most cases of pancreatic cancer are sporadic
  - Cases of familial pancreatic cancer suggest a genetic linkage
  - Gene mutations in hereditary chronic pancreatitis, Peutz-Jeghers syndrome, and hereditary breast cancer (*BRCA2*) are associated with pancreatic cancer

Clinical Presentation
- Most common presenting symptoms are abdominal pain (frequently radiating to the back), weight loss, and jaundice
- Jaundice caused by biliary obstruction commonly found in patients with tumors of the pancreatic head
- On examination, a palpable gallbladder (Courvoisier's sign) may be present but is not sensitive or specific
- Glucose intolerance, venous thrombosis (Trousseau syndrome), and GI variceal bleeding (from compression of the portal system) may occur
- **Most patients present with advanced disease**

Diagnosis and Evaluation
- CT scan (Fig. 27-6)
  - A specific diagnosis of a pancreatic mass can be made with up to 95% accuracy
  - Pancreatic protocol (high-resolution CT with IV contrast and water contrast in the stomach) improves sensitivity
  - Necessary for staging and to rule out metastatic disease
- Serum cancer antigen (CA) 19-9
  - Has a sensitivity of 80% to 90% and specificity of 85% to 95% in patients with signs and symptoms of pancreatic cancer
  - In patients with pancreatic masses on CT scan, high levels may be suggestive of malignancy
  - Can be elevated in colon, gastric, and bile duct cancers
  - **Not considered an appropriate screening test at this time**
- EUS: Can diagnose small tumors (<1–2 cm) not seen by CT scan
  - Provides staging information as well as histology (via EUS-guided FNA) at the same procedure
  - EUS is also useful in diagnosing and localizing pancreatic endocrine tumors, including gastrinomas (associated with Zollinger-Ellison syndrome) and insulinomas (associated with hypoglycemia)
- ERCP
  - Compression of the main pancreatic duct and common bile duct, the "double duct" sign, is suggestive of pancreatic cancer
  - Cytologic sampling and/or biopsy at the time of ERCP is possible, but the yield can be lower than with EUS-guided FNA
  - ERCP is most useful in the setting of biliary obstruction because endoscopic sphincterotomy and biliary stent placement can be done in the same procedure

FIGURE 27-6 CT scan: Mass in the body of the pancreas.

Treatment

- Surgery: Results vary from 0% to 35% 5-year survival in curative resections, with better outcome in ampullary carcinomas (up to 50% survival)
  - Patients who have the best chance for curative resection are those who present with painless obstructive jaundice
  - **Patients with tumors in the body or tail are rarely eligible for resection for cure (because of late presentation)**
- Chemotherapy and chemoradiotherapy: 5-fluorouracil (5-FU) and gemcitabine are the most commonly used chemotherapy agents. Often used as adjuvant therapy after surgery.
- Palliation
  - Endoscopic or percutaneous stenting or biliary bypass at the time of surgery may relieve obstruction and jaundice
  - Pain can be palliated with celiac axis nerve block during surgery or under CT or EUS guidance
  - Chemotherapy with gemcitabine and 5-FU–based chemoradiotherapy are also used for treatment

Biliary Diseases

Overview of Anatomy and Physiology

- Gallbladder (Fig. 27-7)
  - The anatomic parts of the gallbladder are the fundus, body, infundibulum, and neck
  - Accumulates and concentrates bile and stores concentrated bile between meals
  - Filling and emptying of the gallbladder are controlled by neural and hormonal factors, including cholecystokinin (CCK), cholinergic vagal stimulation, motilin, and pancreatic polypeptide
  - In response to hormonal stimulation after meals, the gallbladder releases concentrated bile into the duodenum for activation of digestive enzymes and digestion of dietary lipids

- Extrahepatic biliary tree
  - Main right and left hepatic ducts join to form the common hepatic duct, which joins with the cystic duct to form the common bile duct (CBD); in most patients, the CBD joins with the pancreatic duct to open into the major duodenal papilla
  - Bile flow from liver to duodenum is controlled by gallbladder contraction and sphincter of Oddi activity

GALLSTONE DISEASE

Basic Information

- Definition and epidemiology
  - Cholelithiasis describes presence of microscopic crystals or large stones in the gallbladder
  - Choledocholithiasis refers to presence of gallstones in extrahepatic bile ducts
  - **Women are diagnosed with gallstones two to three times more often than men of the same age**
  - Most gallstones are cholesterol stones (contain >50% cholesterol) that have centers with calcium, pigment, and glycoprotein
  - A minority of gallstones are pigment stones (have <20% cholesterol content) that contain calcium salts of carbonate, phosphate, and bilirubin distributed evenly throughout the stone; these usually form in the setting of hemolysis (e.g., sickle cell anemia), cirrhosis, or chronic biliary infection
- Pathogenesis and risk factors
  - The healthy gallbladder prevents gallstone formation by acidifying bile, absorbing cholesterol, concentrating bile (which in turn promotes micelle formation), and expelling crystals and sludge
  - Risk factors for development of cholelithiasis: see Box 27-2

Clinical Presentation

- Biliary colic: Transient episodes of pain caused by intermittent obstruction of the cystic duct or CBD by a passing stone or sludge
  - The pain typically occurs in the right upper quadrant or epigastrium and can radiate to the shoulder or back. May be associated with nausea and vomiting.

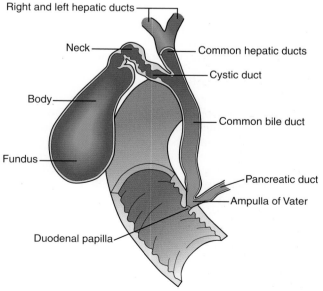

Right and left hepatic ducts

Neck

Common hepatic ducts

Cystic duct

Body

Common bile duct

Fundus

Pancreatic duct

Ampulla of Vater

Duodenal papilla

FIGURE 27-7 Gallbladder and biliary tree.

BOX 27-2	*Risk Factors for the Development of Cholelithiasis*

Genetic predisposition (Pima Indians, other Native Americans, Mexican Americans, Scandinavians)

Older age (>50 yr)

Obesity

Pregnancy

Medications (e.g., oral contraceptives, octreotide, ceftriaxone)

Prolonged total parenteral nutrition

Rapid weight loss

Diseases of the terminal ileum causing decreased reabsorption of bile acids

■ **The pain can be sharp and intense, often related to meals (particularly fatty food)**
- Acute cholecystitis: Results from lasting obstruction of the cystic duct by a gallstone
  - Abdominal pain is more intense and prolonged than that of biliary colic
  - Fevers, chills, nausea, and vomiting commonly accompany the pain
  - Obstructive jaundice may occur when migration of the gallstone into the extrahepatic bile duct with obstruction of the duct occurs; it may also occur when a cystic duct stone erodes into or compresses the adjacent common bile duct (Mirizzi syndrome)
  - Acalculous cholecystitis may be seen in up to 10% of patients with cholecystitis symptoms
    - Usually associated with other underlying illness (e.g., patients in the intensive care unit, those with diabetes)
    - Has a higher morbidity and mortality rate than calculous cholecystitis
  - Chronic cholecystitis—Chronic inflammation and fibrosis of the gallbladder
    - Typically associated with cholelithiasis
    - Can by seen with dyskinesia of the gallbladder
    - Symptoms include biliary colic
  - Complications of cholecystitis
    - Gangrenous cholecystitis: From ischemia of the gallbladder wall; advanced age and diabetes are commonly present
    - Emphysematous cholecystitis may occur with gangrene and infection of the gallbladder with gas-forming bacteria
    - Perforation—Can occur with gangrenous or emphysematous cholecystitis with abscess and sepsis
    - Gallstone ileus: Bowel obstruction caused by large stones that erode into the duodenum from an inflamed gallbladder (Bouveret syndrome) or pass into the small bowel from the bile duct
- Cholangitis: Patients present with spiking fever, right upper quadrant abdominal pain, jaundice, tachycardia, nausea and vomiting
  - Caused by obstruction of the CBD
  - IV antibiotics and IV fluids are essential for management
  - Urgent ERCP with sphincterotomy ± biliary stent placement is helpful for removing obstructing stones and sludge and decompressing the biliary tree
- Gallstone pancreatitis
  - Caused by acute impaction of gallstones in the CBD or at the major papilla
  - Urgent ERCP with sphincterotomy is necessary to remove the impacted stone and to restore adequate drainage from biliary and pancreatic ducts

Diagnosis and Evaluation
- Physical examination
  - Acute cholecystitis
    - Right upper quadrant tenderness with or without peritoneal signs
    - Murphy's sign—inspiratory arrest with right upper quadrant palpation
    - The gallbladder is palpable in less than half of cases

- Acute cholangitis
  - Charcot's triad—fever, right upper quadrant pain, jaundice
  - Reynold's pentad—hypotension, confusion, and Charcot's triad
  - Most patient with cholangitis do not have all the above symptoms
- Leukocytosis and elevated liver function tests commonly noted in cases of acute cholecystitis or cholangitis
- Most common organisms cultured are *Escherichia coli*, *Klebsiella* spp., group D *Streptococcus*, *Staphylococcus* spp., and *Clostridium* spp.
- Lipase and amylase will be elevated in gallstone pancreatitis. Bilirubin and liver function tests may also be elevated
- Radiologic tests can be helpful (Fig. 27-8)

Treatment
See Figure 27-8 for treatment options.

POSTCHOLECYSTECTOMY SYNDROME
Basic Information
- Postcholecystectomy syndrome: Abdominal discomfort, pain, and nausea persisting or presenting after cholecystectomy. Can be associated with abnormal liver function tests, and occasionally with an abnormal amylase and lipase.
- Most common causes of the postcholecystectomy syndrome:
  - Papillary stenosis: Fixed narrowing of the distal CBD and/or pancreatic duct as a result of fibrosis
  - Retained bile duct stone
  - Consequences of the intraoperative bile duct injury (strictures, bile leak)
  - Biliary dyskinesia (also called *sphincter of Oddi dysfunction*): Primary motility disorder of the sphincter of Oddi leading to elevated intraductal pressure

Clinical Presentation
- Persistent or recurrent pain in the right upper quadrant and/or epigastric area that can be accompanied by nausea and vomiting and that resembles symptoms that occurred before cholecystectomy
- Patients with postoperative bile duct strictures can present with pruritus, jaundice, or cholangitis

Diagnosis and Evaluation
- A biliary cause for postcholecystectomy pain should be suspected in the presence of bile duct dilation and abnormalities in liver function tests during painful attacks
- If ductal dilation and laboratory abnormalities are absent, patients may require ERCP with sphincter of Oddi manometry to document an elevated intraductal pressure. There is a high risk of post-ERCP pancreatitis after sphincter of Oddi manometry.
- The less-invasive CCK–hepatobiliary iminodiacetic acid (HIDA) scan correlates well with sphincter of Oddi manometry
- Patients with unexplained pain after cholecystectomy, with normal imaging and labs, should have a careful evaluation for other causes of pain prior to proceeding with ERCP with sphincter of Oddi manometry

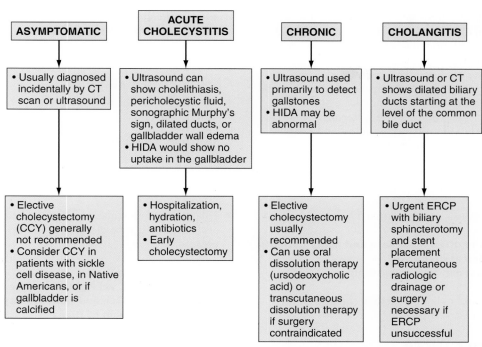

FIGURE 27-8 Diagnosis and treatment of gallstone disease. (CT, computed tomography; ERCP, endoscopic retrograde cholangiopancreatography; HIDA, hepatobiliary iminodiacetic acid.)

Treatment

- Most causes of postcholecystectomy syndrome, particularly those with imaging and lab abnormalities, can be corrected endoscopically during ERCP

CHOLANGIOCARCINOMA

Basic Information

- Rare tumor of the biliary tree that is challenging to diagnose, accounting for 3% of all GI cancers
- Defined as a primary malignant tumor originating from cells resembling biliary epithelium and distinguished from gallbladder cancer. These tumors may arise from
  - Small peripheral intrahepatic bile ducts
  - Larger intrahepatic bile ducts at or near the hilar confluence of the right and left hepatic ducts (Klatskin tumor)
  - Extrahepatic bile ducts (distal bile duct carcinoma)
- Associated risk factors include the following:
  - Primary sclerosing cholangitis (PSC) (lifetime risk of 15%); between 50% and 90% of PSC patients have ulcerative colitis
  - Chronic parasitic infection of the biliary tree with *Clonorchis sinensis, Opisthorchis* spp., *Ascaris,* and other parasites
  - Exposure to thorium dioxide (Thorotrast, a radiocontrast medium used in the 1930s and 1940s)
  - Choledochal cysts (Box 27-3)
  - Oriental cholangiohepatitis—Brown pigment intrahepatic biliary stones develop as a result of chronic inflammation from chronic bacterial infection
  - Multiple biliary papillomatosis
  - Hereditary nonpolyposis colorectal cancer (Lynch syndrome)
  - Increasing age, male gender

BOX 27-3 *Choledochal Cysts*

- Cystic dilations of any segment of the biliary system (intrahepatic and/or extrahepatic)
- Can present with abdominal pain, jaundice, and right upper quadrant mass
- Bile duct obstruction and pancreatitis can occur
- Surgical excision can be indicated to prevent malignant transformation
- Types of choledochal cysts
  Type I—cystic dilation of the common bile duct (most common)
  Type III—choledochocele. Intraduodenal choledochal cyst.
  Type V—Caroli syndrome
  - Autosomal-recessive condition
  - Patients have widespread saccular dilations of the bile ducts
  - Bile collections may become infected
  - Associated with polycystic kidney disease

Clinical Presentation

- **Patients typically present with jaundice, weight loss, abdominal pain, and pruritus; may also have dark urine and acholic stools**
- Physical exam
  - Courvoisier's sign—palpable gallbladder
  - Hepatomegaly may be present
  - Jaundice
- Bilirubin, alkaline phosphatase, γ-glutamyltransferase (GGT) may be elevated. Aspartate aminotransferase (AST) and ALT are often normal early in disease.

Diagnosis and Evaluation

- Transabdominal ultrasonography, CT scan, or MRCP may show biliary dilation, a level of obstruction, and possibly a ductal mass
- Cholangiography (percutaneous or endoscopic via ERCP) will show irregular, tight strictures with proximal dilation and allow for histologic sampling; however, brushings and biopsies may be falsely negative
- EUS can be used to identify small tumors and lymph nodes. Histologic sampling can be performed by FNA.
- CA 19-9 may be elevated but is nonspecific for cholangiocarcinoma and can be falsely negative

Treatment

- The overall prognosis is poor, with a 5% 5-year survival rate
- **The diagnosis is often made late and many patients are unresectable at diagnosis**
- Surgical resection may be possible in up to 20% of patients
- Chemotherapy and radiation therapy can also be used, but long-term survival is poor

GALLBLADDER CANCER

Basic Information

- Rare GI cancer that presents late in life and is usually unresectable when symptomatic
- It is potentially curable when incidentally found or removed by cholecystectomy (seen in up to 2% of gallbladders removed for symptomatic gallstones or cholecystitis)
- Predisposing risk factors include
  - Cholelithiasis—Present in up to 90% of patients with gallbladder cancer. However, the incidence is rare in patients with gallstones.
  - Older age
  - Female gender
  - Obesity
  - Gallbladder adenomas/polyps (particularly those >1 cm in diameter)

- Chronic cholecystitis (e.g., large gallstones)
- Chronic *Salmonella typhi* infection
- Calcified or (porcelain) gallbladder
- Some carcinogenic occupational chemical exposures

Clinical Presentation

- Weight loss, abdominal pain, biliary obstruction, nausea, or right upper quadrant mass

Diagnosis and Evaluation

- Ultrasound may show a mass, thickening of the gallbladder wall, or extraluminal extension of the tumor
- CT and MRCP can also be used to identify gallbladder masses and polyps
- Laboratory studies are less helpful; alkaline phosphatase and bilirubin can be elevated if biliary obstruction is present

Treatment

- **The prognosis is very poor because these cancers are very aggressive and patients usually present with advanced form of disease**
- Surgery for very limited disease may be curative. Overall survival rates for more advanced disease are poor.
- Treatment options are limited for tumors that extend beyond the gallbladder and include aggressive surgery, chemotherapy, and radiation

REVIEW QUESTIONS

For review questions, please go to www.expertconsult.com.

SUGGESTED READINGS

Braganza JM, Lee SH, McCloy RF, McMahon MJ: Chronic pancreatitis, *Lancet* 377:1184–1197, 2011.

Feldman M, Friedman LS, Brandt LJ, et al: *Sleisenger and Fordtran's gastrointestinal and liver disease: pathophysiology/diagnosis/management*, ed 8, Philadelphia, 2006, Saunders Elsevier.

Gupta K, Wu B: In the clinic: acute pancreatitis, *Ann Intern Med* 153:ITC51–ITC55, 2010.

Yamada T, Alpers DH, Kalloo AN, et al: *Textbook of gastroenterology*, ed 5, West Sussex, UK, 2009, Wiley-Blackwell.

Disorders of the Small and Large Intestine

ANNE MARIE LENNON, MB, PhD, MRCPI; and MICHAEL GOGGINS, MD

The small and large bowels are primarily responsible for the absorption of nutrients and fluid and excretion of waste. Diseases that affect the intestinal system are likely to interfere with at least one of these two functions and lead to problems with motility or malabsorption. Diseases that disrupt the mucosal integrity can also cause bleeding, as discussed in Chapter 25.

Diarrhea: General Principles

Basic Information

- Defined as an increase in the fluidity, frequency, or volume of stool output; usually results in increased daily stool weight (>200 g/day in the United States)
- Mechanisms of diarrhea (Table 28-1)
  - Osmotic diarrhea
    - Results from osmotically active solutes that are not absorbed from the gut lumen
    - Higher osmolality in the lumen causes passive water loss across the mucosa of the duodenum and jejunum, overwhelming the absorptive capacities of the ileum and colon
    - **Diarrhea stops when oral intake stops**
    - Volume is usually less than 1 L/day
  - Secretory diarrhea
    - Increased fluid secretion and impaired electrolyte absorption across the intestinal mucosa
    - **Diarrhea continues even when oral intake stops**
    - Stool volume usually large (>1 L/day), watery, without pus or blood
  - Altered motility
    - Increased motility
      - Causes decreased contact time between the gut and digesting food (*chyme*)
      - Leads to less absorption and large amounts of fluid delivered to the colon
    - Decreased motility
      - Causes bacterial overgrowth
      - Leads to impaired bile salt malabsorption
  - Exudative diarrhea
    - Inflamed or ulcerated mucosa permits mucus, blood, and pus to leak into lumen
    - Diarrhea can result directly from the increased osmotic load, increased motility (stimulation of the enteric nervous system), or secretion of the products of inflammation

- Stool volume can be large or small, depending on the part of the bowel affected
- Anorectal dysfunction or injury
  - Leads to the inability to retain feces
  - Characterized by fecal incontinence and small-volume stools
- Many diseases have more than one mechanism (e.g., diseases of malabsorption)

Clinical Presentation

- Acute diarrhea
  - Most cases are infectious (see Chapter 14)
  - Consider medications (e.g., laxatives, magnesium-containing antacids, proton pump inhibitors, colchicine, furosemide)
  - Usually self-limited (<4 weeks' duration)
  - **If abdominal pain and bloody diarrhea occur together in a patient older than 50 years, consider ischemic colitis**
- Chronic diarrhea
  - Lasts longer than 4 weeks
  - Stools can be watery, bloody, contain grease, and be foul-smelling
  - Steatorrhea is defined as more than 7 g of fat per day over 72-hour fecal fat collection while on a high-fat diet
  - Abdominal pain or cramping is often present
  - Associated signs and symptoms that suggest an organic rather than a functional (e.g., irritable bowel syndrome [IBS]) cause are:
    - Fever
    - Weight loss
    - Arthritis
    - Signs and symptoms of malabsorption (Table 28-2)
  - Can result from a number of different etiologies (Table 28-3)

Diagnosis and Evaluation

- History and physical examination
  - Should focus on stool character, associated symptoms, and predisposing conditions (e.g., travel, HIV, family history of inflammatory bowel disease [IBD], antibiotic use)
  - Acute diarrhea in a nonimmunocompromised patient does not require evaluation unless dehydration, bloody stools, fever, or severe abdominal pain is present (see Chapter 14)
- Diagnostic tests for chronic diarrhea

TABLE 28-1	*Mechanisms of Diarrheal Disease*	
Category	**Example Conditions**	**Comments**
Osmotic	Maldigestion of carbohydrates (e.g., lactase deficiency, sucrase deficiency) Ingestion of nonabsorbed solutes (e.g., mannitol, sorbitol) Ingestion of poorly absorbed salts (magnesium hydroxide)	Small stool volume Osmolar gap present Stops with fasting Stool pH <6
Secretory	Bacterial toxins (e.g., cholera, *Escherichia coli*) Hormonal secretagogues (e.g., vasoactive intestinal peptides, serotonin) Gastric hypersecretion (e.g., Zollinger-Ellison syndrome) Laxatives (e.g., senna, phenolphthalein) Bile salt malabsorption	Large volume of stool No osmolar gap Persistent diarrhea with fasting
Abnormal motility	Increased motility—hyperthyroidism, carcinoid, postgastrectomy dumping syndrome Decreased motility—diabetes, hypothyroidism, scleroderma, amyloidosis, postvagotomy syndromes	Bacterial overgrowth motility usually secondary to decreased motility
Exudative	Inflammatory bowel disease Bacterial pathogens (e.g., *Salmonella, Shigella*) Vasculitis Radiation enteritis Severe diverticulitis Ischemic injury	Volume can be small or large
Anorectal dysfunction	Neurologic disease Postsurgical complication Inflammatory bowel disease	Small volume of stools

TABLE 28-2	*Nutrient Malabsorption*	
Location of Normal Absorption	**Nutrient**	**Consequences of Malabsorption**
Proximal small bowel	Iron	Glossitis, pallor Anemia, pica
	Calcium	Bone pain, tetany Osteoporosis
	Folate	Glossitis, pallor Anemia, depression
Distal small bowel	Vitamin A	Night blindness Hyperkeratosis Corneal ulcers
	Vitamin D	Bone pain Muscle weakness Osteomalacia
	Vitamin E	Peripheral neuropathy Retinopathy
	Vitamin K	Bleeding Bruising
	Vitamin B_{12}	Peripheral neuropathy, subacute combined degeneration of the spinal cord Dementia, neuropsychiatric effects Anemia

- General blood studies: complete blood count (CBC) with differential, chemistry panel that includes renal and liver function should initially be obtained
- Use of further testing needs to be guided by history, physical findings, and results of general blood studies
- Stool studies
  - Fecal leukocytes: Suggest inflammatory or infectious process
  - Bacterial culture: Most useful for acute diarrhea

- Ova and parasites
- *Clostridium difficile* toxin assay: Particularly useful if antibiotics recently administered
- 72-hour quantitative stool collection for volume
- Stool electrolyte concentration to calculate osmolar gap
  - Measure stool Na^+ and K^+ concentrations
  - **Osmolar gap = 290 − ([Na^+] + [K^+]) × 2**
  - **Osmolar gap greater than 40 suggests osmotic diarrhea**
  - **Osmolar gap less than 40 suggests secretory diarrhea**
- Qualitative and quantitative fecal fat on a high-fat diet (e.g., 72 hr, 100 g fat/day)
- Stool phenolphthalein (if laxative abuse is suspected)
- Tests for malabsorption
  - D-Xylose test
    - Measures the absorptive capacity of the proximal small bowel
    - Urine and blood are collected after 25 g oral xylose is administered
    - Abnormal test suggests small bowel mucosal disease or bacterial overgrowth
    - It is normal in pancreatic enzyme deficiency
  - Hydrogen breath test
    - Tests for lactose intolerance
    - After ingestion of lactose, the amount of hydrogen in expired air is measured
    - If substantial levels are recorded, lactose intolerance is suggested
    - **This test is generally unnecessary since a therapeutic trial of lactose restriction is more cost-effective**
- Endoscopy
  - Not routinely indicated

TABLE 28-3	*Selected Causes of Chronic Diarrhea*
Category	**Examples**
Infections	Amebiasis Giardiasis *Clostridium difficile* HIV enteropathy *Yersinia, Campylobacter* *Cryptosporidium, Cyclospora* Intestinal schistosomiasis
Inflammatory	Ulcerative colitis Crohn disease Microscopic colitis Eosinophilic gastroenteritis
Hormonal abnormalities/ tumors	Diabetes Hyperthyroidism Adrenal insufficiency Vasoactive intestinal peptide tumors (VIPomas) Carcinoid syndrome Medullary thyroid cancer Gastrinoma Mastocytosis
Nonendocrine neoplasms	Villous adenoma secreting bicarbonate Obstructive colon cancer causing impaction and overflow diarrhea of liquid feces
Steatorrheal causes— maldigestion	Pancreatic exocrine insufficiency Bacterial overgrowth Liver disease
Steatorrheal causes—mucosal malabsorption	Celiac sprue Tropical sprue Whipple disease Ischemia
Structural	Bile salt diarrhea after ileal resection Vagotomy Short-gut syndrome
Osmotic	Laxatives (magnesium) Carbohydrate enzyme deficiencies (e.g., lactase) Sorbitol, lactulose ingestion
Functional	Irritable bowel syndrome
Anorectal dysfunction	Neurologic disease

FIGURE 28-1 Celiac disease (gluten-sensitive enteropathy). **A,** A jejunal biopsy specimen of diseased mucosa shows diffuse severe atrophy and blunting of villi, with a chronic inflammatory infiltrate of the lamina propria. **B,** A normal mucosal biopsy. *(From Kumar V, Fausto N, Abbas A: Robbins and Cotran: Pathologic basis of disease, ed 7, Philadelphia, Elsevier Saunders, 2005, Fig. 17-38.)*

- Colonoscopy and sigmoidoscopy are useful in cases where bloody diarrhea is present
  - Colonic biopsies are needed to diagnose microscopic colitis
- Upper endoscopy with small bowel biopsy helpful in suspected cases of malabsorption, such as celiac disease
- Radiologic studies may also be useful in certain cases
- Capsule endoscopy may be helpful to evaluate the cause of suspected small intestinal diarrhea if radiology and endoscopy are nondiagnostic
- Specific blood and urine studies assist in searching for specific etiologies

Treatment

- Directed at the specific cause
- Treat dehydration
- Avoid caffeine and other secretagogues

- Antimotility agents (e.g., loperamide) can be useful if infection has been ruled out

Diarrheal Diseases

CELIAC SPRUE (GLUTEN-SENSITIVE ENTEROPATHY)

Basic Information

- Predominantly seen in white population
- Causes flattened villi of the proximal small bowel (Fig. 28-1)
- Most patients express human leukocyte antigen (HLA) DQ2 or DQ8, reflecting their genetic predisposition
- **Serology studies suggest celiac disease has a prevalence of approximately 1 in 200 individuals in the United States**
- Recent studies have shown that type 1 diabetes mellitus and celiac disease share common alleles, suggesting that they share biologic mechanisms

Clinical Presentation

- Diarrhea is common but might not be present
- Iron deficiency anemia seen in 50% of adults with celiac disease

FIGURE 28-2 Dermatitis herpetiformis of the elbows. *(From Callen JP: Color atlas of dermatology, ed 2, Philadelphia, WB Saunders, 2000.)*

- Osteomalacia and osteoporosis can develop from vitamin D and calcium malabsorption
- Most adult patients do not present with classic features of malabsorption (e.g., steatorrhea)
- 42% of patients with celiac disease have elevation of aminotransferases
- **Diagnosis is often delayed for many years after the onset of symptoms**
- **Patients often have been given a diagnosis of IBS**
- Associated with a number of diseases:
  - Dermatitis herpetiformis (papulovesicular rash usually on the elbows, knees, buttocks, or scalp; Fig. 28-2)
  - Type 1 diabetes mellitus and other autoimmune disorders
  - Immunoglobulin A (IgA) deficiency; occurs in 2% to 5% of patients with celiac disease compared with less than 5% of the general population
  - Autoimmune hepatitis
  - Autoimmune thyroid disease
  - It is also more common in people with Downs, Turner, or Williams syndrome
  - Increased incidence of small bowel lymphoma

Diagnosis and Evaluation

- Initial screening is usually performed with antibodies
  - Antiendomysial antibody is an IgA antibody that is 85% to 98% sensitive and 97% to 100% specific
  - Tissue transglutaminase (tTG) antibody is an IgA antibody that is 90% to 98% sensitive and 95% to 97% specific
  - Antigliadin antibody (immunoglobulin G [IgG] and IgA) has lower sensitivity and specificity
  - **If there is a high suspicion of disease but negative antibodies, the total serum IgA concentration should be checked to rule out IgA deficiency. In these cases, an IgG-based assay (serum IgG tTG antibody) can be used or an upper endoscopy with biopsies performed.**
- The diagnosis of celiac disease requires a small bowel biopsy, which demonstrates flattened or blunted villi and increased lymphocytes (see Fig. 28-1A). A minimum of six biopsies should be taken from the second and third parts of the duodenum, as histologic changes can be patchy.

- The gold standard for the diagnosis of celiac disease includes a repeat endoscopy with biopsies once the patient is on a gluten-free diet. These biopsies should demonstrate resolution of the histologic changes. This is rarely performed nowadays, with the diagnosis made on positive antibodies, histology consistent with celiac disease, and a response to treatment on a gluten-free diet.

Treatment

- Lifelong completely gluten-free diet—highly effective in resolving symptoms and reversing pathologic abnormalities
- Most relapses are caused by dietary noncompliance or hidden sources of gluten
- Refractory cases can be treated with corticosteroids or other immunosuppressives
- The possibility of early-onset small bowel lymphoma should be considered in refractory cases
- Response to treatment can be monitored using either IgA tTG antibody or IgA antigliadin antibody, with a return to normal baseline expected within 3 to 12 months after initiation of gluten-free diet
- Nutritional deficiencies (iron, calcium, phosphorus, folate, vitamin B_{12}, fat-soluble vitamins) should be identified and treated
- Patients should be screened for osteoporosis

TROPICAL SPRUE

- Suspect in patients with chronic diarrhea and malabsorption after residing in or traveling to a tropical area
- **Most patients have evidence of folate deficiency**
- Infectious agents (e.g., *Klebsiella*) have been implicated
- Pathology from a small bowel biopsy can be similar to celiac sprue, but the patient is unresponsive to a gluten-free diet
- Treatment is with tetracycline and folate

WHIPPLE DISEASE

- Usually seen in middle-aged men
- **Caused by gram-positive bacillus (*Tropheryma whippelii*)**
- Presents with diarrhea, steatorrhea, abdominal pain, weight loss, migratory arthritis, and fever
- Neurologic (dementia, ocular disturbances, meningoencephalitis, cerebellar symptoms), cardiac (congestive heart failure, pericarditis, valvular heart disease), and ophthalmologic features may be present
- The diagnosis is made by showing periodic acid–Schiff (PAS)-positive macrophages containing the small bacillus in any affected tissue (usually small bowel). Antibodies to the protein and polymerase chain reaction (PCR) to the DNA of *Tropheryma whippelii* can also help to establish the diagnosis.
- Treatment is with trimethoprim-sulfamethoxazole for 1 year

BACTERIAL OVERGROWTH SYNDROME

Basic Information

- Caused by
  - Small bowel stasis
    - Anatomic abnormalities (postsurgical, diverticulae)

- Abnormal small bowel motility (scleroderma, diabetes mellitus)
- Abnormal communication (Crohn fistula, resection of the ileocecal valve) between the small bowel and colon
  - Multifactorial (chronic pancreatitis, cirrhosis, achlorhydria, immunodeficiency)
  - 90% associated with intestinal dysmotility syndrome and chronic pancreatitis

Clinical Presentation

- Bloating, flatulence, abdominal pain
- Diarrhea
- Weight loss
- Steatorrhea is caused by impaired micelle formation because of bacterial deconjugation of bile acids in the proximal small bowel
- Dermatitis, arthritis
- Vitamin deficiencies:
  - Vitamin B_{12} deficiency is common
  - Vitamin A deficiency with night blindness
  - Hypocalcemia secondary to vitamin D deficiency
  - Folate may be elevated because it is produced by enteric bacteria

Diagnosis and Evaluation

- The gold standard is small bowel aspirate demonstrating bacterial overgrowth ($>10^5$ colony-forming units/mL)
- Breath tests:
  - Lactose: Hydrogen breath test
    - Lactose is normally broken down in the colon. In bacterial overgrowth, an early hydrogen peak is seen.
    - Low sensitivity and specificity
  - ^{14}C-glycocholate breath test and ^{14}C-D-xylose breath test:
    - Detect the release of radiolabeled carbon dioxide resulting from bacterial deconjugation of bile acid and metabolism of xylose
    - D-Xylose sensitivity and specificity approach 90%
- Normalization of the Schilling test after antibiotics is highly suggestive of bacterial overgrowth (see Chapter 46)

Treatment

- Treat any anatomic abnormality with surgery, if possible
- Treat any underlying diseases and correct nutritional deficiencies
- Broad-spectrum antibiotics (ciprofloxacin, tetracycline, metronidazole, and rifamixin) can be administered for 2 to 3 weeks
  - Bacterial overgrowth often recurs in nonfunctional cases, and repeated cycles of antibiotics or alternating antibiotics are often required

BILE ACID MALABSORPTION

- Bile acids are absorbed in the ileum. Diseases that affect the ileum (i.e., Crohn disease) or where the ileum has been resected will cause bile acid diarrhea.
- Two basic forms of the disease:
  - Bile acid diarrhea

- Associated with limited ileal abnormality or resection
- Impaired bile acid absorption in the ileum leads to chloride and water secretion in the colon
- Steatorrhea does not develop because the liver is able to compensate for the loss of bile acids in the stool
- Responds to cholestyramine
- Fatty acid diarrhea
  - Associated with extensive ileal abnormality/resection
  - Liver is unable to compensate for the loss of bile acids in the stool, so steatorrhea develops
  - Does not respond to cholestyramine
  - May respond to low-fat diet

MICROSCOPIC COLITIS

Basic Information

- Usually occurs in patients in their 50s and 60s
- **Accounts for up to 10% of cases of chronic diarrhea**
- There are two types of microscopic colitis based on histology: collagenous colitis and lymphocytic colitis
  - Lymphocytic colitis is more common
  - Collagenous colitis occurs more frequently in women
- Microscopic colitis is associated with certain drugs, especially nonsteroidal anti-inflammatory drugs (NSAIDs)
- Associated with other diseases, especially celiac disease
- Consider it in the differential diagnosis of patient with celiac disease who is maintaining a strict diet but continues to have diarrhea

Clinical Presentation

- Microcytic anemia
- Diarrhea
- Weight loss
- Abdominal discomfort
- Fatigue

Diagnosis and Evaluation

- Colonoscopy
  - Will be grossly normal endoscopically, but biopsies should be taken from both the right and left colon
  - **Diagnosis is made by histologic examination**
- Histologic criteria for diagnosing microscopic colitis are
  - Increased chronic inflammatory infiltrate in the lamina propria
  - Increased number of intraepithelial lymphocytes (>15–20 lymphocytes per 1000 epithelial cells)
  - Damage of the surface epithelium with flattening of the epithelial cells
  - The presence of subepithelial collagenous band distinguishes collagenous colitis from lymphocytic colitis

Treatment

- Microscopic colitis can resolve spontaneously
- Stop NSAIDs or other associated drugs
- **First-line treatment is budesonide**
- A 5-aminosalicylic acid (5-ASA; mesalamine, sulfasalazine) compound can be tried if budesonide is ineffective

TABLE 28-4	*Selected Diseases Causing Chronic Diarrhea*			
Category/Disease	**Extradiarrheal Manifestations**	**Diagnosis**	**Treatment**	**Comments**
Infections *Giardia lamblia*	Bloating Nausea	Stool examination for ova and parasites of *Giardia* antigen	Metronidazole	Suspect in those with exposure to surface water (e.g., campers)
Secretory Vasoactive intestinal peptide tumors (VIPomas)	Hypokalemia Achlorhydria Non–anion gap metabolic acidosis	Elevated plasma VIP	Somatostatin analogues Surgery	Causes massive diarrhea WDHA syndrome (watery diarrhea, hypokalemia, achlorhydria)
Carcinoid syndrome	Flushing Abdominal pain Wheezing Right-sided valvular disease	Elevated urinary 5-hydroxyindoleacetic acid	Somatostatin analogues	Syndrome generally present when hepatic metastases present
Mastocytosis	Pruritus Flushing Abdominal pain Headache Urticaria pigmentosa—macular lesions that urticate when stroked (Darier's sign)	Elevated 24-hr urine for histamine and metabolites Elevated serum tryptase levels Skin biopsy	Histamine receptor blockers Glucocorticoids	Symptoms can be episodic
Osmotic Lactase deficiency	Abdominal cramps Flatulence	Empirical trial of lactose-free diet Hydrogen breath test	Lactose-free diet	Common disorder Symptoms typically occur after ingestion of dairy products
Inflammatory Microscopic/collagenous colitis	None	Colonoscopy shows grossly normal colon Increased collagen or in basement membrane or lymphocytic infiltrate microscopically	Corticosteroids 5-Aminosalicylic acid	More commonly seen in women over age 50 yr

- Other alternatives include bismuth and oral steroids other than budesonide
- Symptoms of diarrhea will often respond to cholestyramine

OTHER DISEASES

See Table 28-4 for selected diseases that cause chronic diarrhea.

Constipation

Basic Information

- Subjectively defined as difficult-to-pass or hard feces, or bowel movements occurring less frequently than usual
- Objective definition is less than three bowel movements per week
- Increases with age
- Women have a greater incidence than men
- Can result from a number of different conditions (Table 28-5)

Clinical Presentation

- Can be acute or chronic
- New-onset, persistent constipation can be a symptom of underlying organic disease
- Abdominal discomfort may also be present but is less prominent than in patients with constipation-predominant IBS

Diagnosis and Evaluation

- History and physical examination should look for secondary causes of constipation. Rectal examination may point to anorectal dysfunction.
- Blood work should include CBC, electrolytes, Ca^{2+}, thyroid-stimulating hormone (TSH)
- In problematic cases, consider abdominal radiograph, colonic transit studies, colonoscopy (especially in elderly patients), anorectal motility (if anorectal dysfunction is suspected)
- Constipation is often due to slow transit. Occasionally it is due to pelvic floor dysfunction. With pelvic floor dysfunction, straining is a dominant symptom and soft stool and even enemas may be difficult to pass.

TABLE 28-5	*Causes of Constipation*
Functional (most common)	Psychogenic Irritable bowel syndrome Mental illness (e.g., depression, eating disorders) Inactivity Low dietary fiber
Drugs	Side effects from anticholinergics, calcium channel blockers, diuretics, calcium/aluminum antacids, opiates Laxative abuse leading to diminished neurologic function of the colon Metal toxicity (e.g., arsenic, lead, mercury, phosphates)
Endocrine/metabolic	Hypothyroidism Diabetes Hypokalemia Hypercalcemia Uremia Amyloid neuropathy Porphyria

Neurogenic	Colonic pseudo-obstruction
	Occurs postoperatively, with infections, narcotic use, or electrolyte disorders; risk of perforation when cecum >13 cm
	Peripheral nerve injury—cauda equina syndrome
	Hirschsprung disease
	  Can present in adults as chronic constipation
	  Rectal biopsy shows aganglionosis
	Autonomic neuropathy
	CNS disorders (e.g., MS, Parkinson disease, stroke)

Diseases of the large bowel and rectum	Tumors Volvulus, hernia Colitis, proctitis Infection Scleroderma
Anorectal diseases	Fissure Rectal prolapse, rectocele, pelvic floor injury

CNS, central nervous system; MS, multiple sclerosis.

Treatment

- Functional constipation
  - Hydration
  - Exercise
  - Dietary fiber (15–25 g/day)
  - Psychological counseling
  - Consider osmotic laxatives (e.g., polyethylene glycol, lactulose, sorbitol)
  - Reserve stimulant laxatives (e.g., bisacodyl, senna) for acute constipation
  - Pelvic floor dysfunction requires enemas and biofeedback
- Secondary causes
  - Remove offending drugs
  - Treat specific condition

Irritable Bowel Syndrome

Basic Information

- Characterized by chronic recurrent abdominal pain and altered bowel habits in absence of structural disorder

- Patients may have predominant diarrhea (never nocturnal), constipation, or intermittent episodes of the two. Pain is often relieved with defecation.
- Affects 20% of Western adults
- Women more often affected than men
- Second leading cause of work absenteeism (next to the common cold)
- Patient characteristics
  - Diet may be unhealthy: fast foods, low-fiber diet
  - Emotional or psychological factors: Stress is associated with increase in symptoms; sexual abuse is more common in these patients; an increase in anxiety and depression but possibly only in those who seek medical attention
  - Innate sensitivity or susceptibility: Positive family history of irritable bowel, increased occurrence of other disorders with somatization features (e.g., fibromyalgia)
  - Motility disturbance (slower myoelectric rhythm in colon) and abnormal sensitivity to rectal distention have been demonstrated
  - Postinfectious: Infectious gastroenteritis predisposes to the development of IBS
  - Small bowel bacterial overgrowth may cause IBS symptoms and is found in a minority of patients diagnosed with IBS
  - Celiac disease may cause IBS symptoms

Clinical Presentation

- Pain most commonly in left iliac fossa or hypogastrium
- Knotting, burning, cramping sensation
- Distention, bloating, fullness, especially postprandially
- Small-volume stools whether diarrhea or constipation
- **Constipation stools often scybalous (pebble-like); diarrhea often in morning, following normal bowel movements; mucus is common**
- **Relief of pain often with bowel movement**
- Dyspepsia, heartburn, nausea, headaches, urinary frequency, dysmenorrhea can also be seen
- No history of weight loss, awakening from sleep, rectal bleeding, fever, rigidity on examination (if present, think of other disorders)
- No specific findings on examination except for mild abdominal tenderness—more often over sigmoid colon

Diagnosis and Evaluation

- Diagnostic criteria (Rome III criteria) are based on history (Box 28-1). Extensive investigation is usually not necessary.
- CBC, erythrocyte sedimentation rate, stool studies, occult blood examination are normal
- With diarrhea-predominant IBS, need to rule out lactose intolerance, celiac disease, IBD
- In more severe or unresponsive cases, stool volume (should be normal) can be examined and sigmoidoscopy performed
- If constipation is severe, rule out hypothyroidism, hyperparathyroidism, diverticulosis, anorectal dysfunction, and malignancy
- Occasionally, pelvic pain and altered bowel habit with gynecologic conditions, such as endometriosis, can mimic IBS

BOX 28-1 *Diagnostic Criteria for Irritable Bowel Syndrome (Rome III)*

Symptoms of recurrent abdominal pain or discomfort and a marked change in bowel habit for at least six months, with symptoms experienced on at least three days of at least three months. Two or more of the following must apply:
- Pain is relieved by a bowel movement
- Onset of pain is related to a change in frequency of stool
- Onset of pain is related to a change in the appearance of stool.

Treatment

- Educate patient about condition
- High-fiber diet or supplementation, reduce or remove offending foods (e.g., high-fat, high-carbohydrate diet)
- Antispasmodics (e.g., dicyclomine, hyoscyamine) and low-dose tricyclics may be helpful for abdominal pain
- Antimotility agents (e.g., loperamide) may be helpful for diarrhea
- Probiotics may be useful, particularly for postinfectious IBS. Further studies are required to determine the type and dose of probiotics required.
- Gas symptoms may respond to diet changes, simethicone, or bismuth
- Treat depression and anxiety (avoid narcotics and benzodiazepines)
- Drugs
  - Tegaserod, a 5-hydroxytryptamine receptor 4 partial agonist, may be useful for women with constipation-predominant symptoms. It is associated with an increased incidence of ischemic cardiovascular events and is only available in the United States for use in IBS-predominant constipation and chronic constipation, in women less than 55 years of age with no cardiovascular risk factors
  - Alosetron, a 5-hydroxytryptamine receptor 3 agonist, modulates visceral afferent activity from the GI tract and was found to be helpful in IBS in women with diarrhea-predominant symptoms. This drug was withdrawn following its release because of an apparent increased incidence of ischemic colitis; however, it has now been reintroduced

Inflammatory Bowel Disease

Basic Information

- Defined as an idiopathic chronic inflammation of the GI tract: Primarily Crohn disease (CD) and ulcerative colitis (UC)
- **Bimodal peak age distribution: Initial 15 to 25 years, second peak 50 to 80 years**
- Significantly greater incidence in Western developed countries
- Smoking as a risk factor
  - Increased risk in CD
  - Decreased risk of current smokers and increased risk of ex-smokers in UC
- Genetics
  - 10% to 20% of patients with IBD have additional relatives with IBD

- First-degree relatives of patients with IBD are 3 to 20 times more likely to develop the disease than the general population
  - Increased risk of IBD in patients with other autoimmune diseases
  - NOD2/CARD15 mutation is a risk factor for CD but not UC (mutation carriers often do not have disease)
- Crohn disease can affect any part of the bowel from the mouth to the anus. It can have "skip lesions" with a normal section of bowel between diseased sections.
  - 80% of patients have small bowel involvement, usually in the distal ileum
  - 50% have involvement of both the ileum and the colon
  - A small number of patients have involvement of the upper GI tract (esophagus, stomach, proximal small bowel)
  - 30% have perianal disease
- UC affects the large bowel and is continuous from the rectum to the proximal extent of the disease
  - Proctitis: Ulcerative colitis limited to the rectum
  - Distal colitis: Affects the rectum and sigmoid colon
  - Left-sided colitis: Affects area from the rectum to the splenic flexure
  - Extensive colitis: Extends from the rectum past the splenic flexure but does not involve the cecum
  - Pancolitis: Extends from the rectum to the cecum

Clinical Presentation

- Typically characterized by recurrence of a number of symptoms
  - Diarrhea
  - Abdominal pain
  - Weight loss
  - Rectal bleeding
  - Fever
- Causes of exacerbations
  - Usually not identifiable
  - NSAID use, tobacco use (in CD), infections, and medication noncompliance may predispose to attacks
- Extraintestinal manifestations may present without symptoms of abdominal disease (Box 28-2)
- Cancer
  - Colorectal cancer
    - The risk is related to the duration and extent of the disease
    - **Overall risk in UC and extensive colitis from CD is 2% to 5%**
    - **Screen for dysplasia and cancer 8 to 10 years after diagnosis of IBD is made, then every 1 to 2 years**
  - Small bowel cancer increased in CD

Diagnosis and Evaluation

- Laboratory tests
  - Increased C-reactive protein and sedimentation rate; leukocytosis, anemia, and thrombocytosis are commonly seen
  - Stool studies for ova and parasites, culture, and C. difficile should be obtained to rule out infection

BOX 28-2 Extraintestinal Manifestations and Complications of Inflammatory Bowel Disease

Arthritis
  Peripheral arthritis involving large joints
  Spondyloarthropathy/ankylosing spondylitis
Uveitis/iritis
Skin manifestations
Pyoderma gangrenosum
Erythema nodosum
Hepatobiliary manifestations
Primary sclerosing cholangitis (PSC)
  70% of PSC patients have inflammatory bowel disease (IBD)
  All PSC patients should be screened for IBD with colonoscopy
Cholelithiasis
Fistulas (Crohn disease [CD])
  Often involve perianal area, but any area of bowel may be involved, can lead to abscess formation
  Usually extend to skin, bowel, or vagina
Hemorrhage
Bowel obstruction/perforation
  Stricturing can lead to obstruction
  Spontaneous perforation more common in CD
  Toxic megacolon (abdominal distention, diarrhea, colonic dilation on radiograph)
    More commonly seen in ulcerative colitis
    Fever, tachycardia, leukocytosis, anemia
    50% of patients will require surgery
    15% mortality rate
Nutritional manifestations/malabsorption
Malnutrition
Dehydration
Anemia (iron deficiency, vitamin B_{12} deficiency)
Osteoporosis
  Can occur even without corticosteroid use
  Bone density scans should be checked routinely
Thromboembolism
Spontaneous abortion/premature delivery
Protein-losing enteropathy
Nephrolithiasis (calcium oxalate and uric acid stones)
Amyloid
Colorectal carcinoma

FIGURE 28-3 Air-contrast barium enema demonstrating luminal narrowing and loss of haustral markings in the sigmoid and descending colon in a patient with ulcerative colitis. *(From Goldman L, Bennett JC, Ausiello D: Cecil textbook of medicine, ed 22, Philadelphia, WB Saunders, 2004, Fig. 142-1.)*

TABLE 28-6 Differentiating Ulcerative Colitis from Crohn Disease*

	UC	CD
Perianal disease	−	+
Fistula formation	−	+
Small bowel involvement	−	+
Granuloma formation on biopsy	−	+
Transmural inflammation	−	+
Inflammation limited to mucosa	+	−
Continuous colonic inflammation	+	−

*In 10% of patients, ulcerative colitis (UC) and Crohn disease (CD) will be indistinguishable.

- Sigmoidoscopy or colonoscopy is most often used to make the diagnosis and to distinguish between UC and colonic CD (Table 28-6)
- Capsule endoscopy is useful for staging small bowel Crohn disease
- Complications of IBD and therapies, such as malnutrition, osteoporosis, and gallstones, should be sought and treated (e.g., nutritional supplementation, bone densitometry; see Box 28-2)
- Assessment of severity of a disease flare
  - Mild to moderate: Able to tolerate oral diet; no dehydration, toxicity, abdominal tenderness, mass or obstruction
  - Moderate to severe: Failed treatment for mild to moderate disease or symptoms of fever, weight loss, abdominal pain and tenderness, intermittent nausea, vomiting, or anemia
  - Severe: Fulminant—persisting symptoms despite treatment with steroids or high temperature, persistent vomiting, intestinal obstruction, rebound tenderness, cachexia, or abscess

- Peripheral antineutrophil cytoplasmic antibody (p-ANCA) is elevated in 60% of patients with CD or UC. Anti–*Saccharomyces cerevisiae* antibody is elevated in 80% of CD patients. Neither is adequate for diagnosis.
- Radiographic features
  - Barium enema can show mucosal granularity or ulceration (in UC; Fig. 28-3)
  - Small bowel series may show ulcerations in between normal mucosa, fistulas ("cobblestoning"), or strictures (in CD)
  - Magnetic resonance imaging is also helpful in evaluating Crohn disease, particularly of the small intestine

TABLE 28-7	*Medications Used for the Treatment of Inflammatory Bowel Disease*
Medication	**Side Effects**
Sulfasalazine	GI distress Allergy (fever and rash, similar to other sulfa drugs) Folic acid deficiency Hemolysis, neutropenia Male infertility
Other aminosalicylates (mesalamine, olsalazine, balsalazide)	Fewer than sulfasalazine; no hemolysis or infertility; rarely nephritis
Corticosteroids (including budesonide)	Hyperglycemia Cataracts Mood disorders Avascular necrosis Osteoporosis
Metronidazole	Metallic taste Peripheral neuropathy
Ciprofloxacin	GI distress Photosensitivity Elevated transaminases
Azathioprine/6-mercaptopurine	Pancreatitis Leukopenia Elevated transaminases
Cyclosporine	Hypertension Renal failure Tremors Paresthesias Seizures Infections
Methotrexate	Leukopenia Hepatic fibrosis Pneumonitis
Infliximab	Infusion reaction Tuberculosis and other infections related to immunosuppression Lupus-like syndrome

Treatment

- Medical (Table 28-7)
  - 5-ASA medications (sulfasalazine, mesalamine, olsalazine)
    - Mainstay of therapy for mild to moderate cases of UC and CD
    - Inhibit lipoxygenase pathway, prostaglandin cytokine synthesis, free radical scavengers
  - Corticosteroids
    - **Initial therapy for most moderate cases and all severe cases**
    - Can be used intravenously, orally, or as an enema (for isolated rectal involvement or proctitis)
    - Oral budesonide undergoes extensive first-pass metabolism and has fewer side effects
  - Antibiotics (metronidazole, ciprofloxacin)
    - No clear role in treatment of UC
    - Most effective in fistulous and perianal disease of CD
  - Immunosuppressants
    - Usually indicated in steroid-resistant or steroid-dependent patients

- Specific agents
  - Azathioprine/6-mercaptopurine: Most frequently used; these agents are used both to induce and to maintain remission
  - Cyclosporine: Used for UC, not CD; given over 2 to 4 months to induce remission
  - Methotrexate: Mainly used for CD
  - Anti–tumor necrosis factor (TNF) therapies
    - Infliximab: Chimeric mouse/human monoclonal antibody against TNF-α; given as IV infusion; licensed for CD and UC both to induce and maintain remission; also used to treat fistulizing Crohn disease
    - Adalimumab: Recombinant human IgG1 monoclonal antibody against TNF-α; subcutaneous administration every 2 weeks; can be used in patients who have lost response to infliximab
    - Certolizumab: Humanized monoclonal antibody Fab fragment linked to polyethylene glycol, which neutralizes TNF; subcutaneous administration every 4 weeks
    - **Patients need to be screened for tuberculosis (TB; tuberculin skin test and chest radiograph) before starting anti-TNF therapy because patients are at increased risk of developing TB** and other serious infections
    - Lymphoma risk is also slightly increased, as is risk for demyelinating disease, hematologic disease, and liver toxicity
  - Miscellaneous agents
    - Fibrin sealant for fistulas
    - Fish oil (in UC)
- Surgical
  - UC
    - Because UC is limited to the colon, total proctocolectomy cures UC. An ileal pouch can be formed, replacing the rectum. This can be affected by pouchitis.
    - Indications for surgery:
      - Fulminant disease (toxic megacolon)
      - Colitis refractory to medical therapy
      - Dysplasia or concern for colorectal cancer
      - Stricture
      - Massive bleeding
  - Crohn disease (Fig. 28-4)
    - Indications for surgery include obstructive symptoms, refractory severe inflammation, and repair of fistulas
    - More than 40% of patients require surgery within first 10 years of diagnosis
    - Up to 80% of patients will have evidence of recurrence endoscopically, and 10% to 15% will have clinical recurrence
    - There is an increased risk of recurrence in patients who smoke or have perforating disease
    - The aim of surgery is to preserve as much small bowel as possible
    - A stricturoplasty can be performed to treat strictures, avoiding removing large sections of bowel
    - Bile salt diarrhea and fat malabsorption may occur following ileal resection
- Nutritional (enteral therapy)

FIGURE 28-4 Small bowel (SB) of a patient with Crohn disease. Note the stricture in the terminal ileum (*arrows*). *(From Burkitt GH, Quick CRG: Essential surgery, ed 3, New York, Churchill Livingstone, 2002, Fig. 21.8.)*

- Effective therapy in patients with active CD for treating flare and decreasing fistula output
- Useful in children, but adults can find enteral therapy unpalatable
- Not effective as lone therapy in UC

REVIEW QUESTIONS

For review questions, please go to www.expertconsult.com.

SUGGESTED READINGS

Abraham C, Cho JH: Inflammatory bowel disease, *N Engl J Med* 361:2066–2078, 2009.
Green PHR, Cellier C: Celiac disease, *N Engl J Med* 357:1731–1743, 2007.
Longstreth GL, Thompson WG, Chey WD, et al: Functional bowel disorders, *Gastroenterology* 130:1480–1491, 2006.
Mayer EA: Irritable bowel syndrome, *N Engl J Med* 358:1692–1699, 2008.
Schiller LR: Chronic diarrhea, *Gastroenterology* 127:287–293, 2004.

28

Acute and Chronic Liver Disease

JAMES P. HAMILTON, MD

The widespread use of serum liver chemistries has led to an increase in the identification of diseases of the liver. Diseases such as hepatitis C, hemochromatosis, and non-alcoholic fatty liver disease have been found to be quite prevalent in the general population. A systematic approach designed to assess liver function and disease severity via laboratory testing and imaging can direct the need for more invasive evaluation and defined treatment.

Evaluation of Elevated Liver Tests

Basic Information

- Biochemical liver tests lack sensitivity and specificity, but both the pattern and degree of elevation may sometimes give clues to disease processes
- **Persistently or markedly (>10× normal) elevated liver tests should always be fully evaluated**

Clinical Presentation

- Elevated aminotransferases (aspartate aminotransferase [AST] and alanine aminotransferase [ALT]) are usually indicative of hepatic inflammation and hepatocyte necrosis
  - Alcoholic hepatitis, viral hepatitis, drug-induced injury, autoimmune hepatitis, toxic injury, and nonalcoholic fatty liver disease are common causes
  - **The pattern of enzyme elevation (i.e., hepatitic *versus* cholestatic) is a critical first step in the interpretation of liver chemistries**
  - **An AST/ALT ratio of greater than 2 is suggestive of alcoholic liver disease in the appropriate clinical scenario**
  - AST and ALT values greater than 1000 IU/mL are usually indicative of acute viral, toxic, or ischemic hepatitis. Alcoholic hepatitis almost never raises the enzymes above 400 IU/mL.
- Alkaline phosphatase (AP) is elevated in diseases associated with impaired flow of bile, such as cholestatic diseases, infiltrative diseases, biliary tract obstruction, and drug-induced toxic injury
- γ-Glutamyltransferase (GGT) and 5′-nucleotidase are tests that can be used to confirm that the elevation in AP is from the liver and not from another source (e.g., bone)
- Liver function tests (bilirubin, prothrombin time [PT], and albumin) reflect synthetic capacity of the liver
  - Bilirubin is elevated in a variety of hepatocellular and biliary diseases in addition to some nonhepatic causes (e.g., hemolysis)

- PT is prolonged when vitamin K–dependent coagulation factors I, II, V, VII, and X are insufficiently synthesized by the liver. Vitamin K malabsorption in cholestatic liver disease is common.
- Albumin is produced by the liver, has a half-life of 3 weeks, and decreases as synthetic function of the liver fails

Diagnosis: Investigating Elevated Liver Enzymes

- The pattern of elevation dictates the evaluation process and diseases to be considered (Table 29-1)
- A careful history and review of the patient's medications, both prescribed and over the counter, is critical
- Elevated aminotransferases should first be evaluated by serologic and biochemical tests (Fig. 29-1)
- Elevated bilirubin or AP should be evaluated by an ultrasound of the biliary tree and an antimitochondrial antibody (see Fig. 29-1)
- If ascites is present, Doppler studies of hepatic veins should be used to rule out outflow obstruction of the liver (e.g., hepatic vein thrombosis [Budd-Chiari syndrome])
- **Liver biopsy should be considered when diagnostic confirmation is required or if serologic and biochemical tests have not revealed the cause of liver enzyme abnormality**
- Endoscopic retrograde cholangiopancreatography (ERCP) or magnetic resonance cholangiopancreatography (MRCP) can be used to evaluate biliary tract disease
- Computed tomography (CT) scans and magnetic resonance imaging (MRI) can be used in place of or to complement ultrasound

Acute Liver Failure

Basic Information

- *Acute liver failure* (ALF) is defined as hepatocellular dysfunction as evidenced by jaundice with encephalopathy in the setting of no prior liver disease
- Most commonly caused by medications, toxins (mushrooms), or viruses (hepatitis B, herpes)
- **Most commonly implicated drug is acetaminophen, and acetaminophen toxicity is the most common cause of ALF in the United States (40% of reported cases)**
- Other causes of ALF are Wilson disease, Budd-Chiari syndrome, acute fatty liver of pregnancy, autoimmune

TABLE 29-1 *Summary of Common Liver Disorders*

Disease	Liver Test Abnormalities	Diagnostic Testing	Treatment
Autoimmune hepatitis	AST, ALT	ANA, anti–smooth muscle Ab	Prednisone plus azathioprine, transplant
Primary biliary cirrhosis	AP	Antimitochondrial Ab	UDCA, transplant
Primary sclerosing cholangitis	AP	ERCP, p-ANCA	Stenting of strictures, transplant
Alcoholic liver disease	AST/ALT ratio >2:1	History suggestive; improvement with abstention from alcohol	Pentoxifylline, corticosteroids, transplant
Hemochromatosis	AST, ALT	Iron saturation, ferritin, genetic analysis	Transplant
Wilson disease	AST, ALT	AP low, ceruloplasmin low, high 24-hr urine Cu, hepatic Cu high	Chelation, transplant
Hepatitis A	AST, ALT	Anti-HAV IgM	Supportive
Hepatitis B	AST, ALT	HBsAg, anti-HBcAb IgM, HBeAg, HBV DNA	Nucleoside and nucleotide analogues, pegylated interferon alfa, transplant
Hepatitis C	AST, ALT	Anti-HCV, HCV RNA	Interferon, ribavarin, and protease inhibitors, transplant

Ab, antibody; ALT, alanine aminotransferase; ANA, antinuclear antibodies; AP, alkaline phosphatase; AST, aspartate aminotransferase; ERCP, endoscopic retrograde cholangiopancreatography; HAV, hepatitis A virus; HBcAb, hepatitis B core antibody; HBsAg, hepatitis B serum antigen; HBV, hepatis B virus; HCV, hepatitis C virus; HBeAg, hepatitis B early antigen; IgM, immunoglobulin M; p-ANCA, perinuclear antineutrophil cytoplasmic antibody; UDCA, ursodeoxycholic acid.

FIGURE 29-1 Evaluation of elevated liver enzymes. (α_1-AT, α_1-antitrypsin; ALT, alanine aminotransferase; AMA, antimitochondrial antibody; ANA, antinuclear antibody; AST, aspartate aminotransferase; AT, antitrypsin; ERCP, endoscopic retrograde cholangiopancreatography; GGT, γ-glutamyltransferase; MRCP, magnetic resonance cholangiopancreatography; SMA, smooth muscle antibody.)

hepatitis, Reye syndrome, and other idiosyncratic drug reactions (e.g., isoniazid, phenytoin, sulfonamides, propylthiouracil, azoles)
- No specific cause of ALF is identified in approximately 20% of cases

Clinical Presentation

- Patients may present with encephalopathy, which can lead to coma and cerebral edema. Cerebral edema can result in brainstem herniation, which is the leading cause of death in ALF.
- Some patients present with abdominal pain, nausea, lethargy, and massive elevations of serum transaminases (>1000 IU/mL)

- Patients who present with jaundice and then develop encephalopathy after several days have a worse prognosis
- Presentation is often complicated by sepsis, multisystem organ failure (including renal failure and pancreatitis), gastrointestinal bleeding, and coagulopathy
- With progressive coagulopathy, spontaneous hemorrhage is commonly seen
- Widespread hepatocyte necrosis leads to loss of glycogen stores and impaired gluconeogenesis, leading to hypoglycemia

Diagnosis

- Careful history from family and friends, history of toxin exposure, drug use, medications

| TABLE 29-2 | Indicators of Poor Prognosis in Acute Liver Failure (King's College Criteria) |

Acetaminophen Overdose
Arterial pH <7.3 or all of the following:
  PT >100 sec (INR >7.7)
  Cr >3.4 mg/dL
  Grade 3–4 encephalopathy (HE)

Other Causes of ALF
PT >100 sec (INR >7.7) or any three of the following:
  Non-A, non-B hepatitis or drug reaction
  Jaundice >7 days before HE
  Age <10 yr or >40 yr
  PT >50 sec (INR >3.85)
  Bilirubin >17.4 mg/dL

ALF, acute liver failure; Cr, creatinine; HE, hepatic encephalopathy; INR, international normalized ratio; PT, prothrombin time.

- Toxicology screen, including acetaminophen level, should be sent immediately
- Viral serologies, Doppler study of hepatic veins, CT imaging, ceruloplasmin, and 24-hour urinary copper excretion may be helpful in establishing the underlying diagnosis
- Prognosis can be made using King's College criteria (Table 29-2) or the Clichy criteria

Treatment

- Monitor PT, pH, glucose level, liver enzymes, cultures, fluid balance, central venous pressure
- Enteral feeding, dextrose infusion, thiamine
- Prophylactic antibiotics, antifungals
- Proton pump inhibitor or histamine$_2$ receptor antagonist
- **N-Acetylcysteine for all causes, especially acetaminophen toxicity**
- Mechanical ventilation to protect airway in patients with delirium
- Elevate head of bed, hyperventilate initially, induce hypothermia, and mannitol if serum osmolality is less than 320 mOsm to keep intracranial pressure (ICP) low. Avoid procedures that may elevate ICP.
- ICP monitor, when available, should be used to monitor perfusion pressures and ICP
- Continuous venovenous hemofiltration for renal failure
- **Transfuse clotting factors (including recombinant factor VII) only for bleeding or before invasive procedures**
- Disease-specific treatments such as penicillin for mushroom poisoning and acyclovir for herpes hepatitis. Some evidence to support use of acyclovir in idiopathic cases.
- Transfer to transplantation center as soon as possible

Drug-Induced Hepatitis

Basic Information

- 5% of all adverse drug reactions involve the liver
- Approximately 20% to 30% of acute liver failures are drug induced
- Reactions can be dose dependent or idiosyncratic

| TABLE 29-3 | Hepatic Injury Caused by Various Medications |

Injury Pattern	Drug
Nonspecific or viral-like hepatitis	Aspirin, amiodarone, diclofenac, isoniazid, methyldopa, nitrofurantoin, phenytoin, propylthiouracil, sulfonamides
Cholestasis	Carbamazepine, chlorpromazine, co-trimoxazole, haloperidol, tricyclics, estrogens, 17-alpha–substituted steroids
Steatosis	Alcohol, prednisone, tetracycline, valproic acid, amiodarone, zidovudine
Granulomatous hepatitis	Allopurinol, quinidine, sulfonamides, sulfonylurea agents
Veno-occlusive disease	Antineoplastics, azathioprine, pyrrolizidine alkaloids
Adenomas and hepatocellular carcinoma	Estrogens and anabolic steroids

| TABLE 29-4 | Liver Monitoring Schedule for Hepatotoxic Medications |

Medication	Every Month	Every Month for 3 Months, then Every 3 Months	Every 3 Months
Amiodarone			✓
Antiepileptics			✓
Azathioprine	✓		
Diclofenac			✓
HMG-CoA reductase inhibitors			✓
Herbal remedies			✓
All conazoles (e.g., fluconazole)	✓		
Nicotinic acid		✓	
NSAIDs (other)			✓ (3–6 mo)
Tacrine		✓	
Protease inhibitors	✓		

HMG-CoA, 3-hydroxy-3-methylglutaryl coenzyme A; NSAIDs, nonsteroidal anti-inflammatory drugs.

Clinical Presentation

- Usually asymptomatic
- Can follow several patterns of injury: hepatitis, cholestasis, cholestatic hepatitis, and progressive bile duct injury known as "vanishing bile duct syndrome." Some cases can be immune-mediated and hypereosinophilia is present (both in serum and on liver biopsy).
- Most biochemical parameters return to normal after eliminating the offending drug
- Injury pattern can give clue to offending agent (Table 29-3)
- Several medications require regular monitoring (Table 29-4)

Diagnosis

- Thorough history is critical to diagnosis
- Temporal relationship to medication use is critical to the diagnosis
- Rechallenging the patient with the suspected drug is not recommended

Treatment

- Discontinue medication and do not rechallenge
- Biopsy liver if enzymes do not normalize within several weeks or if diagnosis is in question
- Transfer to transplantation center if liver failure ensues (jaundice and encephalopathy)

Herbal Remedies and Natural Products

Basic Information

- Increased use of herbal remedies has led to recognition of potential hepatotoxicity
- Few over-the-counter agents have been put through any rigorous scientific testing
- **Most reactions are idiosyncratic, although some are dose dependent**

Clinical Presentation

- Elevated aminotransferases are the most common presentation
- Can also present with ascites and/or hepatomegaly
- Eosinophilia and rash can be seen
- Cirrhosis or liver failure can occur with ongoing use of offending agent
- Table 29-5 lists herbs and associated hepatic injuries

TABLE 29-5	Herbs and Associated Hepatic Injuries	
Remedy	**Toxic Component**	**Injury**
Gordolobo yerba tea, comfrey	Pyrrolizidine alkaloids	Veno-occlusive disease
Chinese herbal tea	Compositae	Veno-occlusive disease
Jin Bu Huan	*Lycopodium serratum*	Acute hepatitis, steatosis
Germander	Teucrin A	Hepatitis
Chaparral leaf	*Larrea tridentata*	Necrosis, chronic hepatitis
Mistletoe, skullcap, valerian	Unknown	Hepatitis
Natural laxatives	Senna, podophyllin	Elevated aminotransferases
Dai-saiko-to and Sho-saiko-to	*Scutellaria* and others	Hepatitis, fibrosis, steatosis
Kava kava	Kavalactones	Hepatitis

Diagnosis

- Thorough history (patients do not think of herbs as medicines)
- Exclude other forms of liver disease. Liver biopsy findings are often nonspecific.

Treatment

- Discontinue herbal medication and do not rechallenge
- Monitor liver enzymes and biopsy liver if they do not normalize within several weeks

Autoimmune Hepatitis

Basic Information

- Autoimmune hepatitis (AIH) is a diagnosis of exclusion when nonviral, immune-mediated hepatocellular injury is present
- **Should be considered when liver enzymes are elevated and patient has negative viral serologies and no drug injury is implicated**
- Cause of AIH is not known, but pathogenesis likely involves genetic susceptibility with etiologic trigger such as viral infection or medication
- Variant, overlapping, or mixed forms of AIH exist that share features with other autoimmune diseases, such as primary biliary cirrhosis and primary sclerosing cholangitis

Clinical Presentation

- Two established forms of AIH with different autoantibodies (Table 29-6)
  - Both are more common in women, with age of onset in third to fourth decades of life
- Range of presentation varies from mild enzyme elevations to liver failure
- Nonspecific fatigue, lethargy, abdominal pain, rash, and arthralgias may be present
- Concomitant autoimmune diseases (thyroiditis, type 1 diabetes, systemic lupus erythematosus, Sjögren syndrome) are common
- Liver enzyme elevations tend to wax and wane

Diagnosis

- Elevated liver enzymes with negative hepatitis serologies, elevated gamma globulin (especially immunoglobulin G [IgG])

TABLE 29-6	Serologic Features of Autoimmune Hepatitis Variants	
Serologic Features	**Type 1**	**Type 2**
Smooth muscle antibodies	±	−
Antinuclear antibodies	±	−
Liver kidney microsomal antibody	−	+
Anti-actin	±	−
Anti-liver cytosol-1	−	±
Soluble liver antigen/liver pancreas	±	−

29

- Supported by histologic pattern of interface hepatitis, plasma cell infiltrate, and portal tract inflammation
- Autoantibodies usually but not invariably present (see Table 29-6)

Treatment

- Treatment indicated in patients with ALT ≥10 times normal; ALT ≥5 times normal, and gamma globulin ≥2 times normal; or significant inflammation and/or necrosis on liver biopsy
- **Prednisone with or without azathioprine for at least 18 to 36 months (many patients require lifelong therapy)**
- 30% of patients not responsive to this regimen and require more potent immunosuppressives (mycophenolate mofetil, cyclosporine, or tacrolimus)
- Treatment progress is followed by monitoring transaminases, gamma globulin, and liver biopsies
- Presence of soluble liver kidney antibody and human leukocyte antigen (HLA) DR3 haplotype associated with inability to completely wean from immunosuppressive therapy
- Consider liver transplantation for decompensated cirrhosis
- 30% recurrence rate after transplantation

Primary Biliary Cirrhosis

Basic Information

- Immune-mediated destruction of small bile ducts
- Genetic predisposition plus triggering event such as viral infection or medication underlie many cases
- Prevalence in North America is 2 per 100,000
- 6% prevalence in first-degree relatives

Clinical Presentation

- Mean age at diagnosis is 55 years
- **90% of patients are women**
- **Intermittent pruritus, fatigue, and abdominal pain; jaundice late in disease**
- Progresses over 5 to 15 years from diagnosis
- Impaired fat-soluble vitamin (A, D, E, K) absorption leading to osteomalacia, night blindness, etc.
- Elevated total cholesterol without increased cardiac risk (mostly high-density lipoprotein)
- Can lead to cirrhosis, portal hypertension, and hepatocellular carcinoma (HCC)

Diagnosis

- AP almost always elevated
- Aminotransferases typically mildly elevated
- Antimitochondrial antibody is present in 97% of cases
- Antinuclear antibody is also positive in most cases
- Liver biopsy reveals portal tract infiltrates and bile duct injury (Fig. 29-2)

Treatment

- Ursodeoxycholic acid (UDCA, 12–15 mg/kg/day) improves transplant-free survival, improves liver chemistries, and slows histologic progression

- UDCA works by increasing canalicular excretion of toxic bile acids, inhibiting intestinal bile acid reabsorption, and scavenging reactive oxygen species
- Corticosteroids, colchicine, and other immunosuppressants may improve liver chemistries but do not alter disease progression and should not be recommended
- Liver transplantation should be considered once cirrhosis and jaundice develop. The 5-year post-transplantation survival rate is 80% (among the highest for all liver diseases).

Primary Sclerosing Cholangitis

Basic Information

- Autoimmune disease typically seen in young men
- Progressive inflammatory destruction of medium and large bile ducts
- **Most cases (80%) are associated with inflammatory bowel disease, typically ulcerative colitis (UC)**
  - 10% of patients with UC have primary sclerosing cholangitis (PSC)
  - Increased risk of colon cancer in patients with UC and PSC (more than UC alone)
- Increased risk of cholangiocarcinoma
- Prevalence is 1 to 6 per 100,000 in the United States

Clinical Presentation

- Generally asymptomatic but can present with abdominal pain, jaundice, cholangitis, or pruritus
- Mean age at presentation is 30 to 40 years
- Progresses over a mean of 12 years from diagnosis

Diagnosis

- AP is usually elevated, with mild elevation of aminotransferases
- Bilirubin is typically normal, except when common hepatic duct or common bile duct is involved and in late stages of disease
- Diagnosis made by ERCP or MRCP, which demonstrates strictures or beading of the intrahepatic or extrahepatic bile ducts (Fig. 29-3)

FIGURE 29-2 Primary biliary cirrhosis. Note the portal tract inflammation and injury to the bile duct. *(From Kumar V, Fausto N, Abbas A: Robbins and Cotran's pathologic basis of disease, ed 7, Philadelphia, Elsevier Saunders, 2005, Fig. 18-31.)*

FIGURE 29-3 **A,** Primary sclerosing cholangitis. **B,** Endoscopic retrograde cholangiopancreatography showing beading and strictures of the intrahepatic ducts (*arrow*). *(From Feldman M: Sleisenger and Fordtran's gastrointestinal and liver disease, ed 8, Philadelphia, Elsevier Saunders, 2006, Fig. 65-1.)*

- Liver biopsy typically shows pericholangitis and periductular fibrosis but is often not diagnostic in early disease
- Perinuclear antineutrophil cytoplasmic antibody (p-ANCA) positive in two thirds of cases

Treatment

- High-dose (25–28 mg/kg/day) UDCA may actually hasten development of portal hypertension and should not be recommended. Low-dose UDCA has no proven benefit.
- Periodic dilation of strictures via ERCP or percutaneous approach may be necessary
- Annual screening for colon cancer in patients with concomitant UC
- Annual screening for cholangiocarcinoma with serum cancer antigen (CA) 19-9 and MRI/MRCP
- Liver transplantation should be offered to those with advanced liver disease or repeated bouts of cholangitis
- Disease can recur after transplantation

Alcoholic Liver Disease (Alcoholic Hepatitis)

Basic Information

- Chronic liver disease occurs in 15% to 20% of alcoholics
- Variables leading to higher likelihood of alcoholic liver disease include malnutrition and obesity, female gender, concomitant drug toxicity, and coexisting viral hepatitis
- Pathophysiology related to increased reactive oxygen species and inflammatory cytokines (tumor necrosis factor-α)—this is the rationale for anti-inflammatory therapy (see later discussion)

Clinical Presentation

- Physical examination in acute alcoholic hepatitis can reveal fever, malnutrition, jaundice, encephalopathy, tremor, parotid gland enlargement, hepatomegaly, right upper quadrant pain, ascites, spider nevi, and leukocytosis
- Tender hepatomegaly can occur secondary to fatty infiltration
- Can present with portal hypertension and ascites as disease progresses; hepatorenal syndrome is a frequent cause of death in severe acute alcoholic liver disease

Diagnosis

- History of alcohol use (at least 20–40 g/day for 10 years or longer)
- **Patients present with elevated aminotransferases, often with AST/ALT ratio greater than 2:1**
- Bilirubin and PT may be elevated
- GGT and red blood cell mean cell volume are often elevated
- Liver biopsy can be used to stage fibrosis and exclude other forms of liver disease
- Histopathology reveals acute (neutrophilic) and chronic (lymphocytic) inflammatory infiltrate, steatosis, steatonecrosis, or cirrhosis
- Mallory bodies are a classic finding on biopsy but are not specific for alcoholic liver disease

Treatment

- Abstinence is the most crucial component of therapy
- Adequate nutrition is important, although survival benefits using enteral nutrition or parenteral nutrition have not been shown
- Corticosteroids may be of modest benefit in improving short-term survival (see later discussion)
  - The discriminant function (DF), = 4.6 × [PT − control (in seconds)] + serum bilirubin (in mg/dL), determines the need for corticosteroid therapy
  - Score of greater than 32 predicts a greater than 50% 30-day mortality rate and is used to indicate the need for corticosteroid therapy
  - **Long-term survival benefits of corticosteroids have not been shown**
  - Steroids are not recommended for patients with concomitant infection or poorly controlled diabetes
- Pentoxifylline 400 mg three times daily improves short-term survival by decreasing the risk of hepatorenal syndrome and should be considered as a surrogate for

prednisone in patients with severe alcoholic hepatitis (DF >32) in addition to volume repletion, nutritional support, thiamine, and a proton pump inhibitor. Pentoxifylline is not approved by the Food and Drug Administration (FDA) for this indication.
- Nephrotoxins should be carefully avoided (including contrast dye)
- Liver transplantation may be considered if a patient has abstained from alcohol use for the period of time required by the local transplantation program (usually at least 6 months)
- Reversal of portal hypertension and remarkable clinical improvement can be seen after prolonged abstinence

Nonalcoholic Fatty Liver Disease

Basic Information

- **Most common liver disorder causing elevated liver enzymes in the United States**
- Histologically similar to alcoholic liver disease
- Occurs in up to 33% of the U.S. population
- Spectrum of disease ranging from benign hepatic steatosis to steatohepatitis, and can progress to fibrosis and cirrhosis
- **Up to one third of patients with nonalcoholic fatty liver disease (NAFLD) can progress to cirrhosis by the fifth or sixth decade of life**
- Projected to be the leading indication for liver transplantation in the United States by 2025

Clinical Presentation

- The main risk factor is coexisting features of the metabolic syndrome, most notably obesity and diabetes mellitus, but several other risk factors exist (Box 29-1). Insulin resistance is the hallmark of the disease.
- Aminotransferases can be elevated severalfold
- Hepatomegaly typically presents with signs of portal hypertension in more advanced disease

Diagnosis

- Heavy alcohol use should be ruled out by history
- Imaging with ultrasound, CT scan, or MRI often reveals hepatomegaly and suggests fatty infiltration. Ultrasound is limited by body habitus, but is less expensive.
- Liver chemistry elevation pattern not typically helpful in diagnosis
- Histology is the key to diagnosis, revealing either steatosis or steatonecrosis with or without fibrosis (Fig. 29-4)

Treatment

- Weight loss, strict glucose control, treatment of hypertension, and lipid control are recommended (cardiac disease is the leading cause of death in patients with NAFLD)
- Vitamin E (800 IU daily) proven benefit over placebo at improving liver enzymes and reducing hepatic inflammation; the benefit of vitamin E is unknown in diabetics and cirrhotics
- Insulin sensitizers and lipid-lowering agents have not conclusively shown benefit

BOX 29-1 *Risk Factors for Nonalcoholic Fatty Liver Disease*

Obesity
Diabetes mellitus
Hyperlipidemia
Jejunoileal bypass and rapid weight loss
Prolonged total parenteral nutrition
Small bowel bacterial overgrowth
Advanced HIV/AIDS with lipodystrophy
Medications
    Amiodarone
    Corticosteroids
    Tamoxifen
    Perihexiline maleate
    Tetracycline
    Calcium channel blockers
    Methotrexate

FIGURE 29-4 Nonalcoholic fatty liver disease. Liver biopsy specimen showing diffuse steatosis and focal inflammation and necrosis. *(From Feldman M: Sleisenger and Fordtran's gastrointestinal and liver disease, ed 8, Philadelphia, Elsevier Saunders, 2006, Fig. 82-3.)*

- Potentially-offending medications should be discontinued
- Liver transplantation can be an effective option, although risk of recurrence is significant if risk factors remain

Hereditary Hemochromatosis

Basic Information

- Most common autosomal recessive disease of whites, with 1/10 carrier rate
- Mutant *HFE* gene identified on chromosome 6
- **Disease may be present in homozygotes with the *C282Y* or *H63D* mutation, variable penetrance in compound heterozygotes**

- Pathogenesis involves increased intestinal iron absorption, possibly due to decreased production of the hepatic hormone hepcidin, resulting in hepatic accumulation of iron

Clinical Presentation

- Typically presents in men in the fourth to sixth decade of life and in postmenopausal women
- Nonspecific elevation of liver enzymes
- **In addition to the liver, the joints (caused by calcium pyrophosphate deposition), pituitary gland, testes, pancreas, and heart can be affected**
- Symptoms typically include weakness, fatigue, myalgias, arthralgias, loss of libido
- Hepatomegaly may be present, especially early in disease
- As disease advances, patients can develop skin pigmentation, diabetes, cardiomyopathy, or conduction abnormalities
- HCC risk is significant, especially once cirrhosis develops

Diagnosis

- Elevated transferrin saturation greater than 50% and ferritin greater than 300 mg/L are present in more than 95% of cases
- *HFE* mutational analysis to detect *C282Y* or *H63D* mutations
- Liver biopsy for quantification of iron per gram of dry liver weight remains the gold standard; values greater than 71 mmol/g are highly suggestive
- First-degree family members need screening, either through serum transferrin saturation and ferritin or by genetic testing

Treatment

- Phlebotomy of 1 unit of blood weekly until ferritin level falls from more than 200 mg/L to 10 to 20 mg/L, followed by maintenance phlebotomy every several weeks as needed to keep the ferritin below 50 mg/L
- Iron chelation with deferoxamine is an alternative when phlebotomy is restricted by anemia
- Liver transplantation can be considered once cirrhosis has developed.

α₁-Antitrypsin Deficiency

Basic Information

- 1 in 600 births
- Common in patients with Northern European ancestry
- Mutation in α₁-antitrypsin (AAT), a protein that prevents protease enzymes such as elastin from degrading normal host tissue; mutated protein is abnormally folded and cannot exit hepatocytes
- Absolute deficiency of AAT leads to lung disease, and relative deficiency leads to liver and/or lung disease

Clinical Presentation

- Can present with elevated liver enzymes, hepatomegaly, or cirrhosis in children and adults
- Panacinar emphysema may be present alone or in addition to cirrhosis
- May also be associated with panniculitis and Wegener granulomatosis
- Patients are at high risk for the development of HCC

Diagnosis

- Reduced serum levels of AAT
- Phenotype analysis and liver biopsy are key to diagnosis if levels are found to be low
- Phenotype ZZ most typically seen with advanced liver disease
- Liver biopsy positive for periodic acid–Schiff, diastase-resistant globules

Treatment

- IV infusions of AAT derived from pooled plasma or obtained by recombinant DNA methods are under investigation for treatment of pulmonary disease but have not been successfully used for liver disease
- **Liver transplantation is the only viable therapy for the liver disease component and is curative**

Wilson Disease

Basic Information

- Autosomal recessive disorder of copper metabolism
- Defective mobilization of copper from liver resulting in accumulation in the liver, brain, and eyes
- 1 in 30,000 live births

Clinical Presentation

- Typically presents before the age of 40 years
- Can present with Coombs-negative hemolytic anemia, elevated liver chemistries, cholestatic jaundice, or acute liver failure
- AP often inappropriately low
- Some cases present with neurologic abnormalities, including psychosis, coma, or movement disorders

Diagnosis

- Consider in any young patient with acute hepatitis, jaundice, or hemolysis
- **Kayser-Fleischer rings are nearly 100% sensitive if neurologic abnormalities are present (Fig. 29-5)**
- Serum ceruloplasmin is typically low but may be normal because it is an acute-phase reactant
- 24-hour urine copper level greater than 100 µg
- Liver biopsy for quantification of copper revealing greater than 200 µg/g of dry liver weight is the gold standard

Treatment

- Oral chelation with D-penicillamine or trientine is generally used as primary therapy
- Oral zinc may be used to inhibit copper absorption and prevent reaccumulation after treatment with penicillamine or trientine
- Transplantation is curative and should be offered to patients with advanced or acute fulminant disease

Pregnancy-Related Liver Disease

Basic Information

- Complicates less than 0.1% of pregnancies
- Several different disease processes but no clearly defined causes

29

- All tend to be recurrent in subsequent pregnancies except acute fatty liver of pregnancy
- **Children of mothers who had preeclampsia, HELLP (hemolysis, elevated liver enzymes, and low platelet count) syndrome, or acute fatty liver of pregnancy should be screened for long-chain 3-hydroxyacyl coenzyme A dehydrogenase (LCHAD) deficiency because this may be the underlying etiology**

Clinical Presentation

See Table 29-7 for a summary of liver diseases of pregnancy.

Diagnosis

See Table 29-7.

FIGURE 29-5 Kayser-Fleischer ring in a patient with Wilson disease. Note the brown-green pigment around the cornea. *(From Goldman, L, Bennett JC, Aussiello D: Cecil textbook of medicine, ed 22, Philadelphia, WB Saunders, 2004, Fig. 224-1.)*

Treatment

See Table 29-7.

Viral Hepatitis

Overview

- Several human hepatotropic viruses exist, the most significant being hepatitis A, B, and C
- Hepatitis A is commonly found in developing countries with occasional outbreaks in the United States
- Hepatitis B is the most common chronic viral hepatitis worldwide
- Hepatitis C is the most common in the United States

HEPATITIS A

Basic Information

- 38% of the U.S. population has positive antibodies for past infection
- Incubation period of 2 to 6 weeks

Clinical Presentation

- Fecal-oral spread
- Nausea, vomiting, diarrhea
- Children usually are asymptomatic, but adults are often jaundiced
- **Fatal disease can occur in older patients and in those with chronic liver disease, but most cases are self-limited**
- Never becomes chronic, but cases of relapsing and cholestatic disease can occur

Diagnosis

- Acute disease is diagnosed by serum anti–hepatitis A virus (HAV) immunoglobulin M (IgM)
- Immunity conferred by presence of anti-HAV IgG

TABLE 29-7	*Liver Diseases of Pregnancy*				
Disease	**Symptoms/Signs**	**Lab(s)**	**Treatment**	**Mortality Risk: Mother/Fetus**
Hyperemesis gravidarum	N/V, dehydration in 1st trimester	Bilirubin up to 5 × normal AST/ALT 2–3 × normal	Antiemetics, hydration	–/– (Resolves spontaneously)
Intrahepatic cholestasis of pregnancy	Pruritus, jaundice in 2nd or 3rd trimester	Bilirubin up to 10 × normal AST/ALT up to 1000	Cholestyramine, UDCA; deliver if fetal distress	–/Low
Preeclampsia/eclampsia	N/V, HTN, edema, seizures/coma in late 2nd or 3rd trimester	Bilirubin normal AST/ALT can be >1000	Treat HTN and edema; magnesium sulfate; deliver in severe cases	+/Low
HELLP syndrome	RUQ pain, N/V, HTN, edema in late 2nd or 3rd trimester	Bilirubin up to 20 × normal AST/ALT can be >1000 Low haptoglobin Platelets <100 K	Delivery	+/+
Acute fatty liver of pregnancy	RUQ pain, N/V, fatigue, jaundice, hepatomegaly in 3rd trimester	Bilirubin up to 20 × normal AST/ALT up to >1000 Hyperammonemia Azotemia Disseminated intravascular coagulation can develop	Delivery	+/+
Hepatic rupture	Severe abdominal pain, shock in 3rd trimester	Variable	Immediate surgery	+/+

ALT, alanine aminotransferase; AST, aspartate aminotransferase; HELLP, hemolysis, elevated liver enzymes, and low platelet count; HTN, hypertension; N/V, nausea/vomiting; RUQ, right upper quadrant; UDCA, ursodeoxycholic acid.

Treatment

- Supportive care
- **Vaccinate those at risk of exposure, including close contacts of index case**
- Vaccinate travelers to endemic areas, military workers, IV drug users, those with chronic liver disease
- **Immune globulin can be given for passive protection before or within 2 weeks of exposure**

HEPATITIS B

Basic Information

- 5% of U.S. population has serologic markers of past infection, with chronic infection in 0.7%
- More than 400 million people infected worldwide
- **Incubation period of 6 weeks to 6 months**
- Transmitted parenterally and by sexual contact
- **High risk for vertical transmission**

TABLE 29-8		Serologic Diagnosis of Hepatitis B		
HBsAg	**HBsAb**	**HBcAb IgM**	**HBcAb IgG**	**Disease Pattern**
+	−	+	−	Acute infection
+	−	−	+	Chronic or late acute infection
−	−	+	−	Acute infection or window before HBcAb seroconversion (or HBsAb conversion)
−	+	−	+	Past infection
−	+	−	−	Immunized against hepatitis B or remote infection

HBcAb, hepatitis B core antibody; HBsAb, hepatitis B surface antibody; HBsAg, hepatitis B surface antigen; IgG, immunoglobulin G; IgM, immunoglobulin M.

- Likelihood of chronic infection inversely related to age at time of infection

Clinical Presentation

- Symptomatic disease (e.g., abdominal pain, nausea, jaundice) occurs in only 25% of adults
- Many are chronic "carriers" with normal liver chemistries and no evidence of or low levels of viral replication
- The vast majority of adults infected will clear virus spontaneously, whereas 5% develop chronic hepatitis and 1% fulminant hepatitis
- Death caused by HCC and cirrhosis particularly high in those infected as neonates; HCC risk high even in those without cirrhosis
- Reactivation in the setting of immunosuppression (i.e., chemotherapy) may occur in patients who have had prior exposure to hepatitis B (hepatitis B core antibody [HBcAb] IgG positive)
- Extrahepatic manifestations
  - Polyarteritis nodosa that may improve with antiviral therapy
  - Membranous nephropathy or membranoproliferative glomerulonephritis

Diagnosis

- Based on serologic patterns (Table 29-8)
- **Hepatitis B surface antigen (HBsAg) is the first positive marker of acute infection (Fig. 29-6). It usually disappears within 6 months but persists in chronic disease.**
- Screening for chronic infection should utilize HBsAg
- Anti-HBcAb IgM positive with acute infection, whereas anti-HBcAb IgG indicates past infection
- Hepatitis B early antigen (HBeAg) positivity indicates active replication, although this is negative in some strains
- Hepatitis B virus (HBV) DNA positivity indicates active replication and presence of the disease. HBV DNA viral load correlates with risk of HCC.

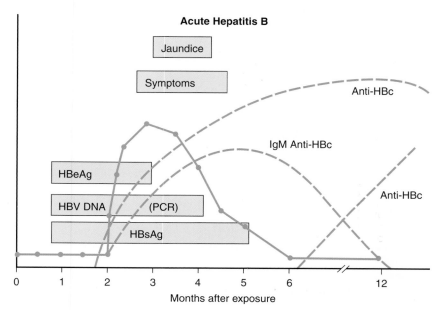

Acute Hepatitis B

FIGURE 29-6 Serologic response to acute hepatitis B infection. (HBc, hepatitis B core antigen; HBeAg, hepatitis B early antigen; HBsAg, hepatitis B serum antigen; HBV, hepatitis B virus; IgM, immunoglobulin M; PCR, polymerase chain reaction.)

- **Presence of anti-HBV surface antibody denotes immunity**
- To determine presence of viral replication in chronic infection, check HBeAg and HBV DNA

Treatment

- Pegylated interferon alfa, lamivudine, adefovir, entecavir, tenofovir, and telbivudine are all FDA approved for treatment of chronic hepatitis B. Entecavir and tenofovir are associated with the most impressive reduction in viral load and lack of resistance.
- Interferon alfa may provide a more durable response but is quite expensive and is associated with more side effects than the others (e.g., flu-like symptoms, cytopenias, elevated liver tests, mood changes)
- **Treatment indicated in HBeAg-negative patients with HBV DNA greater than 2000 IU/mL, in HBeAg-postive patients with HBV DNA greater than 20,000 IU/mL, or liver enzymes greater than 5× the upper limit of normal, or active necroinflammatory disease on liver biopsy**

HEPATITIS C

Basic Information

- RNA virus with incubation from 2 to 26 weeks
- Chronic infections occur in 75% to 85% of cases
- Leads to cirrhosis in 20% to 50% of those infected, usually after about 20 years
- Heavy alcohol use, obesity, or coinfection with HIV accelerates progression of fibrosis
- Most common hepatotropic viral infection in America, with an estimated 4 million anti–hepatitis C virus (HCV) positive
- Risk factors for hepatitis C include IV drug use, transfusions before 1990, high-risk sexual behavior, dialysis, and hemophilia

Clinical Presentation

- Acute disease is often asymptomatic, although profound hepatitis occurs rarely
- Common symptoms of chronic infection include fatigue and periodic right upper quadrant discomfort
- May be complicated by HCC once cirrhosis develops (2–5% risk per year)
- Extrahepatic manifestations include cryoglobulinemia, vasculitis, glomerulonephritis, porphyria cutanea tarda, cardiomyopathy, and lymphoma

Diagnosis

- Hepatitis C antibody develops within 6 months of infection
- Diagnosis of persistent or past infection indicated by anti-HCV positivity
- Aminotransferases may be normal, periodically elevated, or persistently elevated to any degree
  - Aminotransferase levels should not be used as an indication of presence or absence of disease (one third of infected patients will have normal liver enzymes)
- Active viral replication determined by presence of serum RNA
- Most commonly used test to detect RNA is polymerase chain reaction (PCR)

- Liver biopsy is a useful tool to stage disease and render prognosis
- Strain or genotype of the virus and the viral load should be determined if therapy is considered
- Genotype 1 is associated with reduced responsiveness to therapy and is the most common

Treatment

- Standard of care for genotype 1 infection is pegylated interferon, ribavirin, and either telaprevir or boceprevir
- Standard of care for genotype 2 and 3 is pegylated interferon and ribavirin with or without a protease inhibitor for 6 to 12 months, depending on genotype and response to treatment
- Genetic polymorphisms at the interferon locus (IL28b) predict responsiveness to treatment. The CC phenotype is associated with the highest reponse rates and is most common in patients with European ancestry. The TT phenotype is associated with the lowest response rates and is most common in patients with African ancestry.
- **If serum RNA persists after 6 months of therapy, there is nearly no likelihood of cure**
- Multiple side effects exist with therapy, including flu-like symptoms, depression, anemia, thrombocytopenia, leukopenia, rash, and teratogenicity
- Multiple new therapies that directly target the replication machinery of the virus are in development. Sustained viral clearence after treatment with these agents in conjunction with pegylated interferon and ribavirin is greater than 75%.

HEPATITIS D

Basic Information

- Hepatitis D is partial RNA virus and requires the presence of HBV surface antigen for infection and replication

Clinical Presentation

- Can coinfect or superinfect with HBV
- In superinfection, disease is more severe with higher rates of cirrhosis and liver failure
- More common in Mediterranean countries and the Far East

Diagnosis

- Can be diagnosed by presence of hepatitis D virus antigen or anti-HDV
- PCR test available only through research laboratories

Treatment

- Modest benefit from treatment with interferon; however, it is currently recommended because of lack of other effective therapies. Nucleoside or nucleotide analogues used for hepatitis B are not effective.

HEPATITIS E

Basic Information

- RNA virus transmitted by contaminated water supply
- Endemic in India and parts of Asia although increasingly common in the United States
- Two to 8 weeks' incubation

Clinical Presentation

- Generally mild acute disease and often subclinical
- Rarely fatal except in late pregnancy, when mortality can reach 20%
- Disease is never chronic

Diagnosis

- Anti–hepatitis E virus (HEV) IgM and IgG
- Suspect disease in patient presenting with acute hepatitis or unexplained hepatitis/cholestasis and recent travel to endemic areas

Treatment

- Supportive
- Vaccine is in development
- Liver transplantation should be considered for fulminant disease

Liver Lesions

Overview

- Focal lesions of the liver are found frequently, and often incidentally, during abdominal imaging studies for other disorders
- It is important to diagnose these lesions accurately, if possible. Imaging often the key to diagnosis.
- In addition to hepatic malignancy, there are two broad categories of liver lesions: cysts or abscesses, and other benign conditions

Cysts and Abscesses

- Simple cysts (solitary or a few cysts) are found in about 1% of the adult population and are usually congenital and benign
  - Tend to have a uniform fluid density and a thin, regular wall without mass effect or complexity
  - Hydatid cysts are diagnosed by the presence of daughter cysts and the presence of echinococcal serologies. May be calcified.
  - Aspiration of simple cysts usually results in recurrence of the fluid, and needle aspiration of hydatid cyst is contraindicated due to the risk of tracking or rupture
- Hepatic abscesses are usually associated with fever, right upper quadrant pain, or other systemic signs of infection. Typically the sequela of a colonic/intestinal infection.
  - May be pyogenic or amebic
  - Sonogram-guided needle aspiration of pyogenic abscesses can help guide antibiotic treatment and allow placement of a percutaneous catheter for large abscesses
  - Surgery rarely needed
  - Amebic abscesses are usually difficult to diagnose with aspiration and frequently respond to metronidazole treatment

Other Benign Lesions

- Hemangioma
  - Most frequent benign lesion of the liver; occurs in about 4% of the population

- Complications and need for intervention are rare unless they achieve a large size (>5 cm) with replacement of a significant part of the hepatic parenchyma. In such cases, resection may be indicated.
  - Diagnosis requires sonogram, triphasic CT, or MRI, with occasional use of technetium-99m–tagged red blood cell single-photon emission CT (SPECT) studies
- Focal nodular hyperplasia
  - Occurs in 0.4% of the population
  - Lesions have a characteristic central stellate scar that may be seen on sonogram, CT, or MRI
  - Liver biopsies tend to be nondiagnostic, but occasional use of sulfur-colloid hepatic scans is helpful because these lesions contain nonparenchymal cells that take up the sulfur-colloid particles, leading to a contrast pattern equivalent to the hepatic parenchyma (i.e., a disappearing mass lesion)
  - **Treatment or surgical intervention is not required, except in rare cases of diagnostic uncertainty; no risk of malignancy**
  - Not caused by oral contraceptives, but may grow in response to estrogen
- Hepatic adenoma
  - A rare benign tumor, most often seen in the setting of oral contraceptive use in women of childbearing age; has the ability to transform to HCC
  - Can occasionally be associated with diabetes mellitus, glycogen storage disease, or pregnancy
  - Large lesions can cause pain, intraperitoneal bleeding, and occasionally a "mass effect" with replacement of an entire lobe
  - Surgical resection or liver transplantation in extreme cases has been used effectively. Discontinuation of any offending agents (e.g., oral contraceptives, anabolic steroids, etc.) is a cornerstone of treatment. Regular follow-up with imaging studies is recommended to monitor any changes, including malignant degeneration. Surgery often recommended for lesions greater than 4 to 5 cm, due to risk of malignant degeneration.

REVIEW QUESTIONS

For review questions, please go to www.expertconsult.com.

SUGGESTED READINGS

David S, Hamilton JP: Drug induced liver disease, *US Gastroenterol Hepatol Rev* 6:73–80, 2010.

de Alwis NM, Day CP: Non-alcoholic fatty liver disease: the mist gradually clears, *J Hepatol* 48(Suppl 1):S104–S112, 2008.

Ghany MG, Strader DB, et al: Diagnosis, management, and treatment of hepatitis C: an update, *Hepatology* 49:1335–1374, 2009.

Lok ASF, McMahon BJ: Chronic hepatitis B, *Hepatology* 45:507–539, 2007.

Mann MP, Czaja AJ, et al: Diagnosis and management of autoimmune hepatitis, *Hepatology* 51:1–31, 2010.

Seeff LB: Herbal hepatotoxicity, *Clin Liver Dis* 11:577–596, 2007.

Su GL: Pregnancy and liver disease, *Curr Gastroenterol Rep* 10:15–21, 2008.

Complications of Liver Disease

JAMES P. HAMILTON, MD

In the previous chapter, a number of causes of liver disease were described. This chapter focuses on the consequences that can result from those disease entities. Morbidity and mortality from cirrhosis can result from numerous different processes, including infection (spontaneous bacterial peritonitis), encephalopathy, renal failure (hepatorenal syndrome), pulmonary disease, and hepatocellular carcinoma. Liver transplantation offers the only cure.

Overview of Cirrhosis

- Definitions
  - Hepatic fibrosis is a reversible wound-healing response characterized by accumulation of extracellular matrix made up of collagen fibrils
  - **Cirrhosis is defined by global hepatic fibrosis and reduced hepatic synthetic function**
- Pathophysiology
  - Chronic inflammation leads to activation of hepatic stellate cells and is the critical event in the pathogenesis of hepatic fibrosis. These perisinusoidal cells lead to deposition of scar tissue with subsequent vascular and organ contraction.
- Causes: see Table 30-1
- Clinical consequences of cirrhosis: see Table 30-2

Portal Hypertension and Varices

Basic Information

- Definition
  - The most common and morbid consequence of liver disease and cirrhosis
  - **Complications of portal hypertension begin to develop when portal pressure reaches values ≥12 mm Hg (normal, up to 7 mm Hg)**
  - Direct measurement of portal pressure is difficult, but indirect measurement of the hepatic vein pressure gradient (HVPG) is possible by catheterizing the hepatic vein
- Classification of portal hypertension (Fig. 30-1)
  - Presinusoidal: Obstruction proximal to hepatic sinusoids
    - Prehepatic (e.g., splanchnic arteriovenous fistula, splenic vein thrombosis, portal vein thrombosis [idiopathic or associated with hypercoagulable states])
    - Hepatic (e.g., schistosomiasis, sarcoidosis, myeloproliferative disorders)
  - Sinusoidal: Results from chronic liver disease

- Postsinusoidal: Obstruction distal to the hepatic sinusoids
  - Posthepatic (e.g., inferior vena cava obstruction, Budd-Chiari syndrome [hepatic vein thrombosis often associated with hypercoagulable states], cardiac disease)
  - Hepatic (e.g., veno-occlusive disease, perivenular/hepatoportal sclerosis)

Clinical Presentation

- The major complication of portal hypertension is development of portosystemic collaterals, the most clinically significant of which are gastroesophageal varices (Fig. 30-2) and hemorrhoids
- For other clinical consequences of portal hypertension, see Table 30-2

Diagnosis

- Laboratory studies should focus on evaluation of hepatic synthetic function, renal function, and hematologic values. Thrombocytopenia usually develops from splenic sequestration.
- Radiographic studies may aid in the diagnosis and treatment of various conditions
- **Patients with cirrhosis should be screened for varices every 1 to 2 years with upper endoscopy**

Treatment

- Attempts to decrease the portal pressure can be made through several different modalities
  - Noncardioselective β-blockers (propranolol or nadolol) are beneficial for the primary prophylaxis of bleeding in patients with medium and large varices. Patients intolerant to β-blockers should have large varices treated by band ligation.
  - Patients with small varices should be followed with annual endoscopy; there is no benefit from β-blockers.
  - Transjugular intrahepatic portosystemic shunt (TIPS) is very effective at decompression of portal hypertension, and the major side effect is hepatic encephalopathy (Fig. 30-3). TIPS is not safe in patients with severe hepatic dysfunction or heart failure.
  - Surgical decompression (portal-systemic shunt) has not been shown to improve survival in patients with cirrhosis, and is technically very difficult.
- Treatment of acute variceal hemorrhage consists of somatostatin analogues to induce splanchnic vasoconstriction, variceal band ligation, balloon tamponade, and TIPS. Antibiotic therapy reduces risk of infection and rebleeding and is recommended.

TABLE 30-1	*Causes of Chronic or Cirrhotic Liver Disease*
Infections	Viral hepatitis (hepatitis B, C), *Echinococcus* infections, brucellosis, congenital tertiary syphilis, schistosomiasis
Drugs and toxins	Alcohol, methotrexate, isoniazid, vitamin A, amiodarone, perhexilene maleate, α-methyldopa, and others
Metabolic or genetic diseases	Wilson disease, hereditary hemochromatosis, α_1-antitrypsin deficiency, carbohydrate metabolism disorders, lipid metabolism disorders, amino acid disorders, metabolism disorders, porphyria
Biliary obstruction	Chronic biliary obstruction, primary biliary cirrhosis, secondary biliary cirrhosis, cystic fibrosis, congenital biliary cysts
Vascular abnormalities	Veno-occlusive disease, Budd-Chiari syndrome, inferior vena cava obstruction, cardiac disease, hereditary hemorrhagic telangiectasias
Miscellaneous	Autoimmune chronic hepatitis, nonalcoholic steatohepatitis, granulomatous liver disease, sarcoidosis, polycystic liver disease

30

TABLE 30-2	*Clinical Consequences of Cirrhosis*
Synthetic defects	Decreased production of procoagulants, albumin, and fibrinogen
Renal	Sodium retention Hepatorenal syndrome Acute tubular necrosis Renal tubular acidosis
Endocrine	Impotence Anovulation Euthyroid sick syndrome Hepatic osteodystrophy
Cardiopulmonary	Hypotension Portal-pulmonary hypertension Hepatopulmonary syndrome
Oncologic	Hepatocellular carcinoma Cholangiocarcinoma
Portal hypertension	Portosystemic encephalopathy Variceal hemorrhage Ascites Spontaneous bacterial peritonitis Splenomegaly

Ascites

Basic Information

- Ascites is the presence of excess fluid in the peritoneal cavity
- Fluid is formed because of a number of contributing factors, including elevated hydrostatic pressure caused by portal hypertension, increased sympathetic outflow, reduced oncotic pressure caused by hypoalbuminemia, and increased renal sodium reabsorption (Fig. 30-4)

Clinical Presentation

- Patients may be asymptomatic or may complain of early satiety, increased abdominal girth, or respiratory distress
- Physical examination can reveal abdominal distention, bulging flanks, shifting dullness, or a fluid wave if there is greater than 500 mL of fluid present

Diagnosis

- Clinical symptoms and examination may be suggestive
- Laboratory studies
- Blood tests may show evidence of underlying liver disease

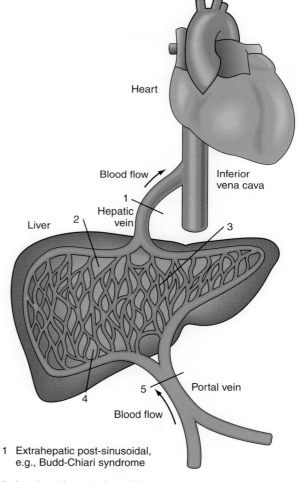

1 Extrahepatic post-sinusoidal, e.g., Budd-Chiari syndrome

2 Intrahepatic post-sinusoidal, e.g., veno-occlusive disease

3 Sinusoidal, e.g., cirrhosis

4 Intrahepatic pre-sinusoidal, e.g., sarcoidosis, schistosomiasis

5 Extrahepatic pre-sinusoidal, e.g., portal vein thrombosis

FIGURE 30-1 Classification of portal hypertension. *(From Boon NA, Colledge NR, Walker BR: Davidson's principles and practice of medicine, ed 20, New York, Churchill Livingstone, 2006, Fig. 23.19.)*

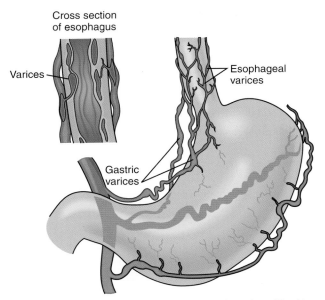

FIGURE 30-2 Esophageal and gastric varices. *(From http://hopkins-gi.nts.jhu.edu/pages/latin/templates/index.cfm? pg=disease4& organ = 2&disease=25&lang_id=1.)*

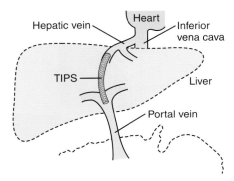

FIGURE 30-3 Transjugular intrahepatic portosystemic shunt (TIPS). A stent is placed from the portal vein to the right hepatic vein, allowing for decompression of the portal system. *(From Boon NA, Colledge NR, Walker BR: Davidson's principles and practice of medicine, ed 19, New York, Churchill Livingstone, 2006, Fig. 23.24B.)*

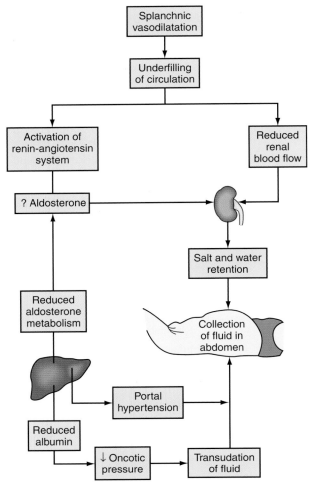

FIGURE 30-4 Pathogenesis of ascites. *(From Boon NA, Colledge NR, Walker BR: Davidson's principles and practice of medicine, ed 20, New York, Churchill Livingstone, 2006, Fig. 23.12.)*

- Ultrasound with Doppler examination is indicated to detect small amounts of fluid and to evaluate for portal vein thrombosis or Budd-Chiari syndrome
- Ascitic fluid analysis
  - Indicated for every patient with new-onset ascites and most patients with ascites admitted to the hospital
  - Tests ordered include cell count with differential, total protein, albumin, Gram stain, culture and sensitivity, cytology (if malignancy suspected), amylase (if pancreatic cause suspected), and triglycerides (if chylous ascites suspected)
  - Serum ascites-albumin gradient (SAAG)
    - **SAAG = serum ascites albumin − ascitic ascites albumin**
    - Levels greater than 1.1 g/dL are more than 90% sensitive for portal hypertension

- Levels less than 1.1 g/dL usually exclude cirrhosis and portal hypertension
- Ascitic total protein levels greater than 3.5 and ascitic albumin levels greater than 2.5 suggest a cardiac cause

Treatment

- Sodium restriction to less than 2 g/day
- Free water restriction only needed if hyponatremia is present
- Diuretic therapy to reduce sodium retention by the kidneys is generally required
  - Spironolactone: Works by inhibition of distal tubular and collecting duct sodium reabsorption and by abrogation of the renin-angiotensin system
  - Loop diuretics function at the ascending limb of the loop of Henle
  - **Generally, a combination of spironolactone or other potassium-sparing diuretic, along with a loop diuretic, is required for complete diuresis**
  - Need to monitor for side effects that may include electrolyte disorders, dehydration, hypotension, and azotemia

- Large-volume paracentesis is still required at times in patients with difficult-to-control ascites or in patients who do not tolerate diuretic therapy. IV albumin (8 g/dL of ascites removed) may be beneficial to prevent post-paracentesis circulatory collapse.
- TIPS can be considered in carefully selected patients, but has not been shown to have a mortality benefit over repeated large-volume paracenteses
- Liver transplantation should also be considered in patients with refractory ascites

Spontaneous Bacterial Peritonitis

Basic Information

- The most important sequela of ascites is the risk for development of spontaneous bacterial peritonitis (SBP)
- Because of the low protein content (including bacterial opsonins) and oncotic pressure of portal hypertensive ascitic fluid, the risk of infection is very high
- Risk factors for developing SBP in cirrhosis include GI hemorrhage, ascitic fluid protein content less than 1 g/dL, and a previous episode of SBP
- **Most infections are caused by transmigration of bacteria through the bowel wall, so enteric gram-negative bacilli are common pathogens (70% of cases)**
- Streptococci and staphylococci make up most of other cases
- Polymicrobial infection may suggest bowel perforation

Clinical Presentation

- Fevers, chills, and generalized abdominal pain can be seen; 33% of patients with cirrhosis and SBP will not have a fever or leukocytosis
- Often a clinical diagnosis is difficult to make because of inconsistent signs and symptoms. Pain is often absent, and the only reliable way to diagnose this condition is by paracentesis.
- Need to suspect SBP in patients with worsening jaundice, encephalopathy, or renal failure

Diagnosis

- The diagnosis of SBP is made based on an ascitic fluid polymorphonuclear (PMN) cell count greater than 250/mL. A very high ascitic PMN count (>1000/mL) suggests bowel perforation.
- Cultures of ascitic fluid taken at the time of paracentesis are often positive if done properly. The preferred method is to inoculate two blood culture bottles with 10 to 20 mL of ascitic fluid.
- Gram stain is commonly negative
- Basic classification of ascitic fluid infection
  - Spontaneous bacterial peritonitis
    - Culture positive
    - Greater than 250 neutrophils
  - Culture-negative neutrocytic ascites
    - Culture negative
    - Greater than 250 neutrophils
  - Monomicrobial non-neutrocytic bacterascites
    - Culture positive
    - Less than 250 neutrophils

Treatment

- The treatment of choice for documented SBP is cefotaxime (1 g IV every 8 hours for a minimum of 5 days)
- Repeat paracentesis at 48 to 72 hours should be done to check response to therapy
- Recurrent episodes of SBP are common, with about 70% of patients experiencing a second infection within 1 year
- **Prophylactic therapy using norfloxacin or trimethoprim-sulfamethoxazole should be initiated in patients with recurrent episodes of SBP**
- Primary prevention indicated in high-risk patients (hospitalized patients with ascitic fluid protein <1 g/dL) and in patients with acute variceal hemorrhage

Hepatorenal Syndrome

Basic Information

- Hepatorenal syndrome is a functional renal failure that occurs in the setting of advanced liver disease and portal hypertension
- It is exhibited by decreased urine production, azotemia, and reduced urinary sodium excretion
- It is seen in up to 10% of patients hospitalized with liver failure
- The exact pathogenesis is not fully understood, but evidence suggests that splanchnic vasodilation leads to reduction in effective circulatory volume. The kidneys compensate by increasing renin, constricting efferent arterioles, increasing sodium resorption, and decreasing urine output. The kidney structure remains essentially normal, and the kidneys will often return to normal function if the liver disease is corrected (e.g., by liver transplantation).
- Risk factors include cirrhosis, alcoholic hepatitis, acute liver failure, recent large-volume paracentesis, infection, GI bleeding, use of diuretics, nephrotoxic agents (i.e., nonsteroidal anti-inflammatory drugs [NSAIDs] and contrast dye), and the presence of orthostatic hypotension

Clinical Presentation

- Hypotension, azotemia, hyponatremia, and progressive oliguria are typically seen
- Hepatorenal syndrome is classified into two types:
  - Type 1: Severe, with rapid lowering of creatinine clearance below 20 mL/min; has virtually 100% mortality; patients will usually have massive ascites
  - Type 2: More insidious, less severe

Diagnosis

- It is typically diagnosed when other causes of kidney failure are excluded
- A number of diagnostic criteria have been developed (Box 30-1)

Treatment

- **No established effective medical therapies are available.** Combinations of midodrine, albumin, and octreotide are commonly used with modest benefit.
- Liver transplantation can be curative
- Renal replacement therapy used as a bridge to transplantation

| BOX 30-1 | *Diagnostic Criteria for Hepatorenal Syndrome* |

BOX 30-1 *Diagnostic Criteria for Hepatorenal Syndrome*

Low glomerular filtration rate (creatinine >1.5 g/dL or 24-hr urine creatinine clearance <40 mL/min) that progresses over days to weeks
Absence of any apparent cause for renal disease
Urine sodium concentration <10 mEq/L and a urine osmolality greater than plasma osmolality
No improvement in renal function with volume with 100 gm albumin IV

BOX 30-2 *Precipitating Factors for the Development of Hepatic Encephalopathy*

Acute hepatitis, progression of liver disease, portal-systemic shunts, portal vein thrombosis
Azotemia
Constipation
Dehydration
Drugs (benzodiazepines, narcotics, sedatives, diuretics)
Electrolyte disorders (hypokalemia, hyponatremia)
GI bleeding
Sepsis

Hepatic Encephalopathy

Basic Information

- Defined as disturbances in behavior and consciousness associated with liver disease and/or portal-systemic shunting
- Associated with acute liver failure, chronic liver disease/cirrhosis, or portosystemic bypass without intrinsic liver disease
- The pathogenesis of hepatic encephalopathy is unknown, but the accumulation of toxins (e.g., ammonia, mercaptans, short-chain fatty acids, phenol) in the systemic circulation because of bypass of the liver (from hepatocellular disease or shunting) is thought to be a major contributing factor
- Precipitating factors for hepatic encephalopathy: see Box 30-2

Clinical Presentation

- Disturbances in behavior and mentation that can progress to coma
- Asterixis, hyperreflexia, abnormal Babinski reflexes can be seen
- Fetor hepaticus: Musty odor emanating from the urine or breath

Diagnosis

- Based primarily on clinical presentation in a patient with acute or chronic liver disease and/or portal-systemic shunting
- Electroencephalography can show symmetrical, high-voltage, triphasic slow waves

| TABLE 30-3 | *Stages of Hepatic Encephalopathy* |

Stage	Clinical Description
0	No alteration in consciousness, intellectual function, personality, or behavior
1	Hypersomnia, insomnia, euphoria or anxiety, short attention span, irritability
2	Lethargy, disorientation, impaired cognition, inappropriate behavior, slurred speech, and ataxia
3	Somnolence, gross confusion, response to noxious stimuli
4	Coma, no response to noxious stimuli

- **Many patients will have elevated ammonia levels, but this is not sensitive or specific for diagnosis**
- Grading of hepatic encephalopathy based on change in mental status (Table 30-3)

Treatment

- Supportive measures: fluid and electrolyte maintenance, pressure sore prevention, aspiration precautions
- Eliminate or treat precipitating factors
  - Treat GI bleeding and SBP or other infections
  - Discontinue sedatives or narcotics (treat with naloxone or flumazenil, if appropriate)
  - Avoid nephrotoxic agents
- Eliminate toxins from the systemic circulation
  - Administer lactulose, nonabsorbable disaccharide that fosters the removal of ammonia in the stool and helps convert ammonia to ammonium ion (which is poorly absorbed); dose is titrated to maintain two to four loose bowel movements per day
  - Rifaximin, neomycin, and metronidazole are antibiotics that diminish GI tract bacterial production of ammonia (only rifaximin is approved by the Food and Drug Administration for this indication)
  - In patients with recurrent hepatic encephalopathy, rifaximin has been shown to reduce recurrences and reduce hospital admissions
- Hepatic support
  - Artificial liver systems have not been successfully developed
  - Liver transplantation

Pulmonary Manifestations of Cirrhosis and Portal Hypertension

Basic Information

- One third of patients with chronic liver disease develop some form of hypoxemia
- Lung disease can take many forms:
  - Parenchymal lung disease
    - Primary biliary cirrhosis—lymphocytic or fibrosing alveolitis and organizing pneumonitis
    - α_1-Antitrypsin deficiency—emphysematous lung disease

- Pleural space disease
  - Hepatic hydrothorax associated with cirrhosis
  - Elevated hemidiaphragms because of ascites or hepatomegaly
- Infected pleural fluid associated with ascites
  - Diseases of the pulmonary circulation
  - Impaired gas exchange
  - Hypoxic vasoconstriction
    - Hepatopulmonary syndrome
      - Hypoxemia related to vasodilation of pulmonary capillary bed resulting in right-to-left shunt
      - **Clinical presentation includes hypoxemia, platypnea (difficulty breathing upon sitting up), and orthodeoxia (decreased oxygen saturation when changing from the lying to sitting position)**
      - Can be diagnosed with contrast-enhanced echo-cardiography or albumin lung perfusion scan
      - Condition is reversed by liver transplantation. Room air arterial oxygen levels less than 50 mm Hg are a contraindication to transplantation, as postoperative survival is drastically reduced.
    - Portopulmonary hypertension
      - Pulmonary hypertension is related to cirrhosis by unclear mechanisms
      - Moderate to severe elevations of right ventricular systolic pressures are a contraindication to transplantation
    - Pulmonary varices

Treatment

- Liver transplantation may result in complete resolution of severe pulmonary manifestation of liver disease, hepatic hydrothorax, and hypoxemia associated with hepatopulmonary syndrome. Pulmonary hypertension may resolve in carefully selected patients following liver transplantation.

Hepatocellular Carcinoma

Basic Information

- Third most common malignancy worldwide, predominantly because of the prevalence of chronic viral hepatitis (hepatitis B and C); the incidence is rising in the United States
- Chronic liver disease of any etiology is a risk factor for development of hepatocellular carcinoma (HCC)
- Aflatoxins, alcohol, hemochromatosis, and anabolic steroids are other potential etiologic factors
- Fibrolamellar HCC is a distinct form of HCC with a characteristic histopathologic and clinical appearance. It typically occurs in younger adults without cirrhosis.
- **Hepatitis C is now associated with HCC in nearly 80% of cases diagnosed in the United States and is almost always found in the setting of established cirrhosis**
- **Hepatitis B may be frequently associated with HCC in the absence of cirrhosis**
  - Caused by the presence of a proto-oncogene
  - Careful radiographic surveillance of chronic hepatitis B carriers should be performed, especially in young adults who may have acquired it vertically at birth or through household contact in early childhood

Clinical Presentation

- Findings may be nonspecific and are often confused with progression of cirrhotic liver disease
- Abdominal pain is the most common symptom
- Examination may reveal a right upper quadrant abdominal mass and/or a bruit over the liver
- Patients who develop symptoms often have advanced disease and a poor prognosis
- **Paraneoplastic syndromes are occasionally seen:**
  - Erythrocytosis—caused by erythropoietin-like activity emanating from tumor cells
  - Hypercalcemia—caused by parathyroid hormone (PTH)–like hormone secretion
  - Acquired porphyria cutanea tarda
  - Carcinoid syndrome
  - Vitiligo

Diagnosis

- Ultrasound, computed tomography, and magnetic resonance imaging are commonly used to image the liver
- α-Fetoprotein (AFP) levels greater than 400 mg/L with an associated hypervascular liver mass are diagnostic
- Liver biopsy is not required when the lesion meets radiologic requirements and the patient has chronic liver disease
- Measurement of serum AFP and ultrasound examination may be used to screen for early HCC in cirrhotic patients
  - Many hepatologists recommend every 6 months
  - A clear benefit to this type of screening has yet to be proven

Treatment

- Surgical resection is indicated in patients with or without well-compensated cirrhosis (Child's class A) and a solitary tumor or disease limited to one half of the liver
- Liver transplantation is indicated in carefully selected patients with advanced cirrhosis and small tumors (Milan criteria: one tumor 2–5 cm or up to 3 tumors all less than 3 cm). The 5-year survival rates are approximately 75%. Metastases (including portal vein invasion) are a contraindication to transplantation.
- Patients with advanced cancers are candidates for locoregional therapy, such as hepatic artery embolization with chemotherapy, cryoablation, radiofrequency ablation, or alcohol ablation. Sorafaneb, an oral chemotherapeutic agent, was recently approved for the treatment of advanced HCC.

Liver Transplantation

Basic Information

- Acceptable indications for liver transplantation may include the following:
  - Acute liver failure
  - Advanced or chronic liver disease
  - Inherited metabolic liver disease
  - HCC using strict selection guidelines (Milan criteria)
- Contraindications to transplantation to be considered (Table 30-4)

30

TABLE 30-4	Contraindications to Liver Transplantation	
Absolute Contraindications	**Relative Contraindications**	
Metastatic cancer of the liver or other organs	Alcoholism (ongoing or untreated)	
Irreversible cardiac or pulmonary disease	Drug abuse (ongoing or untreated)	
Acute infection outside the liver	HIV positivity (performed at selective centers)	
AIDS syndrome	HBV DNA positivity	
	Advanced renal disease	

HBV, hepatitis B virus.

BOX 30-3　MELD Score

Based on the values of serum creatinine (Scr), total bilirubin (Tbil), and INR

Formula

$$\text{MELD Score} = 10\,\{0.957\,\text{Ln(Scr)} + 0.378\,\text{Ln(Tbil)} + 1.12\,\text{Ln(INR)} + 0.643\}$$

General Rules
- Minimum value for any variable is 1
- Maximum value for creatinine is 4
- Maximum MELD score is 40
  An online calculator is available at: www.unos.org/resources/MeldPeldCalculator.asp? index=98

INR, international normalized ratio; MELD, Model for End-stage Liver Disease.

- There are different sources of donor livers:
  - Cadaveric—Most common type of transplantation performed; long waiting times because of liver shortages
  - Living-related donor—Portion of the liver from a friend or relative is transplanted
- After an evaluation is completed, the patient is placed on the liver transplant waiting list with United Network for Organ Sharing (UNOS). The criteria for prioritizing patients for liver transplantation are
  - Status 1: Acute liver failure with stage 3 or 4 encephalopathy and retransplantation or failed liver transplant resulting from primary graft nonfunction or hepatic artery thrombosis
  - Status 2: Model for End-stage Liver Disease (MELD) score ranging from 6 to 40 points
  - Status 7: Inactive but on list
- The waiting time depends on the severity of liver disease as assessed by the MELD score in all patients with chronic liver disease, but there are variations

based on blood type, body size, and geographic regions. The MELD score provides a reliable estimate of short-term survival for patients with a wide range of liver diseases and is based on easily obtainable and objective laboratory parameters (Box 30-3).
- The 5-year survival rate is now close to 80% at well-established liver transplantation centers, and the 1-year survival rate exceeds 85%

REVIEW QUESTIONS

For review questions, please go to www.expertconsult.com.

SUGGESTED READINGS

Bruix J, Sherman M: Management of hepatocellular carcinoma: an update, *Hepatology* 53:1–35, 2010.
Runyon BA: Management of adult patients with ascites due to cirrhosis: an update, *Hepatology* 49:2087–2107, 2009.
Munoz SJ: Hepatic encephalopathy, *Med Clin North Am* 92:795–812, 2008.
Munoz SJ: The hepatorenal syndrome, *Med Clin North Am* 92:813–837, 2008.

SECTION FIVE

Nephrology

Acid-Base Disorders and Renal Tubular Acidosis

STEPHEN D. SISSON, MD

Acid-base disorders are extremely common in clinical medicine and can be seen in numerous disease states. The lungs and kidneys help maintain acid-base equilibrium (in the lungs via CO_2, in the kidneys via bicarbonate [HCO_3^-]; Fig. 31-1). **The body never overcorrects for a single acid-base disorder. When evaluating acid-base status, begin by looking at the serum pH to decide if acidosis or alkalosis is present** (pH <7.4 indicates acidosis; pH >7.4 indicates alkalosis). Then look at the partial pressure of carbon dioxide (Pco_2) and serum HCO_3^- to see which one (or both) is consistent with the pH, to determine if the primary disorder is respiratory or metabolic. **Note that a normal pH does not exclude an acid-base disorder; for instance, with a coexisting metabolic acidosis and metabolic alkalosis, the pH may be normal.**

Metabolic Acidosis

Basic Information

- Primary defect in metabolic acidosis is decreased serum HCO_3^-
- Calculation of the anion gap is used to help narrow differential diagnosis
    - Anion gap calculated as $Na^+ - (Cl^- + HCO_3^-)$
    - **The normal anion gap is 12 ± 2** and is made of phosphates, sulfates, organic acids, and negatively charged plasma proteins
- When metabolic acidosis develops, determining whether the anion gap is elevated, normal, or low will narrow the differential diagnosis

Metabolic Acidosis with Increased Anion Gap

- **The differential diagnosis of the most common causes of an anion gap acidosis is remembered by the mnemonic MUDPILES (Box 31-1)**
- Besides a thorough history and physical examination, **evaluation of serum ketones, serum lactate, toxicology screen, and salicylate level should be considered**

Metabolic Acidosis with Normal Anion Gap

- Also referred to as a non–anion gap acidosis, although an anion gap is present but normal
- In this group, the increased anion is chloride (Cl^-); therefore, the anion gap does not change

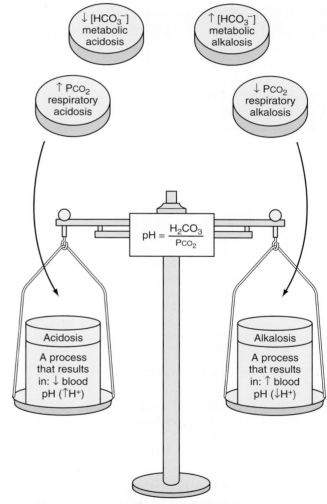

FIGURE 31-1 Acid-base disorders. *(From Baynes JW, Dominiczak MH: Medical biochemistry, ed 2, St. Louis, Mosby, 2004, Fig. 22-5.)*

- **The mnemonic for the most common causes of a normal anion gap acidosis is DURHAM (Box 31-2)**
- **Calculation of the urine anion gap may be helpful in evaluating normal anion gap metabolic acidosis** to differentiate renal tubular acidoses (RTAs) from other causes of normal anion gap metabolic acidosis

- Normal kidney response to acidosis is to excrete acid in the form of NH_4^+, which is balanced by increases in urine chloride, so urine chloride is a marker of urine acid excretion. In type 1 or type 4 RTA, NH_4^+ excretion does not occur, and urine chloride is low.
- **Formula for urine anion gap: Urine (Na + K − Cl)**
  - In a normal patient (without RTA) with metabolic acidosis, the sum of this equation is less than 0
  - If normal anion gap metabolic acidosis exists, and urine anion gap is greater than 0, type 1 or type 4 RTA is likely

Metabolic Acidosis with Decreased Anion Gap

- Low anion gap acidoses are less commonly seen
  - **May be caused by hypoalbuminemia, multiple myeloma, ingestion of bromide**
  - The acid-base disorders in these diseases are of little clinical consequence

Investigation of Coexistent Anion Gap and Normal Anion Gap Metabolic Acidoses

- **An anion gap acidosis and a normal anion gap acidosis may coexist**
- To determine if the metabolic acidosis is caused by more than one process, compare the increase in the anion gap with the decrease in HCO_3^-
  - In pure anion gap metabolic acidosis, the decrease in HCO_3^- equals the increase in the anion gap
  - **If the HCO_3^- decreases significantly more than the anion gap increases, then a coexisting normal anion gap metabolic acidosis is present**

FIGURE 31-2 Pathogenesis of metabolic acidosis in ketogenesis. Acetoacetate, acetone, and β-hydroxybutyrate pass into the bloodstream, producing acidosis. (CoA, coenzyme A.) *(From Kumar P, Clark M: Clinical medicine, ed 5, Philadelphia, Elsevier Saunders, 2005, Fig. 19-12.)*

- Expressed as the "delta-delta equation": Change (Δ) in anion gap = change (Δ) in HCO_3^-
  - Note that the actual values of the HCO_3^- and anion gap are not compared, but rather the change in each of these values from their baseline (baseline HCO_3^- is 24 mEq/dL; baseline anion gap is 12)

Osmolar Gap

- **Metabolic acidosis is occasionally caused by the ingestion of toxic compounds that are osmotically active (e.g., methanol, ethylene glycol, toluene)**
- May be investigated in the clinically appropriate setting by calculating the difference between the measured osmolality and the calculated osmolality; in normal host, difference between measured and calculated osmolality is less than 10
- If this difference is greater than 10 (i.e., measured osmolality >10 units higher than estimated osmolality), there are extra osmotically active compounds in the blood; **compare clinical picture with signs and symptoms of suggested toxin, including methanol (associated with papilledema and retinal hemorrhages), ethylene glycol (associated with calcium oxalate crystals in the urine), toluene (presents first with anion gap metabolic acidosis, then metabolized resulting in normal anion gap metabolic acidosis)**
- Isopropyl alcohol ingestion also results in an osmolar gap, although no acid-base disorder is associated
- Written mathematically, the osmolar gap is calculated as

Osmolality(measured) − Osmolality(calculated)

A

35-year-old male

- Mild polyuria
- Blood pressure 188/104 mm Hg

Plasma biochemistry
- Na 144 mmol/L (132–144)
- K 3.1 mmol/L (3.3–4.7)
- HCO₃⁻ 29 mmol/L (21–27)

Lying at 0900 hr
- Renin activity <0.5 (0.4–1.5)
- Aldosterone 850 pmol/L (30–440)

Standing at 1200 hr
- Renin activity <0.5 (1–2.5)
- Aldosterone 750 pmol/L (110–860)

FIGURE 31-3 Conn's adenoma causing metabolic alkalosis. **A,** Note hypernatremic, hypokalemic metabolic alkalosis. **B,** Computed tomographic appearance of right adrenal adenoma *(arrow)*. **C,** Unilateral uptake of radiolabeled cholesterol in right adrenal gland. **D,** Pathologic specimen following surgical excision. *(From Haslett C, Chilvers ER, Boon NA, et al: Davidson's principles and practice of medicine, ed 19, New York, Churchill Livingstone, 2002, Fig. 16.19.)*

where

$$Osm_{calc} = [2 \times Na] + [Blood\ urea\ nitrogen\ /\ 2.8] + [Glucose\ /\ 18]$$

(normal <10)

Clinical Presentation

- Respiratory compensation in patients presenting with metabolic acidosis
  - The body compensates for metabolic acidosis by creating respiratory alkalosis
  - Pco₂ may be predicted by the following equation (Winter's formula):

$$[1.5(HCO_3^-) + 8] \pm 2 = P_{CO_2}$$

  - Equation only valid when primary disorder is metabolic acidosis; do not use this equation when the primary disorder is not a metabolic acidosis
  - If the measured Pco₂ is not close to what is predicted, a second disorder coexists
    - If the Pco₂ is less than predicted, second disorder is respiratory alkalosis
    - If the Pco₂ is higher than predicted, second disorder is respiratory acidosis

Metabolic Alkalosis

Basic Information

- **The primary defect in a metabolic alkalosis is an increase in the serum HCO₃⁻, implying either a gain of HCO₃⁻ or a loss of acid**
  - **Examples of HCO₃⁻ gain**
    - Administration of sodium bicarbonate (NaHCO₃), baking soda, or medication formulations that include citrate or lactate

- **Examples of acid loss**
  - Gastric losses, such as vomiting or nasogastric suction
  - Renal causes (e.g., side effects from diuretics), as well as administration of nonresorbable anions (e.g., IV penicillin or carbenicillin)
  - Hypermineralocorticoid states

Clinical Presentation

- The presence of a metabolic alkalosis always implies that two events have occurred: (1) initiation of the alkalosis and (2) maintenance of the alkalosis
  - The initiating factors are the gain of HCO₃⁻ or loss of acid described previously
  - The kidneys always are responsible for the maintenance of alkalosis; two states favor maintenance of alkalosis by the kidney
    - **Volume depletion:** The kidney responds to volume depletion by becoming Na⁺ avid, and Na⁺ is resorbed along with an anion (i.e., HCO₃⁻, because urine Cl⁻ is low in volume depletion)
    - **Hypermineralocorticoid states:** Mineralocorticoids stimulate renal hydrogen ion (H⁺) excretion; examples include hyperaldosteronism (Conn syndrome; Fig. 31-3) and Cushing disease

Diagnosis and Evaluation

- **Measurement of spot urine Cl⁻ is helpful in evaluating the cause of the metabolic alkalosis (Box 31-3)**
- Respiratory compensation in primary metabolic alkalosis
  - **Response to metabolic alkalosis requires respiratory acidosis; response therefore limited**
  - In general, the Pco₂ rises 0.5 to 1 mm Hg for every 1-unit increase in serum HCO₃⁻ from a baseline of 24 mmol/L
  - The maximum Pco₂ in compensation is 55 to 60 mm Hg

31

| BOX 31-3 | *Differential Diagnosis of Metabolic Alkalosis* |

Causes of a saline-responsive alkalosis (urine chloride <10 mEq/L)
- NG suction
- Vomiting
- Diuretics
- Posthypercapnia

Causes of a saline-resistant alkalosis (urine chloride >10 mEq/L) are further divided according to BP:
- With elevated BP: Primary aldosteronism, Cushing disease, renal artery stenosis, renal failure plus alkali administration
- With normal BP: Hypomagnesemia, severe hypokalemia, Bartter syndrome, $NaHCO_3$ administration, licorice ingestion (enzymatically inhibits degradation of cortisol)

BP, blood pressure; NG, nasogastric.

Respiratory Acidosis

Basic Information

- **The primary defect in respiratory acidosis is an increase in Pco_2**
- Whereas the lungs can respond rapidly to a metabolic challenge, the kidneys cannot respond immediately to a challenge from the lungs
  - **Respiratory processes (both acidosis and alkalosis) have an acute compensatory phase, in which plasma buffers help maintain pH; and a chronic phase, in which the kidney participates**
  - The acute response takes minutes to hours, whereas the chronic response takes 3 to 5 days
- Prediction of pH and HCO_3^- in respiratory acidosis
  - **Acute respiratory acidosis: For every 10 mm Hg increase in Pco_2, pH decreases by 0.08, and serum HCO_3^- increases by 1**
  - **Chronic respiratory acidosis: For every 10 mm Hg increase in Pco_2, pH decreases by 0.03, and serum HCO_3^- increases by 3 to 4**

Differential Diagnosis

- Differential diagnosis of respiratory acidosis is shown in Box 31-4

Respiratory Alkalosis

Basic Information

- **The primary defect in respiratory alkalosis is a decrease in Pco_2**
- As with respiratory acidosis, there are acute and chronic phases to respiratory alkalosis
  - **Acute respiratory alkalosis: For every 10 mm Hg decrease in Pco_2, HCO_3^- decreases by 2.5**
  - **Chronic respiratory alkalosis: For every 10 mm Hg decrease in Pco_2, HCO_3^- decreases by 5; maximum compensation of HCO_3^- is 15**
  - Although many use the same estimates of pH change seen in respiratory acidosis (i.e., acutely for each

| BOX 31-4 | *Differential Diagnosis of Respiratory Acidosis* |

Chest Cavity
Neurologic disorders (e.g., amyotrophic lateral sclerosis)
Muscular disorders
Kyphoscoliosis (severe)
Pleural effusion
Pneumothorax

Central
Sedation or narcotics
Respiratory center hypofunction (infection, ischemia, infarction)
Obstructive sleep apnea

Lung/Airways
Pneumonia, pulmonary edema, bronchospasm or laryngospasm
Chronic obstructive pulmonary disease
Mechanical obstruction (foreign body/tumor)

| BOX 31-5 | *Differential Diagnosis of Respiratory Alkalosis* |

Systemic
Sepsis
Salicylates
Liver failure
Hyperthyroidism
Pregnancy
High-altitude residence
Hypotension

Central
Ischemia or cerebrovascular accident
Tumor
Infection
Progesterone
Anxiety
Fever

Pulmonary
Pulmonary embolus
Restrictive lung disease
Hypoxemia (e.g., pneumonia, pulmonary edema)

10 mm Hg decrease in Pco_2, pH increases 0.08), the pH changes in respiratory alkalosis are less predictable
  - In respiratory alkalosis the body can return the pH to normal

Differential Diagnosis

- Differential diagnosis of respiratory alkalosis is shown in Box 31-5
  - **Note that sepsis and salicylate toxicity result in both a metabolic acidosis and respiratory alkalosis (Fig. 31-4)**

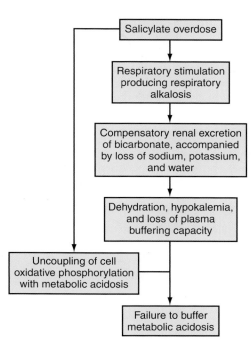

FIGURE 31-4 Salicylate overdose results in metabolic acidosis and respiratory alkalosis. *(From Waller D, Renwick A: Medical pharmacology and therapeutics, ed 2, Philadelphia, WB Saunders, 2005, Fig. 53-9.)*

TABLE 31-1	*Characteristics of Renal Tubular Acidoses*		
	Type 1	**Type 2**	**Type 4**
Basic defect	Distal renal tubular defect in NH_4^+ excretion	Proximal tubular defect in HCO_3^- resorption	Hyporeninemic hypoaldo-steronism
Serum potassium	Low	Low	High
Able to acidify urine to pH <5.5	No	Yes	Yes
Responds to $NaHCO_3$	Yes	No	N/A

Renal Tubular Acidosis

See Table 31-1 for the characteristics of renal tubular acidosis.

Basic Information

- The kidney contributes to maintaining the acid-base equilibrium of the serum by either resorbing or excreting acid (in the form of NH_4^+) and HCO_3^- as needed
- If the kidney does not appropriately excrete acid (NH_4^+) or resorb HCO_3^-, acidosis will develop
- Because a renal tubular defect is responsible when this acidosis occurs, these disorders are termed *renal tubular acidoses*

TYPE 1 RTA
Basic Information

- **Distal renal tubular defect in NH_4^+ excretion, resulting in severe acidosis and an inability to acidify urine below a pH of 5.5, even with an acid challenge**
- Potassium conservation in most patients with type 1 RTA is typically impaired, and **hypokalemia often accompanies this disorder**
- Causes may include
  - Congenital autosomal dominant disorder (most common cause of type 1 RTA)
  - Other genetic disorders (Marfan syndrome, Ehlers-Danlos syndrome)
  - Autoimmune diseases (systemic lupus erythematosus, rheumatoid arthritis, Sjögren syndrome)
  - Medications such as amphotericin, lithium, and high doses of salicylates

- Urinary tract obstruction and the renal defects seen in sickle cell anemia (usually associated with hyperkalemia)

Clinical Presentation

- **Clinical manifestations include hypercalciuria and calcium oxalate stones**
  - Hyperparathyroidism and low vitamin D levels may develop, leading to rickets in children and osteomalacia in adults
  - Other clinical manifestations are related to associated diseases

Diagnosis

- **Diagnosis is made on clinical grounds and confirmed by ammonium chloride (NH_4Cl) administration, which will result in worsening systemic acidosis without drop in urine pH below 5.5**
  - Urine anion gap is also greater than 0

Treatment

- **Treatment consists of $NaHCO_3$,** which is titrated until the serum HCO_3^- and urine calcium excretion normalize

TYPE 2 RTA
Basic Information

- **A proximal renal tubular defect in HCO_3^- resorption leading to a mild acidosis**
- **Able to acidify urine below a pH of 5.5 with an acid challenge**
- Low levels of proximal tubular resorption do occur, which prevent severe acidosis
  - There is no defect in renal H^+ excretion
  - Because potassium often complexes with HCO_3^-, **hypokalemia is common with type 2 RTA**
  - Calcium resorption is also typically impaired, but not as severely as in type 1
- **Commonly seen in conjunction with defective resorption of other molecules, such as glucose and amino acids (as seen in Fanconi syndrome)**
- Other causes: carbonic anhydrase inhibitors, outdated tetracycline, lead and mercury toxicity

Diagnosis and Evaluation

- Diagnosis is suggested on clinical grounds
  - Administration of NH_4Cl results in normal acidification of urine because acid excretion is normal in type 2 RTA
  - **Administration of $NaHCO_3$ results in alkaline urine despite systemic acidosis because renal HCO_3^- resorption does not occur**
  - Urine anion gap is not useful in evaluation, since defect is HCO_3^- resorption, not acid excretion

Treatment

- Treatment is usually not indicated
- If necessary, can try very high doses of HCO_3^-

TYPE 4 RTA

Basic Information

- **Type 4 RTA is an acquired diffuse renal defect in $NH4^+$ excretion, resulting in mild normal anion gap acidosis**
- **Able to acidify urine below a pH of 5.5 with an acid challenge**
- Mechanism in type 4 RTA is not completely understood; the majority of patients with type 4 RTA have low levels of renin and aldosterone (referred to as "hyporeninemic, hypoaldosterone" states)
- **A distinguishing feature is the coexisting inability of the kidney to excrete potassium, leading to high serum potassium (types 1 and 2 RTAs are usually hypokalemic)**
- **Causes include diabetes (the most common cause);** mineralocorticoid deficiency (including Addison disease); therapy with NSAIDs, heparin, or angiotensin-converting enzyme inhibitors

Diagnosis and Evaluation

- Diagnosis usually made on clinical grounds
  - Administration of NH_4Cl results in some acidification of urine because some renal acid excretion occurs; urine pH declines below 5.5
- Urine anion gap is greater than 0

Treatment

- If treatment is desired, a mineralocorticoid may be administered (e.g., fludrocortisone)
- Another option is treatment with furosemide, as long as sodium intake is adequate

REVIEW QUESTIONS

For review questions, please go to www.expertconsult.com.

SUGGESTED READINGS

Androgue HJ, Madias NE: Management of life-threatening acid-base disorders (Part 1), N Engl J Med 338:26–34, 1998.

Androgue HJ, Madias NE: Management of life-threatening acid-base disorders (Part 2), N Engl J Med 338:107–111, 1998.

Battle DC, Hizon M, Cohen E, et al: The use of the urinary anion gap in the diagnosis of hyperchloremic metabolic acidosis, N Engl J Med 318:594–599, 1988.

Narins RG, Emmett M: Simple and mixed acid-base disorders: a practical approach, Medicine 59:161–187, 1980.

Rose BD: Renal tubular acidosis. In Rose BD, editor: *Clinical physiology of acid-base and electrolyte disorders*, ed 3, New York, 1989, McGraw Hill.

Stewart PA: Modern quantitative acid-base chemistry, Can J Physiol Pharmacol 61:1444–1461, 1983.

Electrolyte Disorders

C. JOHN SPERATI, MD, MHS

The maintenance of proper electrolyte concentrations is crucial to normal organ function and regulation of body volume. Alterations in the balance between electrolyte and water content may change electrolyte concentrations, osmolality, body volume status, and cellular function.

Osmolality

- Number of particles (osmoles, Osm) dissolved in solution
- Water moves between body compartments along osmolal gradients from an area of lower osmolality to an area of higher osmolality
- Only *effective* osmoles (substances that do not freely cross cell membranes) induce a water shift
  - Predominant effective osmole: sodium
  - Ineffective osmole (does not induce fluid shift): urea
- The body attempts to regulate osmolality *primarily* via retention or excretion of water, not osmoles (i.e., sodium, Na^+)

Sodium and Water Balance

Sodium

- As the major extracellular cation, Na^+ is the predominant solute contributing to osmolality
  - Na^+ is actively pumped from the intracellular to the extracellular space
  - Na^+ leaves the body primarily through urinary excretion, which is tightly regulated
- Serum osmolality may be estimated using the following equation:

$$\text{Serum osmolality} = [2 \times \text{serum } Na^+ (mEq/L)] + [\text{blood urea nitrogen } (mg/dL)/2.8] + [\text{glucose } (mg/dL)/18]$$

Aldosterone

- Mineralocorticoid produced in the zona glomerulosa of the adrenal glands
- **Major actions are to stimulate Na^+ reabsorption and potassium (K^+) secretion in the renal collecting tubule. Hydrogen (H^+) secretion is increased due to the electronegative lumen generated by Na^+ reabsorption.**
- Aldosterone release is stimulated by:
  - Hyperkalemia
  - Angiotensin II

- The renin-angiotensin-aldosterone axis modulates Na^+ retention and excretion to regulate total body volume (and hence blood pressure)

Water

- Total body water (TBW) represents 60% of body weight in men and 50% in women
  - TBW is distributed:
    - Intracellular ⅔
    - Extracellular ⅓
      - Interstitial ¾ of extracellular
      - Intravascular ¼ of extracellular
- Water losses occur via the kidney, GI tract, skin, and respiratory tract
  - Renal water excretion is tightly regulated via concentration or dilution of urine
  - 500 to 1000 mL/day lost through skin and respiratory tract ("insensible losses")
- Thirst is an essential mechanism for preventing and correcting a water deficit
  - Stimulated by hypovolemia and an elevated serum osmolality

Antidiuretic Hormone (ADH, Vasopressin)

- ADH is the principal hormone regulating osmolality
  - ADH increases water reabsorption from the collecting duct lumen back into the circulation
    - ADH present: concentrated urine; smaller urine volume
    - ADH absent: dilute urine; larger urine volume
- ADH release from the posterior pituitary is stimulated by:
  - Increases in plasma osmolality as small as 1%
  - Pain, nausea, multiple medications
  - Greater than or equal to 10% decrease in effective circulating volume
- See Figure 32-1

HYPONATREMIA

Basic Information

- Serum Na^+ concentration less than 135 mEq/L
- Most common electrolyte disturbance in hospitalized patients
- **Can occur with low, normal, or high total body Na^+; hyponatremia requires the presence of too much water relative to the quantity of total body Na^+**

Clinical Presentation

- Not all hyponatremia is symptomatic (see later information on iso-osmolar hyponatremia)

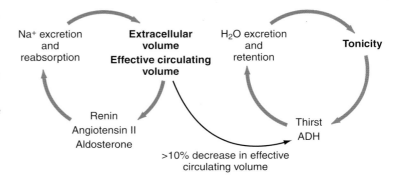

FIGURE 32-1 Regulation of body fluid compartments and osmolality. The renin-angiotensin-aldosterone pathway regulates body volume, while antidiuretic hormone (ADH) regulates osmolality via excretion/retention of water. A greater than 10% decrease in effective circulating volume will stimulate a nonosmotic release of ADH.

TABLE 32-1	Signs and Symptoms of Hyponatremia	
Mild	**Moderate**	**Severe**
[Na$^+$] = 125–135 mEq/L	[Na$^+$] = 120–125 mEq/L	[Na$^+$] <120 mEq/L
Anorexia	Agitation	Seizures
Apathy	Disorientation	Coma
Restlessness	Headache	Areflexia
Nausea		Cheyne-Stokes respirations
Lethargy		Incontinence
Muscle cramps		Death

- Signs and symptoms are due to swelling of the central nervous system (CNS)
  - As serum osmolality falls, water shifts intracellularly to an area of higher osmolality until an osmolal gradient no longer exists
- Signs and symptoms: See Table 32-1

Diagnosis and Evaluation

- Figure 32-2 shows an algorithm for the differential diagnosis of hyponatremia
- Determine osmolality
  - Normal
    - Pseudohyponatremia: Hyperlipidemia and hyperproteinemia can cause an artifactual decrease in measured serum Na$^+$. The true serum Na$^+$ concentration is normal.
      - Asymptomatic; exclude before pursuing evaluation of hyponatremia
  - High
    - Osmotically active particles may pull water into the extracellular space, creating a dilutional hyponatremia
      - Examples: glucose, mannitol, maltose
      - For every 100-mg/dL increase in glucose above 100, serum Na$^+$ decreases around 1.6 to 2.4 mEq/L
  - Low
    - Characteristic of most cases of hyponatremia
- Determine volume status
  - Findings suggestive of hypovolemia
    - Hypotension, tachycardia, dry mucous membranes, skin tenting, absence of edema
  - Findings suggestive of hypervolemia
    - Edema, elevated jugular venous pressure, crackles, S$_3$ heart sound, pulmonary edema

- Evaluate urine indices
  - Can be seen in hypovolemia or hypervolemia (congestive heart failure, cirrhosis)
    - Urine Na$^+$ less than 10 mEq/L
    - Fractional excretion of sodium (FE$_{Na}$) less than 1%:

    $$[(\text{Urine Na}^+ \times \text{serum creatinine})/(\text{Serum Na}^+ \times \text{urine creatinine})] \times 100$$

    - Urine osmolality greater than serum osmolality
  - Suggestive of euvolemia or recent diuretic use
    - Urine Na$^+$ greater than 20 mEq/L
- Special consideration: Syndrome of inappropriate antidiuresis (SIAD)
  - Must exclude known stimuli of ADH release before labeling *idiopathic*
  - Must be clinically euvolemic
  - Urine sodium greater than 20 mEq/L
  - Urine osmolality greater than serum osmolality
  - Causes of SIAD are listed in Box 32-1 (medications, pulmonary disease, and CNS disease are major causes)

Treatment

- Treat underlying cause
  - Hypovolemic hypo-osmolar: Isotonic saline
  - Hypervolemic hypo-osmolar: Fluid restriction, diuresis, dialysis
  - Euvolemic hypo-osmolar: Fluid restriction, consider use of V$_2$ receptor antagonists, address any contributing medical condition
- V$_2$ receptor antagonists ("vaptans")
  - Block the V$_2$ ADH receptor in collecting duct
  - Only for use in euvolemic (SIAD) and potentially hypervolemic disorders
  - Results in aquaresis without significant natriuresis
  - Hyponatremia will reoccur with discontinuation of drug if underlying cause not addressed
  - Demeclocycline is an older therapy to antagonize ADH action that is rarely used
- Severe CNS symptoms (e.g., seizure, obtundation)
  - Raise Na$^+$ concentration 1 to 2 mEq/L/hr with 3% saline until symptoms abate
- Rate of correction is usually proportional to rate at which hyponatremia developed
  - Chronic hyponatremia (>24–48 hours): Raise Na$^+$ concentration 0.5 to 1 mEq/L/hr and no more than 8 to 10 mEq/L in 24 hours

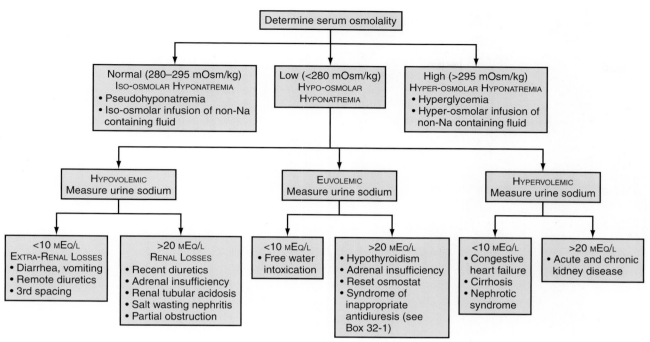

FIGURE 32-2 Differential diagnosis of hyponatremia.

32

| BOX 32-1 | *Causes of Syndrome of Inappropriate Antidiuresis* |

Idiopathic

Pulmonary disease

Ectopic ADH production (e.g., small cell carcinoma of lung)

Infections: meningitis, encephalitis, abscess, VZV

Vascular: subarachnoid hemorrhage, CVA, temporal arteritis

Severe nausea/vomiting

Drugs: SSRIs, narcotics, cyclophosphamide, chlorpropamide

Ecstasy ingestion (aggravated by copious fluid intake)

HIV

Prolactinoma

Waldenström macroglobulinemia

Shy-Drager syndrome

Delirium tremens

Oxytocin

Marathon runner

ADH, antidiuretic hormone; CVA, cerebrovascular accident; HIV, human immunodeficiency virus; SSRIs, selective serotonin reuptake inhibitors; VZV, varicella-zoster virus

- Acute hyponatremia (<24–36 hours): Can raise 1 to 2 mEq/L/hr usually without the need for 3% saline unless severe CNS symptoms are present
- Rapid correction can result in prompt cerebral dehydration and irreversible osmotic demyelination of the CNS (i.e., central pontine myelinolysis, Fig. 32-3)

HYPERNATREMIA

Overview

- Serum Na⁺ concentration greater than 145 mEq/L
- **Thirst is the major defense against the development of hypernatremia**

- Usually requires impaired access to water
- If free access to water is present, consider impaired thirst mechanism
- Most cases occur in hospitalized patients
  - Classic outpatient presentation: Elderly nursing home resident with underlying infection

Clinical Presentation

- Signs and symptoms are due to dehydration of the CNS
  - As serum osmolality rises, water flows from inside cells of the CNS into the extracellular space along the osmolal gradient
- **Patients may experience restlessness, irritability, lethargy, muscle twitching, hyperreflexia, spasticity, and, in severe cases, intracranial hemorrhage**

Diagnosis and Evaluation

- Differential diagnosis of hypernatremia is shown in Figure 32-4
- Special consideration: Diabetes insipidus (DI)
  - Insufficient ADH action leads to polyuria and free water loss
    - Central: Lack of pituitary ADH production
    - Nephrogenic: Renal resistance to ADH action
  - High-normal to high serum Na⁺ concentration with low urine osmolality (<300 mOsm/kg)
  - Differential diagnosis—Rule out polyuria due to:
    - Primary polydipsia
    - Diuretics
    - Osmotic diuresis (e.g., hyperglycemia)
  - Major causes of DI include pituitary tumor or apoplexy, lithium, hypercalcemia, hyperkalemia, and pregnancy

Treatment

- Address underlying cause
- **Overly rapid correction can result in cerebral edema**

FIGURE 32-3 Central pontine myelinolysis (**A**, *arrowheads*) indicate low signal intensity on T1-weighted imaging. **B**, *Arrows* indicate high signal intensity on T2-weighted imaging; *arrowheads* demonstrate normal corticospinal tracts in a patient who presents with serum Na$^+$ 99 mEq/L corrected to 125 mEq/L in 24 hours. *(From Goetz CG: Textbook of clinical neurology, ed 2, Philadelphia, WB Saunders, 2003. In Hart BL, Eaton RP: Images in clinical medicine—osmotic myelinolysis, N Engl J Med 333:1259, 1995.)*

FIGURE 32-4 Differential diagnosis of hypernatremia. NG, nasogastric.

- If evidence of circulatory collapse, first correct hypovolemia with isotonic saline
- To calculate free water deficit:

$$\text{Free water deficit} = \text{TBW} \times [(\text{Serum sodium concentration} / 140) - 1]$$

- Decrease serum Na$^+$ concentration approximately 0.5 mEq/L/hr and no more than 8 to 10 mEq/L in 24 hours

Potassium Disorders

POTASSIUM BALANCE
- K$^+$ is the major intracellular cation
  - Intracellular K$^+$ is maintained at a high concentration by the 3Na,2K-ATPase pump
  - 95% to 98% of total body K$^+$ is stored intracellularly

- 80% of K$^+$ excretion occurs via the kidney, with the remainder in the stool and sweat
  - Renal K$^+$ excretion increased by aldosterone
  - Increased Na$^+$ and water delivery to the distal nephron increases K$^+$ excretion
- Disorders of K$^+$ concentration occur via:
  - Gain or loss in total body K$^+$ stores
  - Shifts between intracellular and extracellular compartments
- Changes in the electrical potential of cellular membranes lead to the major signs and symptoms

HYPOKALEMIA

Basic Information
- Serum K$^+$ concentration less than 3.5 mEq/L
- In the absence of intracellular shifting, **hypokalemia implies low total body K$^+$**
- Most commonly results when K$^+$ losses exceed intake
  - More rarely may result simply from inadequate daily intake

Clinical Presentation
- May result in fatigue progressing to muscle weakness and arrhythmia, followed by tetany or rhabdomyolysis at K$^+$ less than 2.5 mEq/L and then paralysis when less than 2 mEq/L
- Cardiac conduction is affected, resulting in T-wave flattening, the development of U waves, and arrhythmias (e.g., atrial tachycardia, atrioventricular dissociation, ventricular tachycardia, and ventricular fibrillation; Fig. 32-5)
  - Risk of arrhythmia is increased in the presence of high concentrations of digoxin

FIGURE 32-5 Electrocardiogram of patient with hypokalemia. Note flattening of T waves and prominent U waves. *(From Goldberger AL: Clinical electrocardiography: a simplified approach, ed 6, St. Louis, Mosby, 1998.)*

- Hypokalemia may increase the risk of osmotic demyelination when correcting hyponatremia
  - If neurologically stable, correct hypokalemia before correcting hyponatremia

Diagnosis and Evaluation

- Differential diagnosis of hypokalemia is shown in Figures 32-6 through 32-8
- Evaluate for spurious hypokalemia, intracellular shift, and inadequate intake
  - Spurious hypokalemia due to increased uptake after venipuncture when leukocytosis greater than 100,000 cells/mm^3 is present
  - Intracellular shift due to insulin, β-receptor stimulation, or alkalosis
  - Classic example of intracellular shifting is hypokalemic periodic paralysis
    - Autosomal dominant inheritance—mutations in *CACNA1S* (Ca^{2+} channel) or *SCN4A* (Na$^+$ channel)
    - Onset in childhood to adolescence
    - Attacks last for minutes to days and are of longer duration than in hyperkalemic periodic paralysis
    - Acquired form may be seen in thyrotoxicosis
- Renal K$^+$ wasting
  - Urine K$^+$ concentration greater than 25 to 30 mEq/day or spot greater than 20 mEq/L in the presence of normal urine output
- Extrarenal K$^+$ wasting
  - Urine K$^+$ concentration less than 25 to 30 mEq/day or spot less than 15 mEq/L in the presence of normal urine output

Treatment

- Investigate and treat underlying cause
- Nature of treatment determined by degree of hypokalemia and presence or absence of symptoms
- Patients at increased risk of arrhythmia (e.g., digoxin therapy, coronary artery disease) merit more aggressive treatment
- In patients with total body depletion, serum K$^+$ concentration of 3 mEq/L represents loss of approximately 200 to 300 mEq of K$^+$
  - K$^+$ concentration 3 to 3.5 mEq/L: Prevent further K$^+$ loss and consider oral repletion

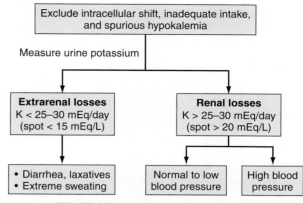

FIGURE 32-6 Approach to hypokalemia.

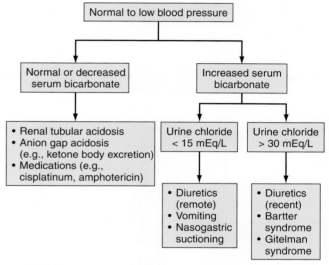

FIGURE 32-7 Renal K$^+$ loss with normal to low blood pressure.

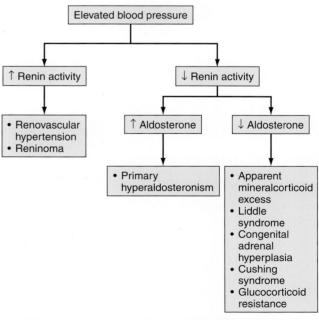

FIGURE 32-8 Renal K$^+$ loss with elevated blood pressure.

- K+ concentration less than 3 mEq/L: Intravenous K+ repletion with cardiac monitoring should be considered
- Hypomagnesemia and hypocalcemia may render correction of hypokalemia more difficult and should be addressed prior to K+ repletion
- In patients with impaired renal function, intravenous K+ repletion can lead to unpredictable serum concentrations and should be utilized with caution

HYPERKALEMIA

Basic Information

- Serum K+ concentration greater than 5.5 mEq/L
- Rarely caused by excess intake alone, as normally functioning kidneys have a substantial excretory capacity

Clinical Presentation

- Mild elevations (5.5–6 mEq/L): Usually asymptomatic
- Greater than 6.5 mEq/L: Progressive weakness, muscle aches, areflexia, paresthesias, electrocardiogram (ECG) changes

- Greater than 7 mEq/L: Paralysis, respiratory failure, life-threatening arrhythmias
- ECG changes are not a sensitive marker for presence or severity of hyperkalemia (Fig. 32-9)
    - 6 to 7 mEq/L: Peaked T waves (height >5 mm)
    - 7 to 8 mEq/L: Widening of QRS complex, prolonged P–R interval with flattening of P wave
- Greater than 8 mEq/L: Atrial standstill, progressive QRS widening and fusion with T wave to form sine wave pattern, ventricular tachycardia and fibrillation

Diagnosis and Evaluation

- Differential diagnosis of hyperkalemia is shown in Figure 32-10
- Evaluate for extracellular shift and pseudohyperkalemia
    - Pseudohyperkalemia may occur with:
        - Hemolysis during venipuncture
        - Leukocytosis greater than 100,000 cells/mm^3 or thrombocytosis greater than 500,000 cells/mm^3. Plasma (as compared to serum) K+ should be normal.

FIGURE 32-9 Electrocardiogram changes in hyperkalemia. The first panel demonstrates peaked T waves, which worsen as the P waves begin to disappear in the second panel. A sine wave configuration is shown in panel 3, as seen in a patient with severe hyperkalemia. *(From Goldberger AL: Clinical electrocardiography: a simplified approach, ed 6, St. Louis, Mosby, 1998.)*

FIGURE 32-10 Differential diagnosis of hyperkalemia. (ACE-I, angiotensin-converting enzyme inhibitor; ARB, angiotensin receptor blocker; NSAIDs, nonsteroidal anti-inflammatory drugs; RTA, renal tubular acidosis.)

- Familial pseudohyperkalemia (autosomal dominant)
- Classic example of extracellular shifting is hyperkalemic periodic paralysis
  - Autosomal dominant inheritance—mutation in SCN4A Na$^+$ channel
  - Onset early in life
  - Attacks more frequent and of shorter duration than with hypokalemic periodic paralysis
- Evaluate for mechanisms of impaired renal excretion
  - Calculate transtubular potassium gradient (TTKG):

$$TTKG = (Urine\ K\ /\ Plasma\ K)\ /\ (Urine\ Osm\ /\ Plasma\ Osm)$$

  - Value less than 5 suggests hypoaldosteronism or K$^+$ secretory defect in setting of urine Na$^+$ greater than 25 mEq/L and urine osmolality greater than plasma osmolality
  - True utility of TTKG, however, is often quite limited

Treatment

- For K$^+$ greater than 6.5 mEq/L or in the presence of ECG changes, administer IV calcium to decrease myocardial excitability
- **Decrease intake of K$^+$**
  - Examine medications and dietary factors high in K$^+$
  - Avoid medications that inhibit K$^+$ secretion
- Shift K$^+$ intracellularly
  - Correct hyperglycemia, if present
    - 10 units of regular insulin administered intravenously with an ampule of 50% dextrose in water (D$_{50}$W) to prevent hypoglycemia
    - Consider IV bicarbonate, although effectiveness is marginal
- Increase K$^+$ elimination from the body
  - Oral or rectal administration of a K$^+$ exchange resin, sodium polystyrene sulfonate (SPS). One gram binds approximately 1 mEq K$^+$ *in vivo*.
  - SPS is ineffective in patients with prior colectomy
  - Loop diuretics may be of utility in a stable patient with mild hyperkalemia
  - Dialysis if severe and life-threatening

REVIEW QUESTIONS

For review questions, please go to www.expertconsult.com.

SUGGESTED READINGS

Androgue HJ, Madias NE: Hypernatremia, N Engl J Med 342:1493–1499, 2000.

Androgue HJ, Madias NE: Hyponatremia, N Engl J Med 342:1581–1589, 2000.

Ellison DH, Berl T: The syndrome of inappropriate antidiuresis, N Engl J Med 356:2064–2072, 2007.

Fried LF, Palevsky PM: Hyponatremia and hypernatremia, Med Clin North Am 81:585–609, 1997.

Mandal AK: Hypokalemia and hyperkalemia, Med Clin North Am 81:611–639, 1997.

Nyirenda MJ, Tang JI, Padfield PL, Seckl JR: Hyperkalemia, BMJ 339:1019–1024, 2009.

Unwin RJ, Luft FC: Shirley DG: Pathophysiology and management of hypokalemia: a clinical perspective, Nat Rev Nephrol 7:75–84, 2011.

32

Acute Kidney Injury

HYUNG M. LIM, MD

Acute kidney injury (AKI) may result from a wide array of renal insults in both hospitalized patients and outpatients. A systematic approach that includes a detailed history, focused physical examination, and supporting laboratory or radiologic evaluation is needed to determine the diagnosis. Supportive care, specifically dialysis, may be needed until renal function returns.

Basic Information

- Definition: AKI is deterioration in renal function manifested by an acute rise in serum creatinine (Cr) and blood urea nitrogen (BUN) caused by the inability to clear water, electrolytes, and nitrogenous wastes, occurring over hours to days
  - Doubling of serum Cr indicates approximately 50% reduction in renal function
  - AKI results in altered urine output, classified as either oliguric (400 mL/day) or nonoliguric (>400 mL/day)
- RIFLE (risk, injury, failure, loss, and ESRD [end-stage renal disease]) criteria
  - Risk: 1.5× increase in the serum Cr *or* glomerular filtration rate (GFR) decrease by 25% *or* urine output less than 0.5 mL/kg/hr for 6 hours
  - Injury: 2× increase in the serum Cr *or* GFR decrease by 50% *or* urine output less than 0.5 mL/kg/hr for 12 hours
  - Failure: 3× increase in the serum Cr *or* GFR decrease by 75% *or* serum Cr more than 4 mg/dL with acute increase of ≥0.5 mg/dL *or* urine output less than 0.3 mL/kg/hr for 24 hours, or anuria for 12 hours
  - Loss: Persistent AKI = complete loss of renal function for more than 4 weeks
  - ESRD: Persistent AKI more than 3 months
- AKIN (Acute Kidney Injury Network)—modified RIFLE criteria
  - Stage 1: Increase in serum Cr of 0.3 mg/dL from baseline *or* Cr increase of 1.5 to 2 times baseline; urine output less than 0.5 mL/kg/hr for more than 6 hours
  - Stage 2: Serum Cr concentration increase of 2 to 3 times baseline; urine output less than 0.5 mL/kg/hr for more than 12 hours
  - Stage 3: Serum Cr concentration increase over 3 times baseline *or* Cr value greater than 4 mg/dL with acute increase of Cr greater than 0.5 mg/dL; urine output less than 0.3 mL/kg/hr for 24 hours or anuria for 12 hours
- Categories of AKI (Fig. 33-1)
  - Prerenal: Reduction in effective circulating volume and renal perfusion or bilateral renal artery occlusion
  - Intrarenal: Vascular, glomerular, or tubular injuries

- Postrenal: Obstruction of urinary tract or bilateral renal veins
- General approach to the evaluation of the patient with AKI: see Figure 33-2
- General principles for treatment of AKI
- **Correct any reversible causes**
- Assess potassium, acid-base status, fluid status, toxin accumulation, and need for dialysis (Table 33-1)
- **Adjust dosage of renally cleared medications**
- Fluid challenge if appropriate
- Discontinue all nephrotoxic drugs
- Avoid angiotensin-converting enzyme (ACE) inhibitors, angiotensin receptor blockers (ARBs), and nonsteroidal anti-inflammatory drugs (NSAIDs)

Prerenal Causes of Acute Kidney Injury

Basic Information

- AKI that is caused by reduction of effective circulating volume or decreased renal blood flow
- **Prerenal causes are the second most common general cause of AKI in the hospital setting (most common is acute tubular necrosis)**
- Patients can present with severe oliguric renal failure
- Once the effective circulating volume has been restored, renal recovery is the general rule

Clinical Presentation

- **True volume depletion**
  - Lack of oral intake or vomiting
  - GI loss: Bleeding or diarrhea
  - Renal loss: Diuretics, hyperglycemia, salt-wasting nephropathy, diabetes insipidus
  - Skin loss: Sweats or burns
- **Reduction in effective circulating volume**
  - Congestive heart failure (cardiorenal syndrome)
  - Cirrhosis
  - Nephrotic syndrome
  - Sepsis and shock
  - **Hepatorenal syndrome: A poorly understood, relentless worsening of renal function in the patient with advanced liver disease, with no other apparent cause (a diagnosis of exclusion)**
    - Pathophysiology includes dilation of the splanchnic bed vasculature, which pools blood and results in a fall in the systemic vascular resistance and blood pressure, with reduced renal perfusion

FIGURE 33-1 Differential diagnosis of acute kidney injury. (GI, gastrointestinal; HUS/TTP, hemolytic uremic syndrome/thrombotic thrombocytopenic purpura; PO, oral.)

FIGURE 33-2 Initial evaluation of the patient with acute kidney injury. *$FE_{Na} = U_{Na}/P_{Na} \times P_{Cr}/U_{Cr} \times 100\%$. †Gadolinium contraindicated in moderate to severe renal failure due to risk of nephrogenic systemic fibrosis. (ATN, acute tubular necrosis; BP, blood pressure; CBC, complete blood count; CPK, creatine phosphokinase; CT, computed tomography; FE_{Na}, fractional excretion of sodium; H&P, history and physical examination; IVP, intravenous pyelogram; LFTs, liver function tests; MRI/MRA, magnetic resonance imaging/magnetic resonance angiography; P_{Cr}, plasma creatinine; P_{Na}, plasma sodium; RBC, red blood cell; U_{Cr}, urine creatinine; U_{Na}, urine sodium; WBC, white blood cell.)

TABLE 33-1	Indications for Dialysis	
Indication	**Findings**	
Volume overload	Congestive heart failure Uncontrolled hypertension Massive edema	
Severe metabolic acidosis	Hyperventilation Hyperkalemia	
Hyperkalemia	Cardiac arrhythmias	
Uremia	Pericarditis; stupor; seizures; asterixis; platelet dysfunction	
Drug toxicity (e.g., lithium, digoxin)	Specific to drug	

- The renin-angiotensin and sympathetic nervous systems are activated, and vasopressin is released, resulting in renal artery vasoconstriction
- **Medications**
  - Diuretics—volume depletion
  - ACE inhibitor/ARB/renin inhibitor—Decreases the formation of angiotensin II or blocks the effects of angiotensin II, thus resulting in efferent arteriolar vasodilation and reduced intraglomerular pressure and reduced GFR
  - NSAID—Inhibits the production of vasodilatory prostaglandins, resulting in afferent arteriolar vasoconstriction and reduced GFR
  - Calcineurin inhibitors (tacrolimus, cyclosporine)—Cause renal artery vasoconstriction, resulting in reduced GFR

Diagnosis

- **BUN/Cr ratio greater than 20:1** because of increased water and urea reabsorption
- Low urine sodium concentration **(usually <20 mEq/L)**
- **Low urine fractional excretion of sodium (FE$_{Na}$ <1%; Table 33-2)**

TABLE 33-2	*Use of Fractional Excretion of Sodium (Fe$_{Na}$) in AKI*	
Causes of AKI		**Fe$_{Na}$* (%)**
Prerenal causes of AKI because of hypovolemia		<1
Prerenal causes of AKI because of decreased effective circulating volume		<1
Acute tubular necrosis, from any cause		>2
Hepatorenal syndrome		<1

*Fe$_{Na}$ = U$_{Na}$/P$_{Na}$ × P$_{Cr}$/U$_{Cr}$ × 100%.
AKI, acute renal failure; P$_{Cr}$, plasma creatinine; P$_{Na}$, plasma sodium; U$_{Cr}$, urine creatinine; U$_{Na}$, urine sodium.

- Urine osmolality greater than 500 mOsm/kg
- Urine Cr/Plasma Cr ratio greater than 40

Treatment

- Volume depletion: **Vigorous IV fluid resuscitation typically improves renal function and urine output within 24 to 48 hours**
- Reduced effective volume: Treatment of the underlying disease process; **maximize cardiac output**
- **Hepatorenal syndrome is best treated by liver transplantation.** Dialysis may be needed in the interim.
  - Peritoneovenous shunt or transjugular intrahepatic portosystemic shunt (TIPS) may prolong renal function but can cause worsening of encephalopathy of liver disease
  - **Omnipressin (an antidiuretic hormone analogue that constricts the splanchnic bed) may be administered with IV albumin, which may improve renal function but can cause ischemia**
  - Midodrine (systemic vasoconstrictor) and octreotide (blocks vasodilator release) may be of some benefit

Intrarenal Causes of Acute Kidney Injury

Table 33-3 lists the intrarenal causes of AKI. Acute glomerulonephritis and vasculitis are covered in Chapter 34.

Acute Tubular Necrosis

See Figure 33-3 for an illustration of acute tubular necrosis.

Basic Information

- **The most common cause of AKI in the hospital setting**
  - Results from ischemic (i.e., prerenal) or nephrotoxic (i.e., intrarenal) injury to renal tubules
  - Damaged tubular cells accumulate in tubular lumen, resulting in occlusion
    - Injury commonly most severe in early proximal tubule and medullary segment

Clinical Presentation

- Appropriate clinical setting, such as ischemic event or exposure to nephrotoxin, precedes deterioration in renal function
- **Clinical course typically progresses, then resolves over 1 to 3 weeks**

Diagnosis

- **BUN/Cr ratio is normal,** usually less than 20:1
- Urinalysis shows **muddy brown granular casts and epithelial cell casts**
- **High urine sodium concentration (usually >40 mEq/L)** is caused by tubular injury and decreased sodium reabsorption
- High urine fractional excretion of sodium (**FE$_{Na}$ >2%; see Table 33-2**)
- Urine osmolality less than 350 to 450 mOsm/kg
- **Urine Cr/Plasma Cr ratio less than 20:1** (measure of tubular water reabsorption)

Treatment

- **Supportive care** until renal function returns
- Avoid nephrotoxins

Interstitial Nephritis

Basic Information

- Results from the infiltration of the interstitial space by inflammatory cells (mostly T cells and monocytes; Fig. 33-4)
- Process **initiated by reaction to medication**
  - β-Lactam antibiotics and cephalosporins are the most common
  - NSAIDs are associated with
    - Either pure interstitial disease or additional glomerular disease **(minimal change disease or membranous glomerulonephritis)**
    - NSAIDs can also cause **acute ischemic renal injury (hemodynamic change), analgesic nephropathy, or papillary necrosis**
    - **Urine sediment may not contain significant eosinophils**
  - **Rifampin** is associated with acute tubulointerstitial disease even with intermittent dosing or after discontinuation of the drug
  - **Sulfonamides** can cause vasculitis

Clinical Presentation

- Acute worsening of renal function after starting a new medication
- **Fever and skin rash are also common**

Diagnosis

- Diagnosis is made based on clinical presentation or renal biopsy and is supported by
  - **Hematuria, pyuria, and white blood cell casts in urine**
  - **Eosinophilia and eosinophiluria are seen in more than 75% of cases**
  - Mild proteinuria also seen

TABLE 33-3	*Intrarenal Causes of AKI*	
Disorder	**Suggestive Features**	**Treatment**
Contrast nephropathy	Appropriate clinical setting, such as recent (<72 hr) contrast radiography	Prevention; supportive measures until recovery of renal function
Interstitial nephritis	Fever; skin rash; WBC casts in urine; eosinophilia and eosinophiluria	Discontinue offending drug; prednisone
Acute glomerulonephritis	Hypertension; fluid retention; hematuria; proteinuria	Differs based on underlying cause of glomerulonephritis
Acute tubular necrosis	Recent hypotensive event; recent exposure to nephrotoxin	Supportive care until renal function returns
Pigment nephropathy	High serum CPK (typically >10,000 IU/L); pigmented casts, hemoglobinuria, but no RBCs in urine	IV hydration; alkalinize urine to pH >6.5
Renal artery atheroembolic disease	Low serum complement; eosinophilia; eosinophiluria; cholesterol crystals on renal or skin biopsy	Supportive measures, but prognosis poor
Renal artery thromboembolic disease	Flank pain, hematuria, elevated LDH	Supportive measures, anticoagulation

AKI, acute kidney injury; CPK, creatine phosphokinase; LDH, lactate dehydrogenase; RBC, red blood cell; WBC, white blood cell.

33

FIGURE 33-3 Acute tubular necrosis. In acute tubular necrosis, kidneys are swollen and pale, particularly in the renal cortex. *(From Stevens A, Lowe J: Pathology, ed 2, St. Louis, Mosby, 2000, Fig. 17.23.)*

FIGURE 33-4 Drug-induced interstitial nephritis, with prominent eosinophilic and mononuclear cell infiltrate. *(From Kumar V, Fausto N, Abbas A: Robbins and Cotran: pathologic basis of disease, ed 7, Philadelphia, Elsevier Saunders, 2005, Fig. 20-44.)*

Treatment
- Discontinuation of offending agent(s)
- **Corticosteroids: Prednisone 1 mg/kg/day**

Contrast-Induced Nephropathy

Basic Information
- **Caused by renal vasoconstriction** from the release of endothelin and adenosine as well as from the high osmolality of the contrast material
- **Also caused by direct tubular injury** by the contrast agent
- Those at greatest risk include those with
  - Underlying renal insufficiency with **plasma Cr greater than 1.5 mg/dL**
  - **Diabetic nephropathy** with renal insufficiency
  - Poor renal perfusion: **Heart failure, dehydration, or liver failure**
  - **Multiple myeloma**
  - High doses of contrast agent
- **Magnetic resonance gadolinium contrast media may also be associated with nephrotoxicity in high concentrations**
  - Use of gadolinium in the setting of advanced renal failure has been associated with nephrogenic systemic fibrosis

Clinical Presentation
- Acute rise of serum BUN/Cr occurs within 24 to 48 hours of IV contrast exposure
- **Cr peaks within 7 days and usually returns to baseline within 10 days**
- Renal failure is usually reversible

Diagnosis
- Clinical diagnosis based on **history of exposure in appropriate time period**
- Imaging of the kidneys, ureter, and bladder reveals enhanced outline of kidneys secondary to retained IV contrast

Treatment

- No specific therapy; supportive measures only
- Maintain renal perfusion with IV hydration, but with risk of volume overload
- Avoid repeated contrast exposure
- **Best treatment is prevention**
  - **IV hydration with normal saline** 1 mL/kg/hr, 12 hours before and after administration of IV contrast agent
  - **Sodium bicarbonate** hydration may also be of benefit before IV contrast
  - N-Acetylcysteine (Mucomyst) 600 to 1200 mg PO twice a day for 2 days, starting 1 day before IV contrast exposure
  - **Minimize** IV contrast volume
  - Use **nonionic contrast or dilute contrast media**
  - Prophylactic dialysis to remove contrast has no proven benefit

Renal Artery Embolic Disease

Basic Information

- AKI results from cholesterol emboli, which lodge in medium or small renal arteries
- Inflammatory reaction causes **intimal proliferation, fibrosis, and irreversible blockages**

Clinical Presentation

- Two common presentations, caused by either thrombo-embolic or atheroembolic event
  - **Thromboembolic: Occurs after myocardial infarction or with atrial arrhythmias,** resulting in complete arterial obstruction and renal infarction
    - Individual notes flank pain, hematuria
    - Lactate dehydrogenase is elevated
  - **Atheroembolic: Occurs spontaneously or following a catheter manipulation in aorta or surgery;** produces incomplete obstruction and renal atrophy; renal function worsens acutely and continues to progress over several weeks
    - Other physical findings include cyanosis, gangrene of toes or feet, livedo reticularis (Fig. 33-5)
    - If pancreatic or mesenteric emboli also occur, abdominal pain may result

Diagnosis

- Clinical suggestion in appropriate setting
- Laboratory findings include **eosinophilia, eosinophi-luria, and hypocomplementemia**
- Cholesterol crystals may be present on renal or **skin biopsy,** or elsewhere in body (Fig. 33-6)

Treatment

- Supportive care only; prognosis is poor
- Consider anticoagulation with thromboembolic disease

Pigment Nephropathy

Basic Information

- Acute renal tubular injury from **myoglobin or hemoglobin**

FIGURE 33-5 Livedo reticularis. Note the characteristic "fishnet stocking" pattern of the rash. (*From Haslett C, Chilvers ER, Boon NA, et al: Davidson's principles and practice of medicine, ed 19, New York, Churchill Livingstone, 2002, Fig. 20.48.*)

FIGURE 33-6 Cholesterol emboli noted in the funduscopic exam. (*From Swash M: Hutchinson's clinical methods, ed 21, Philadelphia, WB Saunders, 2002, Fig. 12.14.*)

- Pathogenesis is **tubular cell injury from free chelat-able iron** (ferrihemate), which results in intrarenal vasoconstriction
- **Obstruction of tubules** with pigment casts, which results in renal failure

Clinical Presentation

- Patient often notes dark urine ("Coca-Cola urine") because of presence of myoglobin/hemoglobin pigments in urine
- Usually **associated with traumatic muscle injuries** (extreme exercises, trauma, seizures, ischemia), **muscle** toxins (drugs, including cocaine and statins), or other causes (infections, electrolyte abnormalities, endocrine, inflammatory myopathies)
  - Release of intracellular electrolytes results in **hyper-kalemia, hyperphosphatemia, and hyperuricemia**
- Sequestration of fluid and calcium into injured muscles leading to **volume depletion and hypocalcemia**

Diagnosis

- AKI in appropriate clinical setting
- Associated with high serum creatine phosphokinase (CPK); **renal injury often associated with CPK greater than 10,000 IU/L**

- Hyperkalemia, hyperphosphatemia, and hypocalcemia also common and support the diagnosis
- Urinalysis reveals pigmented casts (**but no red blood cells**) with myoglobin or hemoglobin in the urine

Treatment

- **Aggressive IV hydration**
- **Alkalinize urine to pH above 6.5** (2–3 ampules of bicarbonate mixed in 1 L of 5% dextrose in water) to prevent formation of ferrihemate from myoglobin or hemoglobin
- Recovery is the general rule, but dialysis may be needed until renal function returns

Postrenal Causes of Acute Kidney Injury

Basic Information

- **Group of disorders resulting from the physical obstruction of the ureters (e.g., obstructing nephrolithiasis, malignancy, retroperitonal fibrosis), bladder (e.g., prostatic hypertrophy, clots, tumors), or renal veins (e.g., renal vein thrombosis, see Chapter 34; Fig. 33-7)**

Clinical Presentation

- If onset sudden, patient will note flank pain
  - **If obstruction complete, anuria results**
- **Partial obstruction may result in polyuria or oliguria**
- Physical examination may note abdominal mass from hydronephrosis, or pelvic mass from distended bladder

Diagnosis

- **Ultrasound is the test of choice to determine the presence of obstruction** because of high sensitivity (90%) and specificity (90%), low cost, and safety
- **IV pyelography is the test of choice to define the location of obstruction** and anatomy of the ureters; however, one must consider the potential toxicity of IV contrast medium and poor visualization of the kidneys with low GFR (Fig. 33-8)
- **Computed tomography is able to diagnose hydronephrosis without IV contrast** and is useful in determining extrinsic mass, hematoma, or stones
- **Nuclear medicine furosemide renogram can provide functional status of the kidneys** and avoid risk of IV contrast; however, anatomic visualization is poor

Treatment

- The most effective treatment is determined by the location of the obstruction. **Emergency relief of the obstruction is indicated if AKI or urosepsis has resulted.**
  - Obstruction distal to the bladder can be relieved by a Foley catheter or a suprapubic catheter
  - Upper urinary tract obstruction can be relieved by either a percutaneous nephrostomy tube or ureteral stent placement

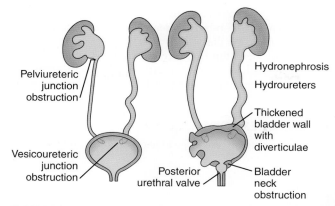

FIGURE 33-7   Postrenal causes of acute kidney injury include any obstruction along the urinary outflow tract. *(From Lissauer T, Clayden G: Illustrated textbook of paediatrics, ed 2, St. Louis, Mosby, 2001, Fig. 16-6a.)*

FIGURE 33-8   *Unilateral urinary outflow tract obstruction. This patient has an obstructing kidney stone at the lower end of the right ureter. This image, taken 2 hours after contrast injection, demonstrates persistent contrast in the right kidney and collecting system as compared with that on the left. (From Haslett C, Chilvers ER, Boon NA, et al: Davidson's principles and practice of medicine, ed 19, New York, Churchill Livingstone, 2002, Fig. 14.38.)*

- Recovery of renal function depends on the duration of the obstruction
  - Postobstructive diuresis: Marked polyuria with loss of water, sodium, potassium, and other electrolytes
    - Replacement fluid should be half-normal saline initially and readjusted according to serum electrolyte changes

33

- Etiology of massive diuresis is volume expansion, urea accumulation, tubular damage, and accumulation of natriuretic factors
  - Prolonged fluid replacement should be avoided, as it will perpetuate postobstructive diuresis by continued replacement of sodium and water

REVIEW QUESTIONS

For review questions, please go to www.expertconsult.com.

SUGGESTED READINGS

Bellomo R, Ronco C, Kellum JA, et al, for the Acute Dialysis Quality Initiative Workgroup: Acute renal failure—definition, outcome measures, animal models, fluid therapy and information technology needs: the Second International Consensus Conference of the Acute Dialysis Quality Initiative (ADQI) Group, *Crit Care* 8:R204–R212, 2004.

Brenner BM, Rector FC: *The kidney*, ed 8, Philadelphia, 2007, Elsevier Saunders.

Mehta RL, Kellum JA, Shah SV, et al, for the Acute Kidney Injury Network: Acute Kidney Injury Network: report of an initiative to improve outcomes in acute kidney injury, *Crit Care* 11:R31, 2007.

Post TW, Rose BD: Diagnostic approach to the patient with acute or chronic kidney disease. (Available at: Up-To-Date Online).

Glomerular Disease

TARIQ SHAFI, MBBS, MHS; and DEREK M. FINE, MD

Glomerular disease includes a group of disorders in which the glomerular filtration barrier is altered. The resultant change in filtration may be accompanied by proteinuria (in nephrotic disorders) or hematuria (in nephritic disorders), or both. Familiarity with the causes of nephrotic and nephritic disorders will guide the history, physical, and laboratory examination of patients presenting with abnormal urinary sediment.

Basic Information

- **Glomerular disease refers to disorders of the glomerular filtration barrier that occur either as a primary disorder or as a result of other diseases, toxins, or infections**
- **The glomerular filtration barrier may be affected so that proteinuria results; if the proteinuria is greater than 3.5 g/24 hr (nephrotic-range proteinuria), a nephrotic syndrome may result**
- **If glomerular filtration barrier is affected so that hematuria results (often accompanied by proteinuria), the disorder is classified as nephritic (glomerulonephritis [GN])**
- Additional clinical features typically accompany nephrotic and nephritic disorders (see following)
- Significant overlap may exist among disorders that result in nephrotic syndrome and GN

Nephrotic Syndrome

Basic Information

- General features of nephrotic syndrome
  - **Nephrotic syndrome is defined by the presence of**
    - **Proteinuria (>3.5 g/24 hr)**
    - **Hypoalbuminemia (<3.0 g/dL)**
    - **Hyperlipidemia**
  - Edema results from hypoalbuminemia
  - Blood pressure is variable depending on the underlying disease
    - Usually normal in minimal change disease and membranous nephropathy
    - Frequently elevated in focal segmental glomerulosclerosis (FSGS)
  - **Urinary loss of anticoagulant proteins (e.g., protein C, protein S, antithrombin III) may result in a hypercoagulable state**
    - **Renal vein thrombosis** may occur with any cause of nephrotic syndrome but is **most common with membranous GN**
    - Renal vein thrombosis often presents as sudden-onset worsening of renal insufficiency, worsening proteinuria, hematuria, or flank pain
  - Loss of immunoglobulins may result in a relative immune-deficient state

Clinical Presentation

- Features of specific causes of nephrotic syndrome—all may be idiopathic or related to secondary causes (Table 34-1)
  - **Minimal change disease**
    - Rapid onset; patient is normal one day and has edema the next
      - Glomerular filtration rate (GFR) remains normal
        - **Massive proteinuria common (>4 g/24 hr)**
        - **Pathologic hallmark is normal-appearing glomeruli on microscopy and generalized loss of foot processes of podocytes on electron microscopy** (Fig. 34-1)
  - **Focal segmental glomerulosclerosis (FSGS)**
    - "Classic" FSGS common in African Americans
    - Slow onset with progressive decrease in GFR if untreated
    - Creatinine normal, but may be elevated at presentation (elevated creatinine indicates poorer prognosis)
    - Proteinuria not massive (2–4 g/24 hr)
    - Includes findings seen with hyperfiltration injury (secondary FSGS)
    - Human immunodeficiency virus (HIV)–associated nephropathy (HIVAN) presents with a collapsing FSGS (vs. classic FSGS)
      - Characterized by a very rapid onset of renal failure (over months) with massive proteinuria
      - Collapsing FSGS may occasionally be seen in non–HIV-infected patients
  - **Membranous GN**
    - **The most common cause of nephrotic syndrome in adults**
    - **Associated with presence of anti-phospholipase A_2 (PLA_2) antibodies**
    - **Slow onset with loss of GFR, usually over years**
    - **Spontaneous remission in one third of patients**
    - Creatinine often normal; if creatinine deteriorates rapidly, consider renal vein thrombosis
    - Proteinuria varies from subnephrotic range to massive (>20 g/24 hr)
- Secondary causes of nephrotic syndrome
  - **Diabetes**

TABLE 34-1 *Diagnosis of Causes of Nephrotic Syndrome*

Cause	Typical Age of Onset	Associated Diseases	Pathologic Findings
Minimal change disease	<12 years or mid-60s	NSAIDs Lymphoma Bee sting	Light microscopy: Normal Immunofluorescence: Normal Electron microscopy: Diffuse podocyte foot process effacement
Focal segmental glomerulosclerosis (FSGS)	Early teens to mid-30s	Hyperfiltration (seen in morbid obesity; may result from nephron loss due to other causes) HIV (collapsing variant) Heroin nephropathy	Light microscopy: Focal and segmental glomerulosclerosis Immunofluorescence: May show nonspecific IgM deposition Electron microscopy: Foot process effacement Collapsing variant seen on light microscopy in those with HIV
Membranous glomerulonephritis	Mid-30s to mid-60s	Adenocarcinoma (breast, bowel, lung) Hepatitis B Systemic lupus erythematosus Drug reaction (NSAID)	Light microscopy: Thickened capillary loops Immunofluorescence: Deposition of immunoglobulin and complement Electron microscopy: Subepithelial immune complex deposition

Membranoproliferative glomerulonephritis	Idiopathic: 8–16 years
	Secondary: More common in adults
		Type I:
		  Hepatitis C
		  Chronic hepatitis B
		  Endocarditis
		  Idiopathic
		Type II (dense deposit disease):
		  Lipodystrophy
		Type III:
		  Can be inherited
			Light microscopy: Glomerular lobulation, capillary wall thickening and mesangial expansion
			Immunofluorescence
			  Type I: C3, early complement components, IgG deposits
			  Type II: ±C3, IgM
			Electron microscopy
			  Type I: Subendothelial electron-dense deposits
			  Type II: Dense "ribbon-like" deposits along basement membrane
			  Type III: Large lucent areas in basement membrane

HIV, human immunodeficiency virus; IgG, immunoglobulin G; IgM, immunoglobulin M; NSAIDs, nonsteroidal anti-inflammatory drugs.

FIGURE 34-1 Electron micrograph of a glomerular capillary wall from a patient with minimal change glomerulopathy, showing extensive foot process effacement (*arrows*) and microvillous transformation (magnification ×5000). *(From Brenner BM: Brenner and Rector's the kidney, ed 7, Philadelphia, WB Saunders, 2004, Fig. 28-4.)*

- Diabetic nephropathy is the most common cause of nephrotic proteinuria
- Earliest evidence of diabetic nephropathy is microalbuminuria (30–300 mg albumin/24 hr), which then progresses to albuminuria (>300 mg/24 hr) and may progress to nephrotic-range proteinuria
- Once overt proteinuria has set in, renal function inevitably declines

- Average time to end-stage renal disease (ESRD) after onset of proteinuria is 10 years
- Progression to ESRD may be delayed by angiotensin-converting enzyme (ACE) inhibitors or angiotensin receptor blockers
- Diabetic nephropathy rarely develops before 10 years' duration of diabetes
- Type 1 diabetics with nephropathy
  - 95% also have retinopathy
  - In a patient with type 1 diabetes and nephropathy, the absence of retinopathy should prompt consideration of nondiabetic etiology of proteinuria/nephropathy
- Type 2 diabetics with nephropathy
  - 50% to 75% have retinopathy
  - Nephropathy in the absence of retinopathy in a patient with type 2 diabetes is therefore more common than with type 1 diabetes, but should still prompt consideration of other causes of nephropathy
  - If retinopathy is present in patients with type 2, almost 100% have nephropathy
- **All diabetic patients with proteinuria should be evaluated for other systemic diseases (e.g., hepatitis B and C, systemic lupus erythematosus [SLE], and monoclonal gammopathy) because up to 20% have either primary or superimposed nondiabetic cause of proteinuria**
- Clinical scenarios in which to consider renal biopsy in diabetics
  - Presence of proteinuria with less than 10 years' duration of diabetes

TABLE 34-2	*Treatment of Idiopathic Nephrotic and Nephritic Disorders*	
Disorder	**Treatment**	**Response**
Minimal change disease	Corticosteroids Cyclosporin or cyclophosphamide or mycophenolate mofetil for relapse	Children respond within 2 wk Adults respond in 4–8 wk, but often relapse
Focal segmental glomerulonephritis	Corticosteroids + ACE-I Cyclosporin or mycophenolate mofetil may be added to steroids	40–60% Response takes 4–13 mo

Membranous glomerulonephritis	ACE-I for all patients
	Low risk for progression (proteinuria <4 g/day + creatinine clearance >80 mL/min):
	    Observation with close follow-up
	Moderate risk for progression (persistent proteinuria between 4 g/day and 8 g/day + creatinine clearance >80 mL/min):
	    Corticosteroids ± cytotoxic agents
	High risk for progression (persistent proteinuria >8 g/day and/or abnormal or declining creatinine clearance):
	    Corticosteroids + cytotoxic agents
		Variable, dependent on prognostic indicators
		One third remit spontaneously without treatment—treatment decisions should be based on persistent proteinuria on 24-hr urine collections

Membranoproliferative glomerulonephritis	Corticosteroids ± cytotoxic agents Antiplatelet agents (aspirin; dipyridamole) may slow disease progression	Spontaneous remission in <10% Prolonged course of slowly deteriorating renal function seen in many

ACE-I, angiotensin-converting enzyme inhibitor.

- Presence of significant hematuria or red blood cell (RBC) casts on urinalysis
- Absence of retinopathy in patients with type 1 diabetes and possibly type 2 diabetes
- Any clinical or laboratory evidence of other systemic disease
- Amyloidosis
  - Systemic disease with extracellular deposition of amyloid in various organs (see Chapter 56)
  - Most common is AL amyloid (primary amyloidosis) with deposits of light-chain immunoglobulin
  - Secondary (AA amyloid) associated with chronic inflammatory or infectious states
  - AL amyloid is caused by plasma cell dyscrasia with overt multiple myeloma in 20% of cases
  - 90% have monoclonal light chains (Bence Jones proteins) in urine or blood
  - Proteinuria is the consistent feature with associated renal insufficiency
  - Nephrotic syndrome in patient older than 50 years—should have a high index of suspicion for AL amyloid
  - Generally poor prognosis, but may respond to chemotherapy

Diagnosis

- **Serologic evaluation: antinuclear antibody, hepatitis B surface antigen, anti–hepatitis C antibody, serum and urine protein electrophoresis, HIV antibody, complement levels**
- **Kidney biopsy needed in most patients**
  - All patients with rapidly rising creatinine, biopsy is urgent
  - Diabetics with consistent time course (>10 years' disease), no other systemic disease or serologic abnormalities, and presence of retinopathy may not require biopsy for diagnosis
  - Nephrotic patients with amyloid diagnosed by biopsy of other organ (e.g., heart, skin, or bone marrow) may not need kidney biopsy

Treatment

- When nephrotic syndrome is secondary to a systemic disease, treat the underlying disorder
- Additional renoprotective measures:
  - Strict blood pressure control (<130/80 mm Hg)
  - Use of ACE inhibitors or angiotensin receptor blockers
  - Aggressive control of cardiovascular risk factors
  - Diabetes control essential in the diabetic patient
- Treatment of idiopathic causes of nephrotic syndrome is described in Table 34-2

Nephritic Disorders

Basic Information

- General features of nephritic disorders (GN)
  - **Nephritic disorders are commonly associated with systemic diseases**
  - **Patients typically present with deteriorating renal function, mild to moderate proteinuria, and an active urine sediment (RBCs and RBC casts in the urine; Fig. 34-2)**
  - Hypocomplementemia suggests lupus nephritis, postinfectious GN, mebranoproliferative GN or cryoglobulinemic GN (present 60–80% of the time in these disorders)
  - Patients may report dark urine
  - Blood pressure is typically elevated; peripheral edema may be seen (which may progress to include ascites or pleural effusions)
  - Urine output may be normal or oliguric

Clinical Presentation

- Features of specific causes of GN
  - When evaluating the patient with a diagnosis of nephritis, consideration should be given to a search for a systemic, infectious, or postinfectious cause because GN is often secondary to another disorder

34

- Systemic diseases associated with GN
  - Frequently present with rapid-onset renal insufficiency in the setting of immune dysregulation
  - The role of complement in evaluation of GN is shown in Figure 34-3
  - The role of immune serologies is shown in Figure 34-4
  - Immunofluorescence (IF) of the kidney biopsy sample is essential in defining the underlying process:
    - Immune complex GN (immune complexes seen on IF)
    - Pauci-immune GN (no immune staining, hence the term *pauci*-immune)

FIGURE 34-2 Red cell casts typically seen in acute glomerulonephritis. *(From Noble J, Greene HL, Levinson W, et al: Textbook of primary care medicine, ed 3, St. Louis, Mosby, 2000, Fig. 144-6.)*

- Anti–glomerular basement membrane (anti-GBM) disease (linear GBM staining)
- Systemic lupus erythematosus (SLE): A secondary cause of proliferative or membranous GN (see Chapter 45)
- **Henoch-Schönlein purpura (HSP)**
  - Manifestations often include purpuric rash (Fig. 34-5), arthralgias, abdominal pain, and renal involvement
  - Commonly follows upper respiratory infection
  - Immunoglobulin A (IgA) deposition seen in renal mesangial cells (looks exactly like IgA nephropathy)
  - Uncommon in adults—more common in children; predominates in males
- **Vasculitis** (includes Wegener granulomatosis, microscopic polyangiitis, and Churg-Strauss syndrome; see Chapter 44)
- **Goodpasture syndrome**
  - Results from production of anti-GBM antibodies
  - The presence of both lung and kidney involvement with linear anti-GBM staining on IF defines the syndrome
  - Pathology reveals "crescent formation" in glomeruli; number of crescents relates to severity and prognosis
  - If pulmonary disease is absent in the presence of anti-GBM antibodies, diagnosis of the kidney-specific anti-GBM disease is made
- Infectious diseases associated with GN
  - Endocarditis
  - Hepatitis B and C
  - Less common: syphilis, malaria

FIGURE 34-3 Role of complement levels in diagnosis of the patient with glomerulonephritis. *Refers to infection of a ventriculoatrial shunt. (IgA, immunoglobulin A; HUS/TTP, hemolytic uremic syndrome/thrombotic thrombocytopenic purpura.) *(Adapted from Madaio MP, Harrington JT: The diagnosis of acute glomerulonephritis, N Engl J Med 309:1299–1302, 1983.)*

Glomerulonephritis

ANCA positive
- If necrotizing pulmonary granulomas seen, then consider Wegener granulomatosis (C-ANCA > P-ANCA)
- If other evidence of systemic vasculitis is seen, consider micropolyangiitis or Churg-Strauss disease (P-ANCA > C-ANCA)
- If no other disorder seen, then consider idiopathic crescentic glomerulonephritis

Anti-glomerular basement membrane
- If anti-GBM antibodies present but no lung disease, then consider anti-GBM glomerulonephritis
- If anti-GBM antibodies present with associated lung disease, then consider Goodpasture syndrome

Immune complex constituents
- If anti-DNA positive, then consider systemic lupus erythematosus
- If anti-streptolysin O antibody titer elevated, consider post-streptococcal glomerulonephritis
- If cryoglobulins demonstrated, consider cryoglobulinemia with glomerulonephritis
- If rash present and recent URI, consider Henoch-Schönlein purpura
- Also test for HCV, HBV, and other serologic evidence of infections associated with glomerulonephritis

FIGURE 34-4 Role of immune serologies in evaluation of the patient with glomerulonephritis. (ANCA, antineutrophil cytoplasmic antibody; C-ANCA; cytoplasmic antineutrophil cytoplasmic antibody; GBM, glomerular basement membrane; HBV, hepatitis B virus; HCV, hepatitis C virus; P-ANCA, perinuclear antineutrophil cytoplasmic antibody; URI, upper respiratory infection.) *(Adapted from Falk RJ: ANCA-associated renal disease, Kidney Int 38:998–1010, 1990.)*

FIGURE 34-5 Typical rash (palpable purpura) on the lower extremities seen in Henoch-Schönlein purpura. *(From Goldman L, Bennett JC, Ausiello D: Cecil textbook of medicine, ed 22, Philadelphia, WB Saunders, 2004, Fig. 475.4.)*

- Postinfectious etiologies associated with GN
  - Includes poststreptococcal GN, endocarditis-related GN, various viral infections
  - With poststreptococcal GN, patients present with hypertension, oliguria, and elevated antistreptolysin O (ASO) antibody titers 7 to 14 days after throat or skin infection with group A *Streptococcus*
    - Certain streptococcal strains more likely to cause GN (types 12 and 49)
    - Presentation can be highly variable—from asymptomatic microscopic hematuria to florid nephritic syndrome

- GN may also occur after staphylococcal (increasingly common in the current era) and other bacterial infections
- **IgA nephropathy (Berger disease)**
  - **Most common cause of GN in adults (although uncommon in African Americans)**
  - **Classic presentation is gross hematuria following upper respiratory infection (majority of patients)**
  - Others present with persistent, microscopic hematuria long after viral upper respiratory infection has been forgotten; less than 10% have a nephrotic presentation
  - Mesangial IgA deposition is seen on biopsy (establishes the diagnosis)
  - In contrast to HSP, rash is not seen and course is usually less aggressive
- Membranoproliferative glomerulonephritis (MPGN)
  - Clinical presentation may be nephrotic, nephritic, or mixed
  - **Most often secondary to hepatitis C infection (type I MPGN)**
  - Idiopathic forms of type I and type II
  - Course varies depending on presentation—from slowly progressive nephrotic syndrome similar to membranous GN to a rapidly progressive GN as is seen with the necrotizing vasculitides
  - Associated with cryoglobulins when related to hepatitis C (essential mixed cryoglobulinemia—type II cryoglobulins)

34

Diagnosis

- Clinical presentation and testing for specific diseases (e.g., ASO titers, hepatitis serologies) may be sufficient to diagnose likely, underlying cause of nephritic syndrome
- The evaluation and testing performed differs based on the clinical scenario
- Immunologic testing may also help narrow differential diagnosis (see Figs. 34-1 and 34-2)

BOX 34-1	*Diseases That May Present with Rapidly Progressive Renal Failure and Mimic Glomerulonephritis*

Cholesterol emboli syndrome (transient hypocomplementemia may be seen in 25%)

Thrombotic microangiopathies—include HUS, TTP, and antiphospholipid antibody syndrome

Scleroderma renal crisis

Myeloma cast nephropathy

Collapsing FSGS (usually associated with HIVAN)

FSGS, focal segmental glomerulosclerosis; HIVAN, human immunodeficiency virus–associated nephropathy; HUS, hemolytic uremic syndrome; TTP, thrombotic thrombocytopenic purpura.

- Some diseases manifest with rapidly progressive renal failure and may mimic GN (Box 34-1)
- Renal biopsy should be performed in the following situations:
  - Diagnosis/prognosis remains unclear
  - Rapidly progressive GN
  - Nephrotic-range proteinuria
  - Subnephrotic-range proteinuria (>2 g/day); use same approach as nephrotic patient
  - Presence of a systemic disease if accompanied by proteinuria or hematuria
  - Progressive renal insufficiency
  - Suspected acute tubular injury not improving after 3 to 4 weeks
  - Course atypical for diabetic nephropathy in diabetic patient

Treatment

- When GN is secondary to a systemic disease or infection, treatment is aimed at the underlying disorder
- Table 34-3 outlines therapy for selected nephritic disorders
- Some patients may require dialysis therapy temporarily or indefinitely

TABLE 34-3	*Treatment of Selected Nephritic Disorders*	
Disorder	**Treatment**	**Response**

Henoch-Schönlein purpura	Supportive care
	  Fluids
	  Pain relief
	Hospitalize for
	  Inadequate oral intake
	  GI bleeding
	  Renal failure
	Glucocorticoids for severe disease (unproven efficacy, but reasonable)
		Excellent prognosis
		Roughly one third relapse within 4 mo
		Acute morbidity: Due to GI bleeding
		Chronic morbidity: Renal involvement; 10% develop ESRD

Goodpasture syndrome	Plasmapheresis (to remove anti-GBM antibodies) + corticosteroids + cyclophosphamide Among those with higher creatinine requiring dialysis: Therapy less likely to be beneficial; most would still use above regimen	Prognosis (patient and kidney survival) correlates with number of crescents on biopsy and level of renal insufficiency on presentation Relapses are uncommon unless patient is also ANCA-positive
Postinfectious GN	Immunosuppressive therapy generally not helpful Rapidly progressive GN with crescents: Consider pulse steroids (though unproven efficacy)	Prognosis generally quite good Spontaneous resolution usually occurs over 3–4 wk

IgA nephropathy	Treat progessive disease (not all disease is progressive)
	ACE inhibitors or ARBs to treat hypertension and reduce intraglomerular pressure
	Corticosteroids may be of use in some patients
	Fish oil (omega-3 fatty acid) use is controversial, but frequently used
	Combined therapy with prednisone and other immunosuppressives may be needed in patients who continue to progress and in those with rapidly progressive disease
		Not all patients progress; some have stable course, some experience remission
		In patients who progress, deterioration is usually gradual
		Predictors of progression
		  Elevated creatinine at diagnosis
		  Increase in blood pressure
		  Protein excretion above 500–1000 mg/24 hr
		ESRD eventually develops in 15% at 10 yr and 20% in 20 yr

ACE, angiotensin-converting enzyme; ANCA, antineutrophil cytoplasmic antibody; ARB, angiotensin receptor blocker; ESRD, end-stage renal disease; GBM, glomerular basement membrane; GI, gastrointestinal; GN, glomerulonephritis; IgA, immunoglobulin A.

REVIEW QUESTIONS

For review questions, please go to www.expertconsult.com.

SUGGESTED READINGS

Falk RJ: ANCA-associated renal disease, *Kidney Int* 38:998–1010, 1990.

Madaio MP, Harrington JT: The diagnosis of acute glomerulonephritis, *N Engl J Med* 309:1299–1302, 1983.

Orth S, Ritz E: The nephrotic syndrome, *N Engl J Med* 338:1202–1211, 1998.

Chronic Kidney Disease and End-Stage Renal Disease

TARIQ SHAFI, MBBS, MHS; PAUL J. SCHEEL, Jr., MD, MBA; and DEREK M. FINE, MD

Chronic kidney disease (CKD) is a rising public health problem in the United States, predominantly because of the increasing prevalence of diabetes and hypertension with resultant renal disease. CKD often leads to end-stage renal disease (ESRD) and the need for renal replacement therapy.

Basic Information

- Definition: Defined by structural or functional abnormalities of the kidney for 3 months or longer, with or without decreased glomerular filtration rate (GFR). Normal GFR is ≥90 mL/min/1.73 m².
- **The National Kidney Foundation has established the following stages of CKD:**
  - **Stage I: Kidney damage (proteinuria, cyst formation, etc.) with normal or increased GFR**
  - **Stage II: Kidney damage with mild decrease in GFR (GFR 60–89 mL/min/1.73 m²)**
  - **Stage III: Moderate decrease in GFR (GFR 30–59 mL/min/1.73 m²)**
  - **Stage IV: Severe decrease in GFR (GFR 15–29 mL/min/1.73 m²)**
  - **Stage V: Kidney failure (GFR 15 mL/min/1.73 m² or dialysis)**
- Some experts recommend dividing Stage III CKD into two categories: stage IIIa (GFR 45–60 mL/min/1.73 m²) and stage IIIb (GFR 30–45 mL/min/1.73 m²)
- Presence of albuminuria or proteinuria is associated with increased risk of death or complications in patients with CKD
- Epidemiology
  - Many patients with CKD progress to ESRD
  - Prevalence increases with age
  - Estimated ESRD prevalence in the United States in 2008 was over 500,000, with an annual incidence of greater than 110,000
- Etiology
  - Diabetes (~40%)
  - Hypertension (~25%)
  - Glomerulonephritis (~10%)
  - Genetic or congenital (e.g., polycystic kidney disease; ~3%)
  - Urologic (~2%)

Clinical Presentation

- Usually asymptomatic until the late stages of renal failure

- **Onset of symptoms is usual indication for initiation of dialysis**
- **Early symptoms: anorexia, nausea, lethargy, fatigue**
- **Late symptoms: pruritis, mental status changes due to encephalopathy, volume overload, chest pain from pericarditis, neuropathy**
- Metabolic abnormalities often seen (Table 35-1)
  - Anemia
  - Secondary and tertiary hyperparathyroidism (associated with hypocalcemia, hyperphosphatemia, and metabolic bone disease)
  - Acidosis
  - Hyperkalemia
- Physical examination findings
  - Asterixis (indicative of encephalopathy)
  - Pericardial friction rub
  - Signs of volume overload
  - Uremic fetor: Foul-smelling breath similar to urine or fish
  - Pallor
  - Calciphylaxis: Calcification of arterioles (Fig. 35-1) seen in patients with ESRD (not just CKD). Also called calcific uremic arteriolopathy.
    - Usually in the setting of a high calcium × phosphorus product
    - Violaceous, indurated skin lesions that may ulcerate
    - Predilection for the lower extremities and trunk

Diagnosis

- Diagnose by estimated or actual GFR, not serum creatinine (Cr) levels
  - Normal GFR is usually greater than 90 mL/min in women and greater than 100 mL/min in men
  - **CKD is underdiagnosed if serum Cr is used as sole measure**
  - **Need to use GFR estimation equations**
    - Modification of Diet in Renal Disease (MDRD) formula is preferred for estimating GFR. It is used for GFR estimation by clinical laboratories and in most clinical trials (available at www.kidney.org).
    - Chronic Kidney Disease Epidemiology Collaboration (CKD-EPI) equation improves GFR estimation compared with MDRD equation in those with GFR above 60 mL/min/1.73 m2 (available at www.kidney.org)

TABLE 35-1	*Manifestations of Chronic Kidney Disease*			
Manifestation	**Mechanism**	**Clinical Features**	**Diagnosis**	**Treatment**
Anemia	Erythropoietin (EPO) deficiency	Onset: GFR 25–50 mL/min Early: Asymptomatic Late: Decrease in functional capacity and quality of life, left ventricular hypertrophy	Rule out other causes of anemia Reticulocyte count Peripheral smear, iron studies Hemoccult stool EPO levels *not* useful	**Goal hemoglobin: 10–12 g/dL** **STEP 1: Assess iron status:** Inadequate iron stores if ferritin <100, TSAT <20% IV iron if stores inadequate with oral iron **STEP 2: Consider erythropoiesis-stimulating agents if hemoglobin <9 g/dL and iron replete** **Erythropoietin:** Start dose: 50–70 units/kg subQ weekly **Darbepoetin:** Start dose: 0.45 µg/kg subQ weekly Caution: patients with cancer Monitor hemoglobin weekly until "in range," then monthly. Avoid hemoglobin >13 g/dL. Follow ferritin and TSAT at least quarterly in CKD, monthly in ESRD
Metabolic bone disease	**Low 1,25-dihydroxyvitamin D** (poor conversion from 25-hydroxyvitamin D) **High phosphate** (low excretion) **Low calcium** (due to low vitamin D) ↓ All lead to secondary hyperparathyroidism (high intact PTH) ↓ Renal osteodystrophy	Onset: GFR 25–40 mL/min Usually asymptomatic Bone pain—late manifestation Risk of fractures	High iPTH High phosphate Low calcium	**Goal iPTH:** 1.5–2 times upper limit of normal for the lab K/DOQI goals: CKD III: 35–70 pg/mL CKD IV: 70–110 pg/mL CKD V or ESRD: 150–300 pg/mL **Goal serum phosphorus** 2.7–4.6 mg/dL (CKD III, IV) 3.5–5.5 mg/dL (CKD V or ESRD) **Restrict dietary phosphorus** <800–1000 mg/day **Phosphate binders** Calcium-based Calcium carbonate Calcium acetate Non–calcium-based (if high calcium × phosphorus product [>72]) Sevelamer Lanthanum carbonate **Check 25-vitamin D levels if iPTH is above goal (CKD III–V):** If <30 ng/mL: Supplement with ergocalciferol (caution if serum phosphorus ≥4.6 mg/dL or albumin-corrected serum calcium ≥ 0.2 mg/dL) **Goal serum calcium:** 8.4–10.2 mg/dL **Vitamin D analogues** Calcitriol Paricalcitol Doxercalciferol **Calcimimetics** Cinacalcet
Acidosis	Inability of kidney to excrete acid load Usually a distal RTA	Chronic acidosis can result in hypercatabolism with poor nutritional status Calcium mobilization from the bone—exacerbation of osteoporosis	Low serum bicarbonate	**Goal serum bicarbonate** >22 mEq/L Start therapy if serum bicarbonate <18 mEg/L **Sodium** citrate 10 mL 3 times daily *or* **Sodium** bicarbonate 650 mg 3 times daily Monitor bicarbonate to avoid alkalosis

Continued

TABLE 35-1	*Manifestations of Chronic Kidney Disease* (Continued)			
Manifestation	**Mechanism**	**Clinical Features**	**Diagnosis**	**Treatment**
Volume overload	Inability of kidney to excrete water and salt	CHF Lower extremity edema	Physical exam Chest radiograph	**Sodium restriction** <2 g/day (<100 mEq on a 24-hr urine collection) **Fluid restriction** <1500 mL/day **Diuretics** Loop—increase dose until maximum; twice-daily dosing Thiazide—add to regimen if patient unresponsive to loop diuretic to overcome distal sodium retention
Hyperkalemia	Inability of kidney to excrete potassium load	Usually asymptomatic May cause paralysis or respiratory failure Cardiac arrhythmias	High serum potassium ECG changes Peaked T waves Flat or absent P wave Wide QRS complex Sine waves	**Acute** Calcium gluconate, insulin/glucose, β-agonist, diuretic, dialysis **Long-term** Dietary restriction (high-potassium foods include orange, potato, tomato, banana, cantaloupe, and many others) Loop or thiazide diuretic Correct concurrent acidosis (see above) Consider discontinuation of β-blockers

CHF, congestive heart failure; CKD, chronic kidney disease; ECG, electrocardiogram; ESRD, end-stage renal disease; GFR, glomerular filtration rate; iPTH, intact parathyroid hormone; K/DOQI, National Kidney Foundation Kidney Disease Outcomes Quality Initiative; PTH, parathyroid hormone; RTA, renal tubular acidosis; TSAT, transferrin saturation.

FIGURE 35-1 Typical skin lesion of calciphylaxis. *(From Dharmadhikari A, Sukkar A, Mani S: Cases from the Osler Medical Service at Johns Hopkins University. Am J Med 114:765–767, 2003, Fig. 1.)*

- **Cockcroft-Gault equation is an alternative:**

$$\frac{(140 - \text{age}) \times \text{lean body weight (kg)}}{\text{Serum Cr (mg/dL)} \times 72}$$

- For GFR in women, multiply equation by 0.85

- Other features that indicate CKD
  - Evidence that low GFR is long-standing (more than one measure over longer than 3 months)
  - Small kidneys on renal ultrasound (normal kidney size is 10 to 12 cm; kidneys are smaller in women)
  - Presence of manifestations of CKD: anemia, secondary hyperparathyroidism, acidosis
- Should rule out reversible causes in any patient with renal insufficiency
  - Obstruction and prerenal causes (see Chapter 33)
  - Treatable glomerular disease (see Chapter 34)
  - Atherosclerotic renal vascular disease (Box 35-1)

Management

- Early recognition of CKD
  - **Early referral to nephrologist shown to improve outcomes**
  - **Consider neprology referral for:**
    - Unexplained proteinuria or hematuria suggestive of glomerulonephritis
    - Rapid decline in GFR (>15 mL/min/1.73 m² per year)
    - All patients with GFR less than 30 mL/min/1.73 m²
  - Allows for early intervention (Fig. 35-2)
- Delay progression of CKD
  - **Angiotensin-converting enzyme (ACE) inhibitors and angiotensin receptor blockers (ARBs)**
    - Mechanism: Decrease intraglomerular pressure and hyperfiltration
    - Problem: May lead to elevation of serum creatinine and potassium

- Creatinine rise is 20% or less: Can continue therapy as there is long-term benefit in preservation of GFR
- If potassium is elevated (goal to maintain ACE inhibitor or ARB therapy)
  - Exclude renal artery stenosis
  - Dietary potassium restriction (major culprits include bananas, cantaloupe, oranges, potatoes, tomatoes)
  - Use of potassium-depleting diuretic (thiazide-type or loop diuretic)

BOX 35-1   *Atherosclerotic Renal Vascular Disease*

Common in patients with evidence of atherosclerotic disease in other vascular beds (20% of these patients)

45% to 50% of renal artery stenosis patients will have bilateral disease

Consider if any of the following are present
New-onset hypertension after age 50 years
Newly difficult-to-control hypertension (requiring >2 medications) in known hypertensive patient
Unexplained increase in creatinine in patient with suspected vascular disease (CAD, PVD, smoker, diabetic)
Hypotension or worsening creatinine after initiation of ACE inhibitor
Flash pulmonary edema without evidence of cardiac cause

Diagnosis
Renal angiography (gold standard)
Magnetic resonance angiography (less invasive, >90% sensitivity and specificity)
CT angiogram (best in those who can tolerate IV contrast)
Doppler ultrasound (accuracy is very user-dependent)

Treatment
Angioplasty and endovascular stenting—may not be better than medical management except in selected cases
Fibromuscular dysplasia—angioplasty is highly effective

Outcomes
Improvement in GFR and slowing of CKD progression
Improved blood pressure control requiring fewer antihypertensives (occasional cure of hypertension)

ACE, angiotensin-converting enzyme; CAD, coronary artery disease; CKD, chronic kidney disease; CT, computed tomography; GFR, glomerular filtration rate; IV, intravenous; PVD, peripheral vascular disease.

- Elimination of potassium-sparing diuretics (triamterene, spironolactone, or eplerenone)
- Consider β-blocker dose reduction (unless essential for other reasons)
- Fludrocortisone in selected patients (Caution: Salt and water retention leading to worsening hypertension)
- Management of hypertension
  - Hypertension is a very important risk factor for acceleration in decline in GFR
  - Adequate control of blood pressure reduces rate of decline in GFR
  - **Further reduction in blood pressure below 130/80 mm Hg (125/75 mm Hg) may have added benefit in patients, especially those with proteinuria (Joint National Committee on Prevention, Detection, Evaluation, and Treatment of High Blood Pressure [JNC 7] guidelines)**
  - ACE inhibitors or ARBs should be first line, given their independent benefits in slowing progression of renal disease
  - Atenolol is cleared by the kidney; therefore, use with caution or consider switch to hepatically cleared β-blocker such as metoprolol
- Dietary protein restriction
  - Mechanism: In theory, reduced protein intake decreases intraglomerular pressure and metabolic demands on kidney
  - Conflicting efficacy data from trials
  - Recommendation (largely opinion-based): Maximum dietary restriction for a patient with CKD would be 0.7 g of protein/kg of body weight/day; many would suggest that 1 g of protein/kg of body weight/day would be more appropriate
  - If patient is placed on protein-restricted diet, must have close follow-up of nutritional status to avoid malnutrition
- Management of glucose in patients with diabetes mellitus and CKD
  - Tight control of patient's blood glucose may slow progression of diabetic nephropathy
  - Goal hemoglobin A_{1c} (Hgb A_{1c}) is 6%

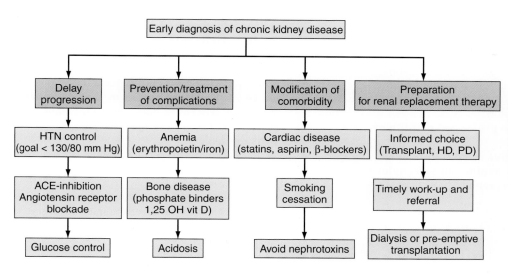

FIGURE 35-2 Management of chronic renal disease. (ACE, angiotensin-converting enzyme; HD, hemodialysis; HTN, hypertension; PD, peritoneal dialysis; 1,25-OH-vit D, 1,25-dihydroxyvitamin D.)

TABLE 35-2	*Drugs to Use with Caution in Renal Insufficiency*	
Drug Name	**Side Effect**	**Mechanism**
Gadolinium-based contrast agents	Nephrogenic systemic fibrosis	Poor clearance with extended half-life and deposition of free gadolinium in tissues. Avoid if GFR <30 mL/min and ESRD. Macrocyclic agent (gadoteridol) safer than linear agents (gadodiamide [Omniscan] or gadopentetate [Magnevist]) if exposure is essential.
Phosphate-containing bowel preps or enemas	Phosphate deposition in kidneys (phosphate nephropathy) or high anion gap acidosis	Poor clearance with renal failure
Aminoglycosides	ARF	Tubular toxicity
Atenolol	Bradycardia	Decreased renal clearance
Gabapentin	Altered mental status and other CNS toxicities	Decreased renal clearance
NSAIDs and COX-2 inhibitors	ARF	Prostacyclin-induced afferent vasoconstriction
Sulfonylureas	Hypoglycemia (glyburide worse than glipizide)	Decreased renal clearance
Metformin	Lactic acidosis (should really avoid in most CKD patients; hold before contrast studies)	Mitochondrial toxicity
Magnesium-containing medications	Hypermagnesemia	Decreased clearance of magnesium
Meperidine	Seizure	Low clearance of toxic metabolite normeperidine
Sucralfate	Aluminum toxicity	High aluminum content with decreased clearance in renal failure, especially ESRD
Potassium supplements or potassium-sparing diuretics	Hyperkalemia	Absorption or retention of potassium

ARF, acute renal failure; CKD, chronic kidney disease; COX-2, cyclooxygenase-2; ESRD, end-stage renal disease; GFR, glomerular filtration rate; NSAIDs, nonsteroidal anti-inflammatory drugs.

- Modify other cardiovascular risk factors (e.g., tobacco use, hypercholesterolemia)
- Avoid nephrotoxins and use renally cleared drugs with caution (Table 35-2)
- Prevent and treat complications of CKD
  - Anemia, metabolic bone disease, acidosis, and volume overload (see Table 35-1)
    - Recent studies suggest increased risk of cardiovascular events (especially stroke) with normalization of hemoglobin (>13 g/dL)
    - Consider iron repletion in all patients and start erythropoiesis-stimulating agents if hemoglobin is below 9 g/dL
  - Other endocrine complications
    - **Decreased GFR leads to prolonged half-life of insulin**
    - **Patients with progressive renal failure need a downward titration of insulin and sulfonylurea dosing to avoid hypoglycemia**
- Avoid additional insults
  - Radiocontrast
    - Risk of acute renal failure 20% to 90%
    - Patients with diabetes at highest risk
    - Choose alternative imaging modality if possible

- **Gadolinium-based contrast agent contraindicated in those with estimated GFR less than 30 due to risk of nephrogenic systemic fibrosis (NSF)—if its use is essential in this high-risk group, use a low dose of a macrocyclic (more stable) agent (gadoteridol)**
- If radiocontrast use unavoidable:
  - **Ensure adequate hydration with isotonic saline or sodium bicarbonate**
  - **Minimize contrast volume**
  - **Utilize nonionic contrast**
  - ***N*-Acetylcysteine 600 mg twice a day for 24 hours before procedure and 48 hours following procedure may reduce incidence of acute renal failure in high-risk groups**
- Avoid volume depletion
  - Tolerated poorly in this patient population
  - May lead to worsening of CKD secondary to acute tubular necrosis
  - Low threshold for IV fluids for hydration
- Avoid iatrogenic complications from medications
  - Adjust dose and interval of all renally metabolized medications
  - See Table 35-2 for specific drugs

- **Renal transplantation**
  - **Preferred treatment of ESRD**
  - Every patient with ESRD should be considered a candidate for transplantation until proven otherwise
  - **Contraindications to transplantation**
    - **Disseminated or untreated cancer**
    - **Recent malignancy (time varies according to cancer type)**
    - **Active infection**
    - **Severe psychiatric disease**
    - **Unreconstructible coronary artery disease or refractory congestive heart failure**
    - **Persistent substance abuse**
    - **Unresolved psychosocial problems**
  - Sources of organs
    - **Living related (best option: Better antigen matches with recipient)**
    - Living unrelated (second best option: But less well matched than related)
    - Deceased donor (less optimal because of cold ischemic times in transport to recipient—may result in cell death and antigen release)
  - **Refer to transplantation center for evaluation when GFR 30 mL/min or less**
  - Patients can be listed for deceased donor transplant when GFR less than 20 mL/min
  - **Treatment goal, for suitable candidate, is to receive a transplant before need for dialysis**
  - Prognosis: The 5-year survival is 80% for deceased donor, 85% for living unrelated donor, and 90% for living related donor
- Dialysis
  - 90% of patients are candidates for either hemodialysis (HD) or peritoneal dialysis (PD)
  - **If therapy prescribed and monitored correctly, HD equals PD in effectiveness**
  - Dialysis initiation: Usually based on combination of GFR level and presence of early symptoms of kidney failure
    - Diabetics: Estimated GFR less than 15 mL/min/1.73 m^2
    - Nondiabetics: Estimated GFR less than 10 mL/min/1.73 m^2
  - Absolute dialysis indications (ideal goal is to avoid these manifestations)
    - **Uremic encephalopathy**
    - **Uremic pericarditis**
    - **Volume overload not responsive to diuretics**
    - **Hyperkalemia despite medical management**
    - **Acidosis despite medical management**
  - Prognosis for dialysis patients is poor in general
    - Median 5-year survival: 33% (1 in 3 dialysis patients will survive for 5 years after starting dialysis)
    - Most common cause of death: Heart disease (usually sudden cardiac death), followed by infection
    - Patients who start dialysis with a catheter have the worst prognosis.

- Peritoneal dialysis (PD)
  - PD is typically performed at home by the patients with or without the help of a partner
  - Can be automated peritoneal dialysis (APD) done over 12 to 13 hours at night or continuous ambulatory peritoneal dialysis (CAPD) performed throughout the day
  - **Major risk is peritonitis; occurs at a rate of 0.5 episodes per patient per year**
  - Preparing patient for PD
    - Electively repair ventral and inguinal hernias
    - PD catheter placement 4 to 6 weeks before initiation of therapy
- Hemodialysis
  - Hemodialysis can be done at home by selected patients but is typically done in a dialysis unit
  - Procedure: Dialyze three times per week for 3 to 5 hours each treatment
  - Requires access to bloodstream (following options in order of preference):
    - Arteriovenous fistula (AVF)
    - Prosthetic bridge graft
    - Dual-lumen catheter
  - AVF preferred access given decreased risk of infection, superior longevity, and high blood-flow rates
  - AVF may take 2 to 8 months to mature, and multiple attempts may be necessary to achieve desired result
  - Once a patient decides on hemodialysis as modality of renal replacement therapy
    - Patient should be referred to vascular surgeon 6 to 12 months before the anticipated need for dialysis; need to place AVF early to mature
    - Phlebotomy and blood pressure measurement should be performed on dominant arm, reserving nondominant arm for dialysis access; preferably use hand veins

REVIEW QUESTIONS

For review questions, please go to www.expertconsult.com.

SUGGESTED READINGS

Kimmel PL: Management of the patient with chronic renal disease. In Greenberg A, editor: *Primer on kidney diseases*, ed 2, San Diego, 1998, Academic Press.

National Kidney Foundation: K/DOQI clinical practice guidelines on chronic kidney disease: evaluation, classification and stratification. (Available at. *www.kidney.org/professionals/doqi/kdoqi/toc.htm*.)

Perazella MA: Current status of gadolinium toxicity in patients with kidney disease, *Clin J Am Soc Nephrol* 4:461–469, 2009.

Post TW, Rose BD: Overview of the management of chronic renal failure. (Available at: Up-to-Date online.)

Winearls CG: Clinical evaluation and manifestations of chronic renal failure. In Johnson RJ, Feehally J, editors: *Comprehensive clinical nephrology*, London, 2000, Harcourt.

35

Selected Topics in Nephrology

MATTHEW FOY, MD; MICHELLE M. ESTRELLA, MD, MHS; and
MICHAEL J. CHOI, MD

Hematuria and nephrolithiasis are among the most common clinical problems in nephrology. The differential diagnosis and associated conditions for both hematuria and nephrolithiasis can be narrowed by a stepwise approach to the clinical presentation.

Hematuria

Basic Information

- Microscopic hematuria
  - Typically discovered on urinalysis in the **asymptomatic** adult
  - Incidence **increases with increasing age;** some series show 2% to 18% of those older than 50 years have microscopic hematuria
  - Definition is variable, but most suggest **more than 3 red blood cells (RBCs) per high-power field** as criterion for microscopic hematuria
  - Urine dipstick testing is highly sensitive for microscopic hematuria but is not specific. **It may indicate the presence of heme despite the absence of RBCs. This may occur with myoglobinuria, intravascular hemolysis, povidone-iodine administration, or the presence of oxidizing agents.**
- Gross hematuria
  - Less common than microscopic hematuria
  - **The presenting symptom in up to 85% of patients diagnosed with bladder cancer and 40% of those with renal cell carcinoma**
  - **Pseudohematuria is the presence of red urine without blood. It may be seen after ingestion of certain foods (e.g., beets, rhubarb) or medications (e.g., pyridium, phenothiazines) or may result from other medical diseases (e.g., porphyria).**
- General approach to the evaluation of the patient with hematuria
  - History: Important details include timing, associated symptoms, social and family history (Table 36-1)
  - Laboratory evaluation: Important details include associated abnormalities in urine (e.g., protein, white blood cells [WBCs]) and appearance of RBCs (Table 36-2)
  - The differential diagnosis of hematuria may be divided between glomerular and nonglomerular causes (Fig. 36-1). Depending on the clinical picture, several radiologic studies may be of diagnostic use (Table 36-3). The general approach to the work-up of hematuria is summarized in Figure 36-2.

- **Anticoagulation alone does not induce hematuria.** Patients on anticoagulation who have hematuria should undergo evaluation unless there is massive bleeding from over-anticoagulation.

Nonglomerular Causes of Hematuria

- Extrarenal disorders
  - **The most common cause of hematuria, with infections and nephrolithiasis the most common disorders**
  - Neoplasms of the bladder, prostate, and ureters may manifest with either microscopic or gross hematuria
- Nonglomerular renal disorders
  - **Autosomal dominant polycystic kidney disease (ADPKD)**
    - Seen in 1 in 500 to 1 in 1000 people
    - Two subtypes: 85% to 95% of cases are *ADPKD1*, located on chromosome 16; the remaining 5% to 15% are *ADPKD2*, located on chromosome 4
    - **Clinical presentation includes gross or microscopic hematuria in 50% of patients; hypertension is common. Many have episodes of flank pain and a palpable abdominal mass on examination (Fig. 36-3).**
    - **Renal cysts are evident on computed tomography (CT) or ultrasound by age 30 years in those with a positive family history**
    - **Intracranial aneurysms seen in less than 10%; screen individual with ADPKD for aneurysm if positive family history or symptoms, or high-risk occupation where loss of consciousness would place patient or others at risk**
    - **Other extrarenal manifestations include hepatic involvement and ovarian cysts, mitral valve prolapse, diverticulosis, and hernias**
  - **Exercise-induced hematuria**
    - Usually **microscopic;** may rarely be associated with **RBC casts**
    - Mechanism unclear, but some suggest bladder trauma or glomerular ischemia cause
    - Seen in both contact and noncontact sports
    - Typically resolves with 1 to 3 days of rest
  - **Papillary necrosis**
    - Results from **ischemic damage** to renal papilla
    - **May be precipitated by sickle cell disease, diabetes mellitus, nonsteroidal anti-inflammatory analgesics (by decreasing vasodilator prostaglandins), urinary tract obstruction, and tuberculosis**

- Diagnosis is by intravenous pyelogram (IVP) or CT urogram, which reveals characteristic changes (Fig. 36-4). Occasionally, necrotic papillary debris can be identified in the urine.

Glomerular Causes of Hematuria

- **The urinalysis serves as an important diagnostic tool in determining a glomerular cause of hematuria by indicating the presence of proteinuria or demonstrating the presence of either dysmorphic RBCs or RBC casts**
  - **Dysmorphic RBCs are thought to form when RBCs passing through the glomerular basement membrane lyse and damage other RBCs, resulting in crenated, misshapen RBCs (>80% dysmorphic RBCs on examination slide is diagnostic of glomerular hematuria; Fig. 36-5)**
  - **RBC casts** result from RBCs adhering to one another in the presence of Tamm-Horsfall protein, forming a "cast" of the tubule (Fig. 36-6)
- **Immunoglobulin A nephropathy, thin basement membrane disease, and Alport syndrome are the three most common glomerular causes of isolated hematuria without significant proteinuria (<500 mg/day)** (Table 36-4; see also Fig. 36-1 and Chapter 34)
- **Evidence of systemic illness (e.g., fatigue, athralgias, hemoptysis, and sore throat) should prompt consideration for collagen vascular disease, other autoimmune disease, postinfectious glomerulonephritis, or viral hepatitis**

Nephrolithiasis

Basic Information

- Incidence: 1% in middle-aged white men
- Stone types
  - Calcium-based (oxalate and phosphate): 75% (pure calcium phosphate: 5%)
  - Uric acid: 10% to 12%
  - Struvite: 10% to 20%
  - Cystine: Less than 1%
  - Other (triamterene, indinavir): Rare

Clinical Presentation

- Patients typically present with **severe flank pain radiating to the groin,** often described as worst pain for men, and worst (other than childbirth) for women

TABLE 36-1	*Historical Details in the Evaluation of the Patient with Hematuria*
Historical Details	
Timing	Transient
	Can be caused by fever, exercise, CHF
	Rule out contamination by menstrual blood
	Initial
	Often implies urethral source
	Terminal
	Often implies bladder source
Associated symptoms	Dysuria
	Suggests urinary tract infection
	Flank pain
	Suggests nephrolithiasis or papillary necrosis
	Weight loss, fatigue
	Suggests vasculitis or cancer
Medications	
Analgesics	Suggests papillary necrosis
Antibiotics, other	Consider acute interstitial nephritis, especially if other evidence of hypersensitivity
Family/Social History	
FH of renal failure	Suggests autosomal dominant polycystic kidney disease (ADPKD)
FH of hematuria in men only	Suggests Alport syndrome (especially if associated with deafness)
SH of tobacco use or dye exposure	Suggests bladder cancer

CHF, congestive heart failure; FH, family history; SH, social history.

TABLE 36-2	*Laboratory Evaluation of the Patient with Hematuria*
Urinalysis	
Clots	
Rules out glomerular source	
Proteinuria, dysmorphic RBCs, RBC casts	
Indicates glomerular source; consider serologic evaluation with ANA, complement levels, cryoglobulins, ANCA, anti-GBM, ASO, hepatitis serologies, and rheumatoid factor	
Pyuria	
Suggests infection or interstitial nephritis; consider urine culture and Hansel's stain for eosinophils	
Urine Cytopathology	
Obtain if bladder cancer suspected	
May detect bladder carcinoma in situ missed by cytoscopy	

ANA, antinuclear antibody; ANCA, antineutrophil cytoplasmic antibody; ASO, antistreptolysin O; GBM, glomerular basement membrane; RBC, red blood cell.

FIGURE 36-1 Causes of hematuria. *Can present with <500 mg/day of proteinuria. (ADPKD, autosomal dominant polycystic kidney disease; CA, cancer; IgA, immunoglobulin A.)

TABLE 36-3	*Imaging Modalities for Evaluation of Hematuria*
IVP	Use when nonglomerular cause suggested Definitive test for medullary sponge kidney disease and papillary necrosis Superior to ultrasound for detection of stones or cancer in the ureters Cannot distinguish between solid and cystic renal masses
Ultrasound	Use when glomerular cause suspected Use when dye allergy or renal insufficiency present Superior to IVP for ADPKD, renal cell CA, small bladder CA Limited in detection of small solid lesions (<3 cm)
CT scan	Superior to IVP for nephrolithiasis Better defines mass that may have been observed with ultrasound More expensive than IVP or ultrasound
CT urogram	Most sensitive test for hematuria Noncontrast CT performed first to look for stones If negative, contrast CT is performed with visualization of kidneys, ureters, and bladder

ADPKD, autosomal dominant polycystic kidney disease; CA, cancer; CT, computed tomography; IVP, intravenous pyelogram.

- Some patients have no symptoms of pain, with the stone discovered during the evaluation of microscopic or gross hematuria

Diagnosis

- Initial step is to image stone and rule out obstruction with CT, ultrasound, or IVP (Fig. 36-7)
  - In the past, IVP was the gold-standard imaging study, but it has been largely replaced by **noncontrast stone protocol CT**
  - IVP and CT urogram remain the best for diagnosing medullary sponge kidney disease (anatomic abnormality with outpouching of collecting ducts leading to urinary stasis)
- Urinalysis and culture should be obtained. **The presence of WBCs may indicate inflammation without infection.** Infected kidney stones need antibiotic treatment and removal.
- Strain urine to capture stone for laboratory analysis of its composition
- **Standard initial studies include serum electrolytes, calcium, phosphorus, and uric acid levels**
- Obtain 24-hour urine collection for stone risk profile if patient has risk factors for stone recurrence

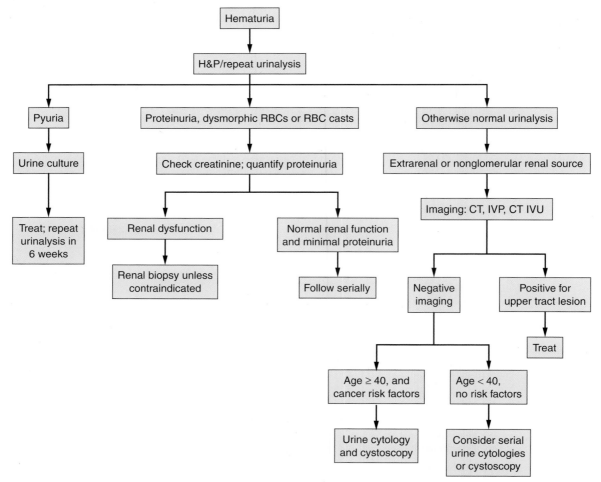

FIGURE 36-2 Algorithm for work-up of microscopic hematuria. (CT, computed tomography; H&P, history and physical; IVP, intravenous pyelogram; IVU, intravenous urogram; RBC, red blood cell.)

FIGURE 36-3 Abdominal distention due to polycystic kidney disease. An enlarged, cystic liver is also present. *(From Haslett C, Chilvers ER, Boon NA, et al: Davidson's principles and practice of medicine, ed 19, New York, Churchill Livingstone, 2002, Fig. 11.8.)*

FIGURE 36-4 Grades II and III reflux in a voiding cystourethrographic study from a young boy who presented with recurrent urinary tract infection. Note early clubbing of the calyces and dilation of the ureter on the left side. *(From Mandell GL, Bennett JE, Dolin R: Principles and practice of infectious diseases, ed 6, Philadelphia, Churchill Livingstone, 2005, Fig. 66-19.)*

FIGURE 36-5 Dysmorphic erythrocytes. These dysmorphic erythrocytes vary in size, shape, and hemoglobin content and reflect glomerular bleeding. *(From Johnson RJ, Feehally J: Comprehensive clinical nephrology, London, Mosby, 2000, Fig. 4.4.)*

FIGURE 36-6 A cast composed entirely of erythrocytes reflects heavy hematuria and active glomerular disease. Crescentic nephritis is likely to be present if erythrocyte casts are greater than 100/mL. *(From Johnson RJ, Feehally J: Comprehensive clinical nephrology, London, Mosby, 2000, Fig. 4.8B.)*

TABLE 36-4	*Glomerular Causes of Hematuria Without Proteinuria*		
Disorder	**Diagnosis**	**Associated Findings**	**Treatment**
IgA nephropathy (Berger disease)	Renal biopsy; IgA immune complex deposits along glomerular mesangium Usually seen in young men (M:F 3:1)	Idiopathic form presents as microscopic hematuria or gross hematuria 1–3 days after URI May be associated with cirrhosis, inflammatory bowel disease Increased serum creatinine at diagnosis, >1 g/day proteinuria, hypertension, and scarring on biopsy portend worse prognosis ESRD in 20% after 20 years	ACEI/ARB if proteinuria present Immunosuppressive agents if creatinine rising rapidly or if urine protein >1 g/day despite ACEI/ARB Fish oil (controversial) if >1 g/day proteinuria
Thin basement membrane disease (benign familial hematuria)	Familial; autosomal dominant; glomerular basement membrane is half normal thickness	90% present with microscopic hematuria; gross hematuria uncommon Proteinuria may be present, usually <1.5 g/day	No treatment needed
Alport syndrome (hereditary nephritis)	Familial, 80% are X-linked due to mutations in genes for type IV collagen	Microscopic or gross hematuria Proteinuria (late) High-tone sensorineural deafness Lenticonus or cataracts ESRD in majority by age 35	Supportive measures

ACEI, angiotensin-converting enzyme inhibitor; ARB, angiotensin receptor blocker; ESRD, end-stage renal disease; IgA, immunoglobulin A; M:F, male:female raio; URI, upper respiratory infection.

FIGURE 36-7 Intravenous pyelogram of a patient with nephrolithiasis, before (**A**) and after (**B**) administration of contrast agent. Multiple kidney stones are noted throughout the urinary collecting system (*black arrows*), with evidence of obstruction (*white arrow*, **B**). Calcified lymph nodes (N) are noted outside the collecting system. *(From Burkitt GH, Quick CRG: Essential surgery, ed 3, New York, Churchill Livingstone, 2003, Fig. 31.3.)*

- Risk factors: **Positive family history in middle-aged white men, malabsorption (e.g., Crohn disease or ulcerative colitis), chronic diarrhea, gout, and procedure required to remove stone**
- The 24-hour urine should be sent for volume, creatinine, calcium, sodium, sulfate or urea nitrogen, oxalate, uric acid, citrate, phosphate, cystine (if suggested), and pH. Saturations or supersaturations for specific stones (e.g., calcium oxalate) are calculated from computer programs.

Treatment

- See Table 36-5 for risk factors and treatment of nephrolithiasis
- There is debate about treatment of the first episode of calcium nephrolithiasis
- **Risk of recurrence after single episode is approximately 50% over the next 10 years**

REVIEW QUESTIONS

For review questions, please go to www.expertconsult.com.

TABLE 36-5	*Nephrolithiasis: Risk Factors and Treatment*		
Stone Type	**Risk Factors**	**Treatment**	**Comments**
Calcium oxalate	*Hypercalciuria* (urine calcium >300 mg/day in men; 250 mg/day in women); most common risk factor (e.g., idiopathic, sarcoidosis, hyperparathyroidism)	Low-sodium diet (urine sodium excretion parallels urine calcium excretion) Thiazide diuretics	Envelope-shaped crystals "Idiopathic" most common cause of hypercalciuria
	Hyperoxaluria (urine oxalate >40 mg/day) (e.g., malabsorption [increased colonic absorption of oxalate])	Avoid calcium limitation as it increases stone risk by leading to decreased intestinal oxalate binding and increased urine oxalate excretion	Baked potatoes, strawberries, okra, spinach, brewed tea, nuts, and chocolate high in oxalate, high-dose vitamin C (>1 g/day)
	Hypocitraturia (urine citrate <320 mg/day vs. <450 mg/day in some labs) (e.g., distal RTA, diarrhea)	Potassium citrate	
	Hyperuricosuria (<800 mg/day for men and <750 mg/day for women)	Decrease purine intake Allopurinol	
Calcium phosphate	Distal (type 1) RTA Primary hyperparathyroidism Alkaline urine	See hypercalciuria treatment	Pure calcium phosphate stones are uncommon
Uric acid	High urine uric acid (e.g., gout, myeloproliferative disorder) Acidic urine	Restrict purine intake; allopurinol Potassium citrate	Radiolucent crystals
Struvite	Urinary tract infection with urease-producing bacteria (e.g., *Proteus*)	Antibiotics Urologic procedure to remove stone	Crystals resemble coffin lids Form staghorn calculi
Cystine	Genetic defect resulting in decreased tubular reabsorption of cystine (urine cystine excretion >400 mg/day)	High fluid intake to decrease urine cystine concentration Alkalinize urine Use medications with sulfhydryl groups to increase cystine solubility (e.g., tiopronin, penicillamine)	Hexagonal greenish-yellow crystals pathognomonic Respond poorly to lithotripsy

RTA, renal tubular acidosis.

SUGGESTED READINGS

Coe FL, Parks JH, Asplin JR: The pathogenesis and treatment of kidney stones, *N Engl J Med* 327:1141–1152, 1992.
Reynolds TM: Chemical pathology, clinical investigation and management of nephrolithaisis, *J Clin Pathol* 58:134–140, 2005.
Yun EJ, Meng MV, Carroll PR: Evaluation of the patient with hematuria, *Med Clin North Am* 88:329–343, 2004.

36

Endocrinology

Diabetes Mellitus

SHERITA H. GOLDEN, MD, MHS

Diabetes is a major health problem. Approximately 8% of the U.S. population, or 17.9 million individuals, have been diagnosed with diabetes, and it is estimated that 5.4 million individuals have undiagnosed diabetes. Type 2 diabetes accounts for 90% to 95% of cases. Significant complications of diabetes include retinopathy, nephropathy, neuropathy, and cardiovascular disease. Approximately 182,000 deaths per year are related to diabetes and its complications, making it the third largest killer in this country. Whereas death from cardiovascular disease has declined over the past two decades, death from diabetes continues to increase.

Diabetes Mellitus

Basic Information

- Diabetes mellitus encompasses several syndromes of altered insulin secretion and/or peripheral resistance that result in hyperglycemia
- Classification of diabetes
  - Type 1 diabetes
  - Type 2 diabetes
  - Gestational diabetes
  - Other specific types
    - Genetic defects: beta cell function, insulin action
    - Disease of exocrine pancreas
    - Endocrinopathies
    - Drug- or chemical-induced
    - Infection-related
    - Other genetic syndromes associated with diabetes
- Pathogenesis of type 1 diabetes mellitus
  - Patients require insulin to prevent hyperglycemia and ketosis
  - Pancreatic beta cell destruction with resulting complete insulinopenia
  - Immune-mediated: Anti–islet cell antibodies and anti-insulin antibodies are humoral markers of islet cell inflammation
  - Idiopathic
- Pathogenesis of type 2 diabetes mellitus
  - Impaired insulin secretion because of beta cell dysfunction
  - Insulin resistance leads to increased hepatic glucose production and decreased peripheral glucose uptake
- Distinguishing between type 1 and type 2: see Table 37-1

Clinical Presentation

- Main symptoms include polyphagia, polydipsia, and polyuria
  - Type 1 diabetes typically presents in the first two decades of life; however, type 1 diabetes can present in adulthood and is then referred to as latent autoimmune diabetes of adulthood (LADA)
  - Type 2 diabetes typically presents after age 40 years

TABLE 37-1	*Distinguishing Between Types 1 and 2 Diabetes Mellitus*	
	Type 1	**Type 2**
Body weight	Lean or normal History of weight loss before presentation	Overweight or obese History of weight gain before diagnosis
Family history	<20% first-degree relatives with diabetes	Strong family history of first-degree relatives with diabetes
Other autoimmune disorders	May be present: Hashimoto thyroiditis, Graves disease, vitiligo, adrenal insufficiency, pernicious anemia	Absent
Glycemic patterns	Greater daily variability Exaggerated hyperglycemic response to stressors and meals	Blood sugars more stable throughout day
Response to oral agents	Nonresponsive	Responsive
Insulin sensitivity	Normal	Very reduced
Islet cell antibodies and/or Glutamic acid decarboxylase (GAD) antibodies	~80% have detectable titers at onset	Not present
C-peptide	Very low or undetectable	Detectable or elevated

TABLE 37-2	*Management of Diabetic Ketoacidosis (DKA) and Nonketotic Hypertonicity (NKH)*	
	Diabetic Ketoacidosis	**Nonketotic Hypertonicity**
Occurrence	Occurs in both type 1 and 2 diabetes	Occurs mainly in type 2 diabetes, but can occur in type 1
Definition	1. Blood glucose >250 mg/dL 2. Low bicarbonate (<15 mEq/L) 3. Low pH (<7.3)	1. Effective osmolarity ≥320 mOsm/L [calculated as 2 × (Na + K) + (glucose/18) + (BUN/2.8)] 2. Blood glucose ≥600 mg/dL 3. pH ≥7.3
Presentation	1. Fatigue, blurred vision, polydipsia, polyuria, weight loss 2. Nausea, vomiting, and vague abdominal pain are common 3. Obtundation, shock, and coma may ensue 4. Kussmaul respirations and fruity breath suggest ketoacidosis	1. Fatigue, blurred vision, polydipsia, polyuria, weight loss 2. Severe dehydration 3. Obtundation, shock, and coma may ensue
Precipitants	Infection, omission, or inadequate use of insulin, new-onset diabetes	Infection, new-onset diabetes, stroke, myocardial infarction, pancreatitis, uremia, burns, subdural hematoma, acromegaly, ectopic ACTH
Treatment	1. Hydration Usually a total of 4–5 L needed 1 L isotonic saline in first hour; add colloid if hypovolemic shock present Switch to hypotonic saline at 200–1000 mL/hr once initial fluid resuscitation complete Add dextrose when glucose <200 mg/dL 2. Insulin therapy Initial priming dose: 0.3–0.4 units/kg regular insulin IV followed by infusion at ~7 units/hr Titrate as needed Continue until pH and serum bicarbonate normal Do not follow serum ketones; as DKA resolves, β-hydroxybutyrate is converted to acetoacetate and acetone, so ketones appear to be increasing In obtunded, hyperosmolar patient, lower glucose to 300 and maintain until patient is alert 3. Electrolyte replacement Hyperkalemia may be seen initially because of insulin deficiency and acidosis, but total body potassium is low After initial liter of normal saline, add 20–30 mEq potassium (⅔ as KCl and ⅓ as KPO₄) to each liter of fluid to correct hypokalemia and hypophosphatemia	1. Hydration 1–2 L fluid in first 2 hr, then 7–9 L over next 2–3 days; give normal saline until blood pressure and urine flow restored, then switch to hypotonic saline Replace half the free water deficit in the first 12 hr and the remainder in the next 24 hr Add dextrose when glucose <250 mg/dL 2. Electrolyte replacement Replace potassium with 20–40 mEq/L once urine flow is normal and serum potassium begins to fall 3. Insulin therapy Additive to fluid therapy but not a primary therapy here; hydration alone can correct hyperglycemia 10-unit bolus of regular insulin IV, then infuse 0.1–0.15 units/kg/hr
Follow-up	Check glucose once every hour for first several hours then every 4 hr while on IV fluids Check electrolytes every 2 hr until normal, then every 4–6 hr while on IV fluids Check venous pH to follow resolution of acidosis	Check glucose once every hour for first several hours, then every 4 hr while on IV fluids Check electrolytes every 2 hr until normal, then every 4–6 hr while on IV fluids
Complications	Cerebral edema ARDS Hyperchloremic acidosis Vascular thromboembolism	Vascular thromboembolism Rhabdomyolysis ARDS

ACTH, adrenocorticotropic hormone; ARDS, acute respiratory distress syndrome; BUN, blood urea nitrogen.

- Acute complications include diabetic ketoacidosis and hyperosmolar hyperglycemic state (Table 37-2)
- Chronic complications
  - Nephropathy (see section on diabetic nephropathy)
  - Retinopathy (see section on diabetic retinopathy)
  - Neuropathy (see section on diabetic neuropathy)
  - Cardiovascular disease (see section on cardiovascular disease)
  - Skin manifestations
    - Acanthosis nigricans (Fig. 37-1)
      - Frequently associated with insulin resistance and obesity; can also be related to underlying malignancy (especially GI and lung)
      - Dark, velvety, thickened plaques occurring in flexural areas (axilla, inguinal crease, back and sides of neck)
      - Treatment
        - Weight reduction, treatment of the diabetes or underlying disorder
        - For severe, odorous lesions: Antibacterial soaps, topical antibiotics
  - Necrobiosis lipoidica (Fig. 37-2)
    - Inflammatory skin condition of unknown etiology; frequently associated with diabetes or impaired glucose tolerance
    - Often asymptomatic lesions; usually occur on the shin

FIGURE 37-1 Acanthosis nigricans occurring in the neck of a patient with severe insulin resistance associated with obesity. (*From Besser GM, Thorner M: Comprehensive clinical endocrinology, ed 3, St. Louis, Mosby, 2002, Fig. 36.7.*)

TABLE 37-3	*American Diabetes Association Recommended Glycemic Targets for Nonpregnant Adults*	
		Glycemic Goals
Preprandial capillary plasma glucose		70–130 mg/dL
Postprandial capillary plasma glucose		<180 mg/dL
Hgb A$_{1c}$		<7%

Hgb A$_{1c}$, glycosylated hemoglobin A$_{1c}$.

Diagnosis and Evaluation

- Four main criteria are used for diagnosis of diabetes (only one of the four is required for diagnosis)
  - Symptoms of diabetes (e.g., polyuria, polydipsia, weight loss, ketoacidosis, hyperosmolarity) plus random plasma glucose greater than 200 mg/dL
  - Fasting plasma glucose of 126 mg/dL or greater or random plasma glucose greater than 200 mg/dL on two separate occasions
  - Two-hour plasma glucose of 200 mg/dL or greater after ingestion of a 75-g glucose load (oral glucose tolerance test [OGTT]) on two occasions
  - Hemoglobin A$_{1c}$ (Hgb A$_{1c}$) ≥6.5%
- Other related conditions
  - Impaired glucose tolerance: 2-hour plasma glucose 140 to 199 mg/dL during OGTT
  - Impaired fasting glucose: Fasting plasma glucose 100 to 125 mg/dL
  - Increased risk for type 2 diabetes: Hgb A$_{1c}$ 5.7% to 6.4%

Treatment

- Treatment objective is glycemic control
  - Glycemic control reduces long-term microvascular complications (e.g., nephropathy, neuropathy, and retinopathy) in both type 1 and type 2 diabetic patients
  - **Goals for glycemic control: see Table 37-3**
  - **Insulin therapy is necessary for type 1 diabetic patients**
  - Oral agents and/or insulin therapy may be used in type 2 diabetic patients
- Insulin therapy
  - Different forms of insulin are characterized by their duration of action (Table 37-4)
  - **Total daily dosage (TDD) of insulin depends on the type of diabetes, diet, exercise, and degree of insulin resistance**
    - Type 1 diabetes: 0.5 unit/kg/day
    - Type 2 diabetes: 0.4 to 1.0 unit/kg/day for patient on only insulin therapy and not on oral agents; daily insulin requirements may be less in patients on insulin-sensitizing agents
  - For both type 1 and type 2 diabetic patients, the insulin regimen should be divided as follows:
    - Determine TDD by multiplying body weight in kilograms by
      - 0.5 to 0.7 unit if patient has type 1 diabetes
      - 0.4 to 1 unit (or more) if patient has type 2 diabetes

FIGURE 37-2 Necrobiosis lipoidica. (*From Swash M: Hutchinson's clinical methods, ed 21, Philadelphia, WB Saunders, 2002, Fig. 8.8.*)

- Indurated, oval plaques with central atrophy and yellow pigmentation; red-brown margins
- Treatment is often suboptimal
  - First-line: Topical or intralesional steroids
  - For ulcers: Cyclosporine, hyperbaric oxygen, infliximab, and others can be tried

TABLE 37-4	*Types of Insulin*		
	Onset of Action	**Peak of Action**	**Duration of Action**
Rapid-acting			
Lispro, aspart, glulisine	5–15 min	1–2 hr	3–5 hr
Regular	30–60 min	2–4 hr	6–8 hr
Intermediate-acting			
Neutral protamine Hagedorn	1–3 hr	5–7 hr	13–18 hr
Long-acting			
Glargine	Within 4 hr	Peakless	>24 hr
Detemir	Within 4 hr	Peakless	18–24 hr

- Determine the basal insulin requirement
  - 40% to 50% of TDD
  - Options for administration
    - Continuous subcutaneous insulin infusion (CSII)
    - Long-acting insulin analogue (glargine or detemir) once daily in the morning or at bedtime
    - Intermediate (neutral protamine Hagedorn [NPH]) twice a day in the morning and at bedtime
- Determine prandial insulin requirement
  - TDD minus basal insulin dose
  - Split to cover meals
    - Lispro, aspart, or glulisine: Divide into three injections (prior to breakfast, lunch, and dinner)
    - Regular: Divide into two injections (before breakfast and dinner)
    - May also give rapid-acting analogues within 30 minutes after meals based on carbohydrate amount consumed
- Correction or supplemental insulin
  - Treats hyperglycemia before meals or between meals
  - Corrects hyperglycemia in NPO patient or in patient receiving scheduled nutritional or basal insulin but not eating discrete meals
  - Sliding scale correction dose based on preprandial blood sugar
    - 1 unit per 50-mg/dL increment over 180 mg/dL (type 1)
    - 1 unit per 30-mg/dL increment over 180 mg/dL (type 2)
- Insulin is the preferable first-line therapy in certain clinical situations
  - Pregnancy: Only insulin is approved for use in pregnancy
  - Polyuria/polydipsia: Indicates severe hyperglycemia that should be rapidly reversed with insulin therapy
  - Ketosis: Indicates insulinopenia
  - Latent autoimmune diabetes of adulthood (LADA)

- Suspect in lean individuals presenting in middle age who do not respond to oral agents
- These individuals really have type 1 diabetes presenting later in life and require insulin therapy
- Insulin antibodies (anti–glutamic acid decarboxylase and anti–islet cell) may be positive within the first year of diagnosis
- Oral antihyperglycemic agents
  - Classes of oral agents: see Table 37-5
  - Multiple factors should be considered in selecting initial oral hypoglycemic agents for patients with type 2 diabetes (Fig. 37-3 gives suggested algorithm)
  - Degree of reduction needed in glycosylated Hgb A_{1c} and/or fasting blood glucose
    - Sulfonlyureas, biguanides (metformin), and thiazolidinediones all lower Hgb A_{1c} 1 to 2 percentage points on average when used as monotherapy
    - Agents targeted at reducing postprandial hyperglycemia, meglitinides, α-glucosidase inhibitors, and dipeptidyl peptidase-4 (DPP-4) inhibitors are less potent, lowering Hgb A_{1c} 0.5 to 1 percentage point when used as monotherapy
  - Body habitus and estimated degree of insulin resistance
    - In obese individuals, insulin resistance is very likely. Thus, an insulin sensitizer (metformin or thiazolidinedione) would be the preferable therapy. Because thiazolidinediones can be associated with weight gain and edema, they are not generally recommended as the agent of first choice.
    - Lean individuals are less likely to be insulin resistant and are more likely to have some β-cell reserve, so a sulfonylurea is a preferable first-line agent
  - Contraindications to agents (see Table 37-5)
    - Metformin is contraindicated in renal insufficiency (creatinine ≥1.4 mg/dL in women and ≥1.5 mg/dL in men), treated congestive heart failure, hypoxemia, hypotension, and binge alcohol use, as these conditions increase the risk of lactic acidosis
    - Thiazolidinediones are contraindicated in classes III and IV congestive heart failure and in individuals with active liver disease
  - Potential for adverse health risks of hypoglycemia inpatients with cerebrovascular or cardiovascular disease
    - Metformin, the thiazolidinediones, acarbose, and DPP-IV inhibitors do not cause hypoglycemia when used as monotherapy
  - Possibility of postprandial hyperglycemia (should be suspected when there is a poor correlation between fasting glucose readings and the Hgb A_{1c})
    - Agents that target postprandial hyperglycemia are the meglitinides, acarbose, and DPP-IV inhibitors
  - Presence of a coexisting lipid disorder
    - Metformin lowers low-density lipoprotein (LDL) and triglycerides and has no effect on high-density lipoprotein (HDL)
    - Compared with rosiglitazone, pioglitazone resulted in a significant reduction in triglycerides, a greater increase in HDL cholesterol, a smaller rise in LDL cholesterol, and a greater increase in LDL particle size

TABLE 37-5	*Oral Agents for Diabetes Mellitus*		
Therapy	**Mechanism**	**Benefits**	**Precautions**
Metformin	Suppresses hepatic glucose output	No weight gain No hypoglycemia when used as monotherapy	GI side effects: nausea, diarrhea (titrate dose upward slowly to minimize) Contraindicated in renal compromise (Cr ≥1.4 in women; Cr ≥1.5 in men; Cr clearance ≤60) Contraindicated in CHF requiring treatment Discontinuation required before contrast dye studies (may restart in 48 hr if normal renal function) Increased risk of lactic acidosis Older age: Use over age 80 yr only if Cr clearance normal Avoid excessive alcohol consumption
Thiazolidinediones Rosiglitazone Pioglitazone	Enhance peripheral muscle sensitivity to insulin	↓ C-peptide and insulin levels No hypoglycemia when used as monotherapy	Monitor LFTs at baseline and every 2 mo for first year Contraindicated in active liver disease and/or LFTs >2.5× upper limit of normal Weight gain (~1–3 kg) Contraindicated in class III/IV CHF Plasma volume expansion (↓ Hct 3–4%) Edema Possible increased MI risk with rosiglitazone
Sulfonylureas Glimepiride Glyburide Glipizide	Increase pancreatic secretion of insulin	Ease of use and familiarity	Weight gain Hypoglycemia Sulfa sensitivity
Metglitinides Repaglinide Nateglinide	Increase pancreatic secretion of insulin	Reduces postprandial hyperglycemia	↓ Compliance due to multiple daily doses with meals Mild hypoglycemia Use cautiously with liver impairment
Acarbose	Delays glucose absorption by inhibition of pancreatic α-amylase and intestinal α-glucoside	No hypoglycemia as monotherapy Reduces postprandial hyperglycemia	GI: Flatulence, cramps, diarrhea Requires multiple dosing with meals Cannot treat hypoglycemia with sucrose
Dipeptidyl peptidase-4 inhibitors Sitagliptin Saxagliptin	Inhibit breakdown of endogenous incretins, resulting in inhibition of postprandial glucagon release, increased satiety, slowed gastric emptying, and stimulation of glucose-dependent insulin release	No hypoglycemia as monotherapy Reduces postprandial hyperglycemia Weight neutral	Pharyngitis, urinary tract infections, possible pancreatitis; long-term safety not established

CHF, congestive heart failure; Cr, creatinine; GI, gastrointestinal; Hct, hematocrit; LFTs, liver function tests; MI, myocardial infarction.
Adapted from Ratner R: *Clinical endocrinology update 1999 syllabus,* Chevy Chase, MD, Endocrine Society, 1999.

- Subcutaneous noninsulin glucoregulatory hormone replacement
  - The incretins, glucagon-like peptide and glucose-dependent insulinotropic polypeptide, are gut-derived hormones released in response to meals
  - Amylin is a beta cell hormone co-secreted with insulin in response to meals
  - **The incretin mimetics, exenatide and liraglutide (glucagon-like peptide-1 analogues), and the amylin agonist pramlintide both stimulate glucose-dependent insulin release in response to meals, inhibit glucagon release, and slow gastric emptying in patients with type 2 diabetes when administered by subcutaneous injection**
  - Dosages and indications
    - Exenatide
      - Exenatide lowers Hgb A_{1c} by 0.4% to 1% when added to sulfonylurea, metformin, thiazolidinediones, or combination therapy
      - Indicated for patients with type 2 diabetes who have not attained adequate glycemic control on maximal sulfonylurea, metformin, and combination therapy
    - Liraglutide
      - Liraglutide lowers Hgb A_{1c} by 0.5% to 1.0% when used as monotherapy and 0.9% to 1.4% when used in combination with metformin, sulfonylureas, or thiazolidinediones
      - Indicated for patients with type 2 diabetes as an adjunct to diet and exercise
    - Pramlintide
      - Pramlintide lowers Hgb A_{1c} by 0.43% when added to insulin alone or insulin in combination with metformin and sulfonylureas
      - Indicated for use in patients with type 1 or type 2 diabetes who have not achieved adequate glycemic control on insulin therapy
      - Mealtime insulin should be decreased by 50% to prevent severe hypoglycemia

Tier 1: Well-validated core therapies

STEP 1   STEP 2   STEP 3

Tier 2: Less well-validated therapies

FIGURE 37-3 A suggested algorithm for initiating oral therapy in type 2 diabetes. [a]Sulfonylureas other than glybencinamide (glyburide) or chlorpropamide. [b]Insufficient clinical use to be confident regarding safety. (CHF, congestive heart failure; GLP-1, glucagon-like peptide-1.) *(From Nathan DM, Buse JB, Davidson MB, et al: Medical management of hyperglycemia in type 2 diabetes: consensus algorithm for the initiation and adjustment of therapy, Diabetes Care, 32:193–203, 2009.)*

- Subcutaneous incretin-based therapies are associated with nausea and vomiting and are contraindicated in patients with gastroparesis. Exenatide and liraglutide may be associated with pancreatitis. Liraglutide cannot be used in patients with a personal or family history of medullary thyroid cancer or in patients with multiple endocrine neoplasia-II syndrome.
- Combination therapy (see Fig. 37-3)
  - Combination therapy (using multiple modalities) is often required even at an early stage to achieve near normoglycemia
    - Combination oral agents
      - Metformin + sulfonylurea
      - Metformin + thiazolidinedione
      - Metformin + sitagliptin
      - Sitagliptin + sulfonylurea
      - Sitagliptin + thiazolidinedione
  - Monotherapy fails because of multiple factors
    - Decreasing beta cell function
    - Obesity
    - Noncompliance with treatment
    - Lack of exercise
    - Intercurrent illness
  - Oral agents can be combined and/or used with insulin therapy to improve glycemic control
    - Methods of adding insulin to an established oral regimen
      - NPH, glargine, or detemir insulin at bedtime
      - 70/30 or 75/25 insulin at evening meal
      - Dose based on weight and blood glucose, but most patients start with 8 to 10 units/day
  - Method of adding oral agents to an established insulin therapy
    - Continue current insulin dosage initially, then decrease the dose by 15% to 25% if hypoglycemia

develops or the fasting blood glucose levels are less than 100 mg/dL
- Exenatide and liraglutide can be added to oral therapy with metformin and/or sulfonylureas in type 2 diabetes
- Pramlintide can be added to insulin therapy in type 1 diabetes and to insulin therapy alone or insulin therapy in combination with sulfonylureas and/or metformin in type 2 diabetes
- Treatment of diabetic ketoacidosis and nonketotic hypertonicity: see Table 37-2

Diabetic Nephropathy

Basic Information

- 20% to 30% of patients with type 1 or type 2 diabetes develop evidence of nephropathy, but a smaller fraction progress to end-stage renal disease (ESRD) in type 2 diabetes
- Native Americans, Mexican Americans, and African Americans have higher risk of developing ESRD than do white individuals
- Natural history is summarized in Figure 37-4

Clinical Presentation

- Patients usually asymptomatic until late in course
- Characterized by proteinuria and rising creatinine

Diagnosis and Evaluation

- Urine microalbumin measurement should be performed annually to screen for diabetic nephropathy after 5 years of disease duration in patients with type 1 diabetes and at diagnosis in patients with type 2 diabetes

FIGURE 37-4 Natural history of diabetic nephropathy. (ESRD, end-stage renal disease; GFR, glomerular filtration rate.)

TABLE 37-6	Definition of Microalbuminuria
Category	**Spot Collection (mg/mg creatinine)**
Normal	<30
Microalbuminuria	30–299
Clinical albuminuria	≥300

TABLE 37-7	Definition of Diabetic Retinopathy
Nonproliferative	Microaneurysms, increased vascular permeability
Preproliferative	Soft exudates representing ischemic infarcts to the retina (cotton-wool spots), beading of retinal veins, tortuosity of retinal capillaries
Proliferative	Neovascularization (fibrous contraction from previous hemorrhage may lead to retinal detachment)
Rubeosis	Neovascularization of the iris
Macular edema	Suspect if hard exudates in proximity of macula

- See Table 37-6 for a definition of microalbuminuria; two of three specimens collected within a 3- to 6-month period should be abnormal before confirming the diagnosis
- **Factors that may increase urinary albumin excretion over baseline values: exercise within 24 hours, fever, infection, congestive heart failure, marked hyperglycemia, marked hypertension, pyuria, hematuria**
- If initial screening tests are negative, patients should undergo annual screen; whether to continue annual screening after microalbuminuria has been diagnosed and appropriately treated is less clear

Treatment

- Pharmacologic therapy
  - Use of angiotensin-converting enzyme (ACE) inhibitors is recommended for all hypertensive and nonhypertensive patients with type 1 diabetes and microalbuminuria or clinical albuminuria
  - Angiotensin II receptor blockers (ARBs) are the agents of first choice in hypertensive type 2 diabetic patients with microalbuminuria or clinical albuminuria
  - Aggressive treatment of hypertension with goal blood pressure of less than 130/80 mm Hg
  - β-Blockers and diuretics are alternatives if ACE inhibitors or ARBs not tolerated or contraindicated
  - Non-dihydropyridine calcium channel blockers should be used as second-line agents
- Behavioral therapy
  - Sodium restriction: Approximately 2000 mg/day

- Weight loss, moderately intense physical activity (30–45 minutes of brisk walking daily), smoking cessation, moderation of alcohol consumption

Diabetic Retinopathy

Basic Information

- Diabetic retinopathy is the leading cause of blindness in adults ages 20 to 74 years, and its presence is strongly related to the duration of diabetes
- Factors that increase the risk of retinopathy
  - Hyperglycemia
  - Presence of nephropathy
  - High blood pressure
  - Pregnancy in patients with type 1 diabetes

Clinical Presentation

- Classification of diabetic retinopathy: see Table 37-7 and Figure 37-5
- Usually asymptomatic unless vitreous hemorrhage occurs (causing visual loss)

Diagnosis and Evaluation

- Ophthalmologic evaluation should be performed starting 5 years after diagnosis of type 1 diabetes and on initial diagnosis of type 2 diabetes (Table 37-8)

37

FIGURE 37-5 **A,** Background and proliferative diabetic retinopathy. **B,** Cystoid macular edema. **C,** Retinal detachment.

- Continue annual screening unless retinopathy warrants more intense follow-up
- Less frequent exams (every 2–3 years) can be considered in those with several normal eye exams

Treatment

- Laser photocoagulation therapy to prevent visual loss
  - Panretinal/scatter photocoagulation therapy is treatment to reduce risk of visual loss in patients with high-risk characteristics (neovascularization, or vitreous hemorrhage with any retinal neovascularization) and in older-onset patients with severe nonproliferative diabetic retinopathy or less than high-risk proliferative diabetic retinopathy
  - Focal laser photocoagulation surgery for eyes with clinically significant macular edema

TABLE 37-8	Ophthalmologic Examination Schedule	
Patient Group	**Recommended First Examination**	**Minimum Routine Follow-Up**
≤29 yr	Within 3–5 yr after diagnosis once patient ≥10 yr of age	Yearly
≥30 yr	At diagnosis	Yearly
Pregnancy in patient with preexisting diabetes	Before conception and 1st trimester	Physician discretion after 1st trimester

Diabetic Neuropathy and Diabetic Foot Disease

- Diabetic neuropathy can take many different forms
- Useful classification
  - Generalized symmetrical polyneuropathies: acute sensory, chronic sensorimotor
  - Focal and multifocal neuropathies: cranial, truncal, focal limb, proximal motor (amyotrophy), coexisting chronic inflammatory demyelinating polyneuropathy (CIDP)
  - Autonomic: cardiac, gastrointestinal, genitourinary
- Chronic sensorimotor distal symmetrical polyneuropathy (DPN) and diabetic autonomic neuropathy (DAN) are the two most common neuropathies
- DPN
  - Up to 50% of DPN cases may be asymptomatic, increasing the patient's risk of insensate foot injuries, which can ultimately lead to ulcers and amputations
  - About 50% of patients have symptoms: Burning pain, electrical or stabbing sensations, paresthesias, hyperesthesia, deep aching pain occurring in the feet and lower limbs; symptoms worse at night
  - Diabetic ulcer (Fig. 37-6)
  - Patients at increased risk for ulcers and amputations
    - Duration of diabetes of 10 years or more
    - Male
    - Poor glucose control
    - Cardiovascular, retinal, or renal complications
    - Peripheral neuropathy with loss of protective sensation
    - Altered foot biomechanics, bony deformity
    - Presence of peripheral vascular disease
    - History of ulcers or amputation
    - Severe nail pathology
  - Diagnosis
    - Careful clinical exam with annual screening by examining pinprick, temperature, and vibration perception (using 128-Hz tuning fork), 10-g monofilament pressure sensation at distal halluces, and ankle reflexes
    - Examination in DPN shows loss of vibration, pressure, pain, and temperature sensation, and absent reflexes
    - Signs of peripheral autonomic (sympathetic) dysfunction: warm or cold feet, distended dorsal foot veins (in absence of peripheral arterial disease), dry skin, calluses in pressure-bearing areas
    - Examine feet for ulcers, calluses, and deformities, and inspect footwear
    - **Rule out other forms of neuropathy: CIDP, vitamin B$_{12}$ deficiency, hypothyroidism, uremia (check B$_{12}$, thyroid function, blood urea nitrogen, and creatinine)**
  - Treatment
    - Optimization of blood sugar control and avoiding extreme blood sugar fluctuations
    - Pharmacologic treatment
      - Tricyclic antidepressant drugs: Amitriptyline, imipramine; use limited by anticholinergic side effects, including fatigue and drowsiness
      - Selective serotonin reuptake inhibitors: Paroxetine, citalopram

FIGURE 37-6   Stage III ulcer beneath second metatarsal head that extends into metatarsal head with presumptive contiguous osteomyelitis. *(From Canale ST: Campbell's operative orthopedics, ed 10, St. Louis, Mosby, 2003, Fig. 82-2.)*

37

-
  -
    -
      - Anticonvulsants: Gabapentin, pregabalin, carbamazepine, topiramate; use limited by drowsiness
      - Opioid or opioid-like drugs: Tramadol, continuous-release oxycodone
      - 5-Hydroxytryptamine and norepinephrine uptake inhibitor: Duloxetine
      - Substance P inhibitor: Capsaicin cream
    - Podiatry referral to reduce the risk of foot ulcers
- Acute sensory neuropathy
  - Follows periods of poor metabolic control or sudden changes in glycemic control ("insulin neuritis")
  - Acute onset of severe sensory symptoms with marked nocturnal exacerbation
  - Few neurologic signs on exam
- Mononeuropathies
  - Focal nerves involved
  - Percent of all diabetic neuropathies
    - Median (5.8%), ulnar (2.1%), radial (0.6%), common peroneal
    - Cranial (0.05%) III, IV, VI, and VII—usually resolve spontaneously
  - Entrapments: Median, ulnar, peroneal, medial plantar
  - Spinal stenosis
  - Diagnosis: Electrophysiologic studies useful in identifying conduction blocks at entrapment sites
- Diabetic amyotrophy
  - Occurs in older patients with type 2 diabetes
  - Severe neuropathic pain, unilateral or bilateral muscle weakness, atrophy in proximal thigh muscles
  - Diagnosis: Needs to be distinguished from CIPD and spinal stenosis; CIPD presents with progressive symmetrical or asymmetrical motor deficits, progressive sensory neuropathy despite optimal glucose control, and elevated cerebrospinal fluid protein
- Diabetic autonomic neuropathy (DAN)
  - Cardiovascular autonomic neuropathy (CAN)
    - Associated with morbidity and increased mortality

- Limits exercise capacity and increases risk of adverse cardiovascular event during exercise
- May lead to sudden death or silent cardiac ischemia
- Presentation: Resting tachycardia (heart rate >100 beats/min), exercise intolerance, orthostatic hypotension (fall in systolic blood pressure >20 mm Hg on standing)
- Diagnosis: Three useful tests
  - R–R variation on electrocardiogram (ECG)
  - Valsalva maneuver
  - Postural blood pressure testing
- Treatment of CAN
  - Graded supervised exercise, ACE inhibitors, and β-blockers for exercise intolerance
  - Mechanical measures, clonidine, midodrine, octreotide to treat postural hypotension
- Gastrointestinal autonomic neuropathy
  - Presentation: Constipation (may alternate with diarrhea), gastroparesis, esophageal enteropathy, fecal incontinence; consider especially in individuals with erratic glucose control
  - Diagnosis: Evaluation with gastric emptying study, barium swallow, or referral for endoscopy
  - Treatment
    - Treat gastroparesis with frequent small meals and prokinetic agents (metoclopramide, domperidone, erythromycin)
    - Abdominal pain, early satiety, nausea, vomiting, and bloating treated with multiple approaches: Antibiotics, antiemetics, bulking agents, tricyclic antidepressants, pancreatic extracts, pyloric Botox, gastric pacing, enteral feeding
    - Constipation: High-fiber diet and bulking agents, osmotic laxatives, lubricating agents; prokinetics should be used with caution
    - Diarrhea: Soluble fiber, gluten and lactose restriction, anticholinergic agents, cholestyramine, antibiotics, clonidine, somatostatin, pancreatic enzyme supplements
- Genitourinary autonomic neuropathy
  - Presentation: Erectile dysfunction, retrograde ejaculation, bladder dysfunction (recurrent urinary tract infections, pyelonephritis, incontinence, palpable bladder)
  - Diagnosis: Medical and sexual history; psychological evaluation; measurement of hormone levels; measurement of nocturnal penile tumescence; assessment of penile, pelvic, and spinal nerve function; cardiovascular autonomic function tests; and measurement of penile and brachial blood pressure
  - Treatment
    - Erectile dysfunction: Sex therapy, psychological counseling, sildenafil, vardenafil, tadalafil, prostaglandin E_1 injection, device, or prosthesis
    - Bladder dysfunction/urinary retention and incontinence: Bethanechol, intermittent catheterization

Cardiovascular Disease

Basic Information

- Atherosclerosis accounts for approximately 80% of all diabetic mortality (75% from coronary atherosclerosis and 25% from cerebral or peripheral vascular disease) and more than 75% of all hospitalizations for diabetic complications
- More than 50% of patients with newly diagnosed type 2 diabetes already have coronary heart disease

Clinical Presentation

- Coronary artery disease may present with chest pain and/or silent ischemia
- Peripheral arterial disease may present with claudication or nonhealing extremity ulcers
- Cerebrovascular disease may present as transient ischemic attacks or stroke. Carotid bruits on physical exam may indicate underlying cerebrovascular disease.

Diagnosis and Evaluation

- Annual screening for dyslipidemia and hypertension
- Recommended diabetic populations to undergo screening with an exercise stress test
  - Symptomatic
    - Typical or atypical cardiac symptoms
    - Abnormal resting ECG
  - Asymptomatic
    - History of peripheral or carotid occlusive disease
    - Sedentary lifestyle, age older than 35 years, and plans to begin a vigorous exercise program

Treatment

- Aggressive management of hypertension and dyslipidemia, smoking cessation, and aspirin prophylaxis
- Blood pressure targets in patients with diabetes: see earlier section on diabetic nephropathy
- Lipid targets in individuals with diabetes: see Table 37-9

TABLE 37-9	*Cholesterol Targets in Patients with Diabetes*			
	MEDICAL NUTRITION TREATMENT		**DRUG TREATMENT**	
Status	**Initiation Level**	**LDL Goal**	**Initiation Level**	**LDL Goal**
With CHD, PVD, or CVD	>100 mg/dL	≤100 mg/dL	>100 mg/dL	≤100 mg/dL
Without CHD, PVD, or CVD	>100 mg/dL	≤100 mg/dL	≥130 mg/dL	≤100 mg/dL

CHD, coronary heart disease; CVD, cerebrovascular disease; LDL, low-density lipoprotein; PVD, peripheral vascular disease.

- In individuals with a prior history of cardiovascular disease (coronary heart, cerebrovascular, or peripheral arterial disease), treat with statin to achieve LDL reduction of 30% to 40%, regardless of baseline LDL; a lower LDL goal of below 70 mg/dL using high-dose statin is also an option
- In individuals without a history of cardiovascular disease who are older than 40 years, treat with statin to achieve 30% to 40% reduction in LDL regardless of baseline LDL
- Treatment options for dyslipidemia: see Chapter 3

REVIEW QUESTIONS

For review questions, please go to www.expertconsult.com.

SUGGESTED READINGS

American Diabetes Association: Diagnosis and classification of diabetes mellitus, *Diabetes Care* 34(Suppl 1):S62–S69, 2011.

American Diabetes Association: Standards of medical care in diabetes, *Diabetes Care* 34(Suppl 1):S11–S61, 2011.

Boulton AJM, Vinik AI, Arezzo JC, et al: Diabetic neuropathies, *Diabetes Care* 28:956–962, 2005.

Efendic S, Portwood N: Overview of incretin hormones, *Horm Metab Res* 36:742–746, 2004.

Kimmel B, Inzucchi SE: Oral agents for type 2 diabetes: an update, *Clin Diabetes* 23:64–76, 2005.

Nathan DM, Buse JB, Davidson MB, et al: Medical management of hyperglycemia in type 2 diabetes: a consensus algorithm for the initiation and adjustment of therapy, *Diabetes Care* 32:193–203, 2009.

37

Thyroid Disease

SHABINA R. AHMED, MD; and DAVID S. COOPER, MD

Thyroid disorders can be classified into two categories: thyroid dysfunction (hyperthyroidism and hypothyroidism, which are generally autoimmune in etiology) and anatomic abnormalities such as goiter, nodules, and cancer. These problems often occur together in the same patient. In addition, they are extremely common, occurring in up to 10% of adults and 20% of women over age 65.

Thyroid Function Testing

- Many of the symptoms and signs of thyroid dysfunction are nonspecific; laboratory testing is an important part of the assessment (Table 38-1)
- Most common tests: thyroid-stimulating hormone (TSH), free thyroxine (T_4), and triiodothyronine (T_3); TSH is the most useful starting point (Fig. 38-1)
- Thyroid function tests in nonthyroidal illness (NTI)
  - NTI results in numerous changes in thyroid hormone metabolism and protein binding
  - Serum TSH may be low or normal in severely ill patients
    - Low values are caused by medications that are used in the intensive care unit that decrease pituitary TSH secretion, such as high doses of glucocorticoids and dopamine, as well as suppressive effects of endogenous cytokines, such as tumor necrosis factor
    - High TSH values are typically seen in the recovery phase of illness, although the levels usually do not rise above 20 mU/L
  - **Therefore, the diagnosis of thyroid disease can be quite difficult in acutely ill individuals**
    - If the TSH is normal, the patient is probably euthyroid
    - If the TSH is increased and the patient is not recovering from an illness, hypothyroidism can be diagnosed
    - If the TSH is low, as occurs in up to 20% of hospitalized patients, the diagnosis of hyperthyroidism should not be made in the absence of supporting clinical and laboratory data
    - Generally, thyroid function tests should be re-evaluated several weeks to months after recovery

Thyrotoxicosis

Basic Information

- Definition: Thyrotoxicosis is a state of increased tissue exposure to elevated circulating thyroid hormone concentrations; it is a syndrome, not a diagnosis

- It is very common; lifetime prevalence is approximately 2% in women, 0.2% in men
- *Thyrotoxicosis* **is the term used to refer to all conditions associated with increased serum levels of thyroid hormone, regardless of the cause**
- *Hyperthyroidism* **usually refers to those diseases in which the thyroid gland is actually synthesizing and secreting excessive thyroid hormones**
- Etiology
  - **Graves disease and toxic multinodular goiter probably account for more than 90% of all hyperthyroidism cases**
  - See Table 38-2 for other causes
- *Subclinical hyperthyroidism* refers to a state of mild thyroid overactivity in which the serum TSH levels are low (subnormal to undetectable) but the levels of free T_4 and T_3 are normal
  - NOTE: In African Americans, the lower limit of normal for TSH may be lower than the established reference ranges, leading to possible misdiagnosis of subclinical hyperthyroidism in healthy individuals
- A low TSH and normal free T_4 are seen physiologically at the end of the first trimester of pregnancy as a result of increased placental secretion of human chorionic gonadotropin, which stimulates the thyroid

Clinical Presentation

- General symptoms and signs (Table 38-3; Figs. 38-2 and 38-3)
  - Reflect an increased metabolic rate and augmentation of adrenergic activity
  - Manifestations of thyrotoxicosis are quite variable and do not necessarily correlate with circulating thyroid hormone concentrations
    - Elderly patients may have few symptoms or may only present with weight loss or atrial fibrillation
    - **"Apathetic thyrotoxicosis": No signs of thyrotoxicosis except for weight loss and depression in elderly persons**
- Most patients with subclinical hyperthyroidism are asymptomatic

Diagnosis and Evaluation

- Often suspected from history and physical
- Drugs such as amiodarone and interferon alfa can cause hyperthyroidism
- Thyroid examination (see Table 38-2)
- Laboratory studies
  - Low TSH (negative feedback with pituitary); usually undetectable (<0.1 mU/L)

TABLE 38-1	Thyroid Function Tests	
Test	**Use**	**Comments**
Thyroid-stimulating hormone (TSH)	Produced by pituitary; stimulates thyroid to produce T_3 and T_4 (which feed back on pituitary) ↑ Suggests hypothyroidism ↓ Suggests hyperthyroidism	Very sensitive; normal TSH effectively excludes disease in asymptomatic patients Exceptions: Patients with severe nonthyroidal illness (NTI), patients on dopamine or high-dose glucocorticoids TSH will be normal or low in central hypothyroidism
Total thyroxine (T_4) and triiodothyronine (T_3)	Helpful to quantitate the degree of hormone deficiency or excess T_3 is active form in tissues T_4 is converted to T_3 in thyroid and peripherally >99% bound to TBG Free fraction (<1%) determines biologic action	Routine assays measure the total levels; need to take into account TBG status

Thyroid-binding globulin (TBG)	Binds T_4 and T_3	Causes of ↑ TBG
		    Drugs (estrogen, oral contraceptives, tamoxifen, heroin, methadone, 5-fluorouracil)
		    Pregnancy
		    Acute hepatitis
		    Congenital
		    Acute intermittent porphyria
		Causes of ↓ TBG
		    Drugs (androgens, glucocorticoids, slow-release nicotinic acid)
		    Severe illness or malnutrition
		    Chronic liver disease
		    Protein-losing states (e.g., nephritic syndrome)
		    Congenital

T_3 resin uptake (T_3RU)	An indirect measure of the binding capacity of patient's serum proteins (measures unoccupied T_4-binding sites) Used in conjunction with serum T_4	↑ T_3RU: Hyperthyroidism, low TBG states ↓ T_3RU: Hypothyroidism, high TBG states
Free thyroxine index (FTI)	Product of serum T_4 and T_3 resin uptake Corrects for changes in binding protein concentration	Highly correlated with free T_4
Free T_4 (fT_4)	Direct measurement of free hormone; bypasses interfering effects of disease or drugs on TBG levels	Preferable over FTI

38

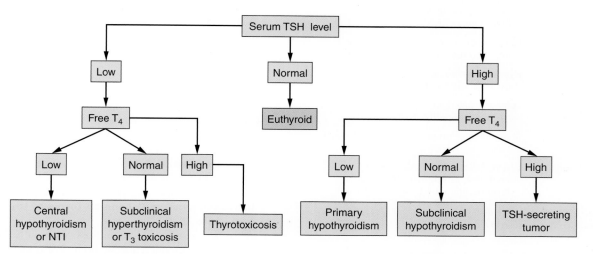

FIGURE 38-1 Sequential thyroid function testing using the serum thyroid-stimulating hormone (TSH) as a starting point. This strategy is useful in asymptomatic individuals. If symptoms are present, both the free thyroxine (fT_4) and TSH should be assessed. (NTI, nonthyroidal illness; T_3, triiodothyronine.)

TABLE 38-2	Causes of Thyrotoxicosis		
Etiology	**Mechanism**	**Thyroid Examination**	**Radioiodine Uptake**
Graves disease	Stimulatory anti-TSH receptor antibodies May be induced by interferon alfa	Diffuse goiter	↑
Toxic multinodular goiter or solitary nodule	Activating gene mutations	Nodule(s), usually >3 cm	↑
Thyroiditis	Follicular destruction causing release of stored hormone; viral (subacute), autoimmune ("silent" or postpartum), or drug-induced (amiodarone)	Tender goiter in subacute; nontender goiter in "silent"	↓
Iodine-induced	Iodine surplus (IV dye or amiodarone-induced thyrotoxicosis type 1)	Nodular or diffuse goiter	↓
Choriocarcinoma	Secretes hCG, a thyroid stimulator	Minimal goiter	↑
Pituitary tumor	TSH overproduction	Minimal goiter	↑
Struma ovarii	Ectopic thyroid tissue in ovarian tumor	Normal	↓ (over thyroid)
Exogenous thyrotoxicosis		Normal in both	↓
Iatrogenic	Oversupplementation of thyroxine		
Factitious	Surreptitious ingestion of thyroxine		

hCG, human chorionic gonadotropin; IV, intravenous; TSH, thyroid-stimulating hormone.

TABLE 38-3	Clinical Manifestations of Thyrotoxicosis
Organ System	**Symptoms and Signs**
Constitutional	Weight loss, heat intolerance
Cardiovascular	Palpitations, atrial arrhythmias, congestive heart failure, systolic hypertension
Respiratory	Dyspnea
Gastrointestinal	Hyperdefecation, increased appetite, nausea
Musculoskeletal	Proximal muscle weakness, osteopenia, hypercalciuria, hypercalcemia, extraocular muscle weakness,* myasthenia gravis*
Neuropsychiatric	Nervousness, anxiety, tremor, insomnia, impaired mentation, delirium, psychosis
Endocrine	Hypomenorrhea, amenorrhea, gynecomastia, decreased libido
Hematologic	Splenomegaly,* enlarged thymus,* lymphadenopathy, neutropenia*
Ophthalmologic	Stare, lid lag,* proptosis,* diplopia,* visual loss*
Dermatologic	Warm, moist, velvety skin; palmar erythema, onycholysis, thinning hair, pruritus, hives, pretibial myxedema,* vitiligo,* thyroid acropachy*

*Denotes findings only seen in Graves disease.

- Rare exception: Patients with TSH-secreting pituitary tumors, in whom the TSH levels are increased or are inappropriately normal in the face of elevations of serum free T_4
- Increased free T_4 or free T_4 index

- Subclinical hyperthyroidism: A low TSH with normal levels of free T_4 and T_3
- Measurement of serum T_3 is also helpful because it can be increased in about 5% of patients with hyperthyroidism when the levels of thyroxine are still normal (T_3 thyrotoxicosis)
- In Graves disease, serum T_3:T_4 ratio is increased because thyroid secretes relatively more T_3 than T_4 compared with the euthyroid state; in various forms of thyroiditis, T_3:T_4 ratio is normal, reflecting the relative amounts of T_3 and T_4 normally present within the thyroid gland
- In Graves disease, circulating antibodies may be present but are not necessary for diagnosis
  - Thyroid-stimulating antibodies (TSAbs) stimulate the TSH receptor
  - May be helpful to measure in pregnancy and in euthyroid patients with Graves eye disease
  - Other antibodies: antithyroperoxidase (anti-TPO) antibodies and antithyroglobulin antibodies (together called *antithyroid antibodies*)
- 24-hour radioiodine uptake test
  - Should not be used as a thyroid function test (can also be increased in hypothyroid patients)
  - **Uptake will be high in Graves disease**
  - **Uptake will be low in diseases associated with excessive release of thyroid hormone, but not increased synthesis, as in all forms of thyroiditis (see Table 38-2)**
  - A thyroid scan should be ordered along with the uptake in cases when a toxic nodule or toxic multinodular goiter is suspected

Treatment

- Treatment of thyrotoxicosis due to Graves disease
  - No ideal treatment for Graves disease: Antithyroid drugs, radioiodine, and surgery are all effective and

FIGURE 38-2 **A,** Computed tomography scan of orbits showing enlarged extraocular muscles. **B,** Patient with typical features of thyroid-associated ophthalmopathy showing lid retraction, exophthalmos, and periorbital edema. Patients may also have diplopia and strabismus due to edema and fibrosis of the extraocular muscles. *(From Souhami R: Textbook of medicine, New York, Churchill Livingstone, 2002, Fig. 17.23B.)*

FIGURE 38-3 Chronic pretibial myxedema in a patient with Graves disease and orbitopathy. The lesions are firm and nonpitting, with a clear edge to feel. *(From Larsen PR, Kronenberg HM, Melmed S, Polonsky KS: Williams' textbook of endocrinology, ed 10, Philadelphia, WB Saunders, 2003, Fig. 82-2.)*

have specific advantages and disadvantages (Table 38-4)

- β-Adrenergic blocking agents
  - Used to control symptoms of palpitations, tremor, heat intolerance, and nervousness
  - Will not alleviate some symptoms (weight loss, myopathy) and are not considered to be a primary mode of therapy
  - Best to use a long-acting agent that is cardioselective (i.e., atenolol)
- Antithyroid drugs
  - **Methimazole (Tapazole) is the drug of choice**
  - Propylthiouracil (PTU), in rare cases, can cause fulminant hepatic failure; *its use should be limited to:*
    - Patients who experienced an allergic reaction with methimazole, and in whom surgery or radioactive iodine is not an option
    - Pregnant patients during the first trimester, after which they should be switched to methimazole (methimazole is not recommended in the first trimester because of its potential to cause rare congenital defects)
    - Patients with life-threatening thyrotoxicosis or thyroid storm, because of PTU's ability to inhibit peripheral conversion of T_4 to T_3
- Both drugs act primarily to diminish thyroid hormone synthesis by interfering with the intrathyroidal use of iodine
- Typical starting doses: Methimazole 10 to 30 mg/day as a single daily dose; PTU 100 mg three times a day

TABLE 38-4	Drugs Used in the Management of Thyroid Storm	
Drug	**Dose**	**Comments**
Propylthiouracil	200–400 mg every 4–6 hr	Must be given PO (or rectally)
Methimazole	30–80 mg/day	Must be given PO (or rectally)
Propranolol	PO: 20–100 mg every 4 hr	The very-short-acting agent esmolol may be used
Hydrocortisone	100 mg every 6–8 hr or equivalent	"Stress doses"—unclear whether use affects outcome
Potassium iodide (SSKI)	3–5 drops 3 times daily	Blocks release of thyroid hormone
Lithium	600–1000 mg daily	May be given orally or by nasogastric tube

- Remission rate less than 50%
- Best used as primary therapy in patients with relatively mild disease (highest likelihood of remission when the drug is discontinued)
  - Dose is adjusted to maintain serum free T_4 and T_3 levels within the normal range
  - Usually takes 4 to 12 weeks to achieve euthyroid state
  - Serum TSH may remain suppressed for 2 to 3 months after the patient has become euthyroid because of the chronic suppressive effects of the previous hyperthyroidism
  - Usually treat for 1 to 2 years, then taper or discontinue to see whether a remission has been achieved; if TSAbs are still positive at this point, remission is unlikely
- **If remission achieved, lifelong follow-up is required because remissions are not necessarily permanent and spontaneous hypothyroidism can also develop many years later**
- Relapse typically occurs in the first 6 months; another course of drug therapy can be undertaken, or the patient may opt for definitive therapy with radioiodine
- Common side effects: rashes, fever, arthralgias, transient leukopenia
- **Major drug reaction is reversible agranulocytosis**
  - Develops in 0.2% to 0.3% of patients
  - Almost always within 90 days of starting the medication
- Radioactive iodine (^{131}I) is the treatment most often used in the United States
  - **Approximately 80% of patients will be cured after a single dose; overall cure rate is greater than 95%**
  - **Works slowly; euthyroid state may not be achieved for 3 to 6 months**
  - May be a transient worsening of thyroid function resulting from radiation-related thyroiditis or an increase in TSAb resulting from thyroid injury

- May need to pretreat elderly patients or those with cardiac disease with antithyroid drugs, which will theoretically deplete the thyroid of hormonal stores
  - Should be stopped 3 to 7 days prior to therapy
- **Hypothyroidism is almost inevitable after radioiodine**
- No immediate side effects and no evidence of long-term sequelae, such as infertility, birth defects, cancer, or other neoplasms either in patients or their offspring
- Only contraindication is pregnancy
- Severe thyroid eye disease is a relative contraindication because radioiodine can exacerbate it; radioiodine can be given with concomitant glucocorticoid therapy to prevent worsening of the ophthalmopathy
- Surgery
  - Rarely used to treat Graves disease in the United States
  - Cure rate greater than 95%
  - Reserved for patients who are allergic to antithyroid drugs, who refuse or cannot take radioiodine (e.g., in pregnancy), patients with a concomitant malignant or suspicious nodule, or patients with very large goiters, who generally have lower success rates with radioiodine
  - Complications may include: Recurrent laryngeal nerve damage, hypoparathyroidism
- Treatment of Graves ophthalmopathy
  - Local symptoms (irritation, tearing, photophobia) can be managed with artificial tears and lubricating eye ointments
  - Ophthalmology consultation for severe degrees of inflammation, diplopia, severe proptosis leading to corneal exposure, or decreased visual acuity
    - May require high-dose glucocorticoids, retro-orbital radiotherapy, and/or surgical decompression of the orbits
  - **Radioiodine may exacerbate ophthalmopathy if severe, especially in patients who smoke**
- Treatment of thyroid storm
  - Represents a rare, exaggerated, or accelerated form of hyperthyroidism
  - **Classic definition of thyroid storm includes fever, severe tachycardia or atrial fibrillation, and altered mental status (agitation, delirium, coma)**
  - Is usually precipitated by a stress (e.g., surgery, infection, childbirth) in a patient with poorly controlled hyperthyroidism
  - Drugs used in thyroid storm treatment (see Table 38-4)
    - **Antithyroid drugs are the mainstay and should be started at least several hours before iodine or iodine-containing drugs are given**
    - PTU may be preferred because of its inhibitory effects on T_4-to-T_3 conversion
  - Supportive measures
    - Attention to fluid and electrolyte balance
    - Search for an underlying cause (e.g., occult infection)
    - Sedatives for agitation

- Cooling blankets and acetaminophen for fever (aspirin should not be used because it binds to thyroid-binding globulin and can displace T_4, causing the free T_4 to rise)
- Treatment of toxic multinodular goiter (Plummer disease) and solitary toxic nodules
  - These entities are less frequent than Graves disease, but they make up a higher proportion of hyperthyroidism in older individuals
  - Little chance for spontaneous remission
  - Antithyroid agents have little role in the management except in preparation for definitive therapy with radioiodine or surgery
  - **Radioactive iodine is the treatment of choice**
  - Surgery is a reasonable therapy, especially in patients with large goiters or nodules and compressive symptoms, such as dysphagia or hoarseness
- Treatment of subclinical hyperthyroidism
  - In untreated patients, may be related to osteopenia and fractures in postmenopausal women and may be a predisposing factor for atrial fibrillation in individuals over age 60 years
  - Recent guidelines recommend treatment in older patients if TSH less than 0.1 mU/L. It is reasonable to treat women who have osteoporosis or patients who have known heart disease with antithyroid drugs or radioiodine.
  - In untreated patients, periodic follow-up is necessary to monitor for the development of overt hyperthyroidism

Hypothyroidism

Basic Information

- **Definition: A clinical state in which the circulating levels of thyroid hormone are insufficient for normal cellular function**
- Extremely common, especially in women
- Prevalence: Approximately 8% in women and 2% in men, most of which is very mild (subclinical)
- **Primary failure of the thyroid due to autoimmune disease (chronic lymphocytic thyroiditis or Hashimoto thyroiditis) is the most common cause of hypothyroidism**
  - Patients will usually, but not always, have positive antithyroid antibodies
  - Anti-TPO antibodies are more sensitive and specific than antithyroglobulin (anti-Tg) antibodies
- Other causes: see Box 38-1
- **Subclinical hypothyroidism**
  - **Refers to a state of mild thyroid dysfunction, in which the serum TSH levels are slightly increased (usually <10 mU/L) and the serum levels of free T_4 and T_3 are normal**
  - Prevalence is up to 15% to 20% in individuals over age 60
    - Recommended to recheck TSH since spontaneous normalization may occur
    - NOTE: slightly elevated TSH levels in the elderly have been associated with a survival benefit, and in this patient population, treatment of subclinical hypothyroidism may be of limited or no clinical benefit
  - Causes similar to those of overt hypothyroidism

BOX 38-1	*Causes of Hypothyroidism*

Associated with Goiter
Chronic lymphocytic (Hashimoto) thyroiditis
Silent (postpartum) thyroiditis (transient)
Subacute thyroiditis (transient)
Iodine deficiency (not seen in North America)
Goitrogenic drugs (lithium, iodine-containing drugs [amiodarone], antithyroid agents, sunitinib [mechanism uncertain])
Congenital biosynthetic enzyme deficiencies

Not Associated with Goiter
Post-thyroidectomy
Post ablation for hyperthyroidism
Congenital absence of the thyroid
Atrophic thyroiditis (variant of Hashimoto thyroiditis)
Following radiation for head and neck tumors

Secondary Hypothyroidism
Pituitary or hypothalamic dysfunction

Peripheral Thyroid Hormone Resistance
Due to defective thyroid hormone receptor

Clinical Presentation

- Symptoms and signs may be nonspecific and overlap with many other conditions (Table 38-5; Fig. 38-4)
- Development of symptoms depends on the severity of disease, its duration, and individual factors, such as the age of the patient (elderly have fewer symptoms than younger individuals)
- Typical patient notes fatigue, mild constipation, cold intolerance, and mild weight gain
  - A weight gain of more than 5 to 10 pounds cannot be attributed to hypothyroidism
- Myxedema coma
  - Typically occurs in patients with long-standing untreated severe hypothyroidism
  - Often precipitated by stress, such as systemic disease, surgery, and sedative drugs or narcotics; occurs more frequently in the winter months
  - Clinical manifestations: Hypothyroidism with mental status changes, such as lethargy, stupor, or seizures, hypoventilation, and hypothermia
  - Mortality may be as high as 50%; should be treated as a medical emergency

Diagnosis and Evaluation

- Laboratory studies
  - **In all forms of hypothyroidism, circulating level of free T_4 will be low**
  - Serum level of T_3 is low as well in severe cases
  - Primary hypothyroidism: Serum level of TSH will be increased (due to the lack of negative feedback inhibition by thyroid hormone on pituitary TSH secretion)
    - Milder cases: TSH may be only slightly increased
    - Severe cases: TSH will be markedly increased (>50 mU/L)

TABLE 38-5	*Clinical Manifestations of Hypothyroidism*
Organ System	**Symptoms and Signs**
Constitutional	Weight gain, cold intolerance, fatigue, weakness, hypercholesterolemia
Cardiovascular	Bradycardia, decreased contractility, pericardial effusion
Respiratory	Hoarseness, dyspnea, hypoventilation, sleep apnea, pleural effusion
Gastrointestinal	Constipation, ileus, macroglossia
Musculoskeletal	Myalgias, arthralgias, nonpitting edema
Neuropsychiatric	Depression, psychosis, carpal tunnel syndrome, delayed reflex relaxation
Endocrine	Growth failure, menorrhagia, galactorrhea (hyperprolactinemia), precocious puberty
Hematologic	Anemia, platelet defect
Dermatologic	Dry skin, pallor, yellowing of skin (carotinemia)

FIGURE 38-4 Advanced hypothyroidism. Note dulled expression, facial puffiness, and periorbital edema. *(From Noble J, Green HL, Levinson W, et al: Textbook of primary care medicine, ed 3, St. Louis, Mosby, 2001, Fig. 97-2.)*

- **Subclinical hypothyroidism: The degree of abnormality is so slight that the free T₄ is still within the broad range of normal, but the TSH level is high (usually 5–10 mU/L)**
- Autoantibodies are not necessary for diagnosis but may be helpful in subclinical hypothyroidism to help predict prognosis (see later discussion)
- Hypothalamic or pituitary disease
  - The free T₄ is low and the TSH levels are either low or normal
  - Stimulation testing with the hypothalamic TSH secretagogue thyrotropin-releasing hormone (TRH) may show a preserved TSH secretory response in hypothalamic disease, whereas the TSH response to TRH is absent in pituitary disease

(TRH is not currently available in the United States)

Treatment

- Synthetic T₄ is the treatment of choice for all forms of hypothyroidism
  - **Replacement dose is roughly 1.6 µg/kg/day, which is in the range of 100 to 200 µg/day for the average adult**
  - Treatment can be initiated with the full dose in younger patients
  - Replacement dose is 10% to 15% lower in patients over age 65 years
  - Should start with lower doses (25–50 µg/day) in elderly patients who may have underlying coronary disease; titrate the dose up gradually
- **Monitoring therapy with the TSH level**
  - **Goal TSH is between 0.5 and 3 mU/L; in elderly patients, the TSH goal may be between 4 and 6 mU/L**
  - **Because of its 7-day half-life, T₄ and TSH blood levels take at least 5 to 6 weeks to reach a steady state**
  - Dose adjustments should be made only every 6 weeks
  - May take weeks or even months for some of the hypothyroid symptoms to resolve
  - Over-replacement, as indicated by a low TSH level, should be avoided (may cause osteopenia in postmenopausal women and may predispose to atrial fibrillation in patients >65 years of age)
  - In hypothyroidism secondary to pituitary or hypothalamic disease, the TSH level cannot be used as a guide to therapy; in this case, the free T₄ level should be maintained in the high-normal range
- Conditions necessitating thyroxine dose adjustment: see Box 38-2
- Treatment of myxedema coma
  - Standard treatment is T₄ given as a loading dose of 300 to 500 µg IV, followed by daily IV doses of 100 to 150 µg
  - If no improvement in patient's clinical status within 1 to 2 days, consider adding IV T₃ (10 µg every 8 hours)
    - Acts more quickly than T₄
    - However, may increase myocardial oxygen consumption and precipitate myocardial infarction or arrhythmias
  - **Scrupulous attention to the patient's ancillary problems: Ventilatory support for hypercarbia or hypoxemia, correction of electrolyte abnormalities (especially hyponatremia), and treatment of possible infection; occult infection should be suspected if the patient is normothermic because hypothyroid patients do not mount a normal febrile response**
  - Sedatives and narcotics are contraindicated because all drugs are metabolized slowly and may have prolonged and unpredictable effects
  - Hypoadrenalism
    - Should be suspected in patients with hypothyroidism caused by autoimmune thyroiditis or in central hypothyroidism and in patients with myxedema coma who may have diminished adrenal reserve

BOX 38-2	*Clinical Situations in Which Thyroxine Doses May Need Adjustment*

Increased Dose

Pregnancy

Malabsorption

Certain drugs that

    Interfere with absorption (sucralfate, aluminum hydroxide, cholestyramine, colestipol, ferrous sulfate, calcium, raloxifene)

    Accelerate thyroxine metabolism (phenytoin, carbamazepine, phenobarbital, rifampin, sertraline, imatinib [Gleevec])

    Increase TBG (estrogen)

    Block T_4 to T_3 conversion in the pituitary gland (amiodarone)

Decreased Dose

Advanced age

Androgen therapy (decreases TBG)

T_3, triiodothyronine; T_4, thyroxine; TBG, thyroid-binding globulin.

- If adrenal insufficiency is not treated first, administration of T_4 may precipitate an adrenal crisis; therefore, it is reasonable to administer hydrocortisone 100 mg every 8 hours IV for several days with rapid tapering as the clinical picture improves or until adrenal insufficiency can be ruled out with a cortisol determination or adrenocorticotropic hormone (ACTH) stimulation test
- Treatment of subclinical hypothyroidism
  - Treatment is controversial, since patients tend to be relatively asymptomatic
  - High rate of progression to overt hypothyroidism in those patients who have positive antithyroid antibodies (5–10% per year)
  - Some untreated patients with TSH levels less than 10 mU/L can revert to a euthyroid state, especially if they are antithyroid antibody negative
  - Treatment may result in an improvement of unfavorable lipid patterns, especially if the TSH level is greater than 10 mU/L
  - Relatively small doses of T_4 (50–100 μg/day) are needed

Thyroiditis

Basic Information

- **Definition: Thyroiditis is a group of diseases characterized by thyroid inflammation**
- Types
  - Chronic lymphocytic (Hashimoto) thyroiditis
    - Most common thyroid disease in the United States; most common cause of hypothyroidism (see previous discussion)
  - Subacute (de Quervain, granulomatous) thyroiditis
    - Fairly uncommon
    - Affects women ages 20 to 50 years, with a female-to-male ratio of 6:1

- Associated with human leukocyte antigen (HLA) Bw35
- Treatment: β-Blockers, nonsteroidal anti-inflammatory drugs (NSAIDs); prednisone if NSAIDs are ineffective
- Silent (painless, postpartum) thyroiditis
  - A variant of Hashimoto thyroiditis
  - Women ages 20 to 60 years, with a female-to-male ratio of 2:1
  - When it occurs after pregnancy, silent thyroiditis is referred to as *postpartum thyroiditis*; approximately 5% of women develop postpartum thyroiditis
  - May cause permanent hypothyroidism in about 25% of patients
  - Treatment: β-Blockers
- Acute bacterial (suppurative) thyroiditis: Rare; occurs in all age groups
- Amiodarone-induced thyroiditis
  - Occurs more than 1 year after starting therapy
  - Treatment: Prednisone
- Etiology: see Table 38-6

Clinical Presentation, Diagnosis, and Treatment

See Table 38-6 for a summary of the presentation, diagnosis, and treatment of thyroiditis.

Goiter and Thyroid Nodules

Basic Information

- Goiter is a chronic enlargement of the thyroid gland
- Thyroid nodules are focal isolated lumps in the thyroid gland
- Thyroid nodules and goiter are extremely common
  - Prevalence on physical examination of one or more thyroid nodules ranges from 1% to 5%
  - **Frequency of small, nonpalpable nodules that are detected by ultrasound examination is as high as 50% to 70% in older persons, especially women**
  - The major clinical significance of thyroid nodules is the possibility of thyroid cancer, which is present in 5% to 10% of thyroid nodules
- Etiology
  - In most patients, the cause of goiter and thyroid nodules is not known
  - Iodine deficiency is the major cause of goiter in the world but probably does not exist in North America
  - Chronic lymphocytic thyroiditis accounts for 10% to 20% of goiters and thyroid nodules
  - Ionizing radiation and genetic factors are also important in the genesis of thyroid nodular disease

Clinical Presentation

- Most patients with thyroid nodules or goiter are asymptomatic and clinically euthyroid
- A large goiter may cause neck discomfort and pressure, dysphagia, hoarseness, and dyspnea (Fig. 38-5)
- Some multinodular goiters are substernal in location and may not be readily palpable, but they can cause significant airway obstruction or superior vena caval compression (with jugular venous distention and facial edema)

TABLE 38-6 *Types of Thyroiditis*

Type	Etiology	Clinical Features	Diagnosis	Treatment
Chronic lymphocytic thyroiditis (CLT)	Autoimmune Antithyroid antibodies: antithyroperoxidase (aka, anti-TPO, antimicrosomal) and antithyroglobulin antibodies May be induced by interferon alfa therapy	Most patients have symptoms of hypothyroidism Often with firm, nontender goiter Pyramidal lobe may be palpable May have other evidence of autoimmunity (prematurely gray hair, vitiligo)	Often see ↑ TSH Radioiodine uptake testing usually not necessary	Thyroxine for hypothyroid patients In euthyroid patients, may use higher doses of thyroxine to shrink goiter
Subacute thyroiditis (SAT)	Probably viral More likely to occur if HLA-Bw35 positive	Gradual or acute onset of thyroid pain; may be severe and disabling Pain may radiate to angle of jaw or ear Often preceded by a viral upper respiratory infection May see systemic symptoms, such as fever, night sweats, fatigue, and weight loss On exam, thyroid is very tender, firm, and irregular Course: Pain and hyperthyroidism for 3–6 wk followed by transient hypothyroidism for several months	Acute inflammatory phase: ↑ T_4, ↓ TSH Radioiodine uptake is low High ESR (>30 mm/hr) or CRP Recovery phase: May see temporary mild ↓ T_4 and ↑ TSH for 1–3 mo	Salicylates or other nonsteroidals for neck discomfort Severe cases: Glucocorticoids are helpful Treat symptoms of hyperthyroidism with β-blocking drugs Full recovery is the rule
Silent thyroiditis (postpartum thyroiditis)	Autoimmune	Symptoms and signs of mild thyrotoxicosis Usually a firm, nontender goiter Triphasic course (as with SAT) May recur with successive pregnancies May present as postpartum depression	Similar to SAT ↑ T_4 and T_3 but T_3 not as high as seen in Graves disease Radioiodine uptake is low	Treat symptoms of hyperthyroidism with β-blocking drugs Glucocorticoids rarely needed for severe hyperthyroidism 25% become permanently hypothyroid
Acute (suppurative) thyroiditis	Bacterial; most commonly *Staphylococcus aureus, Streptococcus pyogenes, Streptococcus pneumoniae,* and *Enterobacter* spp. Typically preceded by an upper respiratory or pharyngeal infection May also be due to opportunistic infections in immunocompromised hosts, especially *Aspergillus* and *Pneumocystis*	Anterior neck pain, fever, dysphagia May see erythema over thyroid or jugular venous phlebitis	Thyroid function usually remains normal Leukocytosis Fine-needle aspiration with stains to identify organism	Antibiotics Surgical drainage if abscess develops
Amiodarone-induced thyroiditis (type 2 amiodarone-induced thyrotoxicosis)	3% of patients on amiodarone Due to a destructive thyroiditis, leading to excess release of T_4 and T_3 More common in men	Thyrotoxicosis features develop rapidly May have recurrence of atrial fibrillation Thyroid is nontender; not enlarged Usually occurs after 1–3 yr of therapy	↑ T_4 and T_3 T_3 may also be normal ↓ TSH ↓ Radioiodine uptake Thyroid Doppler ultrasound will demonstrate "low" blood flow similar to euthyroid state	Prednisone 40 mg daily Slow taper over 2–3 mo

CRP, C-reactive protein; ESR, erythrocyte sedimentation rate; HLA, human leukocyte antigen; T_3, triiodothyronine; T_4, thyroxine; TSH, thyroid-stimulating hormone.

FIGURE 38-5 Dominant left-sided nodule in a multinodular goiter. *(From Souhami R: Textbook of medicine, New York, Churchill Livingstone, 2002, Fig. 17.25.)*

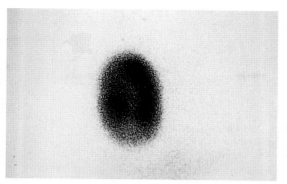

FIGURE 38-6 Toxic adenoma in the right thyroid (a hot nodule) demonstrated with radioiodine uptake scan. Remainder of gland does not take up the isotope. *(From Forbes CD, Jackson WF: Color atlas and text of clinical medicine, ed 3, St. Louis, Mosby, 2003, Fig. 7.63.)*

38

BOX 38-3	*Clinical Features Suggesting Malignancy in a Thyroid Nodule*

History
Rapid growth
Older male or young child
Childhood neck irradiation
Family history of thyroid cancer

Physical Examination
Firm or rock-hard consistency
Ipsilateral cervical adenopathy
Fixation to surrounding structures

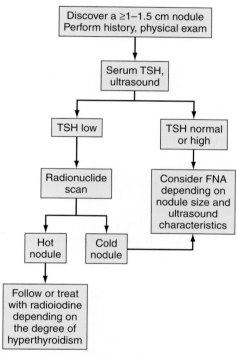

FIGURE 38-7 Evaluation of a thyroid nodule. (FNA, fine-needle aspiration; TSH, thyroid-stimulating hormone.)

- Benign versus malignant nodules
  - The distinction of a benign from a malignant thyroid nodule is almost impossible on clinical grounds
  - A few features favor malignancy (Box 38-3)

Diagnosis and Evaluation

- Diffuse or multinodular goiter
  - Can be seen with a normal TSH (nontoxic goiter), increased TSH (probable chronic lymphocytic thyroiditis), or decreased TSH (Graves disease, toxic multinodular goiter, thyroiditis)
  - Thyroid radionuclide scanning will provide only general information about the size of the thyroid and whether certain areas within the gland concentrate the radioactive tracer (Fig. 38-6)

- Thyroid ultrasound can accurately assess the size of the gland, the overall echotexture of the gland, and the echo characteristics, size, and number of nodules within the gland
- Solitary thyroid nodules
  - Measurement of serum TSH is useful
    - If the value is high, it suggests the presence of chronic lymphocytic thyroiditis
    - If the value is low, it suggests that the nodule is autonomous and one could consider radioiodine scan
    - If TSH is normal or high, an ultrasound should be strongly considered to confirm the presence of the nodule, its size, and its appearance
  - See Figure 38-7 for general approach

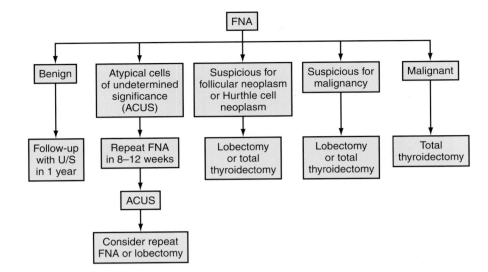

FIGURE 38-8 Management after fine-needle aspiration (FNA) of a thyroid nodule. (U/S, ultrasound.)

- Thyroid ultrasonography cannot reliably differentiate benign from malignant nodules
  - However, certain sonographic features alone and especially in combination have reasonable sensitivity and specificity for predicting malignancy. These include hypoechogenicity, increased blood flow, microcalcifications, and irregular borders.
  - Ultrasound can document the presence and size of a nodule and can define whether a nodule is solitary or whether it is one of many others
  - Good for follow-up of nodule size
- **Fine-needle aspiration (FNA) biopsy is the procedure of choice in the diagnosis of thyroid nodules (Fig. 38-8)**

Treatment

- Therapy of diffuse or multinodular goiters is based on two factors
  - Evidence of thyroid dysfunction
  - Symptoms and/or signs of tracheal, esophageal, or recurrent laryngeal nerve compression
- Pharmacologic therapy
  - Diffuse or multinodular goiters
    - Hypothyroidism is treated with T_4
    - Hyperthyroidism is generally treated with radioiodine
    - The use of T_4 "suppression" therapy in euthyroid patients is controversial but may be effective in some patients with nontoxic goiter
  - Solitary thyroid nodules: Suppression therapy with T_4 is probably of little use
- Nonpharmacologic therapy
  - Diffuse or multinodular goiters: Surgery is usually required for large, obstructive goiters; radioiodine can be used in elderly patients who are not surgical candidates
  - Solitary thyroid nodules
    - Surgery is indicated for malignant and indeterminant nodules and for those nodules that are causing compressive symptoms

- For "hot" nodules that produce hyperthyroidism, radioiodine therapy is the procedure of choice; surgery is also a reasonable option for large (>4 cm) nodules
- In patients with biopsy-proven benign nodules, observation and follow-up ultrasound in 1 year are all that is required in most situations
- Rebiopsy if benign nodule enlarges on follow-up

Thyroid Cancer

Basic Information

- Definition: Primary malignancy arising from thyroid follicular cells or C cells
  - Histologic types: see Table 38-7
  - Papillary and follicular cancer are referred to collectively as *differentiated thyroid cancer* and account for 80% to 90% of all thyroid cancer
- Thyroid lymphomas may develop from lymphocytes within the thyroid gland, especially in individuals with long-standing Hashimoto thyroiditis
- Overall incidence of thyroid cancer in the United States is approximately 10 per 100,000 per year
- Etiology of most cancers is unknown; ionizing radiation is a risk factor for differentiated thyroid cancer
- Medullary thyroid cancer (MTC)
  - About 20% of patients belong to kindreds with multiple endocrine neoplasia-2 syndrome (see Chapter 41)
  - Autosomal dominant

Clinical Presentation

- Patients are usually asymptomatic, and a thyroid nodule is found on routine physical examination or incidentally on imaging done for other purposes (chest computed tomography, neck magnetic resonance imaging, carotid Doppler, positron emission tomography scan, etc.)

Diagnosis and Evaluation

- FNA required for diagnosis
- See Table 38-7 for histologic types

TABLE 38-7	Clinical Features and Therapy of Thyroid Cancer					
Cancer Type	% of All Cancers	Age at Diagnosis (yr)	Rate of Growth	Primary Therapy	Prognosis	Comment
Papillary	70–80	30–60	Slow	Surgery	Excellent	Radioiodine used as adjunct
Follicular	10–15	50+	Slow	Surgery	Good to excellent	Radioiodine used as adjunct
Medullary	10	50+ (younger if MEN-2)	Moderate	Surgery	Fair to good	RET germline mutation in 20% of cases; produces calcitonin
Lymphoma	<5	50+	Moderate	Radiotherapy, chemotherapy	Good	Seen in association with Hashimoto thyroiditis
Anaplastic	<5	60+	Rapid	Surgery, radiotherapy, chemotherapy	Poor	Often prior history of goiter or papillary thyroid cancer

MEN, multiple endocrine neoplasia.

Treatment

- See Table 38-7
- Total thyroidectomy is the primary therapy
- Radioiodine ablation of thyroid remnants after thyroid-ectomy is usually performed in patients with differenti-ated thyroid cancer, especially in those patients at high risk for recurrence
- **Serum markers may be helpful for monitoring for disease recurrence**
  - **Serum thyroglobulin useful in patients with dif-ferentiated thyroid cancer**
  - **Serum calcitonin useful in patients with MTC**
- Factors influencing the prognosis in differentiated cancer include the patient's age (better in patients <50 years of age), the tumor size, the degree of tumor invasiveness, and the presence of distant metastases

REVIEW QUESTIONS

For review questions, please go to www.expertconsult.com.

SUGGESTED READINGS

Bartalena L, Tanda ML: Clinical practice: Graves' ophthalmopathy, N Engl J Med 360:994–1001, 2009.
Biondi B, Cooper DS: The clinical significance of subclinical thyroid dysfunction, Endocr Rev 29:76–131, 2007.
Bogazzi F, Baralena L, Martino E: Approach to the patient with amiodarone-induced thyrotoxicosis, J Clin Endocrinol Metab 95: 2529–2535, 2010.
Brent GA: Clinical practice: Graves' disease, N Engl J Med 358: 2594–2605, 2008.
Cibas ES, Ali SZ, for the NCI Thyroid FNA State of Sciences Confer-ence: The Bethesda System for reporting thyroid cytopathology, Am J Clin Pathol 132:658–665, 2009.
Cooper DS: Antithyroid drugs, N Engl J Med 352:905–917, 2005.
Cooper DS: Clinical practice: subclinical hypothyroidism, N Engl J Med 345:260–265, 2001.
Cooper DS: Hyperthyroidism, Lancet 362:459–468, 2003.
Cooper DS, Doherty GM, Haugen BR, et al: Revised American Thyroid Association management guidelines for patients with thyroid nodules and differentiated thyroid cancer, Thyroid 19:1167–1214, 2009.
Hegedus L: Clinical practice: the thyroid nodule, N Engl J Med 351: 1764–1771, 2004.
Mazzaferri EL, Kloos RT: Current approaches to primary therapy for papillary and follicular thyroid cancer, J Clin Endocrinol Metab 86:1447–1463, 2001.
Roberts CG, Ladenson PW: Hypothyroidism, Lancet 363:793–803, 2004.
Sherman SI: Thyroid carcinoma, Lancet 361:501–511, 2003.
Toft AD: Subclinical hyperthyroidism, N Engl J Med 345:512–516, 2001.

38

Calcium Disorders and Metabolic Bone Disease

REDONDA G. MILLER, MD, MBA

Calcium disorders are common in both inpatients and outpatients. Malignancy accounts for the vast majority of hypercalcemia cases in hospitalized patients. In the outpatient setting, hyperparathyroidism is the leading cause, with an increase in the incidence of asymptomatic primary hyperparathyroidism over the last several decades probably attributable to the frequent use of screening chemistry panels. Metabolic bone disease includes a heterogeneous group of disorders. Given the aging population, osteoporosis is the most prevalent and important of these. Every internist should be familiar with screening and treatment principles of this disease.

Hypercalcemia

Basic Information

- Calcium metabolism
  - Calcium is important for many physiologic processes, including bone matrix crystallization and muscle contraction
  - In the extracellular compartment it circulates in three forms:
    - "Ionized" or the free form: Maintained in very narrow limits (45%)
    - Bound to protein (albumin and globulin) (40%)
    - Bound to anions (bicarbonate, phosphate, citrate) (15%)
  - Parathyroid hormone (PTH), produced by the four parathyroid glands, tightly regulates serum calcium levels
    - PTH level is responsive to level of ionized calcium in the blood as well as to the levels of phosphate and magnesium
    - PTH actions (via G protein–coupled receptor; Fig. 39-1)
  - Vitamin D
    - A fat-soluble steroid obtained from diet or synthesized in skin in presence of ultraviolet light
    - Transported to the liver, where it is 25-hydroxylated to 25-hydroxyvitamin D
    - Then transported to kidney, where it is 1-hydroxylated (under the control of PTH) to 1,25-dihydroxyvitamin D; $1,25(OH)_2D$ (calcitriol) is the active form
    - Actions of $1,25(OH)_2D$ (see Fig. 39-1)

- Definition of hypercalcemia: An abnormal elevation in the ionized calcium (usually >1.32 mmol/L) or total calcium greater than 10.5 mg/dL
  - Moderate hypercalcemia: Levels between 12 and 14 mg/dL; variable clinical manifestations
  - Severe hypercalcemia: Levels of 14 mg/dL or greater; almost always associated with symptoms and requires immediate treatment
    - High levels should always be repeated to confirm, and ionized calcium level also checked
    - **Calcium is bound to albumin (40%); a "normal" total calcium may actually be high if the albumin is low**
      - Formula for approximating the correction: Adjust the total serum calcium level by 0.8 mg/dL for each 1 g by which the serum albumin level is above or below 4 g/dL
    - Acid-base status is also important because alkalosis increases calcium binding to albumin, whereas acidosis decreases it
- Causes of hypercalcemia (Box 39-1; Table 39-1)
  - **The two most common causes are hyperparathyroidism and malignancy, which make up more than 90% of cases**

Clinical Presentation

- The clinical presentation can be variable and often depends on factors other than total calcium level, such as:
  - Age of patient (older patients present more severely)
  - Comorbid conditions
  - Duration of hypercalcemia (the longer the duration, the better tolerated)
  - Rate of increase in calcium concentration (a more rapid increase leads to more severe symptoms)
- Malignancy tends to present most acutely and severely
  - 10% to 20% of cancer patients develop hypercalcemia at some point
  - Associated with a poor prognosis: 50% mortality at 1 month
- Main clinical manifestations of acute hypercalcemia
  - Gastrointestinal: anorexia, nausea, vomiting, constipation (decreased GI motility)
  - Central nervous system: confusion, weakness, lethargy, hyporeflexia, obtundation, coma

39

FIGURE 39-1   Actions of parathyroid hormone (PTH).

BOX 39-1   *Causes of Hypercalcemia*

Primary hyperparathyroidism

Malignancy
   Bone metastases
   Humoral hypercalcemia (related to PTH-rp)
   Conversion of 25(OH) vitamin D to 1,25(OH)$_2$
   vitamin D

Granulomatous disease
   Sarcoidosis
   Tuberculosis

Familial hypocalciuric hypercalcemia

Drugs
   Thiazide diuretics (stimulate renal resorption of calcium)
   Lithium (changes "set point" of PTH release)

Vitamin A or D intoxication

Immobilization

Other
   Thyrotoxicosis
   Pheochromocytoma
   Adrenal insufficiency
   Parenteral nutrition

PTH, parathyroid hormone; PTH-rp, parathyroid hormone–related peptide.

- Cardiovascular: hypertension (if not too dehydrated), shortened Q–T interval, occasional bradycardia, and first-degree atrioventricular block
- Renal: polyuria and polydipsia (via interference with antidiuretic hormone action and inhibition of sodium resorption), azotemia (dehydration and afferent arteriolar constriction)

- Chronic manifestations of hypercalcemia ("stones, bones, abdominal groans, and psychic overtones"); most commonly associated with chronic hyperparathyroidism
  - Osteoporosis with bone pain
  - Nephrocalcinosis
  - Band keratopathy (deposition of calcium phosphate in sun-exposed cornea; Fig. 39-2)
  - Chondrocalcinosis
  - Pancreatitis (calcium deposition in the pancreas)
  - Hypertension

Diagnosis and Evaluation

- Often the cause of the hypercalcemia is readily apparent from a good history and physical examination
- **If not, the first step is to determine between PTH-mediated and non–PTH-mediated forms of hypercalcemia**
  - **Intact PTH (iPTH) is the test of choice**
  - **Diagnosis often suggested by iPTH level (Fig. 39-3)**

Treatment

- Treatment approach for acute, life-threatening hypercalcemia
  - Rapidity and aggressiveness of treatment depend on absolute calcium level and patient's symptoms
    - **All patients should receive aggressive IV fluids as tolerated**
    - Calcitonin, pamidronate, and zoledronate are good first choices (calcitonin will take effect rapidly, but action is short lived; pamidronate and zoledronate will have slower onset but will provide more durable response)

TABLE 39-1	Selected Disorders Associated with Hypercalcemia

Disorder	Pathophysiology	Clinical and Diagnostic Considerations	Treatment
Primary hyperparathyroidism	Oversecretion of parathyroid hormone (PTH) by the parathyroid glands Sporadic, solitary adenoma (85%) Hyperplasia of all 4 glands (10–15%) Carcinoma (<1%)	Most patients are asymptomatic; high calcium found on routine testing Typical symptoms: fatigue, nausea, constipation Associated with osteoporosis Loss of cortical bone > trabecular bone DXA should include forearm measurement for this reason (higher cortical bone percentage) Advanced form: Osteitis fibrosa cystica (rare) Preoperative sestamibi scan is helpful in localizing adenoma if present If hyperplasia of all 4 glands present, consider MEN syndromes Follow patients with serum calcium every 6 mo and yearly creatinine and DXA	All symptomatic patients should undergo surgery Resection of adenoma, if nodule present Removal of 3½ glands if hyperplasia present Minimally invasive surgery if possible Highly consider surgery in asymptomatic patients if: Age <50 yr Calcium >1 mg/dL above upper limit of normal Creatinine clearance <30% of age-matched normal subjects Low bone density Difficult periodic follow-up Medical therapy (if not a surgical candidate) Estrogen and raloxifene will decrease serum calcium and decrease bone resorption Cinacalcet: Calcimimetic that binds to calcium-sensing receptor in parathyroid gland ↓ Sensitivity to serum calcium level ↓ PTH secretion FDA-approved indication for severe hypercalcemia
Malignancy	Three mechanisms Bony metastases resulting in local resorption (e.g., breast, multiple myeloma, prostate, lymphoma, thyroid, lung) Humoral hypercalcemia: Mediated by PTH-related peptide (PTH-rp); analogy with amino terminus of PTH; usually squamous cell carcinomas (e.g., lung); also renal, bladder, ovarian Conversion of 25(OH) vitamin D to active form (e.g., lymphoma)	More likely to present acutely and severely Can measure PTH-rp via sensitive assay	Treat acute, symptomatic hypercalcemia as outlined in text Treat underlying malignancy
Granulomatous diseases	Unregulated synthesis of $1,25(OH)_2$ vitamin D by granuloma-associated macrophages Not sensitive to negative feedback suppression by ↑ calcium	Diseases such as sarcoidosis, tuberculosis, disseminated fungal infections, berylliosis Serum PO_4 often elevated as well; may lead to soft tissue calcification and nephrocalcinosis	Steroids particularly useful Treat underlying disease
Familial hypocalciuric hypercalcemia	Mutation in gene encoding calcium-sensing receptor Kidneys cannot sense calcium level and resorb too much Parathyroid glands also exhibit sensing defect and do not appropriately suppress PTH secretion Autosomal dominant	Clinical manifestations are very benign; most patients asymptomatic May have a family history of unsuccessful neck explorations Urine calcium low (<100 mg/24 hr or urinary calcium/creatinine ratio <0.01) PTH usually normal	No treatment necessary

DXA, dual-energy x-ray absorptiometry; FDA, Food and Drug Administration; MEN, multiple endocrine neoplasia.

- Definitive therapy, however, is to treat the underlying disorder (see Table 39-1)
- **Treatment options for acute, severe hypercalcemia**
  - If severe, acute, symptomatic hypercalcemia is present, institute treatment immediately
  - Saline infusion with diuresis
    - Volume expansion using isotonic saline initially (most patients are severely dehydrated) and delivered at a rapid rate
    - Improves renal blood flow and glomerular filtration rate (GFR) with increased filtration of calcium
    - Once volume is replete, loop diuretic can be added to enhance sodium excretion and protect against volume overload

FIGURE 39-2 Ectopic calcification at the lateral and nasal margins of the right cornea (band keratopathy) in a patient with primary hyperparathyroidism. *(From Forbes CD, Jackson WF: Color atlas and text of clinical medicine, ed 3, St. Louis, Mosby, 2003, Fig. 3.138.)*

- Calcium follows sodium in the proximal tubule; the more sodium excreted, the more calcium excreted
  - Loop diuretics should be used because they also inhibit calcium resorption in the thick ascending limb of the loop of Henle
  - Thiazide diuretics do the opposite and should never be used in hypercalcemia
- Mobilization, if possible (immobility increases bone resorption because of lack of weight bearing)
- Pharmacologic options
  - Bisphosphonates
    - Are the gold standard
    - Bind to hydroxyapatite in bone and inhibit the dissolution of crystals; also inhibit osteoclast activity
    - **Pamidronate or zoledronate are drugs of choice; potent and effective**
    - **Poor oral absorption (<10%) means they must be given parenterally**
    - **Calcium level begins to decline within 2 days and hits nadir at 7 days**
    - Adverse effects include transient, mild increase in temperature and transient leukopenia
  - Calcitonin
    - Inhibits bone resorption and increases renal excretion
    - **Has some analgesic properties and can be effective at relieving bone pain**
    - **Quickest in onset; takes effect within a few hours**
    - Effect is often limited and transient (because of tachyphylaxis)

FIGURE 39-3 Approach to the patient with hypercalcemia. (ACTH, adrenocorticotropic hormone; MEN, multiple endocrine neoplasia; PTH, parathyroid hormone; PTH-rp, parathyroid hormone–related peptide.)

- Very safe; patients may have mild nausea, abdominal cramps, and flushing; because of occasional allergic reactions, initial 1-unit skin test is recommended
- Mithramycin and gallium nitrate: Rarely used because of their serious side effects
- **Glucocorticoids**
  - **Most useful in treating vitamin D–mediated hypercalcemia (i.e., vitamin D intoxication, granulomatous diseases)**
  - **Work via inhibition of 1,25(OH)$_2$D production**
  - Also useful in certain malignancies involving cytokine release (e.g., some myelomas)
  - Usual dose is prednisone 20 to 40 mg/day
- Treatment of other more chronic causes of hypercalcemia (see Table 39-1)

Hypocalcemia

Basic Information

- Causes
  - Defect in action or metabolism of PTH
    - Hypoparathyroidism (after neck surgery, autoimmune, infiltrative diseases)
    - Resistance to action of PTH (pseudohypoparathyroidism)
  - Vitamin D deficiency (often low-normal calcium values) resulting from:
    - Inadequate oral intake
    - GI malabsorptive disorders (celiac disease, pancreatic insufficiency, ileal bypass)
    - End-stage liver or renal disease
    - **May manifest as osteomalacia (Box 39-2)**

- Large-volume blood transfusions (citrate in transfused blood can bind calcium)
- Magnesium depletion (decreased PTH release)
- Acute respiratory alkalosis (increases binding of calcium to albumin)
- Acute pancreatitis (calcium binds to free fatty acids released by lipase)
- Excessive tissue breakdown resulting in calcium binding to excess phosphate (tumor lysis syndrome, rhabdomyolysis)

Clinical Presentation

- Neurologic
  - Numbness, paresthesias (especially perioral), muscle irritability, tetany
  - Chvostek's sign (spasm of the facial nerve when tapped)
  - Trousseau's sign (carpopedal spasm elicited by inflating blood pressure cuff above systolic pressure; Fig. 39-4)
- Cardiovascular
  - Hypotension with decreased contractility
  - Prolonged Q–T interval on electrocardiogram
- Pulmonary
  - Bronchospasm

Diagnosis and Evaluation

- Measurement of serum calcium, phosphate, magnesium, iPTH, vitamin D levels
- Diagnosis often suggested by clinical presentation

Treatment

- Severe cases (symptomatic patients): IV repletion with calcium gluconate or calcium chloride slowly
  - Ensure magnesium is also replete
- Mild cases: Oral calcium carbonate or calcium citrate; usually vitamin D as well

---

BOX 39-2	*Osteomalacia*

Main defect: Undermineralized bone

Cause: Usually calcium ± phosphorus deficiency due to
 Dietary deficiency
 Gastrointestinal malabsorption
 Decreased vitamin D synthesis (liver disease, inadequate sun exposure, drugs such as phenytoin)

Clinical symptoms
 Fatigue
 Diffuse bone pain
 Muscle weakness

Diagnosis
 Labs often reveal low (or low-normal) calcium, significant hypophosphatemia, mildly elevated alkaline phosphatase, low vitamin D levels
 Diagnosis confirmed by bone biopsy (with tetracycline labeling) showing undermineralization

Treatment: Repletion of calcium and vitamin D
 Calcium: 1000–1500 mg by mouth per day in divided doses
 Vitamin D: Often need 50,000 units of ergocalciferol by mouth once or twice weekly for up to 6–12 mo

FIGURE 39-4 Trousseau's sign (carpopedal spasm). *(From Larsen PR, Kronenberg HM, Melmed S, et al: Williams textbook of endocrinology, ed 10, Philadelphia, WB Saunders, 2002, Fig. 26-32.)*

Osteoporosis

Basic Information

- **Definition: A skeletal disorder characterized by compromised bone strength predisposing to an increased risk of fracture**
- Scope of the problem
  - Responsible for 1.5 million fractures per year
  - Lifetime risk for hip fracture of an average 50-year-old woman: 17.5% (with a 1-year mortality rate of 20%)
- Pathophysiology
  - Bone remodeling is a dynamic equilibrium between bone formation (by osteoblasts) and bone resorption (by osteoclasts)
  - Peak bone mass is achieved at age 30 years and is about 30% greater in men than women
  - Around the fourth or fifth decade, women and men start losing bone at a rate of 0.3% to 0.5% per year
  - Loss is accelerated in women with loss of estrogen at menopause (can lose 3–5% per year for up to 5 years)
    - Leads to "postmenopausal" osteoporosis, the most common form
  - Pathology reveals distortion in microarchitecture, loss of trabeculae, and microfractures (Fig. 39-5)
- **Risk factors**
  - **Major risk factors**
    - **Personal history of a fragility fracture**
    - **Family history of osteoporosis or fracture in a first-degree relative**
    - **Thin body habitus (<127 pounds)**
    - **Current smoking**
    - **Current use of glucocorticoid therapy for longer than 3 months**
  - Other risk factors
    - Age
    - Premature menopause (age <45 years) or hypogonadism
    - Predisposition to falls (vision loss, prior cerebrovascular accident, frailty)
    - Heavy alcohol intake
    - Sedentary lifestyle
    - Dietary deficiencies (calcium, vitamin D)
  - Secondary causes (Box 39-3)
    - **Glucocorticoid use is the most common secondary cause**
      - **Only small doses, equivalent to 7.5 mg or higher of prednisone per day, are required for bone loss to occur**
      - **Occurs within 3 to 6 months of use**
    - In men with osteoporosis, consider checking testosterone level (hypogonadism is a fairly common cause)

Clinical Presentation

- Most patients are asymptomatic
- Main causes of symptoms are vertebral and hip fractures
- Physical examination
  - Routine height measurement: Loss of height (>1 inch) may be only clue to vertebral fractures
  - Kyphosis: Decreases thoracic volume and can lead to dyspnea and restrictive lung disease (Fig. 39-6)
  - Look for clues to secondary causes of osteoporosis

Diagnosis and Evaluation

- Radiography: May see increased lucency of bone
  - Not helpful for detecting early disease; osteopenia not evident until approximately 30% of bone is lost

FIGURE 39-5 Cross section of an osteoporotic vertebra showing extensive loss of trabecular bone architecture. *(From Larsen PR, Kronenberg HM, Melmed S, et al: Williams textbook of endocrinology, ed 10, Philadelphia, WB Saunders, 2002, Fig. 27-15.)*

BOX 39-3	*Select Secondary Causes of Osteoporosis*

Endocrine Disorders

Hyperthyroidism
Hyperparathyroidism
Hypogonadism
Excess cortisol production (e.g., Cushing disease)

Bone Marrow Disorders

Multiple myeloma
Leukemia/lymphoma

Gastrointestinal Diseases

Gastrectomy
Malabsorption syndromes

Connective Tissue Diseases

Rheumatoid arthritis
Osteogenesis imperfecta
Ehlers-Danlos syndrome
Marfan syndrome

Drugs

Glucocorticoids
Anticonvulsants
Cyclosporine
Prolonged heparin use

FIGURE 39-6 Radiograph showing radiolucency, compression fractures, and kyphosis in the spine of a patient with osteoporosis. *(From Goldman L, Bennett JC, Ausiello D: Cecil textbook of medicine, ed 22, Philadelphia, WB Saunders, 2004, Fig. 258-4.)*

TABLE 39-2	*World Health Organization Criteria for Diagnosis of Osteoporosis*
T-Score	**Assessment**
> −1	Normal bone mineral density
−1 to −2.5	Osteopenia
< −2.5	Osteoporosis
< −2.5 + fracture	Severe osteoporosis

- Lateral films useful for visualization of spine compression fractures
- Dual-energy x-ray absorptiometry (DXA)
  - Calculates bone mineral density (BMD) on the basis of tissue absorption of photons from a radionuclide source or x-ray tube
  - **Measures BMD both at axial (spine) and at appendicular (hip) sites**
  - **Low BMD highly correlates with increased risk of fracture**
  - Is the gold standard for diagnosis
  - Results expressed as two scores
    - **T-score: BMD expressed as the number of standard deviations above or below the mean BMD of normal young adults (30-year-olds)**
    - Z-score: BMD expressed as the number of standard deviations above or below the mean BMD of adults of the same age and gender
  - **World Health Organization diagnostic criteria based on T-scores: see** Table 39-2
  - **Indications for BMD measurement with DXA scan**
    - **All postmenopausal women 65 years of age or older**
    - **Women under age 65 years with one or more clinical risk factors**
    - **All men 70 years of age or older**
    - **Men under age 70 years with one or more clinical risk factors**
    - **Aid in decision regarding hormone therapy**

- **Radiologic evidence of osteopenia**
- **Prior osteoporotic fracture**
- **Monitoring therapy for osteoporosis**
  - Peripheral devices (e.g., heel ultrasonography, heel or wrist DXA) may not be as accurate but are less expensive and can predict fracture at 1 year; central DXA is preferable if possible
- Biochemical assessment once osteoporosis confirmed by DXA
  - Baseline complete blood count; chemistry panel including calcium, phosphorus, alkaline phosphatase; thyroid-stimulating hormone
    - Useful as a clue to secondary causes
  - Highly consider checking a 25-hydroxyvitamin D level
    - Many adults are deficient (minimal sun exposure, dietary insufficiencies)
    - If less than 30 ng/mL, may need to replete with high-dose ergocalciferol or cholecalciferol (see Box 39-2 on osteomalacia)
  - Other tests are not routinely sent unless history, physical, or initial laboratory test results suggest need: Serum protein electrophoresis (SPEP), urine protein electrophoresis (UPEP), 24-hour urinary calcium, PTH, testosterone (in men)

Treatment

- Traditional indications for instituting therapy (based predominantly on BMD):
  - History of a hip or vertebral fracture
  - History of other fragility fracture with T-score between −1 and −2.5
  - T-score less than −2 with no risk factors present
  - T-score less than −1.5 with at least one risk factor present
- **Newer treatment guidelines from the National Osteoporosis Foundation (NOF) recommend incorporating other risk factors in addition to BMD; treat if**
  - **History of a hip or vertebral fracture**
  - **History of other fragility fracture with T-score between −1 and −2.5**
  - **10-year probability of hip fracture is 3% or greater**
  - **10-year probability of any major osteoporosis-related fracture is 20% or greater**
- 10-year probability of both hip and any major osteoporosis-related fracture is calculated using the FRAX algorithm
  - FRAX is an online tool developed by the World Health Organization

TABLE 39-3	Recommended Daily Calcium and Vitamin D Intake*	
Age (yr)	Calcium (mg/day)	Vitamin D (IU/day)
Adults <50	1000	400–800
Adults ≥50	1200	800–1000

*Adapted from the National Osteoporosis Foundation guidelines.

- Incorporates nine clinical risk factors in addition to BMD
- Tailored to nationality, gender, ethnicity
- All patients with osteoporosis should be prescribed the following:
  - Behavior modification
    - Exercise (particularly modest weight-bearing exercise)
    - Limitation of alcohol intake to moderate levels
    - Smoking cessation if applicable
  - Calcium
    - Recommended dietary requirements (Table 39-3)
    - Average diet in the United States is deficient (roughly 600 mg/day)
    - Major food sources: Milk and dairy products (approximately 300 mg per serving)
    - Nonprescription supplements are helpful in those with deficient diets
      - Supplements better absorbed when taken with meals (presence of acid) and in small doses (500 mg or less at a time)
      - Calcium carbonate has highest calcium content and is cheapest
      - Calcuim citrate may be better absorbed in patients with achlorhydria or in those who take histamine₂-receptor antagonists or proton pump inhibitors
  - Vitamin D
    - Recommended daily requirements (see Table 39-3)
    - Food sources similar to calcium (dairy products)
    - Many calcium supplements also contain vitamin D
- Estrogen
  - At menopause, falling estrogen levels contribute to rapid bone loss
  - Prescribing estrogen will halt bone loss in menopausal women (and result in BMD gain of 3% to 5% in osteoporotic women)
  - The earlier it is started, the bigger the effect on bone density
  - Currently approved only for prevention due to its association with various adverse events and the availability of other options (see below)
- Pharmacologic options for the treatment of osteoporosis (Table 39-4)
  - Therapy must be tailored to individual wants and needs of the patient
  - All approved therapies, except teriparatide, work by inhibiting bone resorption
  - **First-line therapy is often a bisphosphonate because of potency, duration of effect, bone specificity (as opposed to hormonal therapies), and tolerability**

- IV forms (pamidronate, ibandronate, and zoledronic acid) are options for patients who cannot tolerate oral preparations
- Risks to consider:
  - Osteonecrosis of the jaw linked to IV administration in high doses (particularly in cancer patients)
  - Long-term use possibly associated with a very small increase in atypical fractures of the femoral shaft (subtrochanteric or diaphyseal), but doesn't outweigh the known protection against common hip fractures
- Raloxifene and calcitonin: see Table 39-4
- Teriparatide: A recombinant N-terminus of parathyroid hormone
  - Delivered by daily subcutaneous injection
  - Intermittent delivery by injection, as opposed to continuous delivery *in vivo* by parathyroid glands, results in increased bone formation
  - Indicated for "severe" osteoporosis
- Denusomab: Human monoclonal antibody to receptor activator of nuclear factor-kappa beta ligand
  - Inhibits development and activity of osteoclasts
  - Injection every 6 months
- Monitoring therapy
  - Repeat densitometry is the standard method of follow-up
  - **Reassessment by DXA at 2 years is usually reasonable**
    - Need to wait sufficient time to avoid BMD changes that are simply margin of error of the test
    - Possible exceptions: Newly menopausal women, patients on corticosteroids, patients with other secondary causes of low BMD
  - **Treatment is probably successful if repeat DXA documents either modest increase in or stabilization of BMD**
    - Regardless of percent increase in BMD, most medications used for treatment decrease fracture risk by roughly 50%, as they also inprove the quality of the bone

Paget Disease

Basic Information
- Second most common bone disease
- Prevalent in the United Kingdom, Australia, South Africa, and the United States
- Pathophysiology: Chaotic osteoclast function with increased bone remodeling (both formation and resorption)
  - Many large osteoclasts with numerous nuclei
  - New bone formed is structurally weaker
  - Hypervascularity
- Etiology is unclear; possibly linked to a virus or genetic factors

Clinical Presentation
- Pattern of bone involvement
  - **May involve one bone or many bones asymmetrically**

TABLE 39-4	*Pharmacologic Options for Osteoporosis Treatment*					
Medication	**Mechanism**	**Advantages**	**Prevention of Vertebral Fractures**	**Prevention of Hip/Nonvertebral Fractures**	**Side Effects and Precautions**
Raloxifene	Synthetic estrogen receptor agonist and antagonist Inhibits bone resorption	No effect on breast or endometrial tissue (unlike estrogen) Lowers LDL cholesterol	Yes	Not proven	Risk of thromboembolism comparable to estrogen No effect on menopausal vasomotor symptoms
Bisphosphonates (alendronate, risedronate, ibandronate, zoledronic acid)	Structural analogues of inorganic pyrophosphate Bind to hydroxyapatite and inhibit osteoclast activity	Very potent Long half-life: Allows for once-weekly administration (once monthly for risedronate and ibandronate) Zoledronic acid may be administered IV once yearly	Yes	Yes (for alendronate, risedronate, zoledronic acid)	Poor oral absorption Upper GI irritation— have to take with 8 oz water on empty stomach then remain upright with no food for 30 min (60 min for ibandronate)
Calcitonin	Naturally occurring peptide Directly inhibits osteoclast activity	Intranasal administration Well tolerated with few side effects Analgesic effect; useful in compression fractures	Yes	Not proven	Limited effectiveness Tachyphylaxis may develop
Teriparatide	Is the amino terminus (1–34) of PTH Subcutaneous administration causes increase in bone formation with little effect on bone resorption	First drug to result in bone formation Large increases in bone mineral density	Yes	Yes	May see transient hypercalcemia Theoretical risk of osteosarcoma with prolonged use (use currently limited to 2 yr) Disadvantage: Daily subcutaneous administration
Denusomab	Monoclonal antibody to RANK ligand (RANKL) Inhibits osteoclast development and activity	Very potent Long half-life (dosing every 6 mo) Well tolerated	Yes	Yes	No long-term safety data RANKL plays a role in immune function—? higher risk of infections

LDL, low-density lipoprotein; PTH, parathyroid hormone.

- **Most common sites: pelvis, lumbar spine, skull, femur**
- Many patients have no symptoms (>90%)
- **Others experience bone pain, skeletal deformities**
  - **Enlarged skull, particularly frontal and occipital areas (Fig. 39-7)**
  - **Bowed lower extremities (Fig. 39-8)**
  - **Increased risk of fracture, particularly femur, tibia, radius**
  - **Impingement syndromes (e.g., inner ear with hearing loss and vertigo)**
  - Less common and occuring late in course
    - High-output congestive heart failure from numerous vascular shunts
    - Increased risk of osteosarcoma
    - Hypercalcemia during immobilization

Diagnosis and Evaluation

- Lab studies show an isolated increase in alkaline phosphatase (can be quite high: >500 units/L)

- Plain films can reveal all three phases of disease; seeing all three is essentially diagnostic
  - First phase: Osteoporosis from osteolytic activity
  - Second phase (most commonly seen): Mixed phase with both sclerosis and osteolytic activity
  - Third phase: Mainly sclerosis with cortical thickening
- Bone scan: Most sensitive test; can identify areas of increased uptake

Treatment

- **Treatment is recommended for**
  - **All patients with symptoms**
  - **Asymptomatic patients with involvement of the skull, axial skeleton, or weight-bearing long bones (high risk of progression to deformity)**
  - Also highy consider pretreatment prior to surgery on sites of active disease or if alkaline phosphatase greater than two times upper limit of normal
- Analgesics for pain
- **Bisphosphonates for severe disease**

FIGURE 39-7 Radiograph of the skull of a patient with advanced Paget disease showing thickening, disordered new bone formation (cotton-wool patches), and basilar impression. *(From Larsen PR, Kronenberg HM, Melmed S, et al: Williams textbook of endocrinology, ed 10, Philadelphia, 2002, WB Saunders, Fig. 27-22.)*

FIGURE 39-8 Paget disease of the tibia. Note the bowing, marked irregularity of the anterior cortex, and flame-shaped lytic lesion of the posterior cortex. *(From Larsen PR, Kronenberg HM, Melmed S, Polonsky, KS: Williams textbook of endocrinology, ed 10, Philadelphia, WB Saunders, 2003, Fig. 8-14.)*

- First-line therapy
- Requires higher doses than those used for osteoporosis
- Oral agents (risedronate, alendronate)
  - Can use until disease in remission (usual treatment course is 2 months), then discontinue drug with close monitoring of the alkaline phosphatase
- IV agents (pamidronate, zoledronic acid)
  - Single infusion of zoledronic acid provides rapid and sustained response
- Calcitonin is also useful but is not first line
  - Marked decrease in bone resorption, but disease recurs if drug is stopped
  - Significant bone pain relief, even when used intermittently
  - Some patients develop resistance to drug
- Prognosis is good; disease responds well to treatment with an increase in lamellar bone formation and a decrease in pain
- Disease activity can be monitored with biochemical markers (alkaline phosphatase and urine N-telopeptide)

REVIEW QUESTIONS

For review questions, please go to www.expertconsult.com.

SUGGESTED READINGS

Bilezekian JP, Khan AA, Potts JT Jr, et al: Guidelines for the management of aymptomatic primary hyperparathyroidism: summary statement from the third international workshop, *J Clin Endocrinol Metab* 94:335–339, 2009.

Ettinger B, Black DM, Mitlak BH, et al: Reduction of vertebral fracture risk in postmenopausal women with osteoporosis treated with raloxifene, *JAMA* 282:637–645, 1999.

Liberman UA, Weiss SR, Broll J, et al: Effect of oral alendronate on bone mineral density and the incidence of fractures in postmenopausal osteoporosis, *N Engl J Med* 333:1437–1496, 1995.

McClung MR, Geusens P, et al: Effect of risedronate on the risk of hip fracture in elderly women. Hip Intervention Program Study Group, *N Engl J Med* 344:333–340, 2001.

Pecherstorfer M, Brenner K, Zojer N: Current management strategies for hypercalcemia, *Treat Endo* 2:273–292, 2003.

Ralston SH, Langston AL, Reid IR: Pathogenesis and management of Paget's disease of bone, *Lancet* 372:155–163, 2008.

Rosen CJ: Clinical practice: postmenopausal osteoporosis, *N Engl J Med* 353:595–603, 2005.

U.S. Preventive Services Task Force: Screening for osteoporosis: U.S. Preventive Services Task Force recommendation statement, *Ann Intern Med* 154:356–364, 2011.

39

Reproductive Endocrinology

TODD T. BROWN, MD, PhD

This chapter focuses on the reproductive endocrine disorders the internist is most likely to encounter. Common problems for women include amenorrhea and hirsutism. Men may present with symptoms of gynecomastia, impotence, or other features of hypogonadism. Despite their prevalence, patients are often hesitant to discuss these symptoms. Therefore, internists may need to actively inquire about their presence.

Female Reproductive Disorders

FEMALE REPRODUCTIVE PHYSIOLOGY

- Normal menstrual cycle requires cyclic release of gonadotropin-releasing hormone (GnRH) from the hypothalamus, which leads to cyclic secretion of the pituitary gonadotropins: follicle-stimulating hormone (FSH) and luteinizing hormone (LH)
- The ovaries respond to FSH and LH by producing follicles containing ova
- Phases of the normal female menstrual cycle (Fig. 40-1)
  - Follicular phase of menstrual cycle: Ovarian follicle development
    - Estrogen predominantly produced by ovary
    - Causes thickening of uterine endometrium
  - Ovulation: LH surge induces release of egg from ovarian follicle
  - Luteal phase: Progesterone production by corpus luteum induces maturation of secretory endometrium
  - Menses: Decline in estrogen and progesterone results in endometrial shedding

AMENORRHEA

- Oligomenorrhea is defined as infrequent menses (>35 days between cycles or <6–8 periods per year)
- Amenorrhea is the absence of menses; may be physiologic or pathologic
  - Physiologic amenorrhea is normal and occurs with pregnancy, lactation, menopause
  - Pathologic amenorrhea can exist in either a primary or a secondary form
    - *Primary amenorrhea is defined as the persistent absence of menses by age 16 years*
    - *Secondary amenorrhea is the absence of menses for more than 6 months in a patient with a prior history of menses*

PRIMARY AMENORRHEA

Basic Information and Clinical Presentation

- Patients with primary amenorrhea may be grouped into those with and those without secondary sexual characteristics
- Primary amenorrhea with secondary sexual characteristics and normal sexual development
  - Usually indicates presence of ovaries
  - Etiologies include testicular feminization and müllerian defects
  - **Testicular feminization**
    - **Caused by androgen insensitivity**
    - **XY karyotype**
    - Normal male testosterone levels
    - Physical features: Breasts and feminine appearance, absence of axillary or pubic hair, and blind-ending vagina
  - Müllerian defects
    - Usually congenital
    - Physical features: Imperforate hymen, abnormal cervix, absence of vagina
- Primary amenorrhea without secondary sexual characteristics or other signs of puberty
  - Etiologies: see Table 40-1

Diagnosis and Evaluation

- Primary amenorrhea with signs of puberty
  - Many causes can be identified on physical examination and subsequent karyotype if needed
  - If physical examination findings are inconsistent with either testicular feminization or müllerian defects, then perform withdrawal bleed as described in the section on secondary amenorrhea
- Primary amenorrhea without signs of puberty
  - Check gonadotropin (FSH, LH) levels
    - If elevated, check karyotype to rule out Turner syndrome (Fig. 40-2)
    - If low, perform GnRH stimulation testing to assess pituitary function and help differentiate delayed puberty from hypothalamic-pituitary disorder

Treatment

- Primary amenorrhea with signs of puberty
  - For patients with testicular feminization, inguinal testes must be removed at puberty because of risk of malignancy

- For patients with müllerian defects, surgical repair is usually necessary
- Primary amenorrhea without signs of puberty
  - **Treat underlying disorder, if possible (see Table 40-1)**

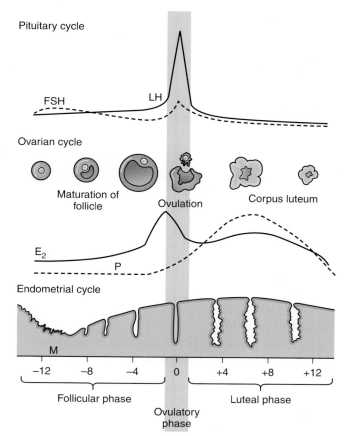

Pituitary cycle

FSH   LH

Ovarian cycle

Maturation of follicle

Ovulation

Corpus luteum

E_2

P

Endometrial cycle

M

−12 −8 −4 0 +4 +8 +12

Follicular phase   Luteal phase

Ovulatory phase

FIGURE 40-1 Hormone levels during the female menstrual cycle. The idealized cyclic changes observed in gonadotropins, estradiol (E_2), progesterone (P), and uterine endometrium during the normal menstrual cycle. The data are centered on the day of the luteinizing hormone (LH) surge (day 0). Days of menstrual bleeding are indicated by M. (FSH, follicle-stimulating hormone.) *(From Goldman L, Bennett JC, Ausiello D: Cecil textbook of medicine, ed 22, Philadelphia, WB Saunders, 2004, Fig. 250-1.)*

- Hormone replacement therapy
  - Start estrogen and progesterone in young patients to preserve bone density, improve well-being, prevent genitourinary atrophy, and promote breast development; long-term safety of hormone replacement in this setting has not been evaluated
  - Oral contraceptives often used for hormone replacement in young patients
- Patients who desire children should be referred to a reproductive endocrinologist

SECONDARY AMENORRHEA

Basic Information

- Most common causes are physiologic (e.g., pregnancy and menopause)
- **Differential diagnosis of pathologic secondary amenorrhea consists of four main disease states:**
  - **Hyperprolactinemia (e.g., prolactinoma, drugs)**
  - **Anovulatory states (e.g., most commonly, polycystic ovary syndrome; Box 40-1)**
  - **Androgen excess (e.g., androgen-secreting tumors)**
  - **Hypothalamic amenorrhea (e.g., physical or emotional stress, anorexia, excessive exercise)**
- Rarely caused by disorders of the outflow tract, such as:
  - Endometrial atrophy from prolonged use of progestins
  - Adhesions and obliteration of the uterine cavity (Asherman syndrome)
  - Endometritis

Clinical Presentation

- **Symptoms and signs of hypoestrogenic state: Hot flashes, vaginal dryness, dyspareunia, osteopenia**
- Findings suggestive of underlying cause
  - Prolactin excess: Breast tenderness, galactorrhea
  - Androgen excess: Hirsutism, acne, increased muscle mass, clitoromegaly

Diagnosis and Evaluation

- **First step always: Rule out pregnancy**
- **Algorithm for evaluation: see Figure 40-3**

TABLE 40-1	*Causes of Primary Amenorrhea Without Secondary Sexual Characteristics*				
Disorder	**Features**	**Diagnosis**	**Fertility**	**Treatment**	
Constitutional delay of puberty	Family history of delayed puberty	Family history Difficult to distinguish from GnRH deficiency	Will be present at maturity	Observation and reassurance	
Pituitary and hypothalamic disorders	Hypogonadotropic hypogonadism Causes include destructive lesions (tumors) or isolated gonadotropin deficiency (Kallman syndrome)	↓ FSH and LH No change in FSH and LH in response to GnRH stimulation	Variable, depending on underlying disorder	If malignancy, consider surgery or radiation Consider hormone replacement	
Turner syndrome (see Fig. 40-2)	45,XO karyotype Physical features include lack of sexual maturation, short stature, webbed neck, shield chest, and valgus deformity of the elbow	↑ FSH and LH XO karyotype	Usually absent unless mosaic of XO and XX cells	Hormone replacement	
Gonadal dysgenesis	Absence of ovaries Congenital	↑ FSH and LH	Absent	Hormone replacement	

FSH, follicle-stimulating hormone; GnRH, gonadotropin-releasing hormone; LH, luteinizing hormone.

- **Mechanics of inducing a withdrawal bleed with progesterone (see Fig. 40-3)**
  - If the endometrium is estrogenized, it should respond to progesterone challenge
  - Give 10 mg medroxyprogesterone daily for 5 to 7 days
  - Withdrawal bleeding should occur within 1 week of completion of progesterone challenge

Treatment

- Treat the underlying disorder (e.g., dopamine agonist for prolactinoma)
- **In young women (younger than 50 years), oral contraceptives are often used (see treatment of primary amenorrhea)**
- In older women (older than 50 years), postmenopausal hormone combinations may be used, but benefits versus risks need to be carefully considered
- In women with normal menopause, postmenopausal hormone therapy (HT) to prevent chronic medical conditions (such as coronary heart disease) is no longer recommended
  - **Indications for HT: Debilitating vasomotor symptoms**

FIGURE 40-2 Girl with Turner syndrome. Note the shield chest, widely spaced nipples, and webbed neck. *(From Lowenstein EJ, Kim KH, Glick SA: Turner's syndrome in dermatology, J Am Acad Dermatol 50:767–776, 2004, Fig. 1.)*

- Other benefits: Preservation of bone mineral density and possible reduced risk of colorectal cancer (but other specific treatments, such as bisphosphonates for osteoporosis, are considered first-line treatments)
- Risks: Results from the Women's Health Initiative demonstrated that HT increases the risk of breast cancer, stroke, and venous thromboembolic disease and has no benefit in preventing heart disease
- **If HT started, lowest dose for shortest duration (preferably <5 years) is generally recommended; reassessment for continued need should be done at least yearly**
- Many forms available (oral, transdermal); none definitively shown to be superior
- If uterus is present, must administer progestin with estrogen to avoid increased risk of endometrial cancer
  - Cycled if patient desires monthly withdrawal bleeding
  - Continuous if withdrawal bleeding is undesirable (more commonly used in postmenopausal women)
- Vaginal spotting and bleeding may be a nuisance side effect
  - Usually resolves within 6 months
  - If heavy or first bleeding occurs 6 months after initiating therapy, endometrial biopsy should be performed to rule out hyperplasia or cancer

HIRSUTISM

Basic Information

- **Hirsutism is defined as the presence of terminal (coarse, pigmented) hairs on parts of a woman's body where terminal hairs are considered to be a male secondary sexual characteristic (e.g., face, chest, back, lower abdomen, inner thighs; Fig. 40-4)**
- **Virilization refers to signs of more severe androgen excess (e.g., deep voice, clitoromegaly, frontal balding, enhanced musculature, hirsutism)**

BOX 40-1   *Polycystic Ovary Syndrome*

Basic Information

Affects up to 10% of women

Thought to be caused by stimulatory effects of excess insulin on ovarian androgen production

Clinical Features

Amenorrhea, hirsutism, acne, obesity, and insulin resistance

Diagnosis

Is a clinical diagnosis; a diagnostic test with high sensitivity and specificity has not been identified

Ovarian ultrasound (for cysts) and LH:FSH ratio (often increased); do not always distinguish these patients from normal

Treatment

Weight loss

Oral contraceptives if fertility is not desired

Metformin or thiazolidinediones (insulin sensitizers) may restore ovulation and fertility, thus confirming the role of insulin resistance, but oral contraceptives considered first line

Antiandrogens for hirsutism (spironolactone)

FSH, follicle-stimulating hormone; LH, luteinzing hormone.

- Hirsutism may occur with or without virilization
- Androgens
  - Testosterone: Derived from the ovaries (25%), adrenals (25%), and peripheral conversion from androstenedione (50%)
    - Most potent androgen
    - Circulates as free (1%) and bound (99%)
  - Dihydroepiandrosterone sulfate (DHEA-S) is predominantly derived from the adrenal cortex (95%)
- Causes of hirsutism include ovarian or adrenal causes, drugs, and physiologic (most common; Box 40-2)

- **Idiopathic familial form (physiologic) is most common cause overall**
- **Most common ovarian cause: Polycystic ovary syndrome (PCOS; see Box 40-1)**
- **Most common adrenal cause: Congenital adrenal hyperplasia (Box 40-3)**

Clinical Presentation

- History
  - Assess onset, duration, and progression of hair growth
  - Look for symptoms of PCOS: weight gain, acne, diabetes, menstrual irregularities

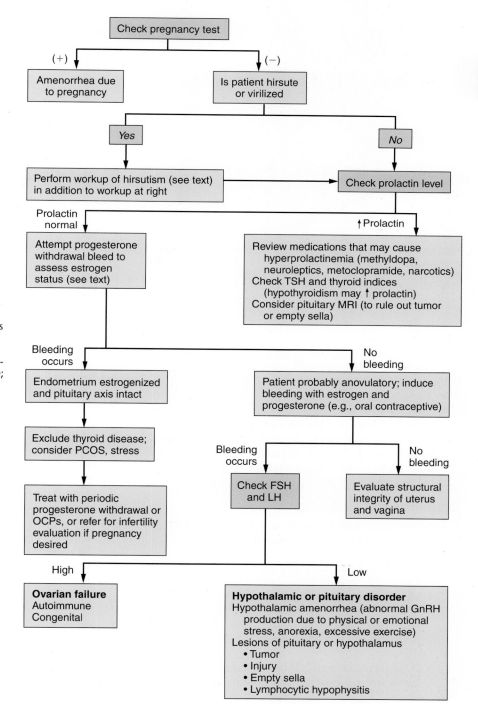

FIGURE 40-3 Algorithm for the diagnosis of secondary amenorrhea. (GnRH, gonadotropin-releasing hormone; LH, luteinizing hormone; OCPs, oral contraceptive pills; PCOS, polycystic ovary syndrome; TSH, thyroid-stimulating hormone.)

FIGURE 40-4 Examples of hirsutism. Male-pattern hair growth on the face (**A**), and on the chest (**B**). *(From Larsen PR, Kronenberg HM, Melmed S, Polonsky, KS: Williams textbook of endocrinology, ed 10, Philadelphia, WB Saunders, 2003, Fig. 16-30.)*

- Inquire about family history of hirsutism (suggesting familial form)
- Inquire about medications that might cause hirsutism (see Table 40-1)
- Physical examination
  - Assess extent of hirsutism
  - Look for signs of virilization (e.g., acne, clitoromegaly, deepened voice, muscle hypertrophy)
  - Look for signs of insulin resistance, including acanthosis nigricans (to suggest PCOS)
  - Look for signs of Cushing syndrome (e.g., dorsocervical fat pad, striae, proximal muscle weakness)

Diagnosis and Evaluation

- **Sudden onset, rapid course, and/or presence of virilization suggestive of a malignancy**
- Laboratory tests
  - Free and total testosterone
    - Often only free (not total) testosterone is elevated
    - Usually only mildly elevated with PCOS
    - Total testosterone greater than 200 ng/dL raises concern for adrenal or ovarian tumor (DHEA-S helpful to distinguish source)
  - DHEA-S
    - If level greater than 500 mg/dL, consider adrenal tumor or late-onset congenital adrenal hyperplasia
  - Prolactin (hyperprolactinemia may cause hirsutism)

| BOX 40-2 | *Causes of Hirsutism* |

Ovarian Causes
Polycystic ovary syndrome
Hyperthecosis (rests of ovarian stromal cells that produce testosterone)
Androgen-producing ovarian tumors

Adrenal Causes
Congenital adrenal hyperplasia
Androgen-producing adrenal tumors
Cushing syndrome

Elevated Prolactin
Unclear mechanism

Medications
Androgens (e.g., danazol)
Cyclosporine
Phenytoin

Physiologic Causes
Idiopathic familial
Postmenopausal

| BOX 40-3 | *Congenital Adrenal Hyperplasia* |

Basic Information
Inherited defects in adrenal cortisol synthesis result in overproduction of other adrenal hormones, including androgens
Late-onset or nonclassic 21-hydroxylase deficiency is the most common form, occurring in 0.1–1% of women

Clinical Presentation
Hirsutism begins at menarche
Menstrual irregularities begin in adulthood

Diagnosis
17-Hydroxyprogesterone will be elevated (stimulation with synthetic ACTH may be necessary to elicit the abnormality)

Treatment
Hydrocortisone will decrease the excess androgen production

ACTH, adrenocorticotropic hormone.

- 17-Hydroxyprogesterone
  - May be elevated in congenital adrenal hyperplasia
  - Adrenocorticotropic hormone stimulation test may be necessary to elicit elevation
- Imaging
  - Abdominal computed tomography or sonogram if adrenal or ovarian tumors are suspected
  - Magnetic resonance imaging (MRI) of the pituitary if prolactin is elevated and no medication is identified as the culprit

Treatment

- Treatment is directed toward correction of the underlying problem (if possible)
- Once a terminal hair has developed, it may not disappear, even if abnormal hormone levels resolve
- Oral contraceptives are generally considered the treatment of choice for hirsutism and androgenic symptoms

BOX 40-4	*Causes of Gynecomastia*

Medications
    ACE inhibitors
    Amiodarone
    Antipsychotics
    Calcium channel blockers
    Diazepam
    Digoxin
    Efavirenz
    HIV nucleoside reverse transcriptase inhibitors
    Ketoconazole
    Omeprazole
    Opiates
    Phenytoin
    Ranitidine
    Spironolactone
    Tricyclic antidepressants
Endocrine disorders
    Hyperthyroidism
    Hypogonadism
    Hormone-secreting tumors
Chronic systemic illness
    Renal disease
    Hepatic disease
Marijuana
Idiopathic

ACE, angiotensin-converting enzyme; HIV, human immunodeficiency virus.

- Spironolactone is useful for inhibiting effects of androgens on hair follicles but primarily prevents worsening of hirsutism
- **Insulin sensitizers, such as metformin or pioglitazone, can induce ovulation, decrease hirsutism, and reduce insulin resistance in women with PCOS, but oral contraceptives are generally the preferred agents**
- Eflornithine cream may inhibit an enzyme needed for hair growth; often used for facial hair

Male Reproductive and Hormonal Disorders

GYNECOMASTIA

Basic Information

- *Gynecomastia* **refers to benign growth of glandular tissue of the male breast**
- **Considered normal in males at three life stages**
  - **Newborn (first 2–3 weeks of life)**
  - **Pubertal**
  - **Elderly**
- Causes of gynecomastia (Box 40-4)
  - Most causes induce gynecomastia by causing a change in the relative amounts of estrogens and androgens (e.g., the ratio favors estrogen excess)
  - Mechanisms include decrease in androgen or androgen effect or increase in estrogen (exogenous or endogenous)
  - Most common causes in adults are medications and alcoholic liver disease

Clinical Presentation

- Confirm gynecomastia: Concentric enlargement of the tissue deep to the nipple
  - May be unilateral or bilateral
  - May be asymmetrical
  - May be associated with pain and tenderness
  - Nipple discharge is rare; if present, consider malignancy
  - Distinguish from obesity by palpating for a ridge of tissue concentric with the nipple
- Assess for sexual dysfunction
- Perform a testicular examination to detect any masses

Diagnosis and Evaluation

- Cause is often clear from history and physical examination
- **Highly consider malignancy if gynecomastia is unilateral, ulcerative, associated with bloody discharge or with axillary adenopathy; in this case, proceed directly to mammography and biopsy**
- Laboratory evaluation (if cause is not clear from the history and physical)
  - Check renal and hepatic function
  - Testosterone level (low level suggests hypogonadal cause)
  - FSH, LH
    - High levels associated with primary testicular failure
    - Low levels associated with exogenous steroids or hypogonadotropic hypogonadism
  - Prolactin (prolactinoma), thyroid-stimulating hormone (TSH; hyperthyroidism), human chorionic gonadotropin (hCG; hCG-producing testicular tumor), estradiol (estrogen-producing testicular tumor)
- Mammogram: Perform if gynecomastia is unilateral or if the mass is not concentric with the nipple

Treatment

- Gynecomastia is primarily a cosmetic problem, although it can be a clue to underlying disease
- Men with gynecomastia may have a slight increase in risk of breast cancer
- **Treatment is aimed at eliminating the underlying disease**
  - If treatment begins in the first few months after symptoms of gynecomastia appear, chance of regression of the gynecomastia is good
  - **Over time, the enlarged breast tissue becomes fibrotic and is not likely to shrink even if hormones return to normal**
- Options
  - Antiestrogens (e.g., tamoxifen) may be useful
  - Surgery may be performed if gynecomastia does not resolve and is bothersome to the patient

MALE HYPOGONADISM

Basic Information

- **Hypogonadism in men is defined as an inappropriately low testosterone level for age**
  - Normal range for men ages 18 to 29 years is approximately 700 to 1300 ng/dL
  - Declines to approximately 150 to 500 ng/dL for men ages 70 to 79 years

40

- **Classification of male hypogonadism**
  - **Primary: Caused by dysfunction of the testes (hypergonadotropic hypogonadism)**
  - **Secondary: Caused by a disorder of the pituitary or hypothalamus that impairs the ability of the pituitary to stimulate testosterone production (hypogonadotropic hypogonadism)**
  - **Testosterone resistance: Inability of the target tissues to respond to testosterone**
- Causes of primary and secondary hypogonadism: see Box 40-5
- Most common cause of primary hypogonadism in men is Klinefelter syndrome (Box 40-6; Fig. 40-5)

Clinical Presentation

- Symptoms
  - Decreased libido
  - Hot flashes if testosterone loss is sudden
- Signs
  - Sparse facial and body hair
  - Gynecomastia
  - Small penis, prostate, and testes
- Related conditions
  - Infertility
  - Osteoporosis
- **If hypogonadal during adolescence, may have complete failure of sexual maturation**
  - **Absence of growth spurt, high-pitched voice, and upper-to-lower body ratio of less than 1**
  - Consider possibility of

FIGURE 40-5 Klinefelter syndrome. Note the narrow shoulders, long upper body segment, and gynecomastia. *(From Ferri FF: Ferri's clinical advisor: instant diagnosis and treatment, ed 8, Philadelphia, Elsevier Mosby, 2006, Fig. 1-133.)*

- Klinefelter syndrome (see Box 40-5 and Fig. 40-5)
- Kallman syndrome (congenital lack of development of the olfactory lobes and GnRH-producing cells leading to anosmia; hypogonadotropic hypogonadism; and, occasionally, cleft palate or color blindness)

Diagnosis and Evaluation

- **Low testosterone is diagnostic**
  - **Total testosterone less than 300 ng/dL is generally considered abnormal at any age when accompanied by clinical symptoms**
  - Check a free testosterone level to rule out an abnormality with sex hormone–binding globulin
- Semen analysis helpful (even if fertility not an issue): If normal, hypogonadism essentially ruled out
- FSH and LH: High in primary hypogonadism, low in secondary hypogonadism
- Other tests should be based on the clinical picture
  - Comprehensive metabolic panel and complete blood counts (to look for undiagnosed chronic disease, such as hepatic or renal failure)
  - Prolactin and brain MRI if pituitary tumor suspected
  - Estradiol, hCG, and testicular ultrasound if testicular tumor suspected
  - Iron studies if hemochromatosis suspected

Treatment

- Treatment of underlying problem if possible
- Androgen replacement with testosterone injection, patch, or gel
  - Contraindication to replacement: History of androgen-dependent tumor (e.g., prostate cancer)
  - **Hematocrit should be monitored regularly given the increased risk of erythrocytosis with testosterone replacement**
  - **Prostate examination and prostate-specific antigen (PSA) testing should be done in men older than 40 years receiving androgen replacement**
- Therapy with FSH and hCG (by injection) may be used in those with hypogonadotropic hypogonadism who desire fertility

ERECTILE DYSFUNCTION

Basic Information

- **Definition: Inability to attain or maintain an erection to achieve penetration**
- Causes
  - Penile disorders
    - Peyronie disease (penile induration): Stems from fibrotic plaques of unclear etiology that can result in penile curvature, painful erections, and impotence; treatment is surgical
    - Trauma
  - Nervous system disorders: Stroke, spinal cord injury, prostatectomy complicated by nerve injury
  - Vascular disorders
    - Atherosclerotic vascular disease
    - **Leriche syndrome (impotence associated with distal aortic atherosclerosis resulting in claudication of the lower back, buttocks, and thighs)**

- Endocrine disorders: Diabetes, hypogonadism
- Psychogenic disorders (common in young men)
- Medications (see Box 40-4 for male hypogonadism), as well as β-blockers, antidepressants, and antipsychotics
- Substance abuse

Clinical Presentation

- Difficulty with obtaining or maintaining an erection
- May or may not have features of hypogonadism (see previous section)

Diagnosis and Evaluation

- History and physical examination
  - Look for clues to an underlying diagnosis (e.g., presence of peripheral vascular disease, complications of diabetes)
  - **Sudden onset of impotence favors psychogenic cause**
- Check testosterone levels, FSH, LH, estradiol
- Psychiatric evaluation if psychogenic cause suspected

Treatment

- Directed at underlying cause
- **Sildenafil, vardenafil, and tadalafil are phosphodiesterase-5 (PDE-5) inhibitors that prolong vasodilation by nitric oxide and are considered first-line drugs after underlying causes have been investigated**
  - Sildenafil and vardenafil should be taken 1 hour before intercourse; duration of effect is approximately 4 hours
  - Tadalafil has a faster onset of action and longer duration (36 hours)
  - **Warn patients about potential side effects**
    - Color vision changes
    - Headaches
    - Sudden blindness from nonischemic anterior optic neuropathy (case reports)
  - **Avoid in patients on nitrates (may induce hypotension) and those with recent or unstable coronary artery disease**
  - All PDE-5 inhibitors are metabolized by cytochrome P450 isozyme 3A4 (CYP3A4); doses should be reduced when combined with inhibitors of CYP3A4 (erythromycin, ketoconazole, protease inhibitors, and grapefruit juice)
- Other treatment options
  - Vasodilators such as prostaglandin E, papaverine, intraurethral alprostadil
  - Vacuum devices (avoid in patients at risk for bleeding)
  - Penile prostheses (associated with risk of infection)

REVIEW QUESTIONS

For review questions, please go to www.expertconsult.com.

SUGGESTED READINGS

Fraser IS, Kovacs G: Current recommendations for the diagnostic evaluation and follow-up of patients presenting with symptomatic polycystic ovary syndrome, *Best Pract Res Clin Obstet Gynaecol* 5:813–823, 2004.

Rosenfield RL: Clinical practice: hirsutism, *N Engl J Med* 353:2578–2588, 2005.

Warren MP, Hagey AR: The genetics, diagnosis and treatment of amenorrhea, *Minerva Ginecol* 56:437–455, 2004.

Neuroendocrine and Adrenal Disease

ROBERTO SALVATORI, MD

Protein hormones, most of which are produced or stored in the pituitary gland, and steroid hormones, many of which are produced in the adrenal glands, have profound impact on growth, development, and metabolism. Overproduction or underproduction of a single or multiple hormones may result in signs or symptoms that range from minimal to life threatening.

Neuroendocrine Disorders

Overview of the Pituitary Gland and Pituitary Masses

- The pituitary gland includes anterior and posterior parts (Fig. 41-1)
  - **Anterior pituitary produces prolactin (PRL), thyroid-stimulating hormone (TSH, also known as thyrotropin), adrenocorticotropic hormone (ACTH), luteinizing hormone (LH), follicle-stimulating hormone (FSH), and growth hormone (GH)**
    - ACTH is synthesized as part of a larger protein, pro-opiomelanocortin. Any stimulation of ACTH production will result in increased production of pro-opiomelanocortin.
  - **The posterior pituitary stores antidiuretic hormone (ADH) and oxytocin, which are produced in the hypothalamus**
- **Pituitary/sellar masses: Neuroendocrine disorders commonly present in the setting of a sellar mass**
  - **Approximately 45% of sellar masses are hormone-secreting pituitary tumors**
  - **Approximately 45% of sellar masses are non–hormone-secreting pituitary tumors**
  - The remainder of sellar masses include craniopharyngiomas, Rathke cleft cysts, meningiomas, metastatic tumors, lymphoma, granulomatous diseases, or the increasingly recognized autoimmune lymphocytic hypophysitis
- **Pituitary tumors smaller than 10 mm are referred to as *microadenomas* (Fig. 41-2). If the adenoma is equal to or larger than 10 mm, it is referred to as a *macroadenoma.***
- Pituitary incidentaloma: A pituitary mass discovered in a patient without endocrine symptoms; prevalence of incidentalomas has increased because of increased use of brain imaging. Often of no clinical consequence.

- **All patients with a pituitary adenoma should be evaluated for hormone hypersecretion syndromes that cannot be excluded by history or physical examination (see following discussion)**
- Incidentally discovered microadenomas grow in less than 10% of cases
  - If nonsecreting, conservative management with periodic magnetic resonance imaging (MRI) studies at progressively increasing intervals is performed
- **Incidental macroadenomas should also be evaluated for hypopituitarism. Visual field testing should be performed as well if the adenoma is close to the optic chiasm.**
  - Further growth occurs in about 50% of macroadenomas
  - Surgery is indicated if optic chiasm is compressed, if the patient is symptomatic (e.g., otherwise not explainable headaches), or if the tumor is growing

Symptoms due to Sellar and Parasellar Masses

- General principles
  - Disorders of the sellar area may present with three classes of signs and symptoms
    - Syndromes of hormone excess (e.g., acromegaly, Cushing disease, hyperprolactinemia)
    - Symptoms of hormone deficit (partial or complete hypopituitarism, discussed in the next section)
    - Compressive symptoms
      - Frontal headaches
      - Visual changes (typically bitemporal hemianopsia)
      - If cavernous sinus invaded by expanding tumor, cranial nerve palsies develop (cranial nerves III, IV, VI)
- The clinical presentation will also vary based on the actions of the hormone that is either undersecreted or oversecreted (Table 41-1; see following discussion)
- Pituitary tumors may exist as part of genetic syndromes
  - In conjunction with other endocrine tumors; this is known as the multiple endocrine neoplasia (MEN)-I syndrome (Box 41-1)
  - As part of the "Carney complex" (autosomal dominant complex of cardiac myxomas, spotty pigmentation of the skin, and various hyperendocrine states, often including growth hormone hypersecretion)

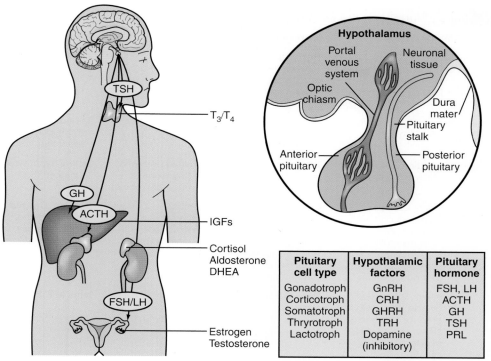

FIGURE 41-1 The hypothalamic-pituitary axis. (ACTH, adrenocorticotropin hormone; CRH, corticotropin-releasing hormone; DHEA, dehydroepiandrosterone; FSH, follicle-stimulating hormone; GH, growth hormone; GHRH, growth hormone–releasing hormone; GnRH, gonadotropin-releasing hormone; IGF, insulin-like growth factor; LH, luteinizing hormone; PRL, prolactin; T_3, triiodothyronine; T_4, thyroxine; TRH, thyroid-releasing hormone. TSH, thyroid-stimulating hormone.) *(From Page C: Integrated pharmacology, ed 3, Philadelphia, Elsevier Mosby, 2006, Fig. 15.2.)*

Pituitary cell type	Hypothalamic factors	Pituitary hormone
Gonadotroph	GnRH	FSH, LH
Corticotroph	CRH	ACTH
Somatotroph	GHRH	GH
Thryrotroph	TRH	TSH
Lactotroph	Dopamine (inhibitory)	PRL

FIGURE 41-2 A magnetic resonance image of pituitary demonstrating the typical appearance of a pituitary microademona. A hypodense lesion is seen in the right side of the gland with deviation of the pituitary stalk away from the lesion (*arrow*). After a biochemical diagnosis of Cushing disease, this patient was cured following transsphenoidal hypophysectomy. *(From Larsen PR, Kronenberg HM, Melmed S, Polonsky, KS: Williams textbook of endocrinology, ed 10, Philadelphia, WB Saunders, 2003, Fig. 14-23.)*

- As the syndrome of familial isolated pituitary adenomas (FIPA) (sometimes isolated familial acromegaly syndrome)
- A thorough family history is indicated for all patients diagnosed with a pituitary adenoma
  - **All patients should be asked about personal or family history of hypercalcemia or kidney stones because hyperparathyroidism is the most common feature of MEN-I, with penetrance close to 100% by age 50**
  - All patients should be examined for perioral hyperpigmentation, tumors of the heart, and hyperendocrine states, which may suggest Carney complex

Pituitary Hormone Excess States

PROLACTINOMA

Basic Information

- PRL is produced by lactotroph cells in the anterior pituitary
- Dopaminergic pathways inhibit PRL production
- Elevations in serum PRL levels may be physiologic (e.g., pregnancy) or pathologic (Box 41-2)
- **Prolactinomas are the most common hormone-secreting pituitary adenomas (see Box 41-2)**

Clinical Presentation

- Elevated PRL levels inhibit gonadotropin secretion (by inhibiting release of luteinizing hormone–releasing hormone) and decrease gonadal responsiveness to gonadotropins (Fig. 41-3)

41

TABLE 41-1	Pituitary Hormones: Key Details			
Hormone	**Major Actions**	**Secretagogue**	**Inhibitor**	**Deficiency Syndrome**
Prolactin (PRL) Growth hormone (GH)	Lactation Linear growth (via insulin-like growth factors)	Thyrotropin-releasing hormone (TRH) Growth hormone–releasing hormone	Dopamine Somatostatin	Inability to lactate Children: Dwarfism Adults: Loss of bone mass, body composition changes, hypercholesterolemia
Adrenocorticotropic hormone (ACTH)	Release of cortisol from adrenal gland	Corticotropin-releasing hormone (CRH)	Glucocorticoids	Secondary adrenal insufficiency (no hyperpigmentation or electrolyte disturbances seen)
Thyroid-stimulating hormone (TSH)	Production and release of thyroid hormones	TRH	Thyroid hormones (thyroxine or triiodothyronine)	Central hypothyroidism (see Chapter 38)
Follicle-stimulating hormone (FSH)	Women: Growth of granulosa cells and estradiol production in ovarian follicle Men: Stimulates seminiferous tubules to produce sperm	Gonadotropin-releasing hormone (GnRH) GnRH is also known as luteinizing hormone– releasing hormone (LHRH)	Inhibin Estradiol Testosterone (PRL inhibits GnRH release)	Children: Delayed puberty Women: Amenorrhea Men: Impotence, testicular atrophy Kallmann syndrome: Gonadotropin deficiency caused by congenital GnRH deficiency
Luteinizing hormone (LH)	Women: Stimulates ovarian theca cells to produce androgens; LH surge stimulates ovulation Men: Stimulates testosterone production in Leydig cells	Same as FSH	Estradiol Testosterone (PRL inhibits GnRH release)	Same as FSH
Antidiuretic hormone (ADH) (arginine vasopressin [AVP])	Makes collecting ducts in renal tubules permeable to water Stimulates thirst	Increases in osmolality Decreases in volume	Decreases in osmolality	Diabetes insipidus
Oxytocin	Contraction of uterine and breast muscles	Estrogen Suckling	None	None

- **Galactorrhea can be seen in premenopausal women and in postmenopausal women if they are taking hormone replacement, but it is rarely seen in men**
- Menstrual irregularities are common and result in women being diagnosed earlier than men. Women most commonly present with microadenomas.
- Men present with decreased libido and impotence or visual loss, and are more likely to present with macroadenomas, sometimes very large (giant prolactinomas)

Diagnosis

- Exclude other causes of elevated PRL levels, particularly antipsychotic medications (see Box 41-2)
  - If PRL level is greater than 200 ng/mL, prolactinoma is very likely
- Obtain MRI of sella
  - High serum PRL level and pituitary mass by MRI typically used to diagnose prolactinoma
    - **However, a sellar mass in the presence of elevated serum PRL levels is not definitive proof of prolactinoma. A large, nonsecreting adenoma may cause elevated PRL levels by compressing the pituitary stalk and inhibiting hypothalamic dopaminergic regulation of PRL.**

- **Suspect this if macroadenoma seen with only moderate elevation of PRL level (i.e., <100 ng/mL)**
- If PRL is elevated but the patient has no clinical symptoms, the presence of "macroprolactinemia" must be suspected. In this condition, PRL molecules bind to circulating immunoglobulins, causing marked increase in serum half-life, but PRL is not biologically active.
- Macroprolactinemia can be identified by repeating serum PRL measurement after precipitating immunoglubulins with polyethylene glycol
- Requires no treatment

Treatment

- Normalization of PRL is usually required to normalize menses and to restore eugonadism
- **First-line treatment is with dopaminergic agonists**
  - **Bromocriptine (Parlodel) and cabergoline are agents most commonly used**
- If medical therapy fails, surgery is performed via transsphenoidal approach
- Radiation used if tumor recurs after surgery (rare)

<table>
<tr><td>

BOX 41-1   *Multiple Endocrine Neoplasia Syndromes*

MEN-I (Autosomal Dominant)

Parathyroid hyperplasia/adenoma (high penetrance)

Pancreatic islet cell hyperplasia/adenoma/carcinoma (usually Zollinger-Ellison syndrome*; insulinoma; or, rarely, glucagonoma)

Pituitary adenomas

MEN-IIA (Autosomal Dominant)

Medullary thyroid carcinoma

Pheochromocytoma

Parathyroid hyperplasia or adenoma

MEN-IIB (Autosomal Dominant)

Medullary thyroid carcinoma

Pheochromocytoma

Mucosal/gastrointestinal neuromas

Marfanoid body habitus

Carney Complex (Autosomal Dominant)

Pituitary tumors (mostly GH secreting)

Cushing syndrome due to bilateral micronodular pigmented adrenal hyperplasia

Thyroid tumors

Atrial myxomas

Perioral hyperpigmentation

</td></tr>
</table>

GH, growth hormone; MEN, multiple endocrine neoplasia.
*Overproduction of gastrin, resulting in recurrent multiple peptic ulcers.

GROWTH HORMONE–SECRETING TUMORS

Basic Information

- **Excess growth hormone (GH) results in gigantism in children, whose epiphyseal bone plates have not closed (Fig. 41-4), or acromegaly in adults (Fig. 41-5)**
- GH acts on tissues both directly and indirectly by stimulating the production of other hormones that stimulate growth (mostly insulin-like growth factor-I [IGF-I])
- Onset of acromegaly is insidious and often missed

Clinical Presentation

- **Most common features are acral growth, excessive sweating, and weakness/fatigue**
  - **Also seen are sleep apnea, arthralgias, hypertension, glucose intolerance or diabetes, teeth malocclusion, and carpal tunnel syndrome**
  - Incidence of colonic polyps two to three times higher than age-matched controls and may correlate with presence of skin tags
- **Characteristic physical appearance includes coarse facial features with frontal bossing; prognathism; and deep, sonorous voice**
  - **Hand, foot, and hat sizes are increased**

Diagnosis

- Because GH levels fluctuate according to a diurnal pattern (and significant overlap exists between normal and abnormal individuals), GH levels alone are not useful to diagnose acromegaly

<table>
<tr><td>

BOX 41-2   *Causes of Elevated Serum Prolactin Level*

Endocrine

Pituitary adenoma

Hypothalamic disease
    Sarcoidosis
    Craniopharyngioma
    Empty sella syndrome

Primary hypothyroidism

Pregnancy

Drugs

CNS active
    Risperidone (associated with very high prolactin levels)
    Phenothiazines
    Haloperidol

Metoclopramide

Antihypertensives
    Methyldopa
    Reserpine
    Verapamil

Estrogens

Opiates

Other

Stress

Nipple stimulation

Chest wall trauma

Renal failure

</td></tr>
</table>

Macroprolactinemia: Artifactual elevation of measured serum prolactin while actual level is normal.
CNS, central nervous system.

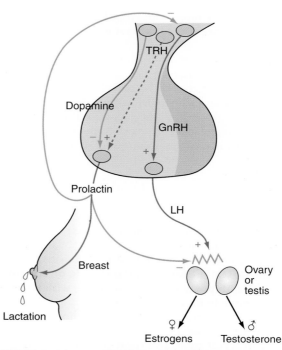

FIGURE 41-3 The control and physiologic effects of prolactin secretion, demonstrating inhibition of luteinizing hormone (LH) secretion and action. (GnRH, gonadotropin-releasing hormone; TRH, thyroid-releasing hormone.) *(From Kumar P, Clark M: Clinical medicine, ed 5, Philadelphia, Elsevier Saunders, 2005, Fig. 18-11.)*

FIGURE 41-4 A 16-year-old patient suffering from gigantism. Growth hormone is raised and bone age is not advanced, indicating that the boy's eventual stature will be abnormally tall. *(From Besser GM, Thorner M: Comprehensive clinical endocrinology, ed 3, St. Louis, Mosby, 2002, Fig. 24B.31.)*

- **IGF-I levels are more consistently elevated in acromegaly and are the initial test of choice in screening for acromegaly**
- To confirm the diagnosis in dubious cases, a glucose suppression test is performed
  - In normal subjects, a 75-g oral glucose load suppresses GH levels to less than 0.4 ng/mL
  - In acromegaly, a 75-g oral glucose load does not suppress GH levels and may paradoxically increase GH levels
- Brain imaging is typically done after serologic evaluation

Treatment

- Goal of treatment is normalization of IGF-I and reduction of GH levels to less than 2.0 ng/mL, because non-cured acromegalic patients have a reduced life expectancy
- **Surgery is initial management in most cases (transsphenoidal approach)**
  - Curative in 50%; cure less likely with macroadenoma
  - **Somatostatin analogues (lanreotide or octreotide) used with postsurgical recurrence, with hormonal response in 60% of patients**
  - Some (20%) may respond to cabergoline (particularly if they co-secrete PRL)
  - GH receptor antagonist (pegvisomant) normalizes IGF-I in 70% to 90% of patients
  - Radiation also used with postsurgical recurrence or surgical failure; it requires several years to be effective

FIGURE 41-5 Acromegaly of the jaw and hand. *(From Regezi JA, Sciubba JJ, Jordan RCK: Oral pathology: clinical pathological correlations, ed 4, Philadelphia, WB Saunders, 2003, Fig. 15-8.)*

HYPERCORTISOLISM

Basic Information

- **Cushing disease: Hypercortisolism as a result of ACTH-producing pituitary adenoma**
- **Cushing syndrome: Hypercortisolism caused by any cause, including pituitary adenoma, adrenal adenoma or carcinoma, ectopic ACTH production, or administration of exogenous glucocorticoids**

Clinical Presentation

- See Figure 41-6 for an example of Cushing syndrome
- Patients present with hypertension, central obesity, moon facies, dorsal fat pad, purple striae on skin, and muscle weakness
- Psychiatric symptoms also common
- Secondary amenorrhea may develop in women, along with hirsutism or other evidence of masculinization
- Osteoporosis also develops in women and men
- Common laboratory abnormalities may include glucose intolerance (or diabetes) and metabolic alkalosis with hypokalemia (in more severe cases)

Diagnosis

- **Diagnosis of hypercortisolism (Fig. 41-7): Begin by measuring 24-hour urine free cortisol or 11 pm salivary cortisol or performing a 1-mg overnight dexamethasone suppression test**
- Plasma ACTH levels differentiate between ACTH-dependent (high or normal plasma ACTH) and ACTH-independent (ACTH levels <10 pg/mL) Cushing
- If ACTH independent, adrenal imaging is necessary
- Localization of source of ACTH in ACTH-dependent conditions (i.e., pituitary versus ectopic ACTH)

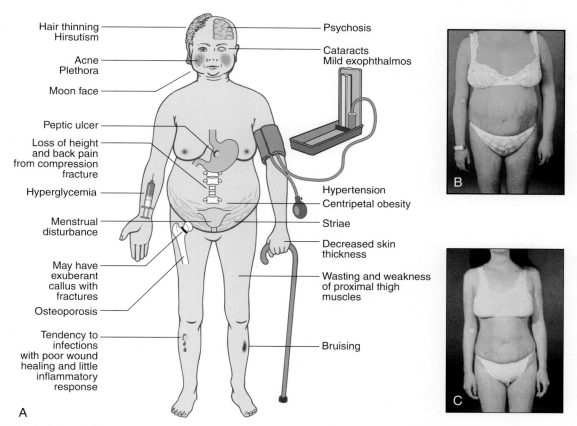

Hair thinning
Hirsutism

Acne
Plethora

Moon face

Peptic ulcer

Loss of height
and back pain
from compression
fracture

Hyperglycemia

Menstrual
disturbance

May have
exuberant
callus with
fractures

Osteoporosis

Tendency to
infections
with poor wound
healing and little
inflammatory
response

A

Psychosis

Cataracts
Mild exophthalmos

Hypertension
Centripetal obesity

Striae

Decreased skin
thickness

Wasting and weakness
of proximal thigh
muscles

Bruising

B

C

FIGURE 41-6 Cushing syndrome. **A,** Clinical features common to all causes. **B,** A patient with Cushing disease before treatment. **C,** The same patient 1 year after successful removal of an adrenocorticotropic hormone–secreting pituitary microadenoma by transsphenoidal surgery. *(From Haslett C, Chilvers ER, Boon NA, et al: Davidson's principles and practice of medicine, ed 19, New York, Churchill Livingstone, 2002, Fig. 16.17.)*

requires sequential testing based on the following principles:
- In normal host, glucocorticoids inhibit ACTH secretion (Fig. 41-8)
- ACTH-secreting pituitary adenomas are partially autonomous but can be inhibited with high dose of glucocorticoids (e.g., dexamethasone)
- In difficult cases of differentiation of pituitary versus ectopic ACTH, bilateral inferior petrosal sinus sampling is done after administration of corticotropin-releasing factor (CRF)

Treatment

- For pituitary source: transsphenoidal resection
- For adrenal source: adrenalectomy
- When surgical cure is not obtainable in Cushing disease, medical adrenalectomy can be transiently achieved with administration of medications that inhibit production of cortisol (e.g., ketoconazole, metyrapone, mitotane). Pituitary radiation and/or bilateral adrenalectomy is sometimes needed.

Syndrome of Inappropriate Antidiuresis

See Chapter 32.

Uncommon Disorders of the Anterior Pituitary

- Pituitary hyperthyroidism, caused by a TSH-producing adenoma, is rare
- Gonadotropin-secreting (i.e., LH, FSH) tumors typically present as macroadenomas and may be asymptomatic
  - Many "nonfunctioning" macroadenomas may actually produce non–biologically active gonadotropins (e.g., α subunits of gonadotropins)

Pituitary Hormone Insufficiency States

Basic Information

- **Hypopituitarism is most commonly caused by pituitary adenoma, with destruction or compression of normal pituitary cells**
  - **With pituitary tumors/mass effect, GH typically is affected first, followed by gonadotropins, then TSH; ACTH is affected last**
  - Order may change with other causes of hypopituitarism (e.g., radiation)

41

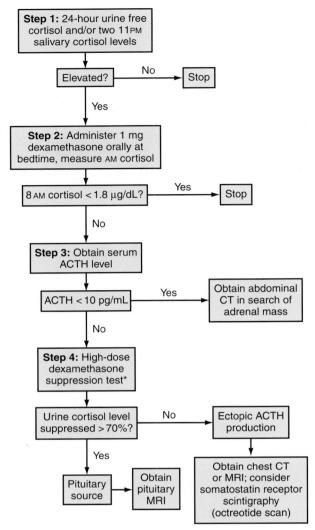

FIGURE 41-7 Evaluation of the patient with suspected hypercortisolism. *Dexamethasone 2 mg every 6 hours for 2 days; collect urine on day 0 and day 2. (ACTH, adrenocorticotropin hormone; CT, computed tomograph; MRI, magnetic resonance imaging.)

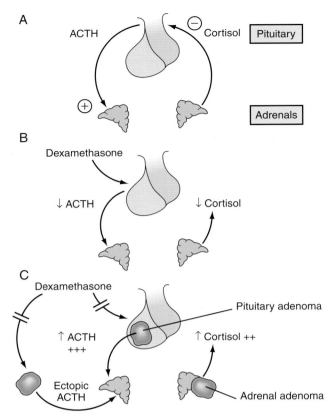

FIGURE 41-8 Dexamethasone suppression test. **A,** Normal feedback mechanism for cortisol production. **B,** Normally, dexamethasone suppresses adrenocorticotropin (ACTH) and hence cortisol production. **C,** In Cushing syndrome resulting from pituitary or ectopic ACTH excess, or adrenal adenoma, dexamethasone has no effect, and cortisol is not suppressed. *(From Souhami R: Textbook of medicine, New York, Churchill Livingstone, 2002, Fig. 17.30.)*

- Other causes of hypopituitarism include pituitary apoplexy (infarction); inflammation of the pituitary (lymphocytic hypophysitis, typically but not exclusively in postpartum women); central nervous system radiation; surgery; head trauma (single or multiple repeated traumas); or replacement of the pituitary or hypothalamus with infectious, granulomatous, or malignant disease (when pituitary metastases are present, often diabetes insipidus occurs)
- Clinical manifestations depend on which hormone or combination of hormones is affected (Fig. 41-9) and to what extent they are affected (see Table 41-1)
- **Pituitary apoplexy: The acute development of pituitary insufficiency, most commonly from sudden hemorrhage or infarction of the pituitary gland**
  - **Most commonly occurs in patients with previously undiagnosed pituitary tumor**

- **Symptoms include sudden headache, visual deficit, ophthalmoplegia** (cranial nerves III, IV, or VI may be affected), and altered mental status
- Most dangerous result is lack of ACTH and therefore acute secondary adrenal insufficiency (see following section on adrenal insufficiency)
- **Sheehan syndrome: Pituitary infarction caused by blood loss during childbirth; presents within first days or week following childbirth; classic presentation is a new mother who is unable to produce milk**

PROLACTIN DEFICIENCY

Basic Information
- **Usually occurs in the setting of other pituitary hormone deficiencies**

Clinical Presentation
- Asymptomatic in men
- Women will note lack of lactation (i.e., with pregnancy)

Diagnosis
- Low serum PRL level in the appropriate host

Treatment
- There is no treatment for PRL deficiency

FIGURE 41-9 A 20-year-old man with idiopathic hypopituitary dwarfism and deficiencies of gonadotropins, thyrotropin, corticotropin, and growth hormone, who had a history of arrested hydrocephalus. Note the extreme atrophy of the genitalia, the absence of body hair, and apparent gynecomastia associated with obesity. *(From Yen SCC, Jaffe RB: Reproductive endocrinology, ed 2, Philadelphia, WB Saunders, 1986, Fig. 24-52.)*

GROWTH HORMONE DEFICIENCY

Basic Information

- Patients with panhypopituitarism have a 99% likelihood of being GH deficient

Clinical Presentation

- Symptoms of GH deficiency depend on the age of onset
  - In children, stunted growth occurs
  - In adults, symptoms of GH deficiency are usually overshadowed by other manifestations of pituitary insufficiency but include a decreased sense of well-being, decreased muscle mass, increased fat mass, osteopenia, and an abnormal lipid profile (increased total and low-density lipoprotein [LDL] cholesterol)

Diagnosis

- To diagnose, a low serum IGF-I is typically seen, but this is not sensitive or specific
- Large overlap exists in serum IGF-I between GH-deficient and normal subjects, particularly in male patients older than 40 years
- If IGF-I is normal but suspicion is high, testing of GH reserve by insulin-induced hypoglycemia or glucagon is used

Treatment

- Although in the past GH deficiency in fully grown adults was not treated, adult patients with severe GH deficiency should be considered for GH replacement therapy to improve muscle mass, bone density, quality of life, and lipid profile

ACTH DEFICIENCY

ACTH deficiency is known as secondary adrenal insufficiency and is discussed in the section on adrenal insufficiency that follows.

Central Hypothyroidism

Basic Information

- A rare cause of hypothyroidism
- As with other disorders noted, most commonly occurs in association with other causes of pituitary insufficiency

Clinical Presentation

- Patient presents with the typical signs and symptoms of hypothyroidism, often milder than primary hypothyroidism (see Chapter 38)

Diagnosis

- **Diagnosed by low serum free thyroxine levels in the setting of low (or inappropriately normal, or even mildly elevated) TSH level**

Treatment

- **TSH cannot be followed for medication dosing in individuals with central hypothyroidism**
- **Treatment is repletion with thyroxine, adjusted to symptoms and serum free thyroxine (T_4) levels**
- **In patients with central hypothyroidism, never replace thyroid hormone before assessing adrenal function because pharmacologically induced euthyroidism may trigger adrenal crisis (thyroid hormones accelerate cortisol catabolism)**

Central Hypogonadism

Basic Information

- Central hypogonadism, or secondary hypogonadism, is caused by insufficient production of LH and/or FSH
- Secondary hypogonadism is less common than primary hypogonadism (primary hypogonadism is testicular or ovarian failure associated with elevated levels of LH and FSH)
- Occurs with other causes of hypopituitarism as well as in other clinical settings
  - **Kallmann syndrome (Fig. 41-10): Lack of GnRH secretion, resulting in central hypogonadism**
    - **Additional features may include neurosensory hearing loss, red-green color blindness, urogenital tract abnormalities, and lack of sense of smell**

Clinical Presentation

- **Determined in large part by the age of onset of secondary hypogonadism**
  - **Prepubertal boys and girls will fail to develop secondary sexual characteristics**
  - **In adults, infertility and decreased sexual drive are common (in both men and women), as well as amenorrhea (females)**

41

- Men whose hypogonadism started before puberty may have eunuchoid body habitus (arm span greater than height; lower body segment longer than upper body segment) and gynecomastia

Diagnosis

- Diagnosed by low sex hormone levels in setting of low (or inappropriately normal) LH and FSH levels

Treatment

- In men, treatment is with testosterone, titrated to normal serum levels
  - If fertility in men is desired, human chorionic gonadotropin (hCG; LH equivalent) and FSH can be administered as intramuscular injections
  - May take several months of therapy to reach normal sperm count
- In women, treatment is with estrogen and progesterone
  - If fertility is desired, hCG and FSH can be administered under the care of a reproductive endocrinologist

Diabetes Insipidus

Basic Information

- **Neurogenic diabetes insipidus (DI): Lack of production and release of ADH from posterior pituitary**
  - **Caused by either hypothalamic disease (e.g., sarcoidosis, tuberculosis, craniopharyngioma) or following neurosurgery;** pituitary adenomas usually do not cause DI unless there has been a surgical treatment
  - Rare forms include familial DI, traumatic DI, or idiopathic DI

- **Nephrogenic DI: Lack of renal response to ADH (no disorder of posterior pituitary implied)**
  - May be congenital or acquired
    - Acquired form may result from hypercalcemia, hypokalemia, or medications (e.g., lithium; nephrogenic DI may persist after discontinuation of lithium)

Clinical Presentation

- **Patients present with impaired renal conservation of water and production of dilute urine**
  - **Polyuria, polydipsia, and sometimes hypernatremia result**

Diagnosis

- Suspect if increased serum osmolarity present, or in an individual who produces high volume (up to 16 L) of inappropriately diluted urine
- Water deprivation test is test of choice in dubious situations (Fig. 41-11)

Treatment

- Treatment of neurogenic DI is deamino-D-arginine vasopressin (dDAVP; a synthetic vasopressin analogue, administered either intranasally or orally)
- Thiazide diuretics are used for treatment of nephrogenic DI to reduce intravascular volume and polyuria

Adrenal Disease

OVERVIEW OF THE ADRENAL GLAND

- The adrenal glands are the major site of synthesis and secretion of steroid hormones

FIGURE 41-10 Grossly eunuchoidal 31-year-old man with Kallmann syndrome. **A,** Before androgen replacement. **B,** After 2 years of androgen replacement. *(From Souhami R: Textbook of medicine, New York, Churchill Livingstone, 2002, Fig. 17.36.)*

- There are three categories of steroid hormones produced in the adrenal glands
  - **Glucocorticoids, such as cortisol (sometimes referred to as *hydrocortisone)***
  - **Mineralocorticoids, such as aldosterone**
  - **Adrenal androgens, such as dehydroepiandrosterone (DHEA)**

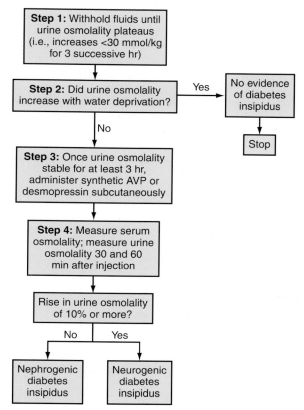

FIGURE 41-11 Water deprivation test. (AVP, arginine vasopressin.)

- Major actions of adrenal hormones are shown in Table 41-2
- Adrenal incidentalomas: Increases in imaging of abdomen result in incidental detection of adrenal mass in 4% to 7% of scans at age greater than 40
  - **Most adrenal incidentalomas (67–94%, depending on the case series) are nonhypersecretory adrenal adenomas**
  - Clinically significant incidentally discovered masses may be hormonally active, malignant, or both
    - In absence of clinical signs or symptoms of Cushing syndrome or hyperaldosteronism (see following discussion), no further biochemical investigation for these disorders is indicated
    - Follow-up imaging always needed
    - If any signs or symptoms of hormone excess are present, further evaluation is needed
  - Pheochromocytoma may be asymptomatic and may be present in the nonhypertensive patient; screening for pheochromocytoma with 24-hour urine total and fractionated metanephrines collection or plasma free metanephrines should always be performed, unless radiologic appearance (very low density by computed tomography [CT], such as <10 Hounsfield units) rules it out
  - **Mass size determines management; size greater than 4 cm increases the suspicion for malignancy**
    - **Biopsy cannot differentiate between benign and malignant primary adrenal tumors; therefore, all masses greater than 4 cm in diameter should be removed**
  - If mass less than 4 cm in diameter, repeat imaging done in 3 to 6 months
    - If no change, imaging repeated annually for 3 years
    - If mass increases in size, surgery should be performed
  - Management is different if patient has known primary cancer that risks spread to adrenals; fine-needle aspiration biopsy may be performed if metastatic disease suspected (after pheochromocytoma is ruled out)

TABLE 41-2	*Adrenal Hormones: Key Details*		
Hormone	**Secretagogues**	**Inhibitor**	**Major Actions**

Cortisol	ACTH	Cortisol inhibits CRH release (and thus ACTH release) in negative feedback loop
		Exogenous steroids also inhibit CRH release
			Increases serum glucose levels
			  Opposes insulin
			  Stimulates hepatic gluconeogenesis
			Creates catabolic protein state
			  Stimulates protein breakdown
			  Stimulates mobilization of amino acid precursors from muscle, bone, skin, and connective tissue
			  Inhibits protein synthesis
			Opposes inflammatory response
			  Opposes increased vascular permeability and other actions of inflammatory mediators
			  Decreases eosinophils and T cells
			  Mobilizes polymorphonuclear lymphocytes

Aldosterone	Renin-angiotensin system activation Hyperkalemia ACTH	Sodium	Stimulates sodium retention, impacting extracellular fluid volume Stimulates potassium excretion
DHEA	ACTH	Inhibitors of ACTH release	Stimulates secondary sexual characteristics in men (or virilization in women)

ACTH, adrenocorticotropic hormone; CRH, corticotropin-releasing hormone; DHEA, dehydroepiandrosterone.

Adrenal Hormone Excess States

CORTISOL EXCESS (CUSHING SYNDROME)

- See preceding section

ALDOSTERONE EXCESS

Basic Information

- **Most common cause is a bilateral adrenal hyperplasia, followed by functional adrenal adenoma (Conn syndrome, Fig. 41-12)**

Clinical Presentation

- **Patients present with hypertension (caused by sodium retention), metabolic alkalosis, and hypokalemia**
- Hypokalemia is not invariably present; may be unveiled by the use of diuretics
- Hypokalemia may result in muscle weakness

Diagnosis

- **Because patients with hyperaldosteronism are typically hypertensive, the diagnosis is suggested by the presence of hypokalemia in the hypertensive patient (although normal potassium does not exclude the diagnosis)**
  - Potassium should be normalized before evaluating for hyperaldosteronism because hypokalemia suppresses aldosterone secretion
- If the patient is taking a potassium-wasting diuretic, this must be discontinued, and potassium supplementation should be given
  - If hypokalemia resolves, hyperaldosteronism is less likely, but it is not ruled out

- **If hyperaldosteronism still considered, screening may be performed with serum aldosterone–plasma renin ratio**
  - If ratio (aldosterone in ng/dL, and plasma renin activity in ng/mL/hr) less than 20, hyperaldosteronism is not suggested
  - If ratio greater than 20, next step is to demonstrate nonsuppressible levels of aldosterone in presence of sodium load
    - 2 L of normal saline administered over 4 hours
    - If aldosterone levels do not suppress to less than 8 ng/dL, hyperaldosteronism is present
    - Alternatively, 24-hour urine aldosterone can be measured during oral salt loading (with simultaneous measurement of urinary sodium)
      - Adrenal imaging then performed to differentiate adrenal adenoma from bilateral adrenal hyperplasia. In patients age greater than 40, adrenal vein sampling is always recommended to determine the source of excessive aldosterone given higher prevalence of bilateral hyperplasia and adrenal incidentalomas.

Treatment

- If hyperaldosteronism is caused by a functional adrenal adenoma (i.e., Conn syndrome), treatment is surgical excision of adenoma
- If hyperaldosteronism is caused by bilateral adrenal hyperplasia, treatment is with a potassium-sparing diuretic (e.g., spironolactone or eplerenone)

ADRENAL ANDROGEN EXCESS

Basic Information

- DHEA and DHEA sulfate are the most common adrenal androgens that may be produced in excess

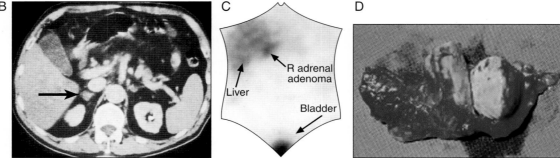

FIGURE 41-12 Conn syndrome. **A,** Characteristic biochemical results, including hypernatremia, hypokalemia, and metabolic alkalosis. Plasma renin activity is suppressed, and aldosterone levels are elevated. **B,** Right adrenal adenoma (*arrow*). **C,** Uptake of radiolabeled cholesterol in right adrenal gland. **D,** Pathologic specimen of the right adrenal gland in part **C.** (*From Haslett C, Chilvers ER, Boon NA, et al: Davidson's principles and practice of medicine, ed 19, New York, Churchill Livingstone, 2002, Fig. 16.19.*)

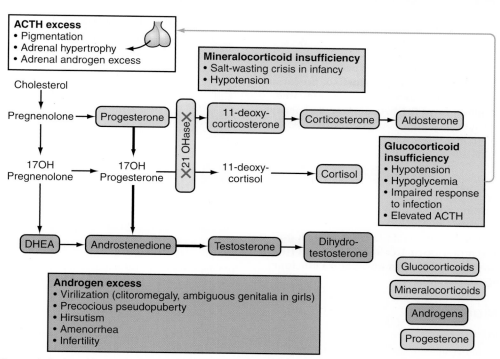

FIGURE 41-13 Congenital adrenal hyperplasia resulting from 21-hydroxylase (21 OHase) deficiency. Note how the enzyme defect results in mineralocorticoid and glucocorticoid deficiency while causing androgen excess. ACTH, adrenocorticotropin hormone; DHEA, dehydroepiandrosterone. *(From Haslett C, Chilvers ER, Boon NA, et al: Davidson's principles and practice of medicine, ed 19, New York, Churchill Livingstone, 2002, Fig. 16.21.)*

- Adrenal androgens may be produced because of adrenal tumors, congenital adrenal hyperplasia (CAH), and Cushing syndrome
  - In the most common form of CAH (21-hydroxylase deficiency, Fig. 41-13), cortisol synthesis is impaired, with overproduction of 17-hydroxyprogesterone and androgens
  - Mineralocorticoid production may also be impaired, resulting in hypoaldosteronism
- Androgen synthesis is intact, resulting in their overproduction

Clinical Presentation

- Classic (complete) forms of CAH present in infancy with hypoadrenalism, electrolyte abnormalities, and ambiguous genitalia (in females)
- Nonclassic (incomplete) forms may present in late childhood or young adulthood
- **Men are typically asymptomatic from overproduction of adrenal androgens**
- **Women present with signs and symptoms of androgen excess (Fig. 41-14), including**
  - Hirsutism (i.e., hair growth in a male pattern, such as on the chest, face, or back)
  - Virilization (e.g., clitoromegaly)
  - Oligomenorrhea, amenorrhea, infertility
  - Acne

Diagnosis

- Clinical manifestations typically prompt evaluation of androgen, cortisol, electrolytes, and ACTH levels

FIGURE 41-14 Ambiguous genitalia of a newborn female infant with virilizing congenital adrenal hyperplasia. An enlarged clitoris (phallic-like structure), genital hyperpigmentation, empty labioscrotal folds, and a single perineal opening into a urogenital sinus were present. *(From Shah BR, Laude TA: Atlas of pediatric clinical diagnosis, Philadelphia, WB Saunders, 2000, Fig. 8-14.)*

41

- Bilateral adrenal enlargement may be noted on imaging in case of CAH. An adrenal mass is seen in case of androgen-producing tumor.
- **If congenital adrenal hyperplasia suspected, 17-hydroxyprogesterone levels (the cortisol precursor that cannot be further metabolized) will be elevated in the most common form (21-hydroxylase deficiency)**
- Adrenal androgen excess often associated with Cushing disease; less commonly it is associated with cortisol-producing adrenal adenomas

Treatment

- If caused by adrenal tumor, treatment is excision of tumor
- If caused by Cushing syndrome, treatment is focused on treatment of Cushing syndrome
- **Congenital adrenal hyperplasia is treated with glucocorticoid and mineralocorticoid replacement (the latter not always needed) as in adrenal insufficiency (see following discussion)**

PHEOCHROMOCYTOMA

Basic Information

- Most pheochromocytomas occur in the adrenal medulla, where catecholamines are produced and stored
- Rarely, pheochromocytomas develop from the wall of the urinary bladder or in the retroperitoneal space
- Pheochromocytoma may occur as part of MEN-IIA or IIB syndrome (see Box 41-1) and is also seen with von Hippel-Lindau disease, neurofibromatosis, or succinyl dehydrogenase genes mutations
- Most pheochromocytomas produce both norepinephrine and epinephrine. Epinephrine-only secreting tumors are rare and are usually seen in the presence of a MEN-II syndrome resulting in an early clinical phenotype characterized by attacks of palpitations, nervousness, anxiety, and headaches rather than hypertension seen with sporadic or other hereditary tumors.

Clinical Presentation

- **Release of catecholamines results in clinical manifestations**
  - **Most common manifestation is hypertension**
  - **Headache, diaphoresis, tachycardia, and anxiety are also common manifestations**
  - Less common are orthostatic hypotension, polycythemia, and congestive heart failure
- **Symptoms classically described as paroxysmal, caused by episodic release of catecholamines from tumor**
  - Pressure on abdomen or urination (if tumor in bladder wall) can precipitate symptoms
  - **Paroxysms more common early in disease; larger tumors lead to more sustained elevations in blood pressure and symptoms**

Diagnosis

- **Diagnosis made by collection of 24-hour urine sample for total and fractionated metanephrines**
- **Yield may be increased in the intermittently symptomatic patient by initiating the urine collection at the onset of a paroxysm**

FIGURE 41-15 A computed tomography scan of the abdomen with IV administration of a contrast agent demonstrating peripartum discovery of pheochromocytoma (*arrow*). (*From Goldman L, Ausiello D: Cecil textbook of medicine, ed 23, Philadelphia, Elsevier Saunders, 2008, Fig. 246-2.*)

- Other tests used include 24-hour urine collection for vanillylmandelic acid (specific but not sensitive) or measurement of plasma free metanephrines
- Once diagnosed, pheochromocytoma must be located
  - Imaging of abdomen with CT or MRI is first step, with attention to adrenal glands (Fig. 41-15)
    - **90% of pheochromocytomas are located in the adrenal glands; those external to the adrenal glands are usually elsewhere in the abdomen (including the bladder)**
  - If initial imaging of abdomen negative, further localization is done, usually with iodinated metaiodobenzylguanidine (MIBG) scan
  - **If a pheochromocytoma is suspected to be malignant, MIBG scan should be performed before surgery to detect metastatic disease**

Treatment

- Treatment consists of surgical excision of tumor
  - **Because surgery can precipitate hormone release, preventive treatment with the α-blocker phenoxybenzamine is given for few weeks before surgery**

Adrenal Hormone Deficiency States

ADRENAL INSUFFICIENCY

Basic Information

- **Adrenal insufficiency may occur because of failure of the adrenal glands (primary adrenal insufficiency) or pituitary disease (secondary adrenal insufficiency)**
  - Autoimmune primary adrenal insufficiency is often associated with other autoimmune disorders (e.g., hypothyroidism, vitiligo)
  - Other causes of primary adrenal insufficiency include infection (e.g., tuberculosis), surgical excision, and bilateral hemorrhage of the adrenal glands

- Hemorrhagic destruction of the adrenal glands is described in disseminated meningococcal infection (Waterhouse-Friderichsen syndrome), as well as with anticoagulation or lupus anticoagulant
- Secondary adrenal insufficiency is much more common than primary adrenal insufficiency and is most often caused by suppression of the hypothalamic-pituitary-adrenal axis by the prolonged (3 weeks or longer) administration of exogenous steroids

Clinical Presentation

- Clinical manifestations of adrenal insufficiency differ based on whether or not the cause is primary or secondary adrenal insufficiency
  - With primary adrenal insufficiency, hypothalamus will respond by increasing CRH production, resulting in increased production of pro-opiomelanocortin (the ACTH precursor) and increased serum levels of ACTH
  - Because of increased production of pro-opiomelanocortin in primary adrenal insufficiency, skin and mucous membrane hyperpigmentation results. Skin hyperpigmentation does not result from secondary adrenal insufficiency.
  - With primary adrenal insufficiency, mineralocorticoid deficiency is also seen and hyponatremia and hyperkalemia result
  - Hyponatremia is less common with secondary adrenal insufficiency and is seen more often if concomitant central hypothyroidism is present
- Clinical manifestations shared by all patients with adrenal insufficiency include weakness, hypotension, nausea, vomiting, diarrhea, and weight loss
  - Acute adrenal insufficiency, which is a medical emergency, can be precipitated in patients with chronic adrenal insufficiency who are exposed to stress (e.g., surgery, infection, gastroenteritis) or by rapid destruction of the adrenal glands (such as with hemorrhage) or pituitary apoplexy

Diagnosis

- In primary adrenal insufficiency, plasma ACTH levels will be elevated, whereas in secondary adrenal insufficiency, plasma ACTH levels will be low (or inappropriately normal)
  - ACTH levels are used in conjunction with other tests to determine presence of primary or secondary adrenal insufficiency
- A random morning cortisol measurement may be insufficient to diagnose partial adrenal insufficiency because normal levels overlap with levels seen in mild adrenal insufficiency
  - However, if a patient is under significant stress (e.g., hypotensive or in the intensive care unit [ICU]) and a random cortisol (taken any time of day) is less than 15 µg/dL, the patient should be considered to be adrenally insufficient unless serum albumin is less than 2.5 g/dL
    - All patients diagnosed with adrenal insufficiency based on a low serum cortisol while in the ICU should be restudied after the acute problem is solved

- A very low serum morning cortisol level (<3 µg/dL) in an ambulatory patient is presumptive evidence of adrenal insufficiency
- Gold-standard test of adrenal function is insulin-induced hypoglycemia or insulin tolerance test (ITT)
  - Test performed by administering insulin (0.1–0.15 units/kg) intravenously, with measurement of cortisol levels during symptomatic hypoglycemia
    - A normal response is considered to be a peak cortisol level greater than 18 µg/dL
  - ITT contraindicated in presence of coronary artery disease, seizure disorder, or age greater than 60 years
- Most commonly used test is ACTH stimulation test
  - Administer ACTH (cosyntropin) 250 mg IV
  - Measure serum cortisol just before injection and 60 minutes following injection
  - If cortisol level 18.5 µg/dL or more at either measure, patient does not have adrenal insufficiency
    - If cortisol levels stay below 18.5 µg/dL, adrenal insufficiency is present, and results are combined with ACTH levels as described previously

Treatment

- Adrenal insufficiency: Treatment differs based on cause of adrenal insufficiency (e.g., primary versus secondary) as well as whether or not adrenal insufficiency is acute or chronic (Fig. 41-16)
  - Usual dose is hydrocortisone 10 to 12.5 mg/m^2/day
  - The lowest dose that improves patient's symptoms should be used
  - Dose should be increased during intercurrent illnesses
  - All patients should wear a medical alert bracelet or necklace stating their adrenal insufficiency status
  - Mineralocorticoid (fludrocortisone 0.05–0.2 mg/day) is used only in primary adrenal insufficiency

HYPOALDOSTERONISM

Basic Information

- Most common presentation is hyporeninemic hypoaldosteronism
  - Common in patients with renal insufficiency and in those with long-standing diabetes
  - Results in type IV renal tubular acidosis (see Chapter 31)
  - Other causes of hyporeninemic hypoaldosteronism include angiotensin-converting enzyme (ACE) inhibitors, NSAIDs, cyclosporine, and heparin
  - AIDS may also be associated with hyporeninemic hypoaldosteronism
- Hypoaldosteronism also occurs in patients with primary adrenal insufficiency and congenital adrenal hyperplasia (see preceding discussion)
  - Rare causes include isolated enzyme defects in synthesis of aldosterone and are usually diagnosed in children

Clinical Presentation

- Hyperkalemia is the major clinical feature of patients with hypoaldosteronism

41

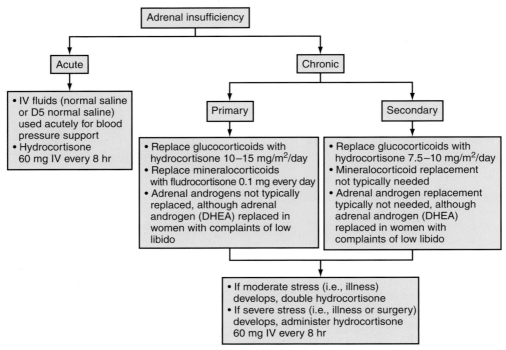

FIGURE 41-16 Treatment of adrenal insufficiency. (D5, 5% dextrose; DHEA, dehydroepiandrosterone; IV, intravenous.)

Diagnosis

- First step is to exclude obvious causes of hyporeninemic hypoaldosteronism (noted previously)
- With these causes excluded, major differential is between hyporeninemic hypoaldosteronism, adrenal insufficiency, congenital adrenal hyperplasia, or rare enzyme defect
  - After patient is upright for 3 hours, check plasma renin activity, serum aldosterone, and serum cortisol levels
    - With hyporeninemic hypoaldosteronism, plasma renin activity and aldosterone levels will be low; cortisol will be normal
    - With adrenal insufficiency, plasma renin activity will be high, whereas serum aldosterone and cortisol will be low
- Further evaluation of the patient with suspected adrenal insufficiency or congenital adrenal hyperplasia is discussed previously

Treatment

- Treatment may or may not be given, based on the cause of hypoaldosteronism and presence or absence of symptoms
- Hypoaldosteronism in the presence of adrenal insufficiency is treated with fludrocortisone (see Fig. 41-16)
- Hypoaldosteronism from hyporeninemic hypoaldosteronism may be treated with fludrocortisone

- If hypertension or fluid retention is present and prevents treatment with fludrocortisone, potassium-wasting diuretics and a low-potassium diet may be used

REVIEW QUESTIONS

For review questions, please go to www.expertconsult.com.

SUGGESTED READINGS

Carroll TB, Findling JW: The diagnosis of Cushing syndrome, *Rev Endocr Metab Disord* 11:147–153, 2010.

Dekkers OM, Pereira AM, Romijin JA: Treatment and follow-up of clinically nonfunctioning pituitary macroadenomas, *J Clin Endocrinol Metab* 93:3717–3726, 2008.

Gordon RD, Laragh JH, Funder JW: Low renin hypertensive states: perspectives, unsolved problems, future research, *Trends Endocrinol Metab* 16:108–113, 2005.

Mathioudakis N, Salvatori R: Adult-onset growth hormone deficiency: causes, complications and treatment options, *Curr Opin Endocrinol Diabetes Obes* 15:352–358, 2008.

Mathioudakis N, Salvatori R: Pituitary tumors, *Curr Treat Options Neurol* 11:287–296, 2009.

Melmed S, Colao A, Barkan A, et al: for the Acromegaly Consensus Group: Guidelines for acromegaly management: an update, *J Clin Endocrinol Metab* 94:1509–1517, 2009.

Molitch ME: Pituitary tumours: pituitary incidentalomas, *Best Pract Res Clin Endocrinol Metab* 23:667–675, 2009.

Salvatori R: Adrenal insufficiency, *JAMA* 294:2481–2488, 2005.

Verbalis JG: Diabetes insipidus, *Rev Endocr Metab Disord* 4:177–185, 2003.

Young WF Jr: Adrenal causes of hypertension: pheochromocytoma and primary aldosteronism, *Rev Endocr Metab Disord* 8:309–320, 2007.

Young WF Jr: Clinical practice: the incidentally discovered adrenal mass, *N Engl J Med* 356:601–610, 2007.

SECTION SEVEN

Rheumatology

Arthritis

ALLAN C. GELBER, MD, MPH, PhD

Arthritis encompasses a number of conditions that in the aggregate are the leading cause of disability in the United States. More than 60% of the population can expect to develop some form of arthritis in their lifetime.

Approach to the Patient with Joint Symptoms

Basic Information

- Strictly speaking, the term *arthritis* refers to joint inflammation, but it is commonly used more loosely to denote more than a hundred musculoskeletal conditions, both inflammatory and mechanical.
- It is important to distinguish true arthritis from conditions that mimic a joint disorder (Box 42-1)

Clinical Presentation

- A careful history and detailed physical examination should be directed at answering the following five key diagnostic questions:
  - Is the process truly **articular?**
  - Is the process **inflammatory** or **mechanical?**
  - What is the pattern of joint involvement?
  - Are there **extra-articular manifestations?**
  - Who is the **host?**
- Features that suggest an articular process
  - Symptoms (pain) localized to the joint(s)
  - Physical findings (swelling, erythema, heat, or tenderness) localized to the joint(s)
  - Joint range of motion is painful
  - Joint range of motion is restricted
- Features that suggest an inflammatory process
  - Morning stiffness longer than 60 minutes (versus worsening in the evening in mechanical processes)
  - Gel phenomenon (stiffness after prolonged inactivity)
  - Symptoms improve with use (versus worsening with use in mechanical processes)

BOX 42-1	*Processes That Mimic Arthritis*
Bursitis	Myositis
Tendinitis	Vasculitis
Fasciitis	Neuropathy
Enthesitis	Thyroid disease
Periostitis	Parathyroid disease
Fibromyalgia	Osteoporosis

- Joint swelling, erythema, heat, or tenderness
- Active constitutional manifestations (e.g., fever, malaise, anorexia or weight loss)
- Relevant patterns of joint involvement
  - **Acute onset** (e.g., microcrystalline) versus insidious onset (e.g., osteoarthritis [OA])
  - **Episodic** (e.g., microcrystalline) versus **migratory** (e.g., disseminated gonococcal infection and acute rheumatic fever) versus **additive** (e.g., rheumatoid arthritis [RA])
  - **Monoarticular** (e.g., microcrystalline and septic) versus **oligoarticular** (e.g., human leukocyte antigen [HLA]-B27 associated) versus **polyarticular** (e.g., RA)
  - **Symmetrical** (e.g., RA) versus **asymmetrical** (e.g., HLA-B27 associated)
  - **Axial** (e.g., HLA-B27 associated) versus **peripheral** (e.g., RA)
- Relevant extra-articular features
  - Constitutional symptoms and signs (i.e., presence of a fever)
  - Mucocutaneous (e.g., photosensitive and other cutaneous eruptions, alopecia, mucosal aphthous ulcers, and Raynaud's phenomenon)
  - Ocular (e.g., conjunctivitis, episcleritis, scleritis, and uveitis)
  - Renal (e.g., glomerulonephritis, renal tubular acidosis, and nephrolithiasis)
  - Neurologic (e.g., focal central and peripheral nerve disease, seizures, and cognitive and psychiatric disorders)
  - Pulmonary (e.g., nodules, infiltrates, interstitial fibrosis, pulmonary embolism and hypertension, alveolar hemorrhage, bronchiolitis, and pleuritis)
  - Gastrointestinal (e.g., inflammatory bowel disease and autoimmune liver disease)
  - Hematologic
    - Anemia (e.g., anemia of "chronic disease" and hemolytic anemia)
    - Leukopenia (e.g., neutropenia in Felty syndrome and lymphopenia in systemic lupus erythematosus [SLE])
    - Thrombocytopenia (e.g., SLE with antiphospholipid antibodies)
- Relevant host factors
  - Age
  - Gender
  - Race
  - Comorbidities
  - Occupational exposures
  - Family history

Diagnosis and Evaluation

- The judicious use of laboratory, synovial fluid, and imaging studies serves to test and confirm the diagnostic hypothesis, to assess the severity and prognosis of the disease process, and to guide therapy
- Obtain relevant laboratory studies as indicated
  - Kidney and liver function
  - Complete blood count with leukocyte differential
  - Urinalysis
  - Erythrocyte sedimentation rate and C-reactive protein
  - Thyroid function
  - Autoantibodies
- Obtain and evaluate synovial fluid as indicated
  - Check synovial fluid leukocyte cell count, Gram stain and culture, and polarized microscopy for crystals
  - White blood cell (WBC) count less than 200/mm^3 (normal), greater than 2000/mm^3 (inflammatory), and greater than 100,000/mm^3 (presumptively septic)
- Obtain relevant imaging studies
  - Conventional radiography is the starting point in imaging studies due to widespread availability, low cost, and high resolution, but may reveal only nonspecific soft tissue swelling in early inflammatory disease
  - Computed tomography (CT) is widely available and a good choice for assessment of the spine and pulmonary parenchyma
  - Magnetic resonance imaging (MRI) has replaced CT in many situations (e.g., disk herniation, sacroiliac joints, osteonecrosis, and soft tissue processes)
  - Arthrography (e.g., evaluation for rotator cuff tears)
  - Angiography (e.g., evaluation for vasculitis)
  - Both mechanical and inflammatory joint disease cause increased tracer uptake so that nuclear medicine scans have a limited role in the evaluation of arthritis
  - Ultrasound is useful in differentiating thrombophlebitis from pseudothrombophlebitis (ruptured Baker cyst), with an expanding role in the assessment of synovitis and erosive joint disease

Osteoarthritis

Basic Information

- **Prototypical and most prevalent mechanical (noninflammatory) joint disorder**
- One third of individuals 65 years and older have radiographic evidence of knee OA
- **Primarily a disease of degenerative cartilage, with secondary bony changes**
- There are a variety of risk factors for OA (Box 42-2)
  - Even though advancing age is a major risk factor for OA, it should not be considered a "normal" part of aging

Clinical Presentation

- Typically presents insidiously in middle-aged or elderly patients
- Most commonly seen in the **hands** (e.g., first carpometacarpal, proximal interphalangeal [PIP], and distal interphalangeal [DIP] joints) and **weight-bearing joints** (e.g., hips, knees, and spine)

- **Joints ache and are painful, worsening with use and at the end of the day**
- Rest and nocturnal pain may be seen with severe disease
- Patients may experience minimal morning stiffness and gelling
- No constitutional or other extra-articular manifestations with primary OA
- May have a variety of clinical presentations that are not mutually exclusive
  - First carpometacarpal joint
  - Interphalangeal joints (often familial and affects primarily older women; Fig. 42-1)
    - **Bouchard nodes** represent bony enlargement of the PIP joints
    - **Heberden nodes** represent bony enlargement of the DIP joints
  - Erosive osteoarthritis
    - Affects the DIP and PIP joints
    - Characterized by recurrent flares of pain, swelling, and tenderness

BOX 42-2	*Risk Factors for Osteoarthritis*

Advanced age
Female gender
Developmental
Collagen polymorphisms
   Types II, IX, and XI
Obesity
Trauma
   Acute and repetitive
Neuropathy
Inflammatory arthritis
Osteonecrosis
Paget disease
Endocrine/metabolic
   Acromegaly
   Alkaptonuria
   Chondrocalcinosis
   Hemochromatosis

FIGURE 42-1 Osteoarthritis of the hands, with Heberden nodes (distal interphalangeal joints) and Bouchard nodes (proximal interphalangeal joints). *(Courtesy of Don R. Martin, MD.)*

- Joint destruction occurs, leading to nonuniform joint space loss and joint deformity
- May be associated with microcrystalline disease and can be confused with RA
  - Hip
    - Symptoms often localize to the groin and anterior thigh
    - Distinguish from trochanteric bursitis (pain over the lateral aspect of the hip)
    - Symptoms provoked by use (e.g., weight-bearing) and internal rotation
    - May be associated with congenital malformations (e.g., hip dysplasia, slipped capital femoral epiphysis, and Legg-Calvé-Perthes disease)
  - Knee
    - All three joint compartments may be affected (e.g., medial tibiofemoral, lateral tibiofemoral, and patellofemoral)
  - Spine
    - Characterized by pain, stiffness, and (sometimes) radicular symptoms
    - Most commonly affects the lower cervical and lumbar spine
  - Diffuse idiopathic skeletal hyperostosis (DISH)
    - Variant of OA with axial and peripheral skeletal manifestations
    - Radiographic diagnosis (Fig. 42-2) characterized by
      - Flowing calcification or ossification along the anterolateral aspect of at least four contiguous vertebrae
      - Relative preservation of the intervertebral disk space at the involved levels (in contrast to classic OA)
      - Absence of apophyseal or sacroiliac joint involvement (in contrast to ankylosing spondylitis)

Diagnosis and Evaluation

- Clinical presentation highly suggestive in classic cases
- History characterized by
  - Insidious onset
  - Absence of inflammatory manifestations
- Physical examination reveals
  - Variable pattern of joint involvement as detailed previously
  - Bony hypertrophy
  - Bony deformity
  - Joint line tenderness
  - Crepitus
  - Limited joint mobility or laxity/pseudolaxity
  - Muscle (disuse) atrophy
- Laboratory findings
  - Renal and hepatic function normal unless impairment results from drug toxicity
  - Normal erythrocyte sedimentation rate (aside from age-associated changes)
  - Seronegative (aside from age-associated changes)
  - **Synovial fluid is noninflammatory with less than 2000 WBCs/mm³**
- Radiographic findings
  - Symptoms and radiographic findings may be discordant (e.g., significant symptoms or functional limitation with minimal radiographic findings, and vice versa)

- May be normal in early disease
- Radiographic hallmarks include
  - Joint space narrowing (often asymmetrical; Fig. 42-3)
  - Subchondral bone sclerosis (or eburnation)
  - Subchondral cysts
  - Joint margin osteophytes

Treatment

- Principles
  - Provide symptomatic relief
  - Maintain and maximize function
  - Minimize medication-associated toxicity
- Nonpharmacologic treatment
  - Patient education, weight loss (if overweight), exercise (low-impact, conditioning, and range of motion), occupational therapy, physical therapy, and assistive devices (e.g., cane)
- Pharmacologic treatment
  - Topical therapy
    - Capsaicin (depletes substance P in sensory nerve endings)
    - Methylsalicylate

42

FIGURE 42-2 Radiographic findings in diffuse idiopathic skeletal hyperostosis (DISH), with flowing ossification along the anterolateral aspect of at least four contiguous vertebral bodies and relative preservation of the disk spaces. *(From Harris ED, Budd RC, Genovese MC, et al [eds]: Kelley's textbook of rheumatology, ed 7, Philadelphia, WB Saunders, 2005, Fig. 51-66.)*

- Oral therapy
  - Acetaminophen (considered first-line oral pharmacologic therapy)
  - Nonsteroidal anti-inflammatory drugs (NSAIDs)
    - Therapeutically equivalent, although individual responses may vary
    - **Nonselective cyclooxygenase (COX)-1 and -2 inhibitors reduce pain and improve function, but carry significant potential for GI and other toxicities**
  - Selective COX-2 inhibitors may be safer with respect to GI toxicity and do not block platelet activity, but have been associated with increased risk for cardiovascular and cerebrovascular morbidity and mortality and are not more effective. Only celecoxib remains available in the United States.
  - Other pure analgesics (e.g., propoxyphene, tramadol, and opioids)
  - Glucosamine and chondroitin sulfate may provide symptomatic relief in some patients, but the results of clinical trials vary. Marketing claims of joint protection and restoration remain unproven.
  - **There is no role for systemic corticosteroid therapy**
  - Intra-articular therapy
    - May provide temporary relief of symptoms when topical and oral regimens are ineffective or not tolerated
    - Joint aspiration may provide temporary relief when a large effusion is present
    - Corticosteroid injections may be particularly helpful in patients who have signs of joint inflammation
    - Hyaluronan injections have demonstrated efficacy, but individual responses are quite variable
- Surgical treatment
  - Arthroscopic débridement is indicated when internal derangements (e.g., meniscal tears) cause joint catching, locking, instability, or pain
  - **Total joint replacement is indicated in patients with symptoms and functional impairment that are unresponsive to medical intervention**
  - Tidal irrigation of joints has not been demonstrated to be effective

Prevention

- Diagnosis and treatment of risk factors for OA may result in prevention of articular damage
- **The relative risk of developing knee OA is higher in obese individuals, so weight loss may have a major role in prevention of disease**

Rheumatoid Arthritis

Basic Information

- **Prototypical and most prevalent inflammatory joint disorder in women**
- Affects 1% of the population
- Peak incidence in the 30s to 50s
- Female-to-male ratio 3:1
- Familial predisposition, with HLA-DR4 association and amino acid motif QKRAA shared epitope susceptibility

Clinical Presentation

- **Additive, symmetrical polyarthritis affecting both small and large joints**
  - **Wrists, metacarpophalangeal (MCP) and PIP joints prominently involved; DIP joints spared**
  - Shoulders, elbows, hips, knees, ankles, and feet commonly involved
  - Cervical spine (atlantoaxial joint) may be involved; lumbar spine is spared
- Presentation is often suggested by its inflammatory character
  - **Fatigue, fever, and weight loss may be present, reflecting systemic nature of the disease**
  - Joint pain, swelling, erythema, heat, and tenderness may develop acutely or insidiously
  - Morning stiffness lasts more than 1 hour, and "gel" phenomenon present after inactivity
- **Untreated, RA can cause joint destruction and disability, beginning in the first year of disease**
  - Ulnar deviation and subluxation of the fingers at the MCP joints, with radial deviation at the wrist

FIGURE 42-3 Radiographic findings in osteoarthritis of the knee, with asymmetrical narrowing of the medial joint space. *(From Harris ED, Budd RC, Genovese MC, et al [eds]: Kelley's textbook of rheumatology, ed 7, Philadelphia, WB Saunders, 2005, Fig. 92-1.)*

- Swan neck deformity (hyperextension of the PIP and flexion of the DIP joints; Fig. 42-4)
- Boutonnière deformity (flexion of the PIP and hyperextension of the DIP joints; Fig. 42-5)
- **Extra-articular manifestations**
  - Rheumatoid nodules
    - Typically appear on extensor surfaces and pressure points (e.g., olecranon process and Achilles tendon) but may also affect internal organs
    - Occur in approximately 25% of patients with RA
    - Associated with rheumatoid factor (RF) seropositivity and more severe disease
    - Nodules are not specific for RA and can occur in other rheumatic diseases
    - Histology marked by central necrosis, surrounded by palisading fibroblasts, and a collagenous capsule with a chronic inflammatory infiltrate
    - **Methotrexate can worsen nodulosis, even as inflammatory joint disease improves**
  - Ocular
    - Episcleritis, scleritis, and scleromalacia perforans
    - Keratoconjunctivitis sicca (secondary Sjögren syndrome)
  - Pulmonary
    - Pleural disease (effusions exudative and pleural fluid glucose typically low)
    - Interstitial lung disease and fibrosis
    - Bronchiolitis obliterans
    - Pulmonary nodules
      - Single or multiple
      - Nodules may cavitate and pleural nodules cause bronchopleural fistulae
      - **Caplan disease (nodules with underlying RA and pneumoconiosis)**
  - Cardiac
    - Pericarditis and effusions are common but rarely symptomatic
    - Constrictive pericarditis, myocarditis, and conduction defects develop rarely
  - Hematologic
    - Anemia due to iron deficiency (NSAID-associated GI loss) and "chronic disease"
    - **Felty syndrome (RA associated with splenomegaly, neutropenia, and leg ulcers)**
    - Thrombocytosis or thrombocytopenia
    - Increased risk for non-Hodgkin lymphoma independent of tumor necrosis factor (TNF) inhibitor use
  - Neurologic
    - Atlantoaxial (C1-C2) instability and subluxation may produce a cervical myelopathy
    - Peripheral neuropathy
      - Compression associated with synovitis (e.g., carpal tunnel syndrome)
      - Ischemic associated with vasculitis (e.g., mononeuritis multiplex)
  - Vasculitis
    - Leukocytoclastic vasculitis, cutaneous ulcers, visceral involvement, and mononeuritis multiplex
    - **Associated with high-titer RF and severe disease**

FIGURE 42-4   Swan neck deformity in advanced rheumatoid arthritis. *(From Harris ED, Budd RC, Genovese MC, et al [eds]: Kelley's textbook of rheumatology, ed 7, Philadelphia, WB Saunders, 2005, Fig. 33-6.)*

FIGURE 42-5   Boutonnière deformity in advanced rheumatoid arthritis. *(From Townsend CM, Beauchamp RD, Evers BM, Mattox KL: Sabiston textbook of surgery, ed 17, Philadelphia, Saunders, 2004, Fig. 73-17.)*

Diagnosis and Evaluation

- Clinical presentation highly suggestive in classic cases
- History characterized by
  - Acute or subacute onset
  - Inflammatory manifestations
- Physical examination reveals
  - Synovitis
  - Symmetrical polyarthritis as detailed previously
- Laboratory findings
  - Renal and hepatic function normal unless the result of drug toxicity
  - Normochromic normocytic anemia
  - Elevated sedimentation rate and C-reactive protein
  - **Rheumatoid factor**
    - Immunoglobulin (Ig)M autoantibody directed against the Fc fragment of IgG
    - IgM-RF is 60% to 80% sensitive and 80% to 90% specific for RA
    - RF is also seen in a wide variety of other rheumatic diseases (Sjögren syndrome, juvenile arthritis, SLE, and cryoglobulinemia) and nonrheumatic diseases (interstitial lung disease, endocarditis, tuberculosis [TB], hepatitis, and malignancy)
    - Prevalence increases with age

- **Anti–cyclic citrullinated peptide (anti-CCP) antibodies**
  - Anti-CCP antibody is 68% to 80% sensitive and 98% specific for RA
  - Anti-CCP is more likely to be present in early RA than is RF

FIGURE 42-6 Radiographic findings in rheumatoid arthritis of the hand, with erosions and ulnar deviation. *(From Harris ED, Budd RC, Genovese MC, et al [eds]: Kelley's textbook of rheumatology, ed 7, Philadelphia, WB Saunders, 2005, Fig. 51-6.)*

- Synovial fluid inflammatory with leukocyte count greater than 2000 WBCs/mm³
- Radiographic findings (Fig. 42-6)
  - May reveal only soft tissue swelling in early disease, but with advanced disease show
    - Periarticular osteopenia
    - **Uniform joint space narrowing**
    - Joint margin erosions
    - Ulnar styloid erosions
    - Atlantoaxial (C1-C2) instability and subluxation
- 1987 Criteria for the classification of RA (Table 42-1)
  - Developed to classify patients for study purposes
  - Need four of the seven criteria to classify patient with RA
  - May still consider the diagnosis of RA if two or more criteria are present
- 2010 Rheumatoid Arthritis Classification Criteria (see Table 42-1)
  - Designed to address criticism of 1987 criteria for their lack of sensitivity in early disease
  - New classification system redefines the current paradigm of RA by focusing on features at earlier stages of disease that are associated with persistent and/or erosive disease.
  - Intent of new criteria is to refocus attention on the important need for earlier diagnosis and institution of effective disease-suppressing therapy to prevent or minimize the occurrence of the undesirable sequelae that currently comprise the paradigm underlying the disease construct "rheumatoid arthritis"

TABLE 42-1　Classification Schemes for Diagnosing Rheumatoid Arthritis

1987 American Rheumatism Association*	2010 American College of Rheumatology/European League Against Rheumatism†	
Morning stiffness (≥1 hr)	Classification criteria for RA (score-based algorithm: add score of categories A–D;	
Arthritis in three or more joint areas (simultaneously)	*A score ≥6/10 is needed for classification of a patient as having definite RA*	
	A. Joint involvement	Score
Arthritis of hand joints (wrist, MCP, or PIP joints)	1 large joint	0
	2–10 large joints (with or without involvement of large joints)	1
Symmetrical arthritis	1–3 small joints (with or without involvement of large joints)	2
Rheumatoid nodules	4–10 small joints (at least 1 small joint)	3
Serum rheumatoid factor	>10 joints (at least 1 small joint)	5
Radiographic changes (consistent with RA)	B. Serology (at least 1 test is needed for classification)	
	Negative RF *and* negative ACPA	0
	Low-positive RF *or* low positive ACPA	2
	High-positive RF *or* high positive ACPA	3
	C. Acute-phase reactants (at least 1 test result is needed for classification)	
	Normal CRP *and* normal ESR	0
	Abnormal CRP *or* abnormal ESR	1
	D. Duration of symptoms	
	<6 weeks	0
	≥6 weeks	1

ACPA, anti–citrullinated protein antibody; CRP, C-reactive protein; ESR, erythrocyte sedimentation rate; MCP, metacarpophalangeal; PIP, proximal interphalangeal; RA, rheumatoid arthritis; RF, rheumatoid factor.
*From Arnett FC, Edworthy SM, Bloch DA, et al: The American Rheumatism Association 1987 revised criteria for the classification of rheumatoid arthritis, *Arthritis Rheum* 31:315–324, 1988
†From Aletha D, Neogi T, Silman AJ, et al: An American College of Rheumatology/European League Against Rheumatism Collaborative Initiative 2010 Rheumatoid Arthritis Classification Criteria, *Arthritis Rheum* 62:2569–2581, 2010.

Treatment

- Principles
  - Provide symptomatic relief
  - Prevent joint destruction
  - Maintain and maximize function
  - Minimize medication-associated toxicity
  - **Tailor approach to the individual patient given heterogeneity in clinical course and outcome**
- Nonpharmacologic treatment
  - Patient education, exercise (low-impact, conditioning, and range of motion), occupational therapy, physical therapy, and assistive devices (e.g., cane, walker)
- **Pharmacologic treatment**
  - NSAIDs
    - Analgesic and anti-inflammatory effects reduce pain and improve function
    - **NSAIDs are not "disease-modifying"**
  - Corticosteroids
    - Anti-inflammatory effect helps to control symptoms and maintain function
    - **Most effective as "bridging therapy" while disease-modifying antirheumatic drugs (DMARDs) take effect**
    - Toxicity (e.g., weight gain, hypertension, glucose intolerance, hyperlipidemia, osteoporosis, etc.) makes prolonged use undesirable, but sometimes it is unavoidable
    - Regimens vary (IV or PO "pulse," daily low dose, and intra-articular)
  - DMARDs (Table 42-2)
    - DMARD use improves long-term outcomes
    - Early use advised for patients with the potential for progressive disease or those with poor prognostic factors
    - **Poor prognostic factors include young women, more than 20 involved joints, rheumatoid nodules, high sedimentation rate, high-titer RF-positive, and radiographic erosions**
    - Time to achieve maximal beneficial effect varies from **4 weeks to 6 months** depending on the agent
    - Often used jointly with NSAIDs or corticosteroids (or both)
    - **Combination therapy (>1 DMARD) used when disease unresponsive to single-agent therapy**

TABLE 42-2	Disease-Modifying Antirheumatic Drugs (DMARDs)		
Drug	**Indication**	**Toxicity/Precautions**	**Monitoring**
Hydroxychloroquine	Mild disease	Nausea, rash, and retinal damage (rare)	Eye exam every 6–12 mo
Sulfasalazine	Mild disease	Nausea, hepatitis, renal, G6PD-associated anemia, myelosuppression, and oligospermia	Initial G6PD; LFTs and CBC monthly ×3, then every 3 mo
Methotrexate (MTX)	First-line DMARD	Stomatitis, nausea, diarrhea, hepatitis, hepatic fibrosis, myelosuppression, interstitial pneumonitis, and teratogenic; requires folate supplementation	Creatinine, LFTs, and CBC monthly until dose stable, then every 2–3 mo
Leflunomide	Alternative to MTX	Stomatitis, nausea, diarrhea, hepatitis, myelosuppression, and teratogenic	LFTs and CBC monthly until dose stable, then every 2–3 mo
Adalimumab	TNF inhibitor, used if MTX ineffective	Injection-site reactions; avoid in patients with active or chronic infections or multiple sclerosis	Baseline PPD
Etanercept	TNF inhibitor, used if MTX ineffective	Injection-site reactions; avoid in patients with active or chronic infections or multiple sclerosis	Baseline PPD
Infliximab	TNF inhibitor, used if MTX ineffective	Infusion reactions; avoid in patients with active or chronic infections or multiple sclerosis	Baseline PPD
Anakinra	IL-1 receptor antagonist used if TNF inhibitors ineffective	Injection-site reactions and neutropenia; avoid in patients with active or chronic infections	Neutrophil count monthly ×3, then every 3 mo
Abatacept	Inhibitor of T-cell activation; used if TNF inhibitors ineffective	Avoid in patients with active or chronic infections; increased adverse respiratory effects in patients with COPD; do not combine with TNF inhibitors or anakinra	Baseline PPD; no live vaccines during treatment
Rituximab	Anti-CD20 monoclonal antibody; used if TNF inhibitors ineffective	Avoid in patients with active or chronic infections; infusion reactions (especially first) common; hepatitis B reactivation reported	Effective contraception required

CBC, complete blood count; COPD, chronic obstructive pulmonary disease; G6PD, glucose-6-phosphate dehydrogenase; IL-1, interleukin-1; LFTs, liver function tests; PPD, purified protein derivative; TNF, tumor necrosis factor.

42

- Gold, D-penicillamine, azathioprine, cyclophosphamide, and cyclosporine C rarely used anymore
- Surgical treatment
  - Synovectomy may be indicated when synovitis fails to respond to medical therapy
  - Joint replacement is indicated when joint destruction occurs despite medical therapy, and the resultant pain is no longer responsive to medical management

Prevention
- RA is not currently preventable

Gout

Basic Information
- **Intensely inflammatory arthritis caused by deposition of monosodium urate crystals**
- Peak incidence in the 50s to 60s
- Most common in postpubertal males (uric acid rises after puberty)
- Incidence rises in postmenopausal females (uric acid rises after menopause)
- Hyperuricemia results from increased production (10%) and diminished excretion (90%; Box 42-3) of uric acid
  - Limit of solubility of uric acid is approximately 7 mg/dL
  - Primary hyperuricemia caused by polygenic factors
  - Secondary hyperuricemia caused by familial or acquired conditions

---

BOX 42-3   Causes of Hyperuricemia

Increased Production
Hypoxanthine-guanine phosphoribosyltransferase deficiency
Glycogen storage diseases
Increased purine intake
Increased nucleic acid turnover
    Myeloproliferative disorder
    Tumor lysis syndrome
    Hemolytic disorder
    Psoriasis
Accelerated adenosine triphosphate degradation
    Tissue hypoxia
    Sustained exercise
Ethanol

Reduced Excretion
Intrinsic renal disease
Drugs
    Diuretics
    Low-dose aspirin
    Cyclosporin A
    Ethambutol
    Pyrazinamide
Ketoacidosis and lactic acidosis
Dehydration
Hyperparathyroidism
Lead nephropathy
Ethanol

Clinical Presentation
- Asymptomatic hyperuricemia
  - Found at some point in about 5% of adult Americans
  - **More than 75% of individuals remain asymptomatic**
- Acute gout
  - Acute onset of intense joint pain, swelling, erythema, and heat
  - Fever (systemic manifestation of inflammation) may be present
  - 50% of patients present with first metatarsophalangeal joint involvement (podagra)
  - **75% to 90% of patients develop podagra at some point in their course**
  - Gout may also affect the ankles, midfoot, knees, wrists, shoulders, and hands
  - Attacks are usually monoarticular or oligoarticular (two to three joints); rarely polyarticular until late in the disease course
  - **Early attacks are self-limited and will resolve over 3 to 10 days, even without treatment**
- Intercritical gout
  - Asymptomatic period between acute attacks
  - May be years in duration
  - Uric acid levels are generally persistently elevated
- Chronic (tophaceous) gout (Fig. 42-7)
  - After years of recurrent attacks, joints develop persistent pain, swelling, and deformity
- Extra-articular disease
  - Tophi
    - Deposits of monosodium urate crystals in soft tissue
    - Typically found in the synovium and subchondral bone, on the pinna of the ear, and over extensor surfaces (e.g., forearm) and pressure points (e.g., Achilles tendon)
    - Typically appear after years of repeated episodes of acute gout
    - May be confused with rheumatoid nodules

FIGURE 42-7 Chronic tophaceous gout involving the hands. *(Courtesy of Don R. Martin, MD.)*

- Renal disease
  - Parenchymal urate nephropathy associated with tumor lysis syndrome (acute) and comorbid conditions (chronic)
  - Nephrolithiasis risk 50% with serum uric acid greater than 13 mg/dL or urinary uric acid excretion greater than 1100 mg/day

Diagnosis and Evaluation

- Clinical presentation highly suggestive in classic cases
- History characterized by
  - Acute onset
  - Intermittent nature with asymptomatic intercritical phase
  - Inflammatory manifestations
- Physical examination reveals
  - Intensely inflammatory arthritis
  - Tophi may be present
- Laboratory findings
  - **Serum uric acid level elevated more than 80% of the time during acute gout, but can be normal**
  - Arthrocentesis (joint aspiration), with synovial fluid examination at onset by polarized microscopy and culture, to rule out septic arthritis and confirm diagnosis of gout
  - Synovial fluid inflammatory with leukocyte count greater than 2000 WBCs/mm³, and as high as 100,000/mm³
  - **Crystals are needle-shaped, negatively birefringent, and may be intracellular (Fig. 42-8)**
  - Crystals may be found in asymptomatic joints (during intercritical period)
- Radiographic findings
  - May reveal only soft tissue swelling in early disease, but with advanced disease show
    - Early relative joint space preservation
    - Joint margin erosions with overhanging edges (**"parrot's beak"**; Fig. 42-9)
  - Uric acid is radiolucent

Treatment

- Acute
  - NSAIDs
    - Effective and rapid, especially if started early
    - Indomethacin has traditionally been used, but there is no evidence that one NSAID agent is superior to another
  - Corticosteroids
    - Effective when NSAIDs are contraindicated
    - Must first rule out infection
    - Carry risk of "rebound" arthritis after taper
    - Administered as an oral taper, parenteral infusion, or intra-articular injection
  - Colchicine
    - Administered PO or IV, but potential for significant toxicity with IV route (GI, hepatic, renal, bone marrow, myopathy, and neuropathy), so use only if NSAIDs or corticosteroids not an option
- Prophylaxis
  - **Low-purine diet, discontinue aspirin and diuretics, and limit alcohol as feasible**

- **Colchicine 0.6 mg once or twice daily reduces or eliminates attacks in approximately 95% of patients**
  - Caution advised in patients with impaired renal function due to risk for toxicity
  - Uric acid–lowering agents
    - Indicated for failure of colchicine prophylaxis or inability to correct hyperuricemia
    - Do not treat asymptomatic hyperuricemia

FIGURE 42-8 Polarized light microscopy demonstrating the strongly negative birefringence of needle-shaped uric acid crystals. *(From Forbes CD, Jackson WF: Color atlas and text of clinical medicine, ed 3, St. Louis, Mosby, 2003, Fig. 3.13.)*

FIGURE 42-9 Radiographic findings in tophaceous gout, with extensive bony destruction of the first metatarsophalangeal joint. *Arrows* indicate erosions; *arrowhead* shows overhanging edge ("parrot's beak"). *(From Harris ED, Budd RC, Genovese MC, et al [eds]: Kelley's textbook of rheumatology, ed 7, Philadelphia, WB Saunders, 2005, Fig. 51-28.)*

42

- **Do not start uric acid–lowering agents during acute gout or without prophylaxis, as any change in the uric acid concentration (up or down) may precipitate an acute gout attack**
- Uricosuric agents (e.g., probenecid and sulfinpyrazone) have limited usefulness in setting of renal impairment
  - Use in patients with reduced uric acid excretion, but need glomerular filtration rate greater than 50 mL/min
  - If used in patients with high excretion, may lead to stone formation
  - Must have no history of nephrolithiasis
  - Must maintain daily fluid intake of more than 2 L to avoid stone formation
  - Must avoid low-dose salicylates
- Xanthine oxidase inhibition (e.g., allopurinol, febuxostat)
  - Blocks xanthine oxidase enzyme in production of uric acid
  - **Indicated for "extreme" hyperuricemia, high frequency of attacks, tophi, stones, and tumor lysis syndrome**
  - Adjust dose for renal function
  - **Lower dose of azathioprine and mercaptopurine by 75% when used in conjunction with allopurinol**
  - Titrate dose to uric acid level of 5 to 6 mg/dL
  - Adverse effects include fever, rash, hepatitis, and leukopenia

Prevention

- Correct causes of hyperuricemia (see Box 42-3)

Calcium Pyrophosphate Dihydrate Deposition Disease

Basic Information

- **Inflammatory arthritis caused by deposition of calcium pyrophosphate dihydrate (CPPD) crystals**
- Incidence increases with age; 50% of population has chondrocalcinosis by 80s
- Most cases are idiopathic, but some are associated with other diseases (Box 42-4)

Clinical Presentation

- Acute (pseudogout)
  - Inflammatory arthritis of large joints

BOX 42-4 **Diseases Associated with Pseudogout**

Osteoarthritis
Gout
Hemochromatosis
Hypothyroidism
Hyperparathyroidism
Wilson disease

- **Knees involved in 50% of cases**
  - Wrists, metacarpophalangeal joints, hips, shoulders, elbows, and ankles also affected
  - Resembles an acute gout attack with monoarticular inflammation
  - Attacks may be recurrent
- Subacute (RA-like) presentation is uncommon
- Chronic (OA-like) presentation is generally more destructive than is typical of OA

Diagnosis and Evaluation

- History characterized by
  - Varied onset and course
  - Inflammation often less intense than in gout
- Physical examination reveals
  - Varied patterns and intensity of disease
- Laboratory findings
  - Synovial fluid inflammatory with leukocyte count greater than 2000 WBCs/mm³ in acute arthritis
  - **Crystals are rhomboid-shaped and positively birefringent (Fig. 42-10)**
- Radiographic findings
  - Chondrocalcinosis (Fig. 42-11)
    - Linear calcifications in the cartilage
    - Most commonly found in the wrist, symphysis pubis, and knee

Treatment

- Acute
  - NSAIDs
  - Corticosteroids
- Chronic
  - NSAIDs
- Prophylaxis
  - Chronic administration of low-dose colchicine or NSAIDs may be effective
  - No CPPD-lowering agents are currently available

Prevention

- Treat associated diseases (see Box 42-4)

FIGURE 42-10 Polarized light microscopy demonstrating the weakly positive birefringence of rhomboidal crystals of calcium pyrophosphate dihydrate. *(From Forbes CD, Jackson WF: Color atlas and text of clinical medicine, ed 3, St. Louis, Mosby, 2003, Fig. 3.14.)*

Seronegative Spondyloarthropathies

Overview

- Four diseases grouped together by overlapping clinical features and molecular evidence of a common etiology
  - Ankylosing spondylitis
  - Enteropathic arthritis
  - Psoriatic arthritis
  - Reactive arthritis
- Common clinical features
  - Enthesopathy (inflammation at the site of ligamentous and tendinous insertion to bone)
  - Inflammatory back disease/sacroiliitis
  - Mucocutaneous manifestations
  - Inflammatory eye disease
  - Inflammatory bowel disease
  - HLA-B27 association
  - RF-seronegative

ANKYLOSING SPONDYLITIS

Basic Information

- Inflammatory arthritis that predominantly affects the axial skeleton
- Affects 0.5% to 1% of whites; less common in blacks
- Peak incidence in the 20s to 30s
- Male-to-female ratio is 5:1

FIGURE 42-11 Radiographic findings of linear calcification of the hyaline cartilage and lateral meniscus in calcium pyrophosphate dihydrate deposition (CPPD) disease. *(From Harris ED, Budd RC, Genovese MC, et al [eds]: Kelley's textbook of rheumatology, ed 7, Philadelphia, WB Saunders, 2005, Fig. 51-30.)*

Clinical Presentation

- **Presents with insidious onset of low back or buttock stiffness**
- Symptoms typically inflammatory (e.g., worse in the morning and with rest; improve with use)
- **Begins as sacroiliitis, progressing to the lumbar spine and cephalad, resulting in vertebral body fusion**
- Thoracic spine disease may present as chest pain
- Extra-axial disease
  - Limb-girdle joints (e.g., shoulders and hips) commonly affected
  - Peripheral joints affected less commonly and usually asymmetrically
  - Enthesopathy (e.g., Achilles tendinitis and plantar fasciitis)
  - Anterior uveitis
  - Aortitis and aortic valve insufficiency
  - Pulmonary fibrosis (apical lung fields)
  - Subclinical colitis

Diagnosis and Evaluation

- Clinical presentation highly suggestive in classic cases
- History characterized by
  - Localization of symptoms to sacroiliac joints and lumbar spine
  - Inflammatory manifestations
  - **Anterior uveitis may be initial manifestation**
- Physical examination reveals
  - Sacroiliac and lumbar spine tenderness
  - Loss of lumbar lordosis
  - Loss of lumbar spine range of motion
    - **Schober test measures lumbar spine distraction with flexion (<5 cm is significant)**
  - Chest expansion is limited in patients with thoracic involvement
- Laboratory findings
  - Inflammatory markers may be elevated
  - **90% of patients are HLA-B27 positive; nearly 100% of those with uveitis or aortitis**
  - **However, HLA-B27 is nondiagnostic, as 6% to 8% of the general white population is positive**
- Radiographic findings
  - Symmetrical sacroiliitis (e.g., iliac margin sclerosis and fusion; Fig. 42-12)
  - Early findings include squaring and sclerosis of the corners of the vertebrae
  - Later findings include ossification of the anterior longitudinal ligament and bridging syndesmophytes resulting in "bamboo spine" (Fig. 42-13)
  - Typical radiographic findings may take months or years to become apparent
  - CT and MRI are sensitive for early sacroiliitis

Treatment

- Nonpharmacologic
  - Thin or no pillow
  - Physical therapy to maintain posture and prevent progressive thoracic kyphosis and loss of mobility
  - Breathing exercises to maintain chest wall expansion
- Pharmacologic
  - NSAIDs

42

FIGURE 42-12 Radiographic findings of sacroiliitis in ankylosing spondylitis, with both erosions and sclerosis along the iliac sides of the sacroiliac joints. *(From Harris ED, Budd RC, Genovese MC, et al [eds]: Kelley's textbook of rheumatology, ed 7, Philadelphia, WB Saunders, 2005, Fig. 51-54.)*

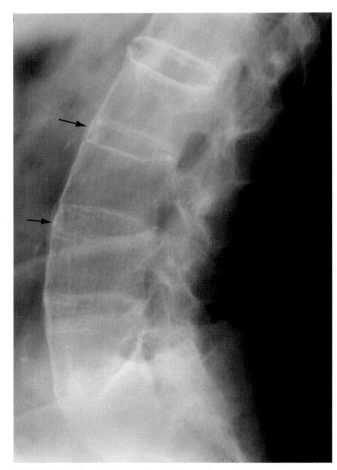

FIGURE 42-13 Radiographic findings of syndesmophytes in ankylosing spondylitis, with bony bridging *(arrows)* extending from the edge of one vertebral body to the next. *(From Harris ED, Budd RC, Genovese MC, et al [eds]: Kelley's textbook of rheumatology, ed 7, Philadelphia, WB Saunders, 2005, Fig. 51-56.)*

- Analgesic and anti-inflammatory effects relieve pain and stiffness
- NSAIDs are not "disease-modifying"
- Indomethacin has traditionally been used, but there is no evidence that one NSAID is superior to another

- Sulfasalazine
  - May slow disease progression
  - Potential for significant toxicity (e.g., GI, hepatic, renal, glucose-6-phosphate dehydrogenase [G6PD] deficiency–associated anemia, myelosuppression, and oligospermia)
- **TNF inhibitors appear to be the first truly "disease-modifying" agents for this disease**
  - Etanercept and infliximab Food and Drug Administration (FDA) approved for this indication

Prevention
- Ankylosing spondylitis is not currently preventable

ENTEROPATHIC ARTHRITIS
Basic Information
- Inflammatory arthritis associated with inflammatory bowel disease (IBD): Crohn disease or ulcerative colitis
- Peripheral arthritis occurs in 10% to 20% of patients with IBD; spondylitis in 10%
- Male-to-female ratio is 3:1 in those with spondylitis

Clinical Presentation
- Axial skeletal disease clinically indistinguishable from ankylosing spondylitis
- Peripheral joint disease most commonly affects the knees, ankles, and feet
- **Peripheral joint disease activity correlates with GI disease activity; axial skeletal disease is independent**
- Extra-axial disease
  - Anterior uveitis
  - Oral aphthous ulcers
  - Erythema nodosum
  - Pyoderma gangrenosum

Diagnosis and Evaluation
- Clinical presentation highly suggestive in classic cases
- History characterized by
  - Coexistence of IBD and arthritis
- Physical examination reveals
  - Manifestations of IBD
  - Inflammatory axial or peripheral joint disease
  - Consider occult IBD in cases of "typical" articular pattern (e.g., isolated knee arthritis) without otherwise symptomatic GI involvement
- Laboratory findings
  - Inflammatory markers may be elevated
  - 50% of patients with spondylitis are HLA-B27 positive
- Radiographic findings are indistinguishable from ankylosing spondylitis

Treatment
- **Treat underlying IBD medically or surgically as indicated**
- NSAIDs must be used cautiously as they may provoke flare of bowel inflammation
- Corticosteroids may be used intravenously, orally, or intra-articularly
- TNF inhibitors
  - Infliximab FDA approved for this indication

Prevention

- Enteropathic arthritis is not currently preventable, beyond treatment of the underlying IBD

PSORIATIC ARTHRITIS

Basic Information

- Inflammatory arthritis associated with psoriatic skin disease
- At least 15% of patients with psoriatic skin disease are affected
- Male-to-female ratio is 1:1

Clinical Presentation

- Psoriasis may precede (70%), present with (15%), or follow (15%) onset of arthritis
- Patterns of joint involvement (not mutually exclusive)
  - Peripheral
    - Symmetrical polyarticular (30–50%; may be clinically indistinguishable from RA, but RF-negative)
    - Asymmetrical oligoarticular (30–50%; "classic" spondyloarthropathy pattern)
    - Distal interphalangeal joints (25%) (frequently associated with nail changes)
    - Arthritis mutilans (5%) (highly destructive)
  - Axial (5%)
    - Sacroiliitis (may be asymptomatic or asymmetrical)
    - Spondylitis (may be discontinuous)
  - Enthesitis
    - Dactylitis ("sausage digit"; Fig. 42-14)
- Extra-articular disease
  - Nail pitting, onycholysis, and "oil drop" sign (yellow-orange discoloration of the nail)
  - Anterior uveitis, aortitis, and pulmonary fibrosis are rare

Diagnosis and Evaluation

- Clinical presentation highly suggestive in classic cases
- History characterized by coexistence of psoriasis and arthritis
- Physical examination reveals
  - Manifestations of psoriatic skin disease
  - Inflammatory axial or peripheral joint disease
- Laboratory findings
  - Inflammatory markers may be elevated
  - 50% of patients with spondylitis are HLA-B27 positive
- Radiographic findings marked by both bony destruction and proliferation
  - Erosive arthritis
  - Osteolysis
  - Sacroiliitis
  - Ankylosis
  - Spondylitis
  - Enthesopathy
  - Periostitis
  - **"Pencil-in-cup" deformity** (i.e., erosion of the distal end of an interphalangeal joint with bony proliferation at the proximal end of the affected joint; Fig. 42-15)

FIGURE 42-14 "Sausage digit" (dactylitis) of the fifth finger in psoriatic arthritis. *(From Harris ED, Budd RC, Genovese MC, et al [eds]: Kelley's textbook of rheumatology, ed 7, Philadelphia, WB Saunders, 2005, Fig. 71-S169.)*

FIGURE 42-15 Bony resorption and osteophyte formation involving the phalanges in psoriatic arthritis creating "pencil-in-cup" changes. *(From Harris ED, Budd RC, Genovese MC, et al [eds]: Kelley's textbook of rheumatology, ed 7, Philadelphia, WB Saunders, 2005, Fig. 72-9.)*

Treatment

- Treat underlying psoriasis as indicated
- NSAIDs
  - Analgesic and anti-inflammatory effects relieve pain and stiffness
- Systemic corticosteroids may provoke flare of skin disease during steroid taper
- Methotrexate effective for both skin and joint disease
- Sulfasalazine
- TNF inhibitors
  - Adalimumab, etanercept, and infliximab all FDA approved for this indication

Prevention

- Psoriatic arthritis is not currently preventable, beyond treatment of the underlying skin disease

REACTIVE ARTHRITIS

Basic Information

- Sterile inflammatory arthritis occurring following a genitourinary or enteric infection
- Reiter disease (arthritis, conjunctivitis, and history of urethritis or enteritis) is the classic triad phenotype
- Etiologic agents: *Chlamydia, Campylobacter, Salmonella, Shigella,* and *Yersinia*
- Typically affects young males
- Male-to-female ratio is 9:1

Clinical Presentation

- **Manifestations typically appear 2 to 4 weeks after genitourinary or enteric infection**
- Patterns of joint involvement
  - Peripheral
    - Lower extremity oligoarthritis (particularly knees, ankles, and feet)
  - Axial
    - Sacroiliitis (may be asymmetrical)
  - Enthesitis
    - Achilles tendinitis
    - Plantar fasciitis
    - Dactylitis ("sausage digit")
- Extra-articular disease
  - Inflammatory eye disease (i.e., conjunctivitis or uveitis)
  - Mucocutaneous manifestations
    - Oral aphthous ulcers
    - Circinate balanitis
    - Keratoderma blenorrhagicum (clinically indistinguishable from psoriasis)
- Epidemiologic association with HIV/AIDS

Diagnosis and Evaluation

- Clinical presentation highly suggestive in classic cases
- History characterized by
  - **Classic triad of arthritis, conjunctivitis, and history of recent urethritis or enteritis**
  - Partial triad raises possibility of forme fruste
- Physical examination as detailed previously
- Laboratory findings
  - Inflammatory markers may be elevated
  - 50% to 80% of patients are HLA-B27 positive; 90% of those with uveitis or sacroiliitis
  - **Urethral swab, or urine nucleic acid detection probe, may be positive for *Chlamydia trachomatis***
  - Stool cultures are usually negative for enteric infections
- Radiographic findings
  - Sacroiliitis
  - Erosions or spurring at insertion of Achilles tendon into plantar fascia (Fig. 42-16)

Treatment

- Disease is usually self-limited, lasting 3 to 12 months
  - Up to 50% of patients may experience relapse (possible reinfection)
  - 15% of patients may experience chronic, destructive, and disabling disease
- NSAIDs

FIGURE 42-16 Calcaneal spur formation at the plantar fascial insertion in reactive arthritis. *(From Harris ED, Budd RC, Genovese MC, et al [eds]: Kelley's textbook of rheumatology, ed 7, Philadelphia, WB Saunders, 2005, Fig. 71-6.)*

- Analgesic and anti-inflammatory effects relieve pain and stiffness
- Doxycycline (3-month course) may be beneficial in patients with persistent disease
- Sulfasalazine may be beneficial in patients with persistent disease
- Methotrexate has been used in patients whose disease is refractory to other measures

Prevention

- Avoidance and early treatment of genitourinary and enteric infections

Septic (Pyogenic/Nongonococcal) Arthritis

Basic Information

- Intensely inflammatory and rapidly destructive arthritis associated with bacterial joint infection
- Populations at risk
  - Chronically ill (e.g., diabetes mellitus, chronic renal failure, and malignancy)
  - Elderly
  - Immunosuppressed (e.g., HIV infection, immunosuppressant medications)
  - Diseased or prosthetic joints
- Routes of infection
  - Direct inoculation
  - Local extension from an adjacent process
  - Hematogenous spread
- Etiology
  - Common agents
    - *Staphylococcus aureus* (~40%)
    - Group A *Streptococcus* (~30%)
    - Gram-negative bacteria (~30%)
  - Injection-drug users may become infected with *Pseudomonas*
  - Sickle cell anemia patients may become infected with *Salmonella*

- **Prosthetic joints are susceptible to infection with *Staphylococcus epidermidis***
- Cat scratches or animal bites may cause *Pasteurella multocida* joint infections

Clinical Presentation

- Most patients present with a monoarticular arthritis
- Oligo- or polyarthritis may be seen with bacteremic route of infection
- Injection-drug users may present with sternoclavicular, sacroiliac, or disk space infections
- Both systemic (fever/chills) and local (joint pain, swelling, erythema, and heat) manifestations
- Distinguish primary cellulitis from skin inflammation attributable to an underlying septic joint

Diagnosis and Evaluation

- Clinical presentation highly suggestive in classic cases
- History as in preceding discussion
- Physical findings as in preceding discussion
- Laboratory findings
  - Synovial fluid analysis is critical
    - Arthrocentesis for cell count, Gram stain, and culture
    - **Highly inflammatory, often with greater than 75,000 cells/mm³ (predominantly neutrophils); 60% to 80% of patients have positive Gram stain**
    - **Synovial fluid leukocyte count greater than 100,000 cells/mm³ is attributed to presumptive septic arthritis until proven otherwise**
    - **Approximately 90% of patients have positive synovial fluid culture**
    - Approximately 50% of patients have positive blood culture
- Radiographic findings
  - May reveal only soft tissue swelling in early disease
  - Joint space narrowing and bony erosions indicate severe and advanced disease
  - CT and MRI may detect fluid in deep joints (e.g., hip and sacroiliac joints)

Treatment

- **Drainage is essential in the management of infected joints**
  - Repeated needle aspiration is adequate for easily accessible joints without loculation
  - Arthroscopy or arthrotomy is required if repeated aspirations do not clear the infection
  - Arthrotomy is indicated as the initial mode of drainage for the hip
- Antibiotics
  - **Broad-spectrum antibiotics must be promptly administered (after arthrocentesis) and continued until the results of the Gram stain and culture are available**
  - Host risk factors (as detailed previously) are taken into consideration with empirical coverage

Prevention

- Avoid risk factors for infection, and treat infections promptly

Disseminated Gonococcal Infection

Basic Information

- Gonococcal (GC) infection is responsible for most cases of septic arthritis in young adults
- Female-to-male ratio is 3:1; women are more likely to have asymptomatic GC infection
- Congenital complement deficiency is a risk factor

Clinical Presentation

- **May present as migratory arthritis or tenosynovitis, with or without rash**
- **May also present as purulent arthritis most commonly involving the wrist, knee, or ankle**
- Systemic manifestations (fevers and chills) may be present
- Macular, papular, or pustular rash may be present on the trunk or extremities

Diagnosis and Evaluation

- Clinical presentation highly suggestive in classic cases
- History characterized by
  - Sexually active young adult
  - Pharyngeal, urethral, cervical, and anal symptoms may be present but are frequently absent
- Physical findings as in the previous discussion
- Laboratory findings
  - Synovial fluid analysis
    - Arthrocentesis for cell count, Gram stain, and culture
    - Highly inflammatory with greater than 2000 WBCs/mm³
    - **Gram stain usually negative**
    - Culture positive in less than 50% of cases
  - Blood and skin lesion cultures rarely positive
  - **Culture pharynx, urethra, cervix, and anus as potential sources of infection**
- Radiographic findings
  - May reveal soft tissue swelling

Treatment

- Repeated needle aspiration may be necessary, but arthroscopy and arthrotomy are rarely needed
- Sensitive to third-generation cephalosporins

Prevention

- Avoid risk factors for infection, and treat infections promptly

Viral Arthritis

Basic Information

- Common agents
  - Parvovirus B19
  - Rubella virus
  - Hepatitis B and C viruses
- Both children and adults affected

Clinical Presentation

- **May present as migratory arthralgias/arthritis or polyarthritis**

- Most commonly affects the wrists, hands, and knees
- Frequently symmetrical
- Rash may be present
- Hepatitis-associated arthritis may precede icterus

Diagnosis and Evaluation

- There may be a history of recent vaccination or exposure to sick contacts

Treatment

- **Most viral arthritides are self-limited, and are best managed supportively**
- Parvovirus may occasionally cause a chronic arthropathy

Prevention

- Avoid risk factors for infection

Lyme Disease

See also Chapter 16.

Basic Information

- Multisystem inflammatory disease caused by the tick-borne spirochete *Borrelia burgdorferi*
- 90% of cases reported from eight states (NY, NJ, CT, RI, MA, PA, WI, and MN)

Clinical Presentation

- Early localized disease (<30 days after infection)
  - Fever, malaise, headache, arthralgias, myalgias, and erythema migrans (50–90%)
- Early disseminated disease (weeks to months after infection)
  - Cardiac (e.g., heart block) and neurologic (e.g., Bell palsy)
- Late disseminated disease (months to years after infection)
  - Cutaneous, neurologic, fibromyalgia-like, and articular (chronic knee arthritis in 10%)

Diagnosis and Evaluation

- **5% of the population has false-positive enzyme-linked immunosorbent assay (ELISA)**
- Confirmation by Western blot

Treatment

- Arthritis treated with
  - Doxycycline (100 mg PO twice daily × 14–21 days)
  - Amoxicillin (500 mg PO three times daily × 21–30 days)
  - Ceftriaxone (2 g IV once daily × 14–28 days)

Prevention

- Avoid risk factors for infection, and treat infections promptly

Tuberculous Arthritis

Basic Information

- Develops in only a small percentage of cases of tuberculosis

Clinical Presentation

- Chronic granulomatous arthritis
  - Monoarticular
  - Usually involves the hips, knees, or ankles
  - Chronic joint pain and swelling
  - Usually not associated with active pulmonary TB
- Poncet disease (tuberculous rheumatism; rare)
  - Symmetrical polyarthritis
  - Seen in conjunction with active disseminated infection

Diagnosis and Evaluation

- Chronic granulomatous arthritis
  - Acid-fast stain and culture of synovial fluid may be positive
  - Synovial biopsy may demonstrate granulomatous inflammation
  - Synovial tissue culture is usually positive
- Poncet disease
  - Acid-fast stain and mycobacterial culture are negative

Treatment

- Six to 9 months of combination antituberculosis therapy

REVIEW QUESTIONS

For review questions, please go to www.expertconsult.com.

SUGGESTED READINGS

Firestein GS, Budd RC, Harris Jr ED, et al editors: *Kelley's textbook of rheumatology*, ed 8, Philadelphia, 2009, Elsevier Saunders.
Hochberg MC, Silman AJ, Smolen JS, et al editors: *Rheumatology*, ed 5, Philadelphia, 2011, Elsevier Saunders.
Klippel JH, Stone JH, Crofford LJ, White PH, editors: *Primer on the rheumatic diseases*, ed 13, Atlanta, 2008, Arthritis Foundation.
Levine SM, Gelber AC: Infectious monoarthritis. In Cheng A, Zaas A, editors: *The Osler medical handbook*, Philadelphia, 2003, Mosby.
Tehlirian C, Gelber AC: Connective tissue diseases. In Nilsson KR Jr, Piccini JP, editors: *The Osler medical handbook*, ed 2, Philadelphia, 2006, Elsevier Saunders.

CHAPTER 43

Office Orthopedics

SABIHA KHAN, MD; and JOHN A. FLYNN, MD, MBA, MEᴅ

Office orthopedics covers a broad spectrum of disorders, many of which are not primarily articular and are variously characterized as "regional, soft tissue, or musculoskeletal pain syndromes." These disorders are common; occur in isolation or as part of a systemic process; involve any of the articular or periarticular soft tissues; cause pain; and may cause progressive functional disability. **In addition, few if any specific diagnostic laboratory tests apply to these disorders, with the diagnosis depending instead on a detailed history and physical examination.**

Shoulder

Figure 43-1 illustrates normal shoulder range of motion.

Basic Information
- Shoulder pain is one of the most common musculoskeletal complaints
- In younger patients (<40 years), symptoms are often caused by acute (e.g., sports-related) injuries
- In older patients, symptoms are more likely caused by chronic, degenerative changes of the rotator cuff
- Table 43-1 compares the most common disorders

Elbow

LATERAL EPICONDYLITIS ("TENNIS ELBOW")
Cause
- Repetitive wrist extension and forearm rotation

Clinical Presentation
- Lateral elbow pain

Diagnosis and Evaluation
- Tenderness over lateral epicondyle
- Pain elicited by resisted wrist extension and forearm supination (Fig. 43-2)

Treatment
- Rest
- Nonsteroidal anti-inflammatory drugs (NSAIDs)
- Steroid injection
- Bracing
- Physical therapy

MEDIAL EPICONDYLITIS ("GOLFER'S ELBOW")
Cause
- Repetitive wrist flexion and forearm rotation

Clinical Presentation
- Medial elbow pain

Diagnosis and Evaluation
- Tenderness over medial epicondyle
- Pain elicited by resisted wrist flexion and forearm pronation (see Fig. 43-2)

Treatment
- Same as for lateral epicondylitis

ULNAR NEUROPATHY
Cause
- Trauma to the ulnar nerve as it traverses the elbow joint

Clinical Presentation
- Posteromedial forearm and fourth and fifth digit and paresthesias

Diagnosis and Evaluation
- Tenderness with percussion over the cubital tunnel
- Decreased sensation in the ulnar nerve distribution

Treatment
- Modification of activity
- NSAIDs
- Splinting
- Surgery is sometimes required for decompression

RADIAL NEUROPATHY
Cause
- Compression of the motor branch of the radial nerve as it traverses the elbow joint between radial head and supinator

Clinical Presentation
- Proximal forearm ache, and possible paresthesias radiating to dorsal radial surface of hand and forearm

Diagnosis and Evaluation
- Reproduction of pain with resisted supination
- Reproduction of pain with elbow flexion while forearm is in supination

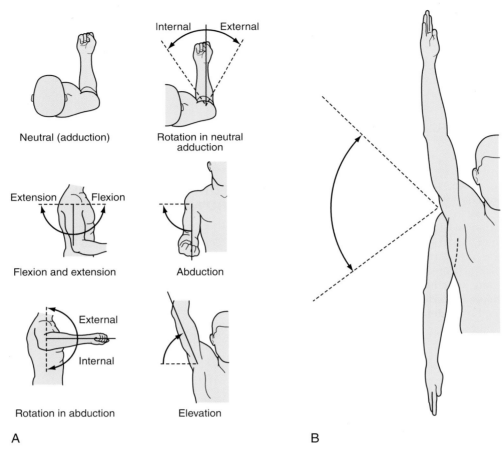

FIGURE 43-1 **A** and **B,** Normal shoulder range of motion. *(From Swash M: Hutchison's clinical methods, ed 21, Philadelphia, WB Saunders, 2001, Fig. 10.30.)*

TABLE 43-1	*Common Disorders of the Shoulder*			
	Rotator Cuff Tendinitis	**Rotator Cuff Tear**	**Adhesive Capsulitis**	**Bicipital Tendinitis**
Cause	Overuse	Trauma Recurrent rotator cuff tendinitis	Prolonged shoulder immobilization	Overuse
Clinical presentation	Anterolateral shoulder pain	Anterolateral shoulder pain	Shoulder pain Loss of motion	Anterior shoulder pain
Diagnosis and evaluation	Pain with Abduction < resisted abduction Internal and external rotation Lateral palpation Positive "impingement test"*	Same as rotator cuff tendinitis Positive "drop test"[†] with full-thickness tear	Painful and limited active and passive motion	Tenderness over bicipital groove Positive "Speed's test"[‡] Positive "Yergason's sign"[§]
Treatment	Rest NSAIDs Steroid injection Physical therapy	Orthopedic evaluation for repair	Physical therapy Steroid injection Possible orthopedics referral	Rest NSAIDs Steroid injection Physical therapy

*Relief of pain after injection of the subacromial bursa.
[†]Unable to maintain active shoulder abduction.
[‡]Pain with resisted shoulder flexion.
[§]Pain with resisted forearm supination.

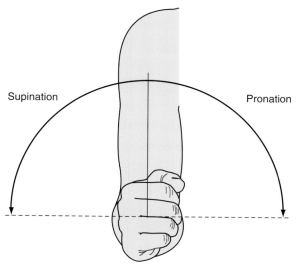

FIGURE 43-2   Forearm pronation and supination. (From Swash M: Hutchison's clinical methods, ed 21, Philadelphia, WB Saunders, 2001, Fig. 10.32.)

FIGURE 43-3   Thenar eminence wasting due to carpal tunnel syndrome. (From Swash M: Hutchison's clinical methods, ed 21, Philadelphia, WB Saunders, 2001, Fig. 10.13.)

- Diagnostic lidocane injection at lateral epicondyle to differentate etiology, as symptoms are similar to lateral epicondylitis

Treatment
- Modification of activity
- NSAIDs
- Splinting
- Surgery is sometimes required for decompression

OLECRANON BURSITIS
Cause
- Trauma
- Infection secondary to overlying cellulitis (most commonly gram-positive bacteria, especially *Staphylococcus aureus*)
- Gout and pseudogout
- Rheumatoid arthritis

Clinical Presentation
- Pain and swelling over olecranon process

Diagnosis and Evaluation
- Inflamed olecranon bursa
- Pain with flexion, but not extension
- Examination of bursa fluid critical to diagnose infection

Treatment
- Rest and treatment of the underlying cause
- NSAIDs for gout
- Drainage and antibiotics for infection

Hand and Wrist

Basic Information
- The hand and wrist are subject to a number of common conditions, many of which may be attributed to overuse or repetitive use (Fig. 43-3)
- Table 43-2 compares the most common disorders

Hip

Figure 43-4 illustrates normal range of motion in the hip.

TROCHANTERIC BURSITIS
Cause
- Overuse
- Trauma
- Associated with obesity

Clinical Presentation
- Deep aching lateral hip pain extending to buttock or lateral knee
- Painful to lie in lateral decubitus position

Diagnosis and Evaluation
- Pain on palpation over greater trochanter
- Pain with resisted hip abduction

Treatment
- Rest
- NSAIDs
- Steroid injection
- Physical therapy

MERALGIA PARESTHETICA
Cause
- Entrapment of lateral femoral cutaneous nerve
- Associated with obesity, pregnancy, diabetes, and tight clothing

Clinical Presentation
- Numbness and paresthesias over anterolateral thigh

Diagnosis and Evaluation
- Anterolateral thigh sensory deficit
- Tender over inguinal ligament

43

TABLE 43-2	Common Disorders of the Wrist and Hand				
	Carpal Tunnel Syndrome	Ulnar Tunnel Syndrome	De Quervain Tenosynovitis	Trigger Finger	Dupuytren Contracture
Cause	Median nerve compression at wrist	Ulnar nerve compression at wrist	Abductor policis longus and extensor policis brevis tendon inflammation	Inflammation and stenosis of digital flexor tendon	Contracture of palmar fascia
Precipitating factors	Overuse Synovitis Hypothyroidism Amyloidosis Acromegaly Pregnancy	Overuse Trauma Ganglion cyst	Overuse Rheumatoid arthritis	Overuse Rheumatoid arthritis	Heredity Alcoholism Diabetes Epilepsy
Clinical presentation	Numbness and paresthesias in median nerve distribution* Nocturnal exacerbation Wasting of thenar eminence (see Fig. 43-3)	Numbness and paresthesias in ulnar nerve distribution†	Wrist pain extending from thumb	Tendon catches with flexion of digit	Unable to fully extend digits
Diagnosis and evaluation	Median nerve Tinel's sign‡ Phalen's sign§ Abnormal nerve conduction test and electromyography	Ulnar nerve "Tinel's sign"‡ Abnormal nerve conduction test and electromyography	Tender over radial styloid Finkelstein test¶	Pain and palpable "catch" with digit flexion Nodule may be palpable	Flexion deformity of fourth > fifth > third > second digits Palpable thickening of palmar fascia
Treatment	Wrist splint NSAIDs Steroid injection Surgical release	Wrist splint NSAIDs Surgical release	Wrist/thumb splint NSAIDs Steroid injection Surgery	Occupational therapy Steroid injection Surgical release	Surgical excision in extreme cases

*First–third fingers and radial half of the fourth.
†Fifth finger and ulnar half of the fourth.
‡Provoke pain and paresthesia with percussion over nerve at the wrist.
§Provoke pain, paresthesia, and numbness with forced wrist flexion (reversed "prayer position").
¶Provoke pain with forced ulnar deviation of the wrist, with thumb enclosed by fist.

Treatment

- NSAIDs
- Treat underlying condition

Hip and Knee

ILIOTIBIAL BAND SYNDROME

Cause
- Overuse of iliotibial band (e.g., running)

Clinical Presentation
- Pain over lateral thigh above the joint line of the knee

Diagnosis and Evaluation
- Tender over lateral femoral condyle
- Pain when standing on flexed knee

Treatment
- Rest
- NSAIDs
- Steroid injection
- Physical therapy

Knee

See Figure 43-5 for ligaments of the knee joint.

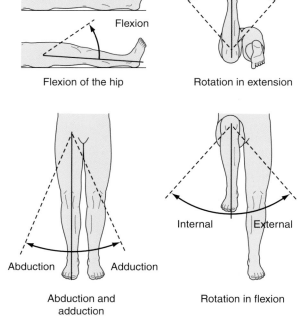

FIGURE 43-4   Normal hip range of motion. (From Swash M: Hutchison's clinical methods, ed 21, Philadelphia, WB Saunders, 2001, Fig. 10.39.)

Basic Information

- The knee, by virtue of its weight-bearing status, is subject to a variety of disorders
- Table 43-3 compares the most common disorders
- McMurray test
  - Flex the knee as much as possible
    - Medial meniscus evaluated by externally rotating the foot and extending the knee
    - Lateral meniscus evaluated by internally rotating the foot and extending the knee
    - A positive test occurs when maneuver provokes pain at the appropriate meniscus; occasionally a click may also be palpated

Ankle

ACHILLES TENDINITIS

Cause

- Overuse, poor training habits, and improper footwear in athletes
- Fluoroquinolone antibiotics
- Associated with spondyloarthritis

Clinical Presentation

- Pain along the Achilles tendon

Diagnosis and Evaluation

- Tenderness and thickening along the tendon
- Dorsiflexion of foot is painful

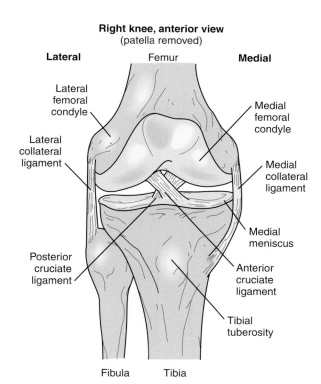

Right knee, anterior view
(patella removed)

Lateral — Femur — Medial

- Lateral femoral condyle
- Lateral collateral ligament
- Posterior cruciate ligament
- Medial femoral condyle
- Medial collateral ligament
- Medial meniscus
- Anterior cruciate ligament
- Tibial tuberosity

Fibula   Tibia

FIGURE 43-5 Anterior view of the knee demonstrating the anterior and posterior cruciate ligaments. *(From Gosling J, Willan PLT, Whitmore I, Harris PF: Human anatomy: color atlas and text, ed 4, St. Louis, Mosby, 2002, Fig. 6.78.)*

Treatment

- NSAIDs
- Heel lift
- Stretching program
- If underlying spondyloarthritis is detected (ankylosing spondylitis, psoriatic arthritis, reactive, or inflammatory bowel disease related), treatment is directed at underlying condition

ACHILLES TENDON RUPTURE

Cause

- Forced dorsiflexion of the foot as the gastrocnemius muscle contracts
- Males affected more than females

Clinical Presentation

- Tearing and popping sensation in the calf

Diagnosis and Evaluation

- Swelling of the calf
- Weakness of foot flexion
- Palpation of gap caused by tendon rupture
- Abnormal Thompson test (failure of the foot to plantar flex when squeezing the gastrocnemius muscle)

Treatment

- Orthopedic evaluation and possible repair

TARSAL TUNNEL SYNDROME

Cause

- Posterior tibial nerve entrapment behind the medial malleolus
- Associated with pes planus (flat feet), ganglion cyst, and lipomata

Clinical Presentation

- Burning pain over the medial and plantar aspects of the foot
- Aggravated by activity

Diagnosis and Evaluation

- Posterior tibial nerve (Tinel's sign) posterior to the medial malleolus
- Decreased sensation over medial and plantar aspects of the foot
- Nerve conduction study if examination equivocal

Treatment

- Orthotics
- Surgery occasionally necessary

Foot

PLANTAR FASCIITIS

Cause

- Overuse, causing inflammation of plantar fascia
- Heel spur
- Associated with spondyloarthritis

43

TABLE 43-3   *Common Disorders of the Knee*

	Chondromalacia Patellae	Meniscal Injury	Collateral Ligament Injury	Anterior Cruciate Ligament Injury	Posterior Cruciate Ligament Injury	Prepatellar Bursitis	Anserine Bursitis	Ruptured Baker Cyst (Pseudothrombophlebitis)
Cause	Patellofemoral cartilage degeneration	Trauma	Overuse Trauma	Twisting injury to knee with foot planted	Hyperextension injury to knee	Overuse Trauma Infection Gout	Overuse Osteoarthritis	One-way flow of knee effusion to gastrocnemius–semimembranosus bursa
Clinical presentation	Anterior knee pain when climbing stairs	Pain Swelling Catching Locking Buckling	Medial or lateral knee pain	Pain Swelling Instability	Pain Swelling Instability	Anterior knee pain Swelling	Anteromedial pain 4–5 cm below joint line	Popliteal fullness Calf pain, swelling, and ecchymosis on rupture
Diagnosis and evaluation	Tender with patellar compression	Tender joint margin Pain with motion Pain with McMurray test	Tenderness over affected ligament Provoke pain with medial or lateral stress in 20° of flexion	Swelling Anterior instability of the tibia at the knee (anterior drawer sign)	Swelling Posterior instability of the tibia at the knee (posterior drawer sign)	Swollen and tender prepatellar bursa Aspirate to diagnose cause	Tender with palpation Pain with knee flexion	Rule out deep venous thrombosis with ultrasound (Fig. 43-6)
Treatment	Quadriceps strengthening exercises NSAIDs Rarely surgery	Rest NSAIDs Physical therapy Possible surgical meniscectomy	Rest Physical therapy Surgery if unstable	Orthopedic evaluation	Orthopedic evaluation	Rest NSAIDs Antibiotic if needed	Rest NSAIDs Steroid injection Physical therapy	Rest Elevation Steroid injection

Clinical Presentation
- Heel and posterior foot pain
- Sensation of "walking on pebbles"
- Classically, with the first steps of the morning and after prolonged sitting
- Improves with use

Diagnosis and Evaluation
- Tenderness on plantar aspect of heel

Treatment
- Stretching
- Orthotics
- NSAIDs
- Steroid injection
- Rarely surgery

MORTON NEUROMA
Cause
- Neuroma formation causing compression of digital nerve in foot

Clinical Presentation
- Pain and paresthesias
- Most commonly between third and fourth toes

Diagnosis and Evaluation
- Tenderness to deep palpation between toes
- Neuroma may be palpable

Treatment
- Metatarsal bar orthotic
- Steroid injection
- Surgical excision of neuroma

Cervical Spine

Figure 43-7 shows normal cervical spine range of motion.

FIGURE 43-6 Arthrogram demonstrating a ruptured Baker cyst. *(From Forbes CD, Jackson WF: Color atlas and text of clinical medicine, ed 3, St. Louis, Mosby, 2003, Fig. 3.28.)*

CERVICAL SPINE STRAIN
Cause
- Overuse
- Poor posture
- Hyperextension injury

Clinical Presentation
- Neck pain and stiffness
- No symptoms or signs of radiculopathy

Diagnosis and Evaluation
- Localized tenderness over cervical musculature
- Absence of neurologic deficits (Table 43-4)

Treatment
- NSAIDs
- Soft cervical collar
- Physical therapy

CERVICAL DISK DISEASE
Cause
- Disk herniation

Clinical Presentation
- Neck pain and stiffness
- Radicular complaints (weakness, numbness, paresthesias along involved nerve root)
- Worse with straining

Diagnosis and Evaluation
- Symptoms exacerbated with neck compression
- Abnormal neurologic examination (Fig. 43-8; see also Table 43-4)

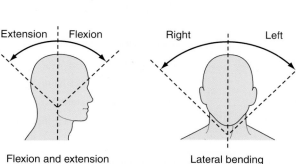

FIGURE 43-7 Normal cervical spine range of motion. *(From Swash M: Hutchison's clinical methods, ed 21, Philadelphia, WB Saunders, 2001, Fig. 10.26.)*

Treatment

- Initially conservative
- NSAIDs
- Soft collar
- Surgical evaluation for intractable pain or progressive neurologic deficits

FIGURE 43-8 Cervical nerve root dermatomal distribution in the upper extremity. *(From Gosling J, Willan PLT, Whitmore I, Harris PF: Human anatomy: color atlas and text, ed 4, St. Louis, Mosby, 2002, Fig. 3.6.)*

Lumbar Spine

Figure 43-9 shows normal lumbar spine range of motion.

Basic Information

- Low back pain is one of the most common musculoskeletal complaints
- 80% of the population experience low back pain at some time in their life
- Low back pain is generally a self-limited condition
  - 50% are better in 1 week
  - 90% are better in 6 weeks
  - Sciatica can have a more protracted course, but 50% recover in 4 weeks

Clinical Presentation

- Acute low back pain (Box 43-1)
- Spinal stenosis
  - Caused by impingement on lumbosacral spinal cord
  - Associated with degenerative arthritis
  - Pseudoclaudication (nonvascular claudication improving with flexion at the waist)

Diagnosis and Evaluation

- Lumbar spine examination (Fig. 43-10; see also Table 43-4)
- Straight leg raise test
  - Sensitive (>90%) but not specific
  - Pain should be radicular
  - Helpful in ruling out sciatica
  - Crossed straight leg raise test less sensitive (25%) but more specific (80%)
- Indications for radiographic evaluation
  - Preceding significant trauma
  - Evolving neurologic findings
  - Suggestion of malignancy or infection
  - Suspect lumbar spinal stenosis
  - Older age
  - Persistent pain

Treatment

- Rest
- Heat and cold
- NSAIDs

TABLE 43-4	*Cervical and Lumbar Spine Neurologic Examination*		
Nerve Root	**Motor Function**	**Sensory Function**	**Reflex**
C5	Deltoid and biceps (elbow flexion)	Shoulder and lateral aspect of arm	Biceps
C6*	Biceps and wrist extensors	Lateral forearm and thumb	Biceps
C7	Triceps (elbow extension)	Middle finger	Triceps
C8	Finger flexors	Medial forearm and little finger	None
T1	Intrinsic muscles of the hand	Medial aspect of arm	None
L4	Quadriceps (knee extension)	Medial aspect of calf and ankle	Quadriceps (knee)
L5	Tibialis anterior (ankle dorsiflexion)†	Dorsum of foot	None
S1	Gastrocnemius (ankle plantar flexion)‡	Lateral aspect of ankle and foot	Gastrocnemius (ankle)

*May be confused with carpal tunnel syndrome.
†Cannot stand on heels.
‡Cannot stand on toes.

FIGURE 43-9 Normal lumbar spine range of motion. *(From Swash M: Hutchison's clinical methods, ed 21, Philadelphia, WB Saunders, 2001, Fig. 10.28.)*

1. Flexion
2. Extension
3. Lateral bending
4. Rotation

FIGURE 43-10 Lumbar nerve root dermatomal distribution in the lower extremity. *(From Gosling J, Willan PLT, Whitmore I, Harris PF: Human anatomy: color atlas and text, ed 4, St. Louis, 2002, Mosby, Fig. 6.10.)*

43

BOX 43-1   *Low Back Pain*

Local Causes

Muscle strain
Lumbar spine osteoarthritis
Degenerative disk disease
Hip osteoarthritis
Vertebral body infection
Vertebral body malignancy
Disk space infection

Distant Causes

Ulcer disease
Pancreatitis
Nephrolithiasis
Prostatitis
Aortic dissection
Subacute bacterial endocarditis
Pelvic pathology

Worrisome Findings

Nocturnal pain
   Cancer
   Infection
Writhing pain
   Aneurysm
   Perforated viscus
Evolving neurologic deficits
   Epidural abscess
   Hemorrhage
   Disk herniation
Fever
   Infection

- Physical therapy
- Surgery may be indicated (e.g., infection, intractable pain, neurologic defects, and spinal stenosis)

REVIEW QUESTIONS

For review questions, please go to www.expertconsult.com.

SUGGESTED READINGS

Biundo JJ: Musculoskeletal signs and symptoms: regional rheumatic pain syndromes. In Klippel JH, editor: *Primer on the rheumatic diseases*, ed 12, Atlanta, 2001, Arthritis Foundation.

Borenstein D: Musculoskeletal signs and symptoms: disorders of the low back and neck. In Klippel JH, editor: *Primer on the rheumatic diseases*, ed 12, Atlanta, 2001, Arthritis Foundation.

Ruddy S, Harris ED, Sledge CB: Musculoskeletal pain and evaluation. In Ruddy S, Harris ED, Sledge CB, editors: *Kelley's textbook of rheumatology*, ed 6, Philadelphia, 2001, WB Saunders.

CHAPTER 44

Vasculitis

PHILIP SEO, MD, MHS

The systemic vasculitides (vasculitis) are autoimmune disorders characterized by inflammation of blood vessels. The vasculitides can affect almost any organ system and often lead to significant morbidity. There are at least 20 recognized individual disorders, differentiated clinically by (1) the size of blood vessel typically involved, (2) their predilection for certain organ systems, and (3) characteristic pathologic features. Classifying the vasculitides by the size of the predominant vessels involved is a valuable method of categorizing these diseases: large-vessel vasculitis predominantly affects the aorta and the great vessels; medium-vessel vasculitis affects predominantly the splanchnic vessels; and small-vessel vasculitis affects the capillaries, arterioles, and venules that provide circulation to the lungs, kidneys, and skin. A widely accepted classification scheme based on blood vessel size is depicted in Box 44-1.

Behçet Disease

Basic Information

- Widest range of blood vessel involvement of all the vasculitides: Small, medium, and large vessels, in both the venous and arterial circulations
- Found most commonly in the regions that once made up the old Silk Route: Turkey, Iran, China, and Japan
- Associated with human leukocyte antigen (HLA)-B51

Clinical Presentation

- **Classic triad of signs is oral ulcers (Fig. 44-1), genital ulcers, and ocular inflammation**
  - Oral ulcers: By themselves, may be seen in a variety of autoimmune diseases
  - Genital ulcers: Commonly heal with scarring and virtually pathognomonic of Behçet disease
  - Ocular inflammation
    - Anterior uveitis: May manifest as a hypopyon (pus in the anterior chamber); asymmetrical pupils may also be present because of synechiae formation between the lens and iris
    - Posterior uveitis: May manifest as retinal vasculitis
  - Folliculitis
  - Erythema nodosum
    - In contrast to erythema nodosum associated with other conditions, they may ulcerate and heal with scarring

- Biopsy often reveals medium-vessel vasculitis rather than septal panniculitis
- **Pathergy: Development of sterile pustules at sites of needle stick; only a minority of patients demonstrate the pathergy phenomenon, but when present, this lesion is highly suggestive of Behçet disease**
- Superficial and deep venous thrombophlebitis
- Cerebral venous thrombosis
- Aseptic meningitis
- Brainstem involvement: May mimic multiple sclerosis because of its tendency to involve white matter
- Arthritis: Typically nondeforming

Diagnosis and Evaluation

- No specific laboratory or histologic findings are diagnostic
- Manifestations may occur simultaneously or be separated by several years
- Diagnosis based on physician observation of the various clinical manifestations and recognition of the characteristic constellation of physical findings, guided by the International Study Group criteria, which require recurrent oral ulceration plus two of the following four manifestations:
  - **Recurrent genital ulceration**
  - **Eye lesions**
  - **Skin lesions**
  - **Positive pathergy test**

Treatment

- A variety of regimens have been used, based on the extent and severity of involvement
  - For mucocutaneous disease
    - Colchicine: First-line therapy for oral ulcers; effective only in milder cases; may be used up to three times per day if tolerated gastrointestinally
    - Topical glucocorticoids: Limited efficacy for oral and genital ulcers
  - For more refractory disease
    - Low-dose systemic glucocorticoids
    - Thalidomide: For mucocutaneous lesions
    - Azathioprine
    - Tumor necrosis factor inhibitors
  - For the most serious disease manifestations, including central nervous system (CNS) and uveitis (because of the risk for blindness)
    - High-dose systemic glucocorticoids
    - Cyclophosphamide

FIGURE 44-2 Digital ischemia in Buerger disease.

BOX 44-1 *Classification of the Vasculitides*

Predominantly or Exclusively Small-Vessel Vasculitides

Immune complex–mediated
  Cutaneous leukocytoclastic angiitis (hypersensitivity vasculitis)
  Henoch-Schönlein purpura
  Urticarial vasculitis
  Cryoglobulinemia*
  Connective tissue disorders*
  Erythema elevatum diutinum
ANCA-associated disorders
  Wegener granulomatosis*
  Microscopic polyangiitis*
  Churg-Strauss syndrome*
Miscellaneous small-vessel vasculitides
  Paraneoplastic
  Infection
  Inflammatory bowel disease

Predominantly or Exclusively Medium-Vessel Vasculitides

Classic polyarteritis nodosa
Cutaneous polyarteritis nodosa
Rheumatoid vasculitis*
Kawasaki disease
Buerger disease (thromboangiitis obliterans)

Predominantly Large-Vessel Vasculitides

Giant-cell (temporal) arteritis
Takayasu arteritis
Cogan syndrome
Behçet disease†

ANCA, antineutrophil cytoplasmic antibody.
*Common overlap of small- and medium-sized blood vessel involvement.
†May involve small-, medium-, and large-sized blood vessels.

FIGURE 44-1 Aphthous oral ulcers in Behçet disease.

Buerger Disease (Thromboangiitis Obliterans)

Basic Information

- Manifestations primarily caused by involvement of medium-sized arteries, but veins affected as well
- Should not be confused with Berger disease (immunoglobulin [Ig]A nephropathy)

Clinical Presentation

- **Typical patient is young male smoker with digital infarction, although it may also occur in female smokers**
- Striking contrast between the severity of digital vasculitis and absence of internal organ disease
- Does not involve smallest vessels (i.e., capillaries) and is therefore more likely to be associated with digital infarction (Fig. 44-2) than with purpura

Diagnosis and Evaluation

- Superficial thrombophlebitis may be the first sign
- Should be considered high on the differential diagnosis when there is severe digital ischemia involving two or more extremities but no other organ dysfunction
- **Angiography reveals distinctive "corkscrew" collateral vessels in blood vessels at the level of the wrists and ankles**

Treatment

- **Smoking cessation is the only effective form of treatment**
- No form of immunosuppression (including glucocorticoids) provides control or cure
- Continued smoking may result in progression of ischemia and the need for amputation

Churg-Strauss Syndrome (Allergic Granulomatosis and Angiitis)

Basic Information

- Characterized by necrotizing inflammation within small arteries, veins, and capillaries
- Classically described as a clinical triad of asthma, hypereosinophilia, and vasculitis

44

Clinical Presentation

- **Typical patient presents with the recent onset of allergy or asthma, followed by eosinophilic tissue infiltration and the subsequent development of symptoms and signs of vasculitis**
- Asthma associated with the Churg-Strauss syndrome may improve as the vasculitic phase begins
- Typical symptoms and signs include
  - **Sinusitis: Nondestructive, in contrast to Wegener granulomatosis**
  - Wheezing
  - **Mononeuritis multiplex: Neuropathy involving named motor and sensory nerves, often acute in onset, which manifests as the inability to dorsiflex the foot or to hyperextend the wrist (i.e., footdrop or wristdrop)**
  - Cutaneous nodules: Cutaneous extravascular necrotizing granuloma
    - May mimic rheumatoid nodules
    - Also known as Churg-Strauss granuloma or Winkelman granuloma
    - Usually occurs over extensor surfaces (e.g., the olecranon)

Diagnosis and Evaluation

- In addition to the characteristic clinical features, distinctive diagnostic features include the following:
  - Fleeting pulmonary infiltrates (30% of cases)
  - **Eosinophilia (up to 60,000 eosinophils/mm³)**
  - Positive antineutrophil cytoplasmic antibody (ANCA) (50% of cases): When present, the antibodies are against myeloperoxidase (MPO-ANCA), which is associated with a peripheral staining pattern (P-ANCA) when using immunofluorescence.
- Biopsy may help confirm the diagnosis

Treatment

- **Usually responds dramatically to glucocorticoids alone**
- Eosinophilia disappears with glucocorticoids; the eosinophilia associated with the idiopathic hypereosinophilic syndromes may be less steroid responsive
- Cyclophosphamide may be required for refractory cases

Cogan Syndrome

Basic Information

- Large-vessel vasculitis (e.g., aortitis) occurs in approximately 10% of patients
- The ocular inflammation and sensorineural hearing loss are presumed secondary to small-vessel vasculitis

Clinical Presentation

- **Typical patient presents with ocular disease (interstitial keratitis) and sensorineural hearing loss**
- Eye and ear disease do not always begin simultaneously, but usually occur within a few months of each other
- Symptoms and signs may include
  - Ocular manifestations
    - Interstitial keratitis (pain, photophobia, decreased visual acuity, and red eye) is most common

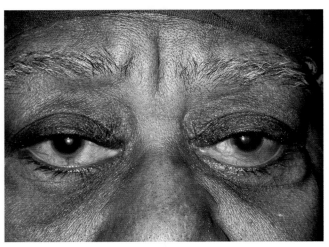

FIGURE 44-3   Scleritis in Cogan syndrome.

- Episcleritis
- Scleritis (Fig. 44-3)
- Retinal disease
- Uveitis
- Sensorineural manifestations
  - Tinnitus
  - Hearing loss
  - Vertigo
  - Oscillopsia
- Constitutional symptoms present in 50% of patients
- 10% of patients present with a large-vessel vasculitis mimicking Takayasu arteritis

Diagnosis and Evaluation

- Diagnosis based on distinctive combination of eye and ear inflammation
- **Important to exclude syphilis and acoustic neuromas**

Treatment

- Topical glucocorticoids used for interstitial keratitis
- Systemic glucocorticoids required for other manifestations
- Sensorineural hearing loss must be treated promptly and aggressively to avoid permanent hearing loss and may require cyclophosphamide

Cryoglobulinemia (Essential Mixed Cryoglobulinemia)

Basic Information

- **Cryoglobulins are immunoglobulins that precipitate out of serum in cold conditions**
- Cryoglobulinemia affects small- to medium-sized arteries, capillaries, and veins

Clinical Presentation

- **Typical patient has hepatitis C virus infection (causes 90% of cases)**
- Symptoms and signs
  - Recurrent purpura
  - Hyperpigmentation that results from repeated bouts of purpura (Fig. 44-4)
  - Brawny induration that mimics venous stasis disease

FIGURE 44-4 Hyperpigmentation and ulceration of the legs due to mixed cryoglobulinemia associated with hepatitis C.

TABLE 44-1	*Subtypes of Cryoglobulinemia*		
	Type I	**Type II**	**Type III**
Monoclonality of immunoglobulin component?	Yes (usually IgG)	Yes (IgM)	No
Rheumatoid factor activity?	No	Yes	Yes
Clinical syndrome	Hyperviscosity	Vasculitis	Vasculitis
Disease association	Hematopoietic malignancy	Hepatitis C Rheumatic diseases Malignancies Idiopathic	Hepatitis C Rheumatic diseases Idiopathic

IgG, immunoglobulin G; IgM, immunoglobulin M.

- Livedo reticularis
- Raynaud's phenomenon
- Digital infarction
- Mononeuritis multiplex (e.g., footdrop)
- Glomerulonephritis (seen only with type II cryoglobulinemia)
- CNS vasculitis (rare)

Diagnosis and Evaluation

- Based on clinical presentation and isolation of cryoglobulins (from blood samples kept at body temperature until transport to the lab)
- Classification (and clinical manifestations) based on properties of cryoproteins present (Table 44-1)
- **Hypocomplementemia is a hallmark of cryoglobulinemic vasculitis because the disorder is mediated by immune complex deposition**
- **Pattern of hypocomplementemia is distinctive: C4 levels are decreased out of proportion to C3**
- Patients with cryoglobulinemia are often initially misdiagnosed as having either rheumatoid arthritis or lupus for the following reasons:
  - Vast majority are positive for rheumatoid factor (IgM component of mixed cryoglobulins has rheumatoid factor activity)

- Majority are antinuclear antibody (ANA) positive
- Hypocomplementemia is also commonly seen in lupus

Treatment

- Interferon-alfa and ribavirin for hepatitis C–related cases
- Glucocorticoids and cyclophosphamide for refractory, organ-threatening cases
- **Plasmapheresis should also be considered in acutely ill patients with severe disease**

Giant-Cell Arteritis (Temporal Arteritis)

Basic Information

- Medium to large arteries of the head and neck affected
- **Never occurs in people younger than 50 years of age**

Clinical Presentation

- Typical patient is elderly person with new-onset headaches and inflamed temporal arteries
- Typical symptoms and signs
  - New headaches of any type
  - **Jaw claudication (most specific symptom) may manifest itself as pain in the face or throat, particularly with chewing**
  - Visual symptoms
    - Possible manifestations include amaurosis fugax, blurriness, or diplopia
    - **Once visual loss occurs in giant-cell arteritis (GCA), it is usually permanent**
  - Large-vessel symptoms (e.g., arm claudication and aortic dissection); symptomatic large-vessel disease occurs in at least 20% of patients with GCA
  - Polymyalgia rheumatica (50% of cases)
- **Atypical manifestations include fever of unknown origin; weight loss; nonproductive cough; and nonspecific pains in the neck, throat, or tongue**

Diagnosis and Evaluation

- Diagnosis based on typical clinical presentation and these additional findings
  - The temporal arteries may be abnormal (swollen, tender, nodular) on examination (Fig. 44-5), but arteries are normal in up to one third of biopsy-proven cases
  - **Elevated erythrocyte sedimentation rate in the great majority of cases (90% of cases >50 mm/hr)**
  - Disruption of internal elastic lamina evident on temporal artery biopsy
    - Giant cells not always present; earliest finding is lymphoplasmacytic inflammation in the adventitia
    - Bilateral temporal artery biopsies that do not reveal GCA have a negative predictive value of 90%
    - **Temporal artery biopsy specimen may be positive for up to 2 weeks (or longer) after treatment with high-dose glucocorticoids is started**
- Despite the importance of the temporal artery biopsy, the diagnosis of GCA and the initiation of treatment ultimately remain clinical decisions

44

FIGURE 44-5   Inflamed temporal artery in giant-cell arteritis.

Treatment

- **Systemic glucocorticoids, initially 1 mg/kg/day**
  - **Glucocorticoid treatment should begin at the time the diagnosis is strongly suspected, without awaiting biopsy results**
- Studies of methotrexate efficacy as a steroid-sparing agent give conflicting results
- Flares occur with tapering of medication in at least 25% to 50% of patients
- GCA tends to run a self-limited course, and glucocorticoids may be tapered off over 1 to 2 years; as many as one third of patients, however, may require chronic low-dose glucocorticoids

Henoch-Schönlein Purpura

Basic Information

- Small arterioles and venules affected
- 90% of cases occur in children
- Majority of cases resolve within a few weeks
- Chronic cases do occur, particularly in adults
- Characterized by IgA deposition in biopsies

Clinical Presentation

- Typical patient is child with recent upper respiratory tract infection, followed by the onset of the typical tetrad of symptoms and signs:
  - Palpable purpura, occasionally with pustular lesions
  - Arthritis
  - Crampy abdominal pain (with or without gastrointestinal bleeding)
  - Hematuria or proteinuria (renal insufficiency in <5% of cases)

FIGURE 44-6   Palpable purpura in hypersensitivity vasculitis.

Diagnosis and Evaluation

- IgA deposition on tissue biopsy specimen
  - Two forms of IgA (IgA1 and IgA2)
  - Henoch-Schönlein purpura (HSP) associated only with abnormalities of IgA1
- Serum and urine protein electrophoresis studies should be performed in chronic cases to exclude IgA paraproteinemia

Treatment

- **Usually self-limited illness that requires no therapy**
- Treatment with glucocorticoids needed only in cases of advancing glomerulonephritis or mesenteric ischemia

Hypersensitivity Vasculitis

Basic Information

- A hypersensitivity response to exogenous antigen
- Postcapillary venules affected

Clinical Presentation

- **Typical patient presents with palpable purpura on shins and buttocks (dependent regions)**
- An array of skin lesions may be seen but are not distinctive for hypersensitivity vasculitis
  - Nonpalpable purpura
  - Palpable purpura (Fig. 44-6)
  - Livedo reticularis
  - Urticaria
  - Erythematous papules or plaques
  - Vesiculobullous lesions
  - Nodules
  - Ulceration
  - Necrotic lesions
- **Vasculitic lesions occur in "crops" (i.e., lesions of approximately same age, corresponding to time of exposure to inciting antigen)**
- Hypersensitivity vasculitis usually starts 7 to 14 days after exposure to the offending agent
- In the case of drug-induced hypersensitivity vasculitis, no new lesions appear after roughly 3 weeks after removal of the offending agent

Diagnosis and Evaluation

- High index of clinical suspicion necessary
- Impossible to distinguish skin lesions from those of HSP without immunofluorescence testing of biopsy specimens, confirming IgA1 deposition in HSP
- Important to exclude underlying systemic involvement (e.g., pulmonary, renal, peripheral nerve)

Treatment

- Colchicine or dapsone may be tried for milder cases
- Systemic glucocorticoids may help, although symptoms may rebound with glucocorticoid taper.
- Leg elevation and compression stockings may be helpful

Microscopic Polyangiitis

Basic Information

- Small- and medium-sized arteries and veins affected (distinct from polyarteritis nodosa, which involves only medium-sized arteries)

Clinical Presentation

- **Typical patient presents with pulmonary-renal syndrome**
  - Alveolar hemorrhage caused by pulmonary capillary alveolitis, *and*
  - Rapidly progressive glomerulonephritis caused by necrotizing, crescentic renal lesion
- More common than Goodpasture syndrome as cause of pulmonary-renal syndrome
- Typical symptoms and signs
  - Glomerulonephritis
  - Weight loss
  - Mononeuritis multiplex
  - Fever
  - Pulmonary hemorrhage

Diagnosis and Evaluation

- **May mimic Wegener granulomatosis clinically, but no granulomatous inflammation evident on pathology**
- Associated with ANCA in most cases (70%), usually directed against myeloperoxidase (MPO) that on immunofluorescence staining demonstrates a P-ANCA (perinuclear) pattern (Table 44-2)

Treatment

- Glucocorticoids and cyclophosphamide
- It is appropriate to use cyclophosphamide from the outset of treatment in microscopic polyangiitis

Polyarteritis Nodosa

Basic Information

- Medium-sized muscular arteries affected (veins spared)
- **The classic medium-vessel vasculitis**
- May be found in patients chronically infected with hepatitis B

TABLE 44-2	Correlation Between Immunofluorescence and Enzyme Immunoassay in Patients with ANCA-Associated Vasculitis	
Immunofluorescence Pattern	Enzyme Immunoassay	Disease Association
C-ANCA	Anti–proteinase-3 (90%*)	Wegener granulomatosis
P-ANCA	Antimyeloperoxidase (90%†)	Wegener granulomatosis Microscopic polyangiitis Churg-Strauss syndrome Renal-limited vasculitis

C-ANCA, cytoplasmic antineutrophil cytoplasmic antibody; P-ANCA, protoplasmic antineutrophil cytoplasmic antibody.
*90% of vasculitis patients who are C-ANCA positive have antibodies to proteinase-3.
†90% of vasculitis patients who are P-ANCA positive have antibodies to myeloperoxidase.

Clinical Presentation

- **Typical patient presents with subacute onset of multisystem inflammatory illness**
- Typical symptoms and signs
  - Constitutional symptoms
  - Livedo reticularis
  - Cutaneous nodules or ulcers, particularly over distal lower extremities
  - Intestinal angina (abdominal pain after eating)
  - Mononeuritis multiplex
  - Hypertension
  - Congestive heart failure
  - Elevated hepatic transaminases
  - Aneurysms of involved blood vessels (Fig. 44-7)
  - Classic polyarteritis nodosa (PAN) spares the lung

Diagnosis and Evaluation

- **Biopsy of affected organ or tissue**
- Blind tissue biopsy rarely useful
- **Mesenteric angiogram may reveal aneurysms even in the absence of gastroinstestinal symptoms**
- Classic PAN is ANCA-negative (i.e., proteinase-3 [PR-3] and MPO-ANCA assays are negative in this disease)

Treatment

- Glucocorticoids
- Cyclophosphamide

Takayasu Arteritis

Basic Information

- Involves large arteries, including the aorta and branches of the aortic arch (Fig. 44-8)

Clinical Presentation

- **Typical patient is a young (<40 years old) woman**
- Typical symptoms and signs

FIGURE 44-7 Angiogram demonstrating renal microaneurysms in polyarteritis nodosa.

FIGURE 44-8 Angiogram demonstrating subclavian artery narrowing in Takayasu arteritis.

- Nonspecific complaints in the prepulseless (inflammatory) stage
- Symptoms and signs of extremity or organ ischemia, although loss of digit or limb very rare
  - Postural dizziness
  - Visual disturbance
  - Claudication
  - Intrascapular back pain
  - Absence of distal pulses in one or more extremities (arms more often than legs)
  - Asymmetrical (or undetectable) blood pressures

- Because of subclavian artery involvement, at times the only way to measure blood pressure accurately is during aortic catheterization
- **Hypertension (usually caused by renal artery stenosis)**
- Bruits
  - Subclavian arteries nearly always involved
  - **Auscultate for bruits above and below clavicle**
- Erythema nodosum–like lesions (20% of cases)

Diagnosis and Evaluation

- **Angiography reveals stenoses that are long, smooth, and concentrically tapered (in contrast to short, irregular, and eccentric vascular narrowing caused by atherosclerotic disease)**
  - Involves thoracic aorta more than abdominal aorta (10–15% of cases affect the latter)
  - Exuberant collateral circulation in extremities is characteristic, often making mechanical revascularization attempts (stents, balloon dilation, bypass) unnecessary
- Magnetic resonance angiography is potentially useful in gauging disease activity through demonstration of thickening of aorta and its branches, and through perivascular edema; the full application of this technique to large-vessel vasculitis, however, remains incompletely understood

Treatment

- Glucocorticoids, if there is evidence of active inflammation

Wegener Granulomatosis

Basic Information

- Small- to medium-sized arteries, veins, and capillaries affected

Clinical Presentation

- **Typical patient is middle-aged individual with long-standing upper respiratory tract or ear complaints (often lasting months or years), who develops symptoms and signs of a systemic inflammatory illness**
- Typical symptoms and signs
  - Skin: Palpable purpura and nodules (often over elbows); nodules are identical to Churg-Strauss granulomas
  - Eye: Episcleritis, scleritis, peripheral ulcerative keratitis, uveitis, and orbital pseudotumor
  - Ear: Conductive hearing loss caused by serous otitis media or granulomatous inflammation in middle ear; less commonly, sensorineural hearing loss
  - **Nose: Septal perforation and saddle-nose deformity (Fig. 44-9)**
  - Trachea: Subglottic stenosis
  - **Lungs: Nodular lesions (with a tendency to cavitate) and pulmonary hemorrhage (Fig. 44-10)**
  - Cardiac: Pericarditis (rare)
  - Kidney: Segmental, necrotizing crescentic glomerulonephritis; the glomerulonephritis that occurs in ANCA-associated vasculitis (Wegener granulomatosis, microscopic polyangiitis, and Churg-Strauss syndrome) is pauci-immune (i.e., characterized by the deposition of few immunoreactants—such as IgG, IgM, C3—within the kidney)

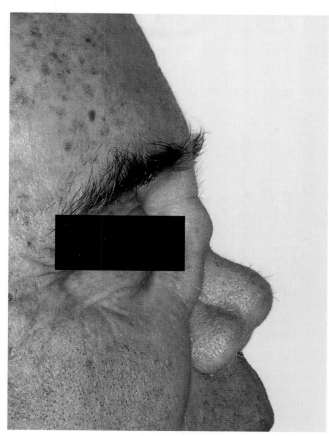

FIGURE 44-9   Saddle-nose deformity in Wegener granulomatosis.

FIGURE 44-10   Computed tomography scan demonstrating nodular and cavitary pulmonary lesions in Wegener granulomatosis.

- CNS: Chronic meningitis and cranial nerve lesions
- Peripheral nerve: Mononeuritis multiplex
- Extremities: Arthralgias or myalgias and frank arthritis (often rheumatoid factor positive)

Diagnosis and Evaluation

- Diagnosis based on three histopathologic hallmarks
  - Granulomatous inflammation
  - "Geographic" (extensive) necrosis
  - Vasculitis
- **Majority of cases associated with cytoplasmic anti-neutrophil cytoplasmic antibody (C-ANCA) pattern on immunofluorescence staining (see Table 44-2), usually caused by antibodies to proteinase-3 (PR-3)**
  - The sera of 10% to 15% of patients with Wegener granulomatosis, however, may demonstrate P-ANCA pattern, typically caused by antibodies to MPO
  - PR-3 and MPO-ANCA never occur in the same patient
  - Despite rigorous testing, 10% of patients with severe Wegener granulomatosis and 20% of those with limited disease may be ANCA negative

Treatment

- Limited disease: Systemic glucocorticoids and methotrexate
- Severe (organ- or life-threatening) disease: Systemic glucocorticoids and (daily) cyclophosphamide
- **Disease appears to accelerate when serum creatinine begins to rise; detection of renal involvement signals medical emergency that must be treated swiftly**
- ANCA serologies useful in making the diagnosis, but serial testing of ANCA titers not useful in predicting disease flares
- Reflecting dramatic improvements in treatment, there is now 90% survival at 5 years

REVIEW QUESTIONS

For review questions, please go to www.expertconsult.com.

SUGGESTED READINGS

Langford CA: Vasculitis, *J Allergy Clin Immunol* 125:S216–S225, 2010.

Sakane T, Takeno M, Suzuki N, Inaba G: Behçet's disease, *N Engl J Med* 341:1284–1291, 1999.

Seo P, Stone JH: ANCA-associated vasculitis, *Am J Med* 117:39–50, 2004.

Seo P, Stone JH: Large-vessel vasculitis, *Arthritis Care Res* 51:128–139, 2004.

Seo P, Stone JH: Small-vessel and medium-vessel vasculitis, *Arthritis Care Res* 57:1552–1559, 2007.

Stone JH, Calabrese LH, Hoffman GS, et al: Vasculitis: pearls and myths, *Rheum Dis Clin North Am* 27:677–728, 2001.

44

Selected Topics in Rheumatology

CAROL M. ZIMINSKI, MD

Clinical presentation is the key element in the diagnosis of rheumatic diseases. The diagnosis of a specific disorder is suggested by a particular constellation of what may individually be nonspecific signs and symptoms. The diagnosis is then confirmed by obtaining a detailed history, physical examination, and appropriate laboratory and imaging studies.

Systemic Lupus Erythematosus

Basic Information

- **Systemic lupus erythematosus (SLE) is the prototypical autoimmune disease, in which the production of autoantibodies is associated with a multisystem inflammatory process**
- Epidemiology and risk factors
  - Incidence greatest from ages 18 to 45 years
  - Female-to-male ratio is 9:1
  - Four times more prevalent in African American women than in white women
  - Regulation of the clearance of immune complexes is a common feature of many associated genes
    - Human leukocyte antigen (HLA) associations: DR2 and DR3
    - Congenital deficiency of complement components: C1, C2, and C4
- Pathogenesis
  - **Cardinal feature is the production of autoantibodies directed against nuclear, cytoplasmic, and cell-surface antigens**
  - Process is antigen-driven and T cell–dependent
  - Antigens to which patients with SLE respond are packaged in "blebs" on the cell surface during the process of apoptosis (programmed cell death)
  - Mechanisms of tissue injury involve both immune complex deposition and cell-specific antibodies
    - Most commonly identified immune complex is double-stranded DNA (dsDNA)–anti-dsDNA that can form in the circulation and deposit in the kidney, or form *in situ*
    - Cell-specific antibodies do not usually destroy cells directly but mark cells for premature destruction by the reticuloendothelial system (e.g., hemolytic anemia, leukopenia, and thrombocytopenia)
  - A recent study from the Department of Defense found that 115 of 130 patients with SLE had at least one autoantibody present before diagnosis (mean, 3.3

years). In 78%, antinuclear antibodies (ANAs) were present in a titer of ≥1:120. Anti-dsDNA was found in 58%.
  - Implication of these data is that **SLE is the culmination of compound and complex autoimmune abnormalities that may begin simply, then spread and multiply until manifesting as clinical disease**

Clinical Presentation

- Cutaneous lupus
  - Common presenting feature
  - **Rash occurs at some time in 90% of cases of SLE**
  - Most rashes are photosensitive
  - Types
    - Malar "butterfly" rash (nonscarring) over cheeks and bridge of nose (Fig. 45-1)
    - Discoid lesions (often scarring) are deeper, but rarely (around 5%) evolve to systemic lupus (Fig. 45-2)
    - Subacute cutaneous lupus (nonscarring) presents with annular, polycyclic lesions (Fig. 45-3); occasional arthritis and serositis; but no central nervous system (CNS) or renal disease
    - Bullous lupus (blistering rash) is rare
- Lupus arthritis
  - Episodic and migratory
  - Distribution often symmetrical, similar to rheumatoid arthritis
  - **Rarely erosive or destructive**
  - Jaccoud arthropathy characterized by reversible, nonerosive, "swan neck" deformities
- Lupus nephritis
  - Occurs in one half to two thirds of SLE patients
  - More common in African Americans
  - Associated with antibodies to native dsDNA
  - Diffuse proliferative glomerulonephritis is the most serious form and can lead to rapidly progressive renal failure
- Drug-induced lupus (Box 45-1)
- Age effect
  - "Young" SLE manifests with more adenopathy; splenomegaly; and cutaneous, CNS, and renal disease
  - 10% of SLE patients have an onset at 50 years of age or older. Their disease is milder, with more serositis and pulmonary manifestations, but it rarely is associated with CNS and renal disease.

FIGURE 45-1　Malar "butterfly" rash demonstrating the typical distribution over the bridge of the nose and cheeks, sparing the nasolabial folds. *(Courtesy of Carol M. Ziminski, MD.)*

FIGURE 45-3　Subacute cutaneous lupus. The annular polycyclic lesions have an erythematous, slightly scaling border with central clearing. The distribution in light-exposed areas suggests photosensitivity. *(Courtesy of Carol M. Ziminski, MD.)*

FIGURE 45-2　Discoid lupus lesions typically occur over exposed areas, such as the face or scalp. This patient demonstrates characteristic features including telangiectasias, erythema, follicular plugging, atrophy, and postinflammatory hypo- and hyperpigmentation. *(Courtesy of Carol M. Ziminski, MD.)*

BOX 45-1	*Drug-Induced Lupus*

Many drug associations (e.g., hydralazine, procainamide, sulfonamides, and INH)

Primarily older patients

No CNS or renal disease

ANA (antihistone) (+); anti-native DNA (−)

Clinical features improve after discontinuing drug, though ANA may persist for years

ANA, antinuclear antibody; CNS, central nervous system; INH, isoniazid.

Diagnosis and Evaluation

- SLE often suggested based on initial presentation with fever, rash, and polyarthritis
- **Diagnosis clinical but aided by the American College of Rheumatology SLE criteria (Table 45-1)**
- The initial criteria date from 1982 and were reevaluated and revised in 1997
- Serology: see Table 45-2

TABLE 45-1	*Criteria for the Classification of Systemic Lupus Erythematosus*
1. Malar rash	
2. Discoid rash	
3. Photosensitivity	
4. Oral ulcers	
5. Nonerosive arthritis	
6. Pleuritis *or* Pericarditis	
7. Renal disorder	Persistent proteinuria >0.5 g/day or >3+ if no quantitation, *or* Cellular casts—RBC, hemoglobin, granular, tubular, or mixed
8. Neurologic disorder	Seizures *or* Psychosis—in absence of offending drugs or known metabolic derangements (e.g., uremia, ketoacidosis, or electrolyte imbalance)
9. Hematologic disorder	Hemolytic anemia—with reticulocytosis *or* Leukopenia: <4000/mm^3 on two or more occasions *or* Lymphopenia: <1500/mm^3 on two or more occasions *or* Thrombocytopenia: <100,000/mm^3, absent offending drugs
10. Immunologic disorder	Anti-DNA: to native (double-stranded) DNA *or* Anti-Sm: Presence of antibody to Smith nuclear antigen *or* Postive finding of antiphospholipid antibodies on: 1. An abnormal serum level of IgG or IgM anticardiolipin antibodies 2. A positive test result for lupus anticoagulant using a standard method, or 3. A false-positive serologic test for syphilis test result for at least 6 months confirmed by *Treponema pallidum* immobilization or fluorescent treponemal antibody absorption test
11. Antinuclear antibody	Abnormal titer of antinuclear antibody by immunofluorescence or an equivalent assay at any point in time, and in the absence of drugs known to be associated with the "drug-induced lupus" syndrome

IgG, immunoglobulin G; IgM, immunoglobulin M; RBC, red blood cell.
Presence of at least 4 of 11 criteria is sensitive and specific for diagnosis of SLE.
Patients may not achieve four criteria until several years into course of disease.
Criteria developed for enrollment of patients in research studies; therefore, should not be adhered to rigorously for diagnosis in the individual patient.
From Tan EM, Cohen AS, Fries JF, et al: The 1982 revised criteria for the classification of systemic lupus erythematosus (SLE), *Arthritis Rheum* 25:1271, 1982; and Hochberg MC: Updating the American College of Rheumatology revised criteria for the classification of systemic lupus erythematosus [letter], *Arthritis Rheum* 40:1725, 1997.

Treatment

- Rationale for treatment
  - Survival 85% to 90% at 10 years and 68% at 20 years, with treatment
  - 50% have relapsing-remitting course
  - Poor prognostic signs: poverty, advanced age, male gender, and increased creatinine at onset
  - Bimodal mortality curve
    - **Early deaths caused by active disease (renal and CNS) or infection**
    - **Late deaths caused by accelerated coronary artery disease;** imaging techniques to measure carotid intimal-medial thickness and coronary artery calcification have shown coronary artery calcification and carotid plaques in women with SLE, presumably the result of both disease and side effects of corticosteroid therapy
- Principles
  - **Treat the disease, not the serologic activity**
  - Use the lowest effective dose of steroids or immunosuppressives for the shortest time necessary
  - Minimize morbidity/mortality of SLE and its therapy by reducing risk factors or treating hypertension, hyperlipidemia, coronary artery disease, osteoporosis, and osteonecrosis
  - In all patients with SLE, traditional cardiovascular risk factors (high blood pressure, hyperlipidemia, elevated fasting blood glucose levels, cigarette smoking, obesity, lack of exercise) should be addressed
- Pharmacotherapy
  - Cutaneous manifestations: sunscreen, topical steroids, and hydroxychloroquine
  - Arthritis: nonsteroidal anti-inflammatory drugs (NSAIDs), hydroxychloroquine, and low-dose steroids
  - Fever and serositis: NSAIDs and low-dose steroids
  - Major organ system involvement (e.g., hematologic, myopathy, renal, and CNS): high-dose steroids and immunosuppressives (mycophenolate mofetil, cyclophosphamide)
- Infections
  - Prednisone (>20 mg/day) and other immunosuppressives increase risk for fatal infections
  - **50% of fatal infections involve opportunistic organisms (e.g., *Pneumocystis jiroveci* and *Candida*)**

Antiphospholipid Syndrome

Basic Information

- Antiphospholipid syndrome (APS) results from the long-term persistence of serum antiphospholipid antibodies, a family of autoantibodies that may be seen in

TABLE 45-2	Serology in the Rheumatic Diseases	
Autoantibody	**Disease Association**	**Comment**
ANA	SLE Polymyositis/dermatomyositis Scleroderma CREST syndrome Sjögren syndrome Mixed connective tissue disease	Antibody to multiple nuclear antigens (see below) Immunofluorescence: Multiple patterns (see below) (+) in 95–99% of SLE (+) in 10–20% of healthy young women
Antihistone	SLE Drug-induced lupus	Antibody to DNA/protein complex Immunofluorescence: Homogeneous
Anti-native DNA	SLE	Antibody to double-stranded DNA Immunofluorescence: Rim (+) in 70% of SLE More specific for SLE than ANA, but less sensitive Associated with renal disease
Anti-Smith (Sm)	SLE	Antibody to nuclear ribonucleoprotein Immunofluorescence: Speckled (+) in 20–30% of SLE More specific for SLE than ANA, but less sensitive
Anti-RNP	SLE Mixed connective tissue disease	Antibody to nuclear ribonucleoprotein Immunofluorescence: Speckled
Anti-Ro/La	SLE Subacute cutaneous lupus Neonatal lupus Sjögren syndrome	Antibody to nuclear ribonucleoprotein Immunofluorescence: Speckled Associated with Photosensitivity Congenital heart block
Anti-Scl 70	Diffuse scleroderma	Antibody to DNA topoisomerase I Immunofluorescence: Nucleolar (+) in 40% of patients with scleroderma
Anticentromere	CREST syndrome	Antibody to centromere/kinetochore Immunofluorescence: Centromere (+) in >50% of patients with CREST
Anti-PM-Scl	Polymyositis/scleroderma overlap	Antibody to nuclear protein Immunofluorescence: Nuclear or nucleolar
Anti-Jo-1	Polymyositis Dermatomyositis	Antibody to histidyl-tRNA synthetase Immunofluorescence: Diffuse Associated with interstitial lung disease
Anti-SRP	Polymyositis	Antibody to signal recognition particle (cytoplasmic ribonucleoprotein) Associated with resistance to therapy
Anti-Mi-2	Dermatomyositis	Antibody to nuclear protein Immunofluorescence: Homogeneous Associated with V (anterior neck/upper chest rash) and "shawl" (posterior neck/shoulder rash) signs

ANA, antinuclear antibody; CREST, calcinosis, Raynaud syndrome, esophageal dysmotility, sclerodactyly, telangiectasia; SLE, systemic lupus erythematosus; tRNA, transfer RNA.

patients who have a hypercoagulable state marked by arterial or venous thromboses, recurrent pregnancy loss, or thrombocytopenia
- Interference with coagulation *in vitro* contrasts with the thrombogenic effect *in vivo*
- **50% of cases of APS are seen in patients who have no associated diseases ("primary"). Most other cases are seen in patients with SLE ("secondary").**
- Antibodies may be produced transiently after infections (e.g., human immunodeficiency virus [HIV]) or following exposure to certain drugs (e.g., chlorpromazine and procainamide)

Clinical Presentation
- Cutaneous: Livedo reticularis (see Fig. 65-37), splinter hemorrhages, leg ulcers, and gangrene
- Hematologic: Thrombocytopenia and hemolytic anemia (especially with anticardiolipin immunoglobulin [IgM])
- Venous thrombosis: Superficial or deep venous thrombophlebitis, retinal vein thrombosis, cerebral venous thrombosis, Budd-Chiari syndrome, and pulmonary hypertension
- Neurologic: Transient ischemic attacks, ischemic cerebral infarction, chorea, and transverse myelitis
- Gynecologic: Recurrent pregnancy loss (antiphospholipid antibodies found in up to 10% of women with three or more consecutive pregnancy losses)

Diagnosis and Evaluation

- **Patients may have antiphospholipid antibodies but not develop the thrombotic manifestations required for the diagnosis of the APS**
- Diagnosis is based on the presence of at least one of the following autoantibody types:
  - Biologic false-positive serologic test for syphilis
  - Lupus anticoagulant
    - IgM or IgG that prolongs phospholipid-dependent coagulation *in vitro* by binding to the prothrombin activator complex, impairing conversion of pro-thrombin to thrombin
    - Assayed by phospholipid-dependent coagulation tests (e.g., activated partial thromboplastin time and Russell viper venom time)
  - Anticardiolipin antibodies (ACAs)
    - Directed against the complex of phospholipid and β_2-glycoproteins
    - High-titer ACA IgG is most strongly associated with thrombosis and pregnancy loss
    - Low titers are found in up to 5% of healthy young women
  - Autoantibodies cannot be assayed in patients taking heparin or warfarin

Treatment

- Directed by clinical features
- Serologic abnormalities alone
  - **No treatment, although some advocate low-dose aspirin prophylaxis**
- Patients who have had a thrombotic event
  - Heparin, then warfarin with target international normalized ratio of 3 to 4
  - Some suggest the addition of low-dose aspirin to warfarin for those who have had an arterial event
  - Steroids, rather than anticoagulation, with thrombocytopenia (e.g., platelets <50,000/mm^3)
  - Warfarin is not used during pregnancy because of potential teratogenicity
  - Prednisone and aspirin, or subcutaneous heparin and aspirin, have been used successfully in pregnancy with APS

Scleroderma and Systemic Sclerosis

Basic Information

- **A multisystem autoimmune disease characterized by vasculopathy, excessive collagen deposition, and tissue fibrosis**
- Epidemiology
  - Usual onset in 20s or 30s
  - Female-to-male ratio is between 3:1 and 4:1
  - More common in African Americans than whites

Clinical Presentation

- Raynaud's phenomenon (Fig. 45-4)
  - One of earliest clinical manifestations
  - Classic phases: White (ischemic), leads to blue (cyanotic), leads to red (hyperemic)
  - Primary Raynaud's phenomenon
    - Occurs in the absence of another rheumatic disease

FIGURE 45-4 Raynaud's phenomenon manifested by digital cyanosis in a patient with scleroderma. *(Courtesy of Carol M. Ziminski, MD.)*

FIGURE 45-5 Nail-fold capillary microscopy showing busy capillaries. *(From Habif TB: Clinical dermatology: a color guide to diagnosis and therapy, ed 4, St. Louis, Mosby, 2004, Fig. 17-24.)*

- Benign and common
- Onset: 14 to 35 years
- Affects 5% to 10% of young women
  - Secondary Raynaud's phenomenon
    - Occurs in the setting of another rheumatic disease (e.g., scleroderma or SLE)
    - Should be considered if
      - Onset in childhood or after age 35 years
      - Patient is male
      - Abnormal nail-fold capillary loops are present (Fig. 45-5)
      - Episodes cause digital tip ulceration or gangrene
      - Patient has symptoms and signs of another disease
- Organ system manifestations (Table 45-3)

TABLE 45-3	*Organ System Manifestations in Scleroderma*				
Cutaneous	**Gastrointestinal**	**Pulmonary**	**Renal**	**Cardiac**

Early
  Edematous phase
  (scleredema); may
  last several months
Subsequent
  Induration and skin
  tightening; may
  last several years
Late
  Atrophic changes
  Also telangiectasias,
  calcification, and
  pruritis
	Esophageal dysmotility,
	  with reflux
	Gastroparesis, with early
	  satiety
	Watermelon stomach
	Small bowel involvement,
	  with pseudo-obstruction
	Colonic involvement,
	  with wide-mouthed
	  diverticulae
		Interstitial pneumonitis
		  with bibasilar interstitial
		  infiltrates
		Pulmonary hypertension
		May manifest as cough or
		  dyspnea
			Renal crisis presents with
			  malignant hypertension
			  and rapidly progressive
			  renal failure
			Biopsy reveals transmural
			  microangiopathy (not
			  vasculitis) with intimal
			  proliferation, medial
			  hypertrophy, and
			  adventitial fibrosis
				Cardiomyopathy
				  with contraction
				  band necrosis
				  or myocardial
				  fibrosis
				Pericarditis

Diagnosis and Evaluation

- **Skin changes suggest the diagnosis, but internal organ involvement determines survival**
- Clinical subsets
  - Limited scleroderma (CREST syndrome)
    - **C**alcinosis
    - **R**aynaud's phenomenon
    - **E**sophageal dysmotility
    - **S**clerodactyly (Fig. 45-6)
    - **T**elangiectasia
  - Diffuse scleroderma (progressive systemic sclerosis)
    - Scleroderma involving not only the fingers but also the dorsum of the hand proximal to the metacarpophalangeal joints or on forearms, legs, face, and trunk, *or*
    - Sclerodactyly associated with either digital pulp pitting (Fig. 45-7) or basilar pulmonary fibrosis
  - Localized scleroderma: Morphea and linear scleroderma
- The presence of a tendon friction rub is highly specific (although not sensitive) for the diagnosis of scleroderma
- **Autoantibodies are found in most affected patients: ANA positive in up to 98% of patients (see Table 45-2)**
- Bronchoalveolar lavage may identify patients with active inflammatory pulmonary disease, who may benefit from immunosuppressive agents

Treatment

- **There is no cure for scleroderma, but many of its problems and complications can be treated (Table 45-4)**
- In the future, therapy may focus on inhibiting the release of cytokines that induce fibrosis
- Many of the major advances in management today are directed toward preventing damage to endothelial cells
- **There is no role for systemic steroids except in pneumonitis or myositis**
- Poor prognostic factors
  - Older age
  - Male gender

FIGURE 45-6 Scleroderma. Digital flexion contractures due to thickened, indurated skin (sclerodactyly). *(Courtesy of Carol M. Ziminski, MD.)*

- African American race
- Diffuse scleroderma
- Early visceral involvement

Polymyositis and Dermatomyositis

Basic Information

- **Immune-mediated inflammatory myopathy affecting striated muscle and resulting in symmetrical proximal (i.e., shoulder and pelvic girdle) weakness**
- Incidence 1 in 100,000
- Bimodal distribution of incidence: Ages 10 to 15 years and 45 to 60 years
- Female-to-male ratio is 2:1

Clinical Presentation

- Muscle manifestations
  - Weakness is pathognomonic
    - **Proximal and symmetrical weakness**
    - May also affect the neck, pharyngeal, respiratory, and trunk muscles, but spares the facial muscles

FIGURE 45-7 Scleroderma. Pitting scars on the pulps of the index and middle fingers due to microvascular disease. *(Courtesy of Carol M. Ziminski, MD.)*

FIGURE 45-8 Dermatomyositis. Gottron papules manifested by a rash accentuated over interphalangeal joints, with variable manifestations including erythematous or violaceous induration, papules, or nodules. *(Courtesy of Carol M. Ziminski, MD.)*

TABLE 45-4	*Management of Scleroderma*
Manifestation	**Intervention**
Raynaud's phenomenon	Cold avoidance Calcium channel blockers
Digital ulcers	Intravenous iloprost (prostaglandin analogue)
Interstitial pneumonitis	Steroids Cytotoxic agents (e.g., cyclophosphamide)
Gastroesophageal reflux	Proton pump inhibitors
GI immotility	Prokinetic agents (e.g., metoclopramide)
GI bacterial overgrowth/malabsorption	Broad-spectrum antibiotics
Pulmonary hypertension	Endothelin receptor antagonist (bosentan) Phosphodiesterase-5 inhibitors (sildenafil, tadalafil) Prostocyclin analogues (epoprostenol, ilioprost) Lung transplantation
Renal crisis	ACE inhibitor

ACE, angiotensin-converting enzyme; GI, gastrointestinal.

- Dysphagia may occur (due to involvement of striated pharyngeal muscle)
- Muscle pain (25% of cases)
- Cutaneous manifestations
  - **Heliotrope rash: Periorbital edema with violaceous discoloration of eyelids**
  - Erythematous, sometimes scaling rash may occur over face, upper chest (V sign), and upper back ("shawl" sign)
  - **Gottron papules: Erythematous or violaceous scaling papules over knuckles** (Fig. 45-8)
  - Mechanic's hand: Scaling skin over palms, with "dirty" discoloration of creases

- Calcinosis (especially in children)
- Vasculitis
- Pulmonary involvement with interstitial lung disease occurs in 30% to 50% of patients
- Clinical patterns
  - Polymyositis (PM)
  - Dermatomyositis (DM)
  - Juvenile DM
  - Myositis associated with another rheumatic disease
  - Myositis associated with malignancy

Diagnosis and Evaluation

- **Clinical suspicion based on presentation with symmetrical proximal muscle weakness**
- Elevated muscle enzymes
  - **Creatine phosphokinase is the most specific and sensitive for muscle injury**
  - Aldolase, aspartate aminotransferase, alanine aminotransferase, and lactate dehydrogenase may also reflect muscle inflammation
- Autoantibodies may allow better definition of subsets but may not be widely available (see Table 45-2)
  - Tests are positive for ANAs in 20% to 30% of patients with PM, more frequently in patients who have myositis in the setting of other rheumatic diseases
  - Approximately 30% of patients have antibodies directed against cytoplasmic ribonucleoproteins; found only in myositis and are known as myositis-specific antibodies
  - Antigens define three subgroups of patients who differ in clinical features and prognosis (Table 45-5)
- Complement system
  - PM: No evidence of complement activation
  - DM: Vascular deposition of complement membrane attack complex
- Electromyography (EMG) reveals inflammatory myopathy with short duration, low-amplitude and polyphasic potentials, and irritative features
- Muscle biopsy may confirm the diagnosis

TABLE 45-5	Syndromes Associated with Myositis-Specific Autoantibodies	
Autoantibody	**Clinical Features**	**Prognosis**
Aminoacyl-tRNA synthetases (anti-Jo-1, PL-7, and others)	Acute onset Interstitial lung disease Arthritis Hyperkeratotic rash ("mechanic's hands") HLA-DR3, -DR52	Variable Significant mortality
Signal recognition peptide	Hyperacute onset Cardiac involvement Onset in autumn More prevalent in black women	Poor 5-year mortality rate 75%
Components of histone acetylase complexes (Mi-2)	Dermatomyositis Shawl sign of rash Cuticular overgrowth	Good

HLA, human leukocyte antigen; tRNA, transfer RNA.

- Negative in up to 30% of cases, but abnormal EMG supports diagnosis of myositis in appropriate clinical setting
- PM: Inflammatory cell infiltrate found between muscle fibers, with varying stages of muscle fiber necrosis and regeneration, but vessels spared
- DM: Inflammatory cells surround the small endomysial vessels
- Magnetic resonance imaging adds important dimension and is noninvasive
  - T1-weighted images provide excellent anatomic detail, useful in assessing changes resulting from damage and chronicity
  - T2-weighted images with fat suppression or STIR (short tau inversion recovery) sequences identify edema, which is indicative of active inflammation
- Differential diagnosis
  - Drugs: Colchicine, penicillamine, "statins," corticosteroids, and zidovudine
  - Endocrine: Hypothyroidism
  - Malignancy-associated: Perform age-appropriate cancer screening
  - Neuromuscular: Muscular dystrophies and myasthenia gravis
  - Inclusion body myositis (Box 45-2)
  - Infections
    - Viral: Coxsackie virus, influenza, and HIV
    - Parasitic: *Trichinella*
    - Protozoan: *Toxoplasma*
  - Other: Electrolyte disorders and metabolic myopathies

Treatment

- **High-dose steroids (80% response)**
- Methotrexate and azathioprine useful as steroid-sparing agents
- Intravenous immune globulin (IVIG) is sometimes used successfully in dermatomyositis refractory to steroids because IVIG can inhibit complement activation
- **Search for and treat associated malignancy**

BOX 45-2	Inclusion Body Myositis

Basic Information

Unique subset of the inflammatory myopathies

Typical patient is a man older than 50 years

Clinical Presentation

Weakness may be both proximal and distal, and less symmetrical

Typical course is chronic, with slow progression over years, or even decades

Diagnosis and Evaluation

Consider in setting of atypical distribution of weakness

Mild elevation in creatine phosphokinase (up to 5× normal)

Muscle biopsy specimen reveals characteristic rimmed vacuoles with inclusions and occasional ragged red fibers

Treatment

Poor response to steroids

45

Polymyalgia Rheumatica

Basic Information

- **Clinical syndrome marked by proximal limb-girdle muscle pain and stiffness**
- May be prodrome for rheumatoid arthritis
- **May be associated with giant-cell arteritis (see Chapter 44)**
- Epidemiology
  - Rarely diagnosed at ages younger than 50 years
  - Female-to-male ratio is 2:1
  - Predominantly whites (especially patients of northern European descent)

Clinical Presentation

- Proximal limb-girdle pain and morning stiffness in the appropriate host
- Constitutional manifestations include fever, malaise, and weight loss

Diagnosis and Evaluation

- **Examination reveals muscle tenderness but no true muscle weakness**
- Laboratory features
  - Elevated erythrocyte sedimentation rate
  - Elevated C-reactive protein
  - Normochromic normocytic anemia
  - Elevated platelets

Treatment

- Steroids
  - Treatment of choice
  - Low-dose (10–20 mg of prednisone daily)
  - Rapid and dramatic symptomatic improvement is characteristic
  - Taper guided by symptoms
- NSAIDs may give partial relief of symptoms in mild cases

Fibromyalgia Syndrome

Basic Information

- **Chronic syndrome marked by multifocal musculoskeletal pain and fatigue, in the setting of a noninflammatory physical examination and laboratory studies**
- Epidemiology
  - May affect 2% of population
  - Peak age 30 to 50 years
  - 80% to 90% of patients are female

Clinical Presentation

- May include the following
  - Chronic, diffuse pain
  - Morning stiffness
  - Subjective swelling
  - Raynaud-like symptoms
  - Sleep disturbance
  - Fatigue
  - Headache
  - Dry mouth
  - Paresthesias
  - Irritable bowel syndrome
  - Urinary urgency
  - Dysmenorrhea
  - Anxiety
  - Depression

Diagnosis and Evaluation

- Criteria for the diagnosis of fibromyalgia were approved by the American College of Rheumatology in 2010 (Table 45-6): A patient satisfies diagnostic criteria for fibromyalgia if the following three conditions are met:
  - Widespread pain index (WPI) ≥7 and symptom severity (SS) scale score ≥5 (or WPI 3–6 and SS scale score ≥9)
  - Symptoms have been present at a similar level for at least 3 months
  - The patient does not have a disorder that would otherwise explain the pain
- Consider possible contributing events
  - Physical trauma: physical abuse or motor vehicle accident
  - Emotional trauma: sexual abuse
  - Infections: hepatitis C, Lyme disease, parvovirus, and HIV

TABLE 45-6 **Fibromyalgia Diagnostic Criteria**

Criteria
A patient satisfies diagnostic criteria for fibromyalgia if the following 3 conditions are met:
1. Widespread pain index (WPI) ≥7 and symptom severity (SS) scale score ≥5 or WPI 3–6 and SS scale score ≥9.
2. Symptoms have been present at a similar level for at least 3 months.
3. The patient does not have a disorder that would otherwise explain the pain.

Ascertainment
1. WPI: note the number of areas in which the patient has had pain over the last week. In how many areas has the patient had pain? Score will be between 0 and 19.

Shoulder girdle, left	Hip (buttock, trochanter), left	Jaw, left	Upper back
Shoulder girdle, right	Hip (buttock, trochanter), left	Jaw, right	Lower back
Upper arm, left	Upper leg, left	Chest	Neck
Upper arm, right	Upper leg, right	Abdomen	
Lower arm, left	Lower leg, left		
Lower arm, right	Lower leg, right		

2. SS scale score:
    Fatigue
    Waking unrefreshed
    Cognitive symptoms
For the each of the 3 symptoms above, indicate the level of severity over the past week using the following scale:
    0 = no problem
    1 = slight or mild problems, generally mild or intermittent
    2 = moderate, considerable problems, often present and/or at a moderate level
    3 = severe: pervasive, continuous, life-disturbing problems
Considering somatic symptoms* in general, indicate whether the patient has:
    0 = no symptoms
    1 = few symptoms
    2 = a moderate number of symptoms
    3 = a great deal of symptoms
The SS scale score is the sum of the severity of the 3 symptoms (fatigue, waking unrefreshed, cognitive symptoms) plus the extent (severity) of somatic symptoms in general. The final score is between 0 and 12.

*Somatic symptoms that might be considered: muscle pain, irritable bowel syndrome, fatigue/tiredness, thinking or remembering problem, muscle weakness, headache, pain/cramps in the abdomen, numbness/tingling, dizziness, insomnia, depression, constipation, pain in the upper abdomen, nausea, nervousness, chest pain, blurred vision, fever, diarrhea, dry mouth, itching, wheezing, Raynaud's phenomenon, hives/welts, ringing in ears, vomiting, heartburn, oral ulcers, loss of/change in taste, seizures, dry eyes, shortness of breath, loss of appetite, rash, sun sensitivity, hearing difficulties, easy bruising, hair loss, frequent urination, painful urination, and bladder spasms.
From Wolfe F, Clauw DJ, Fitzcharles M-A, et al: The American College of Rheumatology preliminary diagnostic criteria for fibromyalgia and measurement of symptom severity, *Arthritis Care Res* 62:600–610, 2010.

Treatment

- Goals
  - Decrease pain
  - Decrease distress
  - Improve sleep
  - Increase energy level
  - Improve function
  - Treat associated symptoms, including anxiety and depression
- Methods
  - Patient education and reassurance
  - Stress reduction
  - **Aerobic conditioning exercise**
  - Pharmacologic intervention
    - **Low-dose tricyclic antidepressant (e.g., amitriptyline or nortriptyline)**
    - Cyclobenzaprine
    - Anticonvulsants (e.g., pregabalin)
    - Serotonin reuptake inhibitors (e.g., fluoxetine)
    - Dual-receptor inhibitors inhibit serotonin and norepinephrine (e.g., venlafaxine, milnacipran)
- **Pitfalls**
  - Psychosocial issues not addressed
  - Benefit of exercise undervalued
  - Exercise program too rigorous or advanced too quickly
  - Tricyclic therapy discontinued prematurely
  - Unrealistic expectations for improvement

REVIEW QUESTIONS

For review questions, please go to www.expertconsult.com.

SUGGESTED READINGS

Erkin D, Salmon JE, Lockshin MD: Antiphospholipid antibody syndrome. In Firestein GS, Budd RC, Harris ED Jr, et al editors: *Kelley's textbook of rheumatology*, ed 8, Philadelphia, 2009, Elsevier Saunders, pp 1301–1310.

Hellmann DB: Giant cell arteritis, polymyalgia rheumatic, and Takayasu's arteritis. In Firestein GS, Budd RC, Harris ED Jr, et al editors: *Kelley's textbook of rheumatology*, ed 8, Philadelphia, 2009, Elsevier Saunders, pp 1409–1425.

Hochberg MC: Updating the American College of Rheumatology revised criteria for the classification of systemic lupus erythematosus [letter], *Arthritis Rheum* 40:1725, 1997.

Nagaraju K, Lundberg IE: Inflammatory diseases of muscle and other myopathies. In Firestein GS, Budd RC, Harris ED Jr, et al editors: *Kelley's textbook of rheumatology*, ed 8, Philadelphia, 2009, Elsevier Saunders, pp 1353–1380.

Tassiulas IO, Boumpas DT: Clinical features and treatment of systemic lupus erythematosus. In Firestein GS, Budd RC, Harris ED Jr, et al editors: *Kelley's textbook of rheumatology*, ed 8, Philadelphia, 2009, Elsevier Saunders, pp 1263–1300.

Wolfe F, Clauw DJ, Fitzcharles M-A, et al: The American College of Rheumatology preliminary diagnostic criteria for fibromyalgia and measurement of symptom severity, *Arthritis Care Res* 62:600–610, 2010.

Wolfe F, Rasker JJ: Fibromyalgia. In Firestein GS, Budd RC, Harris ED Jr, et al editors: *Kelley's textbook of rheumatology*, ed 8, Philadelphia, 2009, Elsevier Saunders, pp 555–566.

45

SECTION EIGHT

Hematology

Anemia

BIMAL H. ASHAR, MD, MBA

Anemia, a reduction in the proportion of red blood cells (RBCs), is one of the most common conditions seen by internists. Although patients are often asymptomatic, the presence of anemia is indicative of an underlying disorder. From a laboratory perspective, anemia is somewhat arbitrarily defined by the World Health Organization as a hemoglobin (Hgb) concentration of less than 12 g/dL in women and less than 13 g/dL in men. Others have proposed slightly different defining values that vary by age and race. If previous hemoglobin values are available, a significant downward trend should be indicative of anemia regardless of absolute hemoglobin values. This chapter provides a general framework for approaching patients with anemia in order to uncover their underlying disorders.

Overview

Basic Information

- Normal erythropoiesis (Fig. 46-1)
  - Regulated by the production of erythropoietin (EPO) in the kidney
    - EPO production increases as a result of hypoxia, as sensed by the kidney
    - EPO then stimulates RBC production by the bone marrow
- Mechanisms of anemia
  - Decreased production of RBCs (hypoproliferation)
  - Increased destruction of RBCs (hemolysis)
  - Acute blood loss (hemorrhage)

Clinical Presentation

- Often asymptomatic
- When symptomatic, weakness and fatigue are the most common
- Angina, congestive heart failure, dyspnea, tachycardia, and cerebral insufficiency can occur
- **Severity of symptoms is dependent on rapidity of development of anemia, degree of anemia, and the ability of the body to compensate**

Diagnosis

- Laboratory evaluation begins with a complete blood count (CBC)
  - Hgb and hematocrit (Hct) values determine the presence of anemia
  - White blood cell (WBC) and platelet counts should be examined to determine the presence or absence of pancytopenia
  - Mean corpuscular volume (MCV): Serves as an estimate of RBC size

  - RBC count: Low in most cases of anemia but can be normal or high in some conditions (e.g., thalassemia trait)
  - Red cell distribution width (RDW): Estimates the degree of variation in red cell size
- Reticulocytes: Immature RBCs
  - Correct the reticulocyte count for the degree of anemia as follows:

  Reticulocyte index = Percent reticulocytes ×
  (Patient's hematocrit / normal hematocrit)

  - **A reticulocyte index greater than 2% suggests hemolysis or acute blood loss**
  - **A recticulocyte index less than 2% suggests a hypoproliferative process**
- Peripheral smear
  - Can help confirm the MCV and potentially identify mixed disorders (e.g., concomitant iron deficiency and folate deficiency presenting with a normal MCV)
  - Can be suggestive of specific diagnoses (see Chapter 51)
- Basic approach to anemia: see Figure 46-2

Treatment

- Blood transfusions
  - **Not routinely indicated in asymptomatic patients**
  - Transfusion is currently recommended for patients with
    - Rapid acute blood loss
    - Cardiovascular disease and an Hgb less than 8 g/dL
    - Symptomatic patients with an Hgb between 7 and 9 g/dL
    - Stable patients with an Hgb less than 7 g/dL
  - Can cause a number of immunologic reactions (Table 46-1)
- Erythropoiesis-stimulating agents (ESAs)
  - Beneficial for patients with renal failure and Hgb levels less than 11 g/dL, but target Hgb levels on therapy should be 10 g/dL to 12 g/dL
  - Increases quality of life in some patients with anemia of chronic disease (e.g., caused by rheumatoid arthritis)
  - Controversy exists regarding risks and benefits in cancer patients
    - Recommended for symptomatic patients with anemia (Hgb ≤10 g/dL) resulting from chemotherapy for nonhematologic malignancies
    - Not routinely recommended for patients with anemia caused by a nonhematologic malignancy who are not receiving chemotherapy

- Reduces the need for postoperative transfusion in some patients
- May ultimately reduce transfusion requirements in critically ill patients
- Side effects

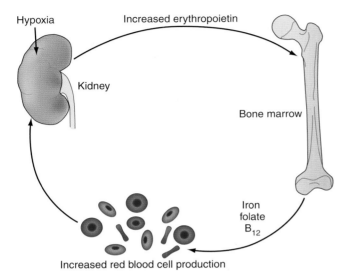

FIGURE 46-1 Regulation of red cell production. *(Adapted from Hoffman R, Heidrick E, Benz E, et al: Hematology: basic principles and practice, ed 4, Philadelphia, Churchill Livingstone, 2005, Fig. 29-2.)*

- Hypertension
- Increased risk of cardiovascular events and death if target hemoglobin is kept greater than 13 g/dL
- Arthralgias
- Thrombosis
- Seizures (rare)
- Polycythemia—if Hct not followed closely
- Some data suggest that it can lead to greater disease progression of certain solid tumors
- Anemia
- Iron deficiency can occur if iron levels are not monitored and repleted when necessary
- Pure RBC aplasia has been reported

Microcytic Anemia

Basic Approach

- Obtain and interpret iron studies (Table 46-2)
  - Serum iron: Not very helpful by itself because there is significant variation in values
  - Total iron-binding capacity (TIBC): Reflects the total amount of transferrin (iron transport protein) available in the blood; is a measure of aggregate iron-binding sites; elevated if iron is low
  - Transferrin saturation: Normally between 20% and 45%

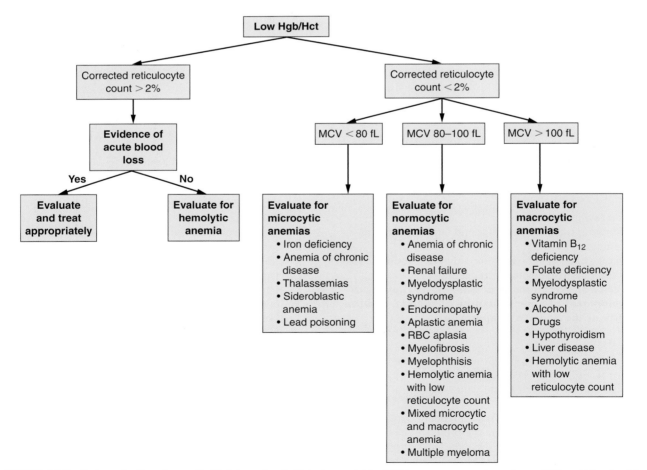

FIGURE 46-2 Basic evaluation of anemia. (Hct, hematocrit; Hgb, hemoglobin; MCV, mean corpuscular volume; RBC, red blood cell.)

- **Ferritin: Correlates with total iron stores; can be normal in iron deficiency if there is concomitant inflammation; even with inflammation, level is usually less than 100 mg/L**

TABLE 46-1	*Immunologic Blood Transfusion Reactions*
Reaction	**Description**
Febrile nonhemolytic	Fever ± chills 1–6 hr after start of transfusion Sometimes can be confused with acute hemolytic reactions so transfusion may need to be temporarily halted Treat with antipyretics and/or meperidine (if chills predominate)

Acute hemolytic	Caused by preformed antibodies in patient's serum that bind and lyse transfused cells
	Most cases are caused by ABO incompatibility
	Can present with fevers and chills with or without flank pain, hypotension, DIC shortly after starting the transfusion
	Management includes
	  Discontinuing the transfusion
	  Notifying the blood bank
	  Starting IV fluids
	  Obtaining blood for direct antiglobulin test, plasma free hemoglobin, coagulation times, renal function

Delayed hemolytic	Caused by an amnestic response in patients who have previously undergone transfusion and have developed low levels of alloantibodies that go undetected during crossmatch Seen 2–10 days after transfusion Direct and indirect antiglobulin tests are positive with identification of the antigen Treatment is supportive
Anaphylactic	Anaphylaxis and shock seconds to minutes after start of the transfusion Commonly caused by anti-IgA antibodies in patients who are IgA deficient Treat by stopping the transfusion, administering epinephrine, and supporting airway and blood pressure
Urticarial	Can continue transfusion after treating with diphenhydramine
Transfusion-related acute lung injury (TRALI)	Dyspnea, hypoxemia, and pulmonary infiltrates that develop within 6 hr after the end of transfusion of a blood product Can cause death in some cases but usually resolves within 96 hr with adequate supportive care (which may include intubation)
Post-transfusion purpura	Causes thrombocytopenia 5–10 days after transfusion of any blood product containing platelets Usually occurs in women Treat with IV immune globulin

DIC, disseminated intravascular coagulation; IgA, immunoglobulin A; IV, intravenous.

- Serum transferrin receptor level: Measure of tissue iron; levels typically go up in iron deficiency but do not change in anemia of chronic disease
- Look at the peripheral smear
- Consider Hgb electrophoresis if studies suggest thalassemia or other hemoglobinopathy
- Bone marrow biopsy with iron staining: Gold standard if etiology unclear

IRON DEFICIENCY ANEMIA

Basic Information

- Present in 2% of the population
- Etiologies
  - **Blood loss is the most common cause**
  - Decreased iron intake
  - Increased iron utilization (e.g., with EPO therapy, chronic hemolysis)
  - Atransferrinemia: Rare autosomal recessive disorder
  - Malabsorption
    - From partial gastrectomy: Iron deficiency develops almost 50% of time
    - From malabsorption syndromes (e.g., celiac sprue) if the disease affects the proximal small intestine

Clinical Presentation

- Paresthesias
- Sore tongue, cheilosis
- Brittle nails or koilonychias ("spoon nails")
- Pica—desire to eat unusual substances (e.g., ice, clay, starch)

Diagnosis

- **Iron studies classically show reduced iron, increased TIBC, reduced transferrin saturation, and reduced ferritin**
- Peripheral smear should show hypochromic, microcytic cells (Fig. 46-3)
- Evaluation of iron-deficient patients
  - Search for evidence of blood loss (e.g., uterine bleeding, gastrointestinal [GI] bleeding, genitourinary [GU] bleeding)
    - If there are no clinical signs or symptoms suggesting a potential cause, start with GI evaluation (esophagogastroduodenoscopy [EGD]/colonoscopy)
    - If EGD and colonoscopy are negative, small bowel capsule endoscopy may be helpful

TABLE 46-2	*Interpretation of Iron Studies*			
	Serum Iron	**TIBC**	**Transferrin Saturation**	**Ferritin**
Iron deficiency	↓	↑	↓	↓ or N
Anemia of chronic disease	↓	N or ↓	N or ↓	N or ↑
Thalassemia trait	N	N	N	N or ↑
Sideroblastic anemia	N or ↑	N or ↑	N or ↑	N or ↑

N, normal; TIBC, total iron-binding capacity.

46

FIGURE 46-3   Iron deficiency anemia. Hypochromic, microcytic blood cells (smaller than the lymphocyte in the center). *(From Goldman L, Bennett JC, Ausiello D: Cecil textbook of medicine, ed 22, Philadelphia, WB Saunders, 2004, Fig. 167-1.)*

- Consider malabsorption if the evaluation for blood loss is negative

Treatment

- Transfusions: Only if there is hemodynamic compromise or acute hemorrhage
- Oral iron
  - Normal dose for iron deficiency is 150 to 200 mg elemental iron daily in divided doses
    - Oral preparations vary in the amount of elemental iron per tablet (i.e., ferrous sulfate typically has 65 mg elemental iron per 325-mg pill while ferrous gluconate may have between 28 and 36 mg of elemental iron per 325-mg pill)
  - Vitamin C administration (250 mg before taking iron) may improve absorption
  - Should see reticulocytosis within 7 days
  - Correction of anemia in about 6 weeks if dose is adequate
  - **If anemia does not improve, consider noncompliance or insufficient dosing, malabsorption, incorrect diagnosis, coexisting disease (e.g., anemia of chronic disease), or continued blood loss**
- Parenteral iron
  - May be indicated in refractory cases
  - Four formulations currently available for use:
    - Iron dextran (IV or IM): Easy to use because total dose can be given in one infusion, but anaphylaxis occurs in 1% of patients
    - Ferric gluconate (IV) and iron sucrose (IV): Need repeat infusions (over weeks) to deliver total dose, but side effects and risk of anaphylaxis lower
    - Ferumoxytol: Approved for the treatment of iron deficiency anemia in adults with chronic kidney disease. Anaphylaxis and hypotension can occur. May transiently interfere with ability to interpret magnetic resonance images.

ANEMIA OF CHRONIC DISEASE

Basic Information

- **Most cases are actually normocytic, not microcytic**
- Etiologies
  - Malignancy
  - Chronic infections (e.g., osteomyelitis, tuberculosis, AIDS)
  - Chronic inflammatory disorders (e.g., rheumatoid arthritis [RA], systemic lupus erythematosus [SLE], ulcerative colitis)
  - Congestive heart failure
- Mechanisms
  - Decreased RBC survival
  - Impaired EPO production
  - Impaired marrow response to EPO
  - Impaired mobilization of iron (i.e., increased iron uptake and retention within the reticuloendothelial system)

Clinical Presentation and Diagnosis

- Iron studies (see Table 46-2)
- Peripheral smear usually shows normocytic, normochromic cells but can be microcytic in 30% to 40% of cases; **MCV is rarely less than 75 fL**
- Bone marrow biopsy may be helpful if the diagnosis is unclear; it should reveal normal or increased iron stores
- Soluble transferrin receptor (sTfR) level may help distinguish pure anemia of chronic disease from anemia of chronic disease with concomitant iron deficiency in patients with normal ferritin levels
  - If the sTfR/log ferritin (sTfR/log ferritin index) is greater than 2, iron deficiency probably coexists with anemia of chronic disease
  - If the sTfR/log ferritin index is less than 1, iron deficiency is likely not present with anemia of chronic disease

Treatment

- Treat the underlying disorder (if possible)
- Transfusion rarely indicated because anemia is usually not severe
- EPO/darbepoietin has been shown to increase quality of life and reduce the need for transfusion in some patients with anemia of chronic disease but is very costly and may be harmful in some cases (e.g., treatment of anemia due to certain solid tumors)
  - Goal is to not exceed hemoglobin values of 12 g/dL

THALASSEMIA

Basic Information

- Defined as a decrease in production of one of the two globin chains
  - Normal Hgb A has two α and two β chains ($\alpha_2\beta_2$)
  - In β-thalassemia, there is partial or complete suppression of β-globin chain synthesis resulting in a relative excess of α-globin chains
  - In α-thalassemia, there is suppression or absence of α chains resulting in a relative excess of β chains
- Seen predominantly in people of African, Asian, or Mediterranean descent
- There are a number of genetic variations seen clinically
  - β-Thalassemia
    - β-Thalassemia major: Presents in the first year of life; patients are transfusion dependent
    - β-Thalassemia intermedia: Regular transfusions unnecessary until second, third, or fourth decade; can develop iron overload independently of transfusions

TABLE 46-3	Clues to Differentiating Thalassemia Trait from Iron Deficiency Anemia	
	Thalassemia Trait	Iron Deficiency Anemia
RBC count	N or ↑	↓
MCV	Lower than would be expected with iron deficiency	↓
RDW	N	↑
Ferritin	N or ↑	↓
Bone marrow iron	N	↓

MCV, mean corpuscular volume; N, normal; RBC, red blood cell; RDW, red cell distribution width.

FIGURE 46-4 β-Thalassemia trait. Hypochromic, microcytic red blood cells with frequent targeting. Mild anemia. *(From McPherson RA, Pincus MR: Henry's clinical diagnosis and management by laboratory methods, ed 21, Philadelphia, Elsevier Saunders, 2006, Fig. 31-27.)*

- β-Thalassemia minor (β-thal trait): Causes mild anemia and significant microcytosis
- α-Thalassemia
  - Hydrops fetalis and Hgb Barts: Usually fatal in utero
  - Hgb H: Significant anemia, hemolysis, splenomegaly are usually diagnosed in late childhood
  - α-Thalassemia trait (α-thalassemia minor): Causes mild anemia and significant microcytosis
  - Asymptomatic carrier (α-thalassemia minima): No significant anemia

Clinical Presentation and Diagnosis

- Most cases of clinically severe anemia present in childhood
- Patients with thalassemia trait are commonly asymptomatic
- Several clues may be present that can help distinguish thalassemia trait from iron deficiency anemia (Table 46-3)
- Peripheral smear can show basophilic stippling, microcytosis, and target cells (Fig. 46-4)
- Hgb electrophoresis can be helpful in some cases
  - Normal: Hgb A ($\alpha_2\beta_2$) 97%; Hgb A_2 ($\alpha_2\delta_2$) 2% to 3%; Hgb F ($\alpha_2\gamma_2$) 0% to 1%
  - **β-Thal trait: Increased Hgb A_2 and Hgb F**
  - α-Thal trait: Usually normal but may possibly show a decreased Hgb A_2 concentration

Treatment

- Thalassemia trait: None indicated
- β-Thalassemia intermedia, β-thalassemia major, and Hgb H
  - Chronic transfusion
  - Splenectomy
  - Treatment for iron overload
  - Management of complications, including leg ulcers, pulmonary hypertension, gallstones, aplasia

SIDEROBLASTIC ANEMIAS

- Consist of inherited or acquired defects that result in impaired heme biosynthesis
- **Characterized by iron-positive granules surrounding the nucleus of RBCs (ringed sideroblasts) in the bone marrow**
- Hereditary sideroblastic anemia
  - Most cases are X-linked and present in childhood
  - Usually presents with a fairly stable anemia
  - **Iron overload develops in all patients because of increased absorption of iron**
  - Iron studies show an increased transferrin saturation and ferritin level
  - Genetic studies should help confirm the diagnosis
  - Anemia responds to pyridoxine in most cases
  - Need to treat iron overload with phlebotomy or chelation
- Acquired idiopathic sideroblastic anemia
  - Usually occurs in older individuals
  - Anemia is usually normocytic or macrocytic
  - Iron studies reveal overload
  - Risk of transformation to acute leukemia
  - **Considered one of the myelodysplastic syndromes** (MDS; see Chapter 50)
  - Typically does not respond to treatment with pyridoxine
- Reversible sideroblastic anemia
  - Can be caused by a number of different precipitants, including alcohol, isoniazid, and chloramphenicol
  - Anemia improves with removal of the drug
- Lead poisoning
  - It is controversial whether it truly causes sideroblastic changes
  - Some causes include ingestion of lead-based paint, ingestion of contaminated dietary supplements, consumption of moonshine from lead-lined stills, and inhalation of fumes
  - **Clinical manifestations include microcytic anemia, autonomic and motor neuropathy, and abdominal pain**
  - Diagnosed by finding elevated blood lead levels
  - Treat with edetate disodium (EDTA) chelation

Normocytic (Nonhemolytic) Anemia

- Basic approach
  - Can result from a number of different processes (see Fig. 46-2)
  - Clues to the diagnosis may be present in the history, physical, and other laboratory tests

46

- The presence of pancytopenia suggests a primary bone marrow disorder
- An elevated creatinine level suggests the possibility of anemia caused by renal insufficiency or failure
- The presence of cancer, infection, or other inflammatory disorder suggests the presence of anemia of chronic disease

ANEMIA OF CHRONIC DISEASE

See the previous discussion of anemia of chronic disease in the Microcytic Anemia section.

ANEMIA OF RENAL INSUFFICIENCY OR FAILURE

- Usually manifests when creatinine clearance falls to below 50 mL/min
- **The primary abnormality is EPO deficiency**
- Uremia can also contribute to anemia
  - Can cause blood loss usually through the GI tract
  - Decreases RBC survival
- Folate deficiency, aluminum overload, and hyperparathyroidism (causing bone marrow fibrosis) can all potentially contribute to anemia
- Treatment
  - Standard of care is now subcutaneous or IV ESA (erythropoietin or darbepoietin)
  - ESAs can potentially delay the progression of renal disease in patients with renal insufficiency and anemia
  - **Goal is to maintain Hct between 33% and 36% (Hgb between 11 and 12 g/dL)**
  - Iron therapy indicated for ferritin levels below 100 mg/L

APLASTIC ANEMIA

- Characterized by pancytopenia and a reticulocyte index less than 2
- Fanconi anemia (short stature, café-au-lait spots, GU abnormalities, microphthalmia, mental retardation, and skeletal abnormalities seen in association with aplastic anemia) is the most common congenital form
- Most acquired cases are idiopathic, but a number of other causes have been described (Box 46-1)
- Usually occurs between the ages of 15 and 25 years, with a second peak after age 60 years
- Thought to be an autoimmune disease
- Bone marrow is hypocellular with fat replacement of bone marrow elements (Fig. 46-5)
- Cytogenetic studies may help to distinguish from hypocellular MDS (i.e., abnormalities can be seen in MDS but not in aplastic anemia)
- Treatment
  - Withdraw the offending agent (if identified)
  - Support with transfusions as needed; mild forms of disease may not need definitive treatment
  - **Bone marrow transplantation (BMT) is the treatment of choice in all patients under the age of 45 years with severe aplastic anemia when there is a human leukocyte antigen–matched donor**
  - Immunosuppression with antithymocyte globulin plus cyclosporine plus corticosteroids is used when BMT not possible

- Is associated with future development of myelodysplasia and paroxysmal nocturnal hemoglobinuria in 10% to 15% of patients

PURE RED CELL APLASIA

- Characterized by selective absence of RBCs in the marrow
- Can be idiopathic or associated with a number of conditions
  - Thymoma
  - Lymphoproliferative disease (e.g., chronic lymphocytic leukemia [CLL], large granular lymphoma, chronic myelogenous leukemia)
  - Collagen vascular disease
  - Drugs (similar to aplastic anemia)
  - EPO
    - Can induce antibodies to EPO, resulting in anemia
      - Most cases have been seen with subcutaneous administration from a formulation not sold in the United States, although cases in the United States have been reported
  - Parvovirus B19

BOX 46-1 *Causes of Aplastic Anemia*

Drugs
  Antiepileptic drugs (e.g, carbamazepine, phenytoin, valproic acid)
  Chemotherapeutic agents
  Chloramphenicol
  Gold
  Nifedipine
  Sulfonamides
  Phenylbutazone
Chemicals (e.g., benzene, insecticides)
Radiation
Viruses
  Parvovirus B19
  Non-A, non-B, non-C hepatitis
  HIV, Epstein-Barr virus, cytomegalovirus
Connective tissue disease
Paroxysmal nocturnal hemoglobinuria

FIGURE 46-5 Bone marrow biopsy from a patient with aplastic anemia. (*From Kumar V, Fausto N, Abbas A: Robbins and Cotran's pathologic basis of disease, ed 7, Philadelphia, WB Saunders, 2004, Fig. 13-27.*)

- Usually a transient process in normal hosts
- Can cause severe transient aplastic crisis in patients with underlying hemolytic disorders
- Can cause chronic aplasia in immunodeficient patients
- CBC reveals anemia with normal WBC and platelet counts
- Bone marrow reveals few or absent erythroid precursors
- **Computed tomography scan should be ordered to look for thymoma in all idiopathic cases**
- Treatment
  - Initial treatment is supportive with transfusions, if needed
  - Cases caused by parvovirus infection may respond to IV immune globulin
  - Cases caused by thymoma may respond to tumor removal
  - Immunosuppressive drugs are used in refractory cases (e.g., corticosteroids, cyclosporine, cyclophosphamide)

Macrocytic Anemia

- Basic approach
  - Confirm that the anemia is hypoproliferative (reticulocyte index <2%)
  - Consider the two basic types of macrocytic anemia: Megaloblastic and nonmegaloblastic
  - The history and physical examination can suggest certain etiologies
    - Use of certain medications (e.g., methotrexate, hydroxyurea, zidovudine, phenytoin, triamterene, imatinib, sunitinib)
    - Alcohol use
    - History of GI surgery (i.e., gastrectomy, ileal resection)
    - Signs or symptoms of liver disease
    - Signs or symptoms of hypothyroidism
  - Clues on the peripheral smear
    - Macro-ovalocytes: Suggestive of megaloblastic anemias (Fig. 46-6)
    - Hypersegmented neutrophils (more than six lobes)

FIGURE 46-6 Megaloblastic anemia. Macrocytes, macro-ovalocytes, and a hypersegmented neutrophil.

- Have a high sensitivity and specificity for megaloblastic anemias (see Fig. 46-6)
  - Can appear before macrocytosis or anemia
- Target cells: Can be suggestive of liver disease
- Pseudo Pelger-Huët anomaly: Hyposegmented neutrophils suggestive of myelodysplasia
- Laboratory evaluation
  - **A very high MCV (>110 fL) is suggestive of vitamin B_{12} or folate deficiency**
  - Vitamin B_{12} and folate levels
  - Liver function tests
  - Thyroid-stimulating hormone
- Bone marrow examination is necessary if etiology is unclear or if MDS is being considered

MEGALOBLASTIC ANEMIA

- Characterized by abnormal nuclear maturation of red cell precursors (megaloblasts) in the bone marrow
- Causes include vitamin B_{12} deficiency, folate deficiency, myelodysplastic syndromes (occasionally), and chemotherapy

VITAMIN B_{12} (COBALAMIN) DEFICIENCY
Basic Information

- Vitamin B_{12} is absorbed in the terminal ileum
- Parietal cells in the stomach secrete intrinsic factor that facilitates absorption
- **Deficiency usually takes years to develop**
- Most cases result from food-cobalamin malabsorption whereby stomach acids are unable to cleave vitamin B_{12} bound to food
- Numerous other causes exist (Table 46-4)

Clinical Presentation

- Symptoms of anemia are nonspecific
- **Neurologic symptoms may be present before anemia develops**
  - Symmetrical paresthesias
  - Ataxia, spasticity
  - Memory loss, irritability, dementia
- Asymptomatic patients may present with only laboratory abnormalities
  - Pancytopenia
  - Elevated low-density lipoprotein and indirect bilirubin caused by destruction of cells within the bone marrow

Diagnosis

- Peripheral smear may show macro-ovalocytes and hypersegmented neutrophils
- Serum vitamin B_{12} level is the standard diagnostic test, but it might not accurately represent true tissue levels in some patients
- Metabolic testing may be useful in patients who present with clinical evidence of deficiency and borderline serum levels (200–300 pg/mL)
  - Methylmalonic acid: Elevated levels are sensitive and specific for vitamin B_{12} deficiency in patients with normal renal function; this elevation is not seen in folate deficiency
  - Homocysteine: Elevated levels are very sensitive but not specific; elevations are also seen in folate deficiency

46

TABLE 46-4	*Etiologies of Vitamin B$_{12}$ Deficiency*
Pernicious anemia	Autoimmune disease that results in achlorhydria and the absence of intrinsic factor Associated with other autoimmune processes (e.g., vitiligo, hypothyroidism, Addison disease) Associated with increased risk of gastric cancer Anti–intrinsic factor antibodies are specific but not sensitive for the diagnosis Anti–parietal cell antibodies are sensitive but not specific for the diagnosis
Gastrectomy	Can result in deficiency in intrinsic factor Can cause impaired ability to cleave cobalamin from food
Atrophic gastritis	Thought to be a major cause of subclinical deficiency in elderly patients Results in inability to cleave cobalamin from food Can be associated with *Helicobacter pylori* infection
Intestinal disorders (e.g., ileal resection, Crohn disease, celiac disease, tropical sprue, bacterial overgrowth syndromes)	Look for other signs of malabsorption Can coexist with iron deficiency
Pancreatic insufficiency	Look for signs of chronic pancreatitis
Diet	Strict vegans have decreased intake of vitamin B$_{12}$
Medications (e.g., metformin, proton pump inhibitors)	Cause impaired intestinal absorption

TABLE 46-5	*Schilling Test*

Stage I: Oral radioactive free B$_{12}$ is given, followed by intramuscular unlabeled B$_{12}$ to saturate tissue receptors and displace bound radiolabeled B$_{12}$. A 24-hr urine is then obtained to look for absorbed oral B$_{12}$. If <9% of the administered oral dose is found in urine, the test is considered abnormal.

Stage II: Oral radioactive B$_{12}$ plus oral intrinsic factor is given, followed by intramuscular unlabeled B$_{12}$. A 24-hr urine is again obtained. Excretion should correct to >9% if the problem is an intrinsic factor deficiency (e.g., pernicious anemia).

Stage III: Done if the first two stages are abnormal. A gluten-free diet (to diagnose celiac sprue), administration of antibiotics (to diagnose bacterial overgrowth), or administration of pancreatic enzymes (to diagnose pancreatic insufficiency) is done before repeating stage I.

TEST INTERPRETATION

Condition	Stage I	Stage II
Normal	Normal	
Dietary deficiency (veganism)	Normal	
Inadequate dissociation of cobalamin from food* (e.g., atrophic gastritis)	Normal	
Pernicious anemia	Low	Normal
Gastrectomy	Low	Normal
Ileal resection/ malabsorption	Low	Low
Bacterial overgrowth of the ileum	Low	Low
Pancreatic insufficiency	Low	Low

*A modified version of stage I of the test can be done to diagnose food-cobalamin malabsorption. This test utilizes radiolabeled B$_{12}$ bound to food rather than free B$_{12}$. Patients with food-cobalamin malabsorption should have abnormally low urine B$_{12}$ excretions.

- Antibody testing for the diagnosis of pernicious anemia (see Table 46-4)
- The Schilling test can be done if a cause for the deficiency is not evident (Table 46-5) but is rarely necessary

Treatment

- Intramuscular vitamin B$_{12}$ injections are usually the initial treatment of choice for pernicious anemia
- Oral vitamin B$_{12}$ can be equally effective in raising serum levels
  - Must be given in very large doses (1–2 mg/day) in patients with pernicious anemia
  - Lower oral doses (250 μg/day) may be sufficient to treat food-cobalamin malabsorption
  - Consider the risk of noncompliance if choosing the oral route
- Other routes (intranasal, sublingual, topical) are less well studied
- Hematologic abnormalities should normalize within 2 months
- Neurologic abnormalities normalize within 6 months

FOLATE DEFICIENCY

- **Can develop rapidly (within months)**
- Causes
  - Nutritional deficiency
  - Alcoholism
  - Malabsorption (e.g., celiac sprue, tropical sprue)
  - Excess demands (e.g., pregnancy, chronic hemolytic states)
  - Drugs that interfere with folate metabolism (e.g., methotrexate, phenytoin, trimethoprim)
- Pancytopenia, elevated lactate dehydrogenase (LDH), and elevated bilirubin can occur
- The peripheral smear will be identical to that seen in vitamin B$_{12}$ deficiency
- Red cell folate levels may more accurately measure true tissue status because normal serum folate levels are a reflection of short-term intake
  - It is reasonable to use serum folate levels as an initial screen for deficiency since the test is less expensive and readily available
- Treat with oral folic acid (1–2 mg/day is usually sufficient)

BOX 46-2 *Effect of Alcohol on Red Blood Cells*

Macrocytosis without anemia can occur with regular intake of as little as a half-bottle of wine per day
Anemia may result from a number of different mechanisms
   Direct toxic effect on the bone marrow
   Iron deficiency caused by GI bleeding
   Folic acid deficiency
   Liver disease causing splenic sequestration hemolysis
   Liver disease resulting in acanthocyte (spur cell) formation and hemolysis

MYELODYSPLASTIC SYNDROMES

- Peripheral smear can have ovalocytes, but hypersegmented neutrophils are not typically seen
- Bone marrow may or may not show megaloblastic changes
- Vitamin B_{12} and folate levels should be normal
- See Chapter 50 for diagnostic and treatment information

CHEMOTHERAPEUTIC AGENTS

- Hydroxyurea and azathioprine are examples
- Peripheral smear should not show hypersegmented neutrophils
- Bone marrow may or may not show megaloblastic changes

NONMEGALOBLASTIC MACROCYTIC ANEMIA

- Alcohol is the most common cause and may affect red cells through several different mechanisms (Box 46-2)
- Hypothyroidism, multiple myeloma, liver disease, aplastic anemia, drugs, and MDS may also present with macrocytic anemia

Hemolytic Anemia

Basic Approach

- Defined as the premature destruction of RBCs
- Occurs by two different mechanisms:
  - Extravascular hemolyis: RBCs are prematurely removed from the circulation by the liver and spleen (most cases)
  - Intravascular hemolysis: RBCs lyse in the circulation
- Laboratory studies
  - **Reticulocyte index is greater than 2%**
  - Indirect bilirubin is elevated
  - LDH is elevated
  - Haptoglobin is low or absent; haptoglobin binds free Hgb and is then taken up by the reticuloendothelial system; during hemolysis the rate of haptoglobin catabolism exceeds the liver's ability to produce it, resulting in a low or absent level
  - Urine hemosiderin: Present in intravascular hemolysis only
  - Urine Hgb: Present in severe intravascular hemolysis; urine dipstick test is positive for blood but no RBCs seen on microscopic examination

FIGURE 46-7 Direct antiglobulin (Coombs') test. (IgG, immunoglobulin G.)

- Direct antiglobulin test (direct Coombs' test; Fig. 46-7)
  - Useful in diagnosing immune hemolytic anemia (>95% sensitivity) where there is antibody coating a patient's RBCs
  - Done by mixing the patient's erythrocytes with antihuman globulin (which contains antibody to immunoglobulin G [IgG] and C3)
  - If agglutination occurs, the test is positive and the diagnosis of immune hemolysis is made
  - **Once a positive test is found, further testing is done to determine whether IgG and/or C3 are coating the patient's erythrocytes**
- Indirect antiglobulin test (indirect Coombs' test)
  - Useful to detect antibodies present in a patient's serum
  - Helpful in detecting alloantibodies that were induced by prior transfusion or by fetal transfer of RBCs to the mother
- The peripheral smear can assist in developing a systematic approach to patients (Fig. 46-8)

IMMUNE HEMOLYTIC ANEMIA

- Autoimmune hemolytic anemia (a positive direct antiglobulin [Coombs'] test)
  - Warm-antibody autoimmune hemolytic anemia
    - Autoantibodies optimally reactive at 37°C
    - **Almost always has IgG identified on red cell surface (Table 46-6)**
    - May also have C3 identified
    - Most cases are idiopathic
    - Can be a complication of an underlying disease
      - Lymphoproliferative disorder: CLL, lymphoma
      - Collagen vascular disease: SLE, RA
      - Ulcerative colitis
      - Congenital immunodeficiency

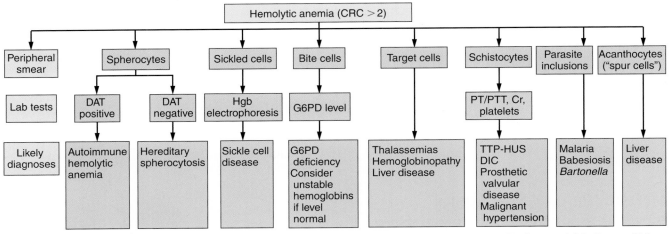

FIGURE 46-8　Basic approach to hemolytic anemia. (Cr, creatinine; CRC, corrected reticulocyte count; DAT, direct antiglobulin test; DIC, disseminated intravascular coagulation; G6PD, glucose-6-phosphate dehydrogenase; Hgb, hemoglobin; PT/PTT, prothrombin time/partial thromboplastin time; TTP-HUS, thrombotic thrombocytopenic purpura–hemolytic uremic syndrome.)

TABLE 46-6	*Interpretation of Antiglobulin Tests in Immune Hemolytic Anemia*		
Condition	**DAT-IgG**	**DAT-C3**	**IAT**
Warm Ab	+	±	± No specific Ab
Cold agglutinin	−	+	± No specific Ab
Drug—methyldopa	+	−	± No specific Ab
Drug—PCN, ceph	+*	−	± No specific Ab
Drug—quinine, sulfa	−	+	± No specific Ab
Delayed transfusion reaction	+	±	+ With alloantibody found

Ab, antibody; ceph, cephalosporins; DAT, direct antiglobulin (Coombs') test; IAT, indirect antiglobulin test; IgG, immunoglobulin G; PCN, penicillin.
*Positive only during exposure to drug.

- Findings include anemia, reticulocytosis, splenomegaly, and spherocytosis
- Rarely patients may have separate antibodies directed at platelets causing concomitant thrombocytopenia (Evan syndrome)
- Treatment
    - Initial: Support with blood transfusions plus prednisone 1 mg/kg/day with or without IV immune globulin (IgG)
    - Splenectomy: If refractory to prednisone
    - Immunosuppressives and/or cytotoxic agents: If refractory to splenectomy and prednisone
- Cold agglutinin syndrome
    - **Caused by an immunoglobulin M (IgM) complement-fixing antibody that binds to C3 on the red cell surface at low temperatures (4°C)**
    - Patients may have worsening of hemolysis and acrocyanosis when exposed to the cold
    - Direct antiglobulin (Coombs') test is positive for C3
    - Associated with a number of infections

- *Mycoplasma* pneumonia self-limited hemolysis can occur 5 to 10 days after recovery from infection
- Infectious mononucleosis (Epstein-Barr virus)
- Also associated with lymphoproliferative disorders and monoclonal gammopathy
    - Disease may be mild and chronic
    - Reticulocytosis may be minimal
- Diagnosed by IgM cold agglutinin antibody titers
    - Low titers (<1:32) can be found in normal serum
    - **Most patients with disease have titers in excess of 1:1000 at 4°C**
- Treatment is usually supportive, but chlorambucil and cyclophosphamide have been used, especially in patients with monoclonal gammopathy
- Paroxysmal cold hemoglobinuria
    - Very rare disorder historically associated with tertiary syphilis
    - Most cases in adults are autoimmune
    - Caused by IgG (Donath-Landsteiner) antibody that can induce hemolysis (and often hemoglobinuria) with cold exposure
    - Direct antiglobulin test can be positive with anti-C3 during episodes of hemolysis but negative between episodes
    - Initial treatment is with prednisone
- Drug-induced hemolytic anemia
    - Drug-independent autoantibody induction
        - Presents identically to warm-antibody hemolytic anemia
        - Seen with methyldopa, procainamide, ibuprofen
        - Red cells coated with IgG but not C3
        - Hemolysis decreases weeks after cessation of drug
    - Drug-dependent drug adsorption
        - Antibody is directed against the drug and the membrane protein to which it is attached
        - Direct antiglobulin test is positive for IgG during the period of drug administration
        - Seen most commonly with cephalosporins and high-dose penicillin
    - Drug-dependent immune complex

- Drugs loosely bind to RBC membrane with formation of antibodies reacting to both drug and membrane components
- Results in stimulation of complement cascade
- Direct antiglobulin test is positive for C3 but not IgG
- Seen most commonly with cephalosporins, quinine, quinidine, sulfa drugs
  - Nonimmunologic protein adsorption
    - Hypothesized that drug induces change in RBC membrane properties
    - Associated with prolonged exposure to high-dose cepahalothin, although other drugs have been implicated as well
- Transfusion-related hemolysis (see Table 46-1)

NONIMMUNE HEMOLYTIC ANEMIA (DIRECT COOMBS' TEST NEGATIVE)

- Inherited nonimmune hemolytic anemia
  - RBC membrane disorders
    - Hereditary spherocytosis
      - More common in patients of northern European ancestry but occurs in all racial groups
      - Clinical manifestations include anemia, splenomegaly, and jaundice
      - Disease severity can range from mild (no anemia) to death in utero
      - Gallstone formation is common
      - Aplastic crises can develop during viral infections (e.g., parvovirus)
      - The mean corpuscular hemoglobin concentration (MCHC) is commonly elevated
      - Diagnosis is suspected in patients with clinical evidence of hemolytic anemia, spherocytes on peripheral smear (Fig. 46-9), and a negative direct antiglobulin test
      - An abnormal osmotic fragility test confirms the diagnosis (hemolysis occurs at progressively diluted salt concentrations)
      - Treat with supportive care (e.g., transfusions) and folic acid
      - Splenectomy (with or without cholecystectomy) is the treatment of choice in symptomatic patients
    - Hereditary elliptocytosis
      - Similar in presentation to spherocytosis
      - More than 75% of cells are elliptical
  - RBC enzyme defects
    - Glucose-6-phosphate dehydrogenase (G6PD) deficiency
      - G6PD helps protect Hgb from oxidation on exposure to a drug or toxin that results in the generation of free radicals
      - The World Health Organization has classified different G6PD variants based on the magnitude of enzyme deficiency and the severity of hemolysis (class I, most severe, to class V, which is not clinically significant)
      - Drugs that have been implicated include primaquine, sulfa drugs, dapsone, and nitrofurantoin
      - Favism is the acute hemolysis seen in some patients with G6PD deficiency after ingestion of fava beans

FIGURE 46-9 Hereditary spherocytosis. *(From Stevens A, Lowe J: Pathology, ed 2, St. Louis, Mosby, 2000, Fig. 15.23.)*

- Patients present with an acute hemolytic reaction of varying severity 2 to 4 days after exposure to a drug
- Infections and diabetic ketoacidosis can also trigger hemolysis
- Can see "bite" cells on peripheral smear
- Can also see Heinz bodies (precipitated Hgb) with a reticulocyte stain
- **Diagnosis is made by measuring the level of the G6PD enzyme, but this may be normal when there is active hemolysis**
- Treatment is supportive
  - Sickle cell disorders (SS, Sβ-thal, SC)
    - Characterized by a chronic hemolytic state in which vaso-occlusion is caused by a deformity of RBCs
    - Sickle trait rarely has clinical implications
    - Hgb SC disease is usually milder than Hgb SS disease
    - Functional asplenia results from SS disease
    - Most common presentation is acute pain crisis but can affect virtually every organ system (Table 46-7)
    - The most life-threatening complications include acute chest syndrome, stroke, and infections
    - **Pulmonary hypertension occurs in about 30% of adults with sickle cell disease and is a strong predictor for near-term mortality**
    - Hgb electrophoresis establishes the diagnosis
    - Treatment
      - Pain crises: Hydration and analgesics (avoid meperidine); transfusion usually not needed
      - Acute chest syndrome: Antibiotics, oxygen, exchange transfusion
      - Stroke: Exchange transfusion

- Hematopoietic cell transplantation may be potentially curative, but criteria for this option are still being developed
- Prevention of complications
  - Vaccination: Pneumococcal, *Haemophilus influenzae* type b, *Meningococcus*, influenza
  - Folate and iron may be necessary to keep up with cell turnover
  - Regular retinal examinations
  - **Hydroxyurea: Has been shown to decrease the incidence of acute chest syndrome, decrease the number of pain crises, decrease transfusions, and possibly decrease mortality**
  - Preoperative transfusion: To an Hgb level of 9 to 11 mg/dL can improve outcome in surgical patients

TABLE 46-7	Clinical Manifestations of Sickle Cell Disease
Organ System	**Type of Complication**
CNS	Stroke Subarachnoid hemorrhage
Eye	Retinopathy Hyphema

Lung	Acute chest syndrome
	  Most common cause of death in adults
	  Patients present with fever, chest pain, and an infiltrate on chest radiography
	  Treat with antibiotics and oxygen
	  Exchange transfusion indicated if there is progressive hypoxemia
	 Fat emboli
	 Restrictive lung disease
	 Pulmonary hypertension/cor pulmonale

Heart	MI CHF (rare)
Renal	Nephrotic syndrome Hypertension Chronic renal failure Hyposthenuria Hematuria Hyperuricemia
Urologic	Priapism
Bone	Joint effusions Avascular necrosis
Skin	Hyperpigmentation Leg ulcers
Liver/GB	Acute/chronic liver disease Gallstones
Infectious disease	Pneumonia (*Streptococcus pneumoniae*, *Haemophilus influenzae*) Osteomyelitis (*Salmonella* spp., *Staphylococcus aureus*) Urinary tract infection Sepsis
Heme	Chronic hemolytic anemia Splenic sequestration crisis Acute aplastic crisis

CHF, congestive heart failure; CNS, central nervous system; GB, gallbladder; MI, myocardial infarction.

- Acquired nonimmune hemolytic anemia
  - Splenomegaly (sequestrational hemolysis)
    - Can lead to destruction of normal RBCs
    - Causes include lymphoproliferative disorders, myeloproliferative disorders, inflammatory diseases, infection, portal hypertension, and hemolytic anemia
  - March hemoglobinuria
    - Intravascular hemolysis with hemoglobinuria
    - Seen after prolonged physical activity
    - Anemia is usually not present
  - Microangiopathic hemolytic anemia
    - Cardiac hemolysis
      - Occurs in about 10% of patients with mechanical aortic valve replacements
      - Severity of the anemia is variable but can cause significant hemoglobinuria
      - Hemosiderin can be detected in the urine
      - Schistocytes seen on peripheral smear
      - Need to watch for iron deficiency because of Hgb loss in urine
      - New-onset (or worsening) hemolysis in a patient with a prosthetic valve warrants an evaluation with an echocardiogram to assess for perivalvular leak and valve failure
    - Thrombotic thrombocytopenic purpura–hemolytic uremic syndrome (see Chapter 47)
    - Disseminated intravascular coagulation (see Chapter 48)
  - Direct toxic effects on RBCs
    - Infections
      - Parasites: Malaria, *Babesia*, *Bartonella*
      - *Clostridium welchii*: Produces a phospholipase that can lead to membrane rupture
    - Snake and spider bites
    - Copper: Seen in Wilson disease
  - Paroxysmal nocturnal hemoglobinuria
    - Caused by an acquired mutation of the X-chromosome gene *PIGA*
    - Ultimately found in 10% to 20% of patients with aplastic anemia
    - Mutation results in impaired synthesis of glycosyl phosphatidylinositol–anchored proteins (GPI-APs)
    - Clinical presentation includes hemolytic anemia (intravascular), venous thrombosis (particularly at unusual sites), and/or deficient hematopoiesis
    - Some patients may also develop esophageal spasm and/or erectile dysfunction from a deficiency in nitric oxide during hemolytic episodes
    - Laboratory features
      - Normocytic anemia usually; can be microcytic if iron deficiency develops from loss of Hgb in the urine
      - Hemoglobinuria: Present only intermittently
      - Hemosiderinuria: Present in virtually all patients
      - Leukopenia and thrombocytopenia: Usually mild but can develop into aplastic anemia
    - Diagnosis
      - Flow cytometry is the test of choice, with demonstration of deficiency of GPI-APs CD55 and CD59

- Treatment
  - Supportive care with iron, folate, and blood transfusions
  - Humanized monoclonal antibody against complement protein C5 (e.g., eculizumab) reduces the need for transfusion, ameliorates (but does not eliminate) the anemia, and improves quality of life
    - Does not affect the underlying stem cell disorder
    - Treatment is lifelong
    - **Increases the risk of *Neisseria meningitides* infection, so need to vaccinate before therapy begins**
  - Prednisone may decrease hemolysis
  - Androgenic hormones may be beneficial
  - Anticoagulation if thrombosis is present
  - BMT should be considered if a donor is available and severe disease is present

REVIEW QUESTIONS

For review questions, please go to www.expertconsult.com.

SUGGESTED READINGS

Brodsky RA, Jones RJ: Aplastic anaemia, *Lancet* 365:1647–1656, 2005.

Gladwin MT, Vichinsky E: Pulmonary complications of sickle cell disease, *N Engl J Med* 359:2254–2265, 2008.

Johnson CS: The acute chest syndrome, *Hematol Oncol Clin North Am* 19:857–879, 2005.

Parker CJ: Bone marrow failure syndromes: paroxysmal nocturnal hemoglobinuria, *Hematol Oncol Clin North Am* 23:333–346, 2009.

Rees DC, Williams TN, Gladwin MT: Sickle-cell disease, *Lancet* 376:2018–2031, 2010.

Rund D, Rachmilewitz E: Beta-thalassemia, *N Engl J Med* 353:1135–1146, 2005.

Sawada K, Hirokawa M, Fujishima N: Diagnosis and management of acquired pure red cell aplasia, *Hematol Oncol Clin North Am* 23:249–259, 2009.

Weiss G, Goodnough LT: Anemia of chronic disease, *N Engl J Med* 352:1011–1023, 2005.

46

CHAPTER 47

Platelet Disorders

ELIZABETH A. GRIFFITHS, MD; and SOPHIE M. LANZKRON, MD, MHS

Platelet disorders may result in life-threatening consequences. They may be due to an isolated defect in the platelet's role in clot formation or evidence of systemic disease. A stepwise approach in the evaluation of a patient with a suspected platelet disorder is essential to make the diagnosis and initiate treatment.

Basic Information

- Normal platelet function requires four steps to result in clot formation: Activation, adhesion, aggregation, and secretion (Fig. 47-1)
- Platelet dysfunction can be categorized as caused by quantitative defects (i.e., the number of platelets), by qualitative defects (i.e., how well they function), or by both
  - Quantitative assessment of platelets is performed by machine counters and by visualization of the peripheral smear
    - **Automated tests identifying thrombocytopenia should be confirmed with visual inspection of a peripheral smear**
    - Bleeding complications may be associated with thrombocytosis if the platelets produced are dysfunctional or if there is an acquired von Willebrand factor (vWF) deficiency
  - Qualitative assessment for defects in platelet function is evaluated by obtaining a bleeding history, bleeding time, platelet function analyzer (PFA-100), and aggregometry (see following discussion)

Clinical Evaluation

- The medical history
  - Clues in the history suggestive of platelet dysfunction include the following:
    - **Bleeding that is limited to superficial sites such as skin or mucosa (hemarthroses are uncommon with platelet disorders and usually represent defects in the clotting cascade)**
    - **Bleeding that starts immediately after trauma or surgery**
    - Excessive menstrual bleeding
    - Other family members with bleeding histories suggest an inherited platelet disorder
    - Many medications may result in thrombocytopenia or dysfunctional platelets; medication (and toxin) exposure should be reviewed in any patient with a suspected platelet disorder
    - Disorders of platelet excess (e.g., thrombocytosis) are most commonly reactions to other illnesses (e.g., acute hemorrhage, iron deficiency, infection), which should be sought in the history (see following discussion)

- The physical examination
  - **Clues in the physical examination suggestive of platelet dysfunction include the following:**
    - **Petechiae**
    - **Mucosal bleeding**
    - Splenomegaly
      - May suggest an underlying bone marrow process or liver disease that may be causing platelet abnormalities

Laboratory Evaluation

- Peripheral blood smear (Fig. 47-2)
  - Great importance for evaluating both qualitative and quantitative deficiencies in platelets
  - Used to confirm platelet number
    - Spuriously low platelet counts may occur as a result of interaction between ethylenediaminetetraacetic acid (EDTA) and platelet glycoproteins, leading to platelet aggregation. Repeating the platelet count drawn in a citrated (rather than an EDTA) tube will verify that the platelet count is normal.
  - Used to evaluate platelet morphology; both the size of platelets and the presence of platelet granularity may aid in the diagnosis
    - Many disorders can produce large platelets, but platelets that approximate the size of red blood cells (RBCs) are seen almost exclusively in the context of inherited platelet disorders
- Bleeding time
  - Reflects quantitative and qualitative platelet disorders as well as some vascular defects that are related to interactions with platelets
    - **Bleeding time does not involve the clotting cascade**
      - Most common technique is Ivy technique, in which a blood pressure cuff is inflated to 40 mm Hg and a small, standardized incision is made in the forearm with a lancet; filter paper or cotton is used to absorb blood at regular intervals, and the time until cessation of bleeding is recorded
    - **Bleeding time is not useful in predicting bleeding risk, does not predict excessive surgical bleeding, and cannot predict bleeding risk in patients who have ingested aspirin**
  - Patients with uremia often have a bleeding diathesis and platelet dysfunction. No controlled study has demonstrated that patients with uremia and prolonged bleeding time have more surgical bleeding than those with normal bleeding time.

FIGURE 47-1 Steps in normal platelet function. (ADP, adenosine diphosphate; GP, glycoprotein; vWF, von Willebrand factor.)

Step 1: Activation	Initiated by Vessel wall damage Collagen Thrombin Epinephrine ADP	Results in Platelet development of pseudopods Platelet release of arachidonic acid
Step 2: Adhesion	Initiated by Platelet activation	Results in vWF forming links between GPIb/IX on platelets and collagen
Step 3: Aggregation	Initiated by Arachidonic acid, which is converted to thromboxane A$_2$	Results in Platelet beginning release of granular contents Platelets clumping when linked together by GPIIb/IIIa
Step 4: Secretion	Initiated by Thromboxane A$_2$	Results in Alpha and dense granules releasing contents Support of the coagulation cascade and formation of the fibrin clot

47

FIGURE 47-2 Normal platelets in a normal peripheral blood smear. *(From Young B, Stevens A, Heath JW, Lowe JS: Wheater's functional histology, ed 5, Philadelphia, Churchill Livingstone, 2006, Fig. 3.10.)*

- The PFA-100 is an *in vitro* test that evaluates platelet function
  - It is now being used in lieu of a bleeding time as it is more convenient and less invasive
  - **As with the bleeding time, the PFA-100 has not been shown to predict bleeding risk**
- Classic platelet aggregation assays
  - Platelet-rich plasma or whole blood is exposed to adenosine diphosphate (ADP), epinephrine, collagen, and ristocetin. The patterns of aggregation suggest specific platelet defects.

- Ristocetin activity
  - Ristocetin is an antibiotic that induces platelet agglutination in the presence of vWF
  - This test is abnormal in patients deficient in vWF (i.e., von Willebrand disease) or in the receptor for vWF (glycoprotein Ib/IX; i.e., Bernard-Soulier syndrome)
- **Laboratory testing for liver disease, hepatitis C, human immunodeficiency virus (HIV), and pregnancy should be sent as all of these can manifest as thrombocytopenia**

Inherited Disorders of Platelets

Basic Information

- **Inherited platelet disorders are rare**
- There are four major inherited platelet disorders (Table 47-1)
- Glanzmann thrombasthenia and Bernard-Soulier syndrome are autosomal recessive
- Gray platelet syndrome (Fig. 47-3) and storage pool disease are of poorly defined inheritance patterns, in part because of their heterogeneous nature

Clinical Presentation

- Bleeding abnormalities may be present at birth or may become evident later in life
- Aspirin may exacerbate bleeding abnormalities
- **Common early manifestations include easy bruising, gingival bleeding, and epistaxis**
- **Menorrhagia with menarche is also common**
- Bleeding with trauma may be severe and life threatening
  - Patients with gray platelet syndrome or storage pool disease often have only mild bleeding manifestations

| TABLE 47-1 | *Inherited Platelet Disorders* |

Platelet Disorder	Defect	Bleeding Time	Aggregation with Ristocetin?	Confirmatory Test	Treatment	Notes
Glanzmann thrombasthenia	Platelets lack functional GP IIb/IIIa receptor (needed to bind fibrinogen and cross-link platelets)	Prolonged	Yes	Flow cytometry, demonstrating absence of receptor	Local measures to stop bleeding; ε-aminocaproic acid. If severe bleeding, transfuse platelets (at risk of developing IIb/IIIa antibodies)	Platelets are normal in quantity and appearance
Bernard-Soulier syndrome	Platelets lack GP Ib/IX complexes (needed to bind subendothelial vWF)	Markedly prolonged	No	Flow cytometry, demonstrating absence of receptor	Local measures; ε-aminocaproic acid; platelet transfusion	Thrombocytopenia common
Gray platelet syndrome	Deficiency of α granules	Prolonged	Yes	Electron microscopy demonstrates absence of α granules	DDAVP; ε-aminocaproic acid; platelet transfusions rarely needed	Large, pale platelets Thrombocytopenia
Storage pool disease	Deficiency of dense granules	Normal or prolonged	Yes	Electron microscopy confirms absence of dense granules	DDAVP; ε-aminocaproic acid; cryoprecipitate; platelet transfusions rarely needed	First wave of platelet aggregation occurs, but second wave does not

DDAVP, desmopressin; GP, glycoprotein; vWF, von Willebrand factor.

FIGURE 47-3   Gray platelet syndrome. *(From Lewis SM, Bain BJ, Bates I: Dacie and Lewis practical haematology, ed 10, Philadelphia, Churchill Livingstone, 2006, Fig. 5-97.)*

Diagnosis

- **Bleeding time is prolonged in all these disorders, except some mild forms of storage pool disease**
- Ristocetin aggregation
  - Absent in Bernard-Soulier syndrome and von Willebrand disease
  - Present in Glanzmann thrombasthenia
- For other results of diagnostic testing, see Table 47-1

Treatment

- Treatment is determined by severity of bleeding; **mild bleeding episodes are treated with local measures (e.g., compression)**
- **Platelet transfusion should be reserved for major episodes of bleeding because transfusion increases risk of alloimmunization and development of platelet receptor antibodies**
- Aminocaproic acid and tranexamic acid
  - Antifibrinolytic agents
  - Useful for treatment of all inherited platelet disorders
- Desmopressin (DDAVP)
  - Analogue of arginine vasopressin but with no activity on blood pressure or vasoconstriction
  - Through an unclear mechanism, increases plasma levels of factor VIII and vWF
  - Effective for treatment of gray platelet syndrome and storage pool disease

Acquired Disorders of Platelets

Basic Information

- **Acquired platelet disorders more common than inherited platelet disorders**
  - Acquired platelet disorders may result from medications, medical disorders, or hematologic disorders (including immune disorders; Table 47-2). These

TABLE 47-2	*Common Acquired Platelet Disorders*
Category of Disorder	**Examples**
Medication-related	Aspirin NSAIDs Heparin Penicillin Quinine/quinidine GP IIb/IIIa inhibitors Clopidogrel/ticlopidine
Medical disease–related	Uremia Liver disease Cardiopulmonary bypass
Hematologic or immunologic disease–related	Paraproteinemia ITP TTP HELLP syndrome Myeloproliferative disorders Myelodysplasia Disseminated intravascular coagulation
Infection-related	HIV CMV, EBV, Hantavirus, *Mycoplasma* Viral hepatitis

CMV, cytomegalovirus; EBV, Epstein-Barr virus; HELLP, hemolysis, elevated liver enzymes, and low platelet count; GP, glycoprotein; HIV, human immunodeficiency virus; ITP, idiopathic thrombocytopenic purpura; NSAIDs, nonsteroidal anti-inflammatory drugs; TTP, thrombotic thrombocytopenic purpura.

should all be considered in the history, physical, and laboratory evaluation of the patient with a suspected acquired platelet disorder.

Clinical Presentation

- Clinical presentation varies but typically results in bleeding
- Exceptions include the following:
  - Heparin-induced thrombocytopenia (HIT) type 2 is associated with thrombosis (Table 47-3)
  - Myeloproliferative disorders, in which patients may have bleeding or thrombosis
- Medication-related platelet disorders (Box 47-1; see also Table 47-3) may result in immediate increase in risk of bleeding by deactivating platelets or delayed impact on bleeding risk if pathogenesis includes development of autoantibodies
- Medical disease–related platelet disorders (specifically liver disease; Table 47-4) may result in apparent thrombocytopenia caused by sequestration but no clinical bleeding disorder. Other causes are included in Table 47-4.
- **Hematologic/immunologic disease–related platelet disorders might be associated with normal numbers of abnormally functioning platelets, decreased platelet counts, or both**

47

TABLE 47-3	*Medication-Related Platelet Disorders*	
Medication	**Mechanism**	**Notes**
Aspirin	Irreversibly acetylates COX-1 and COX-2	COX-1 needed for production of thromboxane A_2, which is needed for platelet aggregation Impact present for lifetime of platelet (7–10 days)
NSAIDs	Reversibly acetylate COX-1 and COX-2	Impact present only for half-life of drug
Heparin	HIT type 1: Nonimmune-mediated; begins a few days after initiation of heparin and will spontaneously resolve if heparin is continued HIT type 2: Immune-mediated development of antibodies against heparin:platelet factor 4 complex; **begins 5–10** days after initiation of heparin	Type 2 associated with thrombosis (type 1 is not) Suspect a type 2 process if the platelet count falls by >50% within 5–10 days of heparin initiation **Heparin must be discontinued immediately in HIT type 2** **Anticoagulation with a direct thrombin inhibitor should be started immediately if HIT type 2 is suspected** An earlier onset of thrombocytopenia is possible if there has been exposure to heparin in the prior 3 mo Thromboses can present 40 days after heparin exposure Type 2 HIT confers significant risk of in-hospital mortality
Penicillin	Binds covalently to platelet membrane and acts as hapten	Typically occurs on reexposure to drug, with rapid drop in platelets Treated by discontinuing drug
Clopidogrel/ ticlopidine	1. Induce platelet clumping in the microvasculature and results in TTP 2. Inhibits ADP-induced platelet aggregation	1. Treated by discontinuing the drug and plasmapheresis Peripheral blood smear is essential for diagnosis 2. Impact present for lifetime of platelet (7–10 days)
GP IIB/IIIa inhibitors	Bind directly to the GP IIb/IIIa receptor, exposing neoantigens that are bound by preformed antibody. Thrombocytopenia occurs rapidly following initiation of the drug.	Treated by discontinuing the drug. Platelets should recover at a rate of about 20,000/day (rate of bone marrow production). Peripheral blood smear should be performed to demonstrate isolated thrombocytopenia without schistocytes May be safely treated with platelet transfusions
Quinine/quinidine, procainamide, gold salts	Induce production of autoantibodies to platelet membrane	Treated by discontinuing drug May require treatment with IVIG or steroids

ADP, adenosine diphosphate; COX, cyclooxygenase; GP, glycoprotein; HIT, heparin-induced thrombocytopenia; IVIG, intravenous immune globulin; NSAIDs, nonsteroidal anti-inflammatory drugs; TTP, thrombotic thrombocytopenic purpura.

BOX 47-1   *Select Medications Associated with Platelet Dysfunction*

Aspirin
NSAIDs
Quinine/quinidine
Calcium channel blockers
Ticlopidine
Clopidogrel
Nitroglycerin
Nitroprusside
Thrombolytic agents
β-Lactam antibiotics
Abciximab
Heparin
Dextran
Lepirudin
Alcohol
Dipyridamole
Antipsychotics
Prostacyclin

For a complete list of drugs associated with thrombocytopenia, see Pedersen-Bjergaard U, Andersen M, Hansen PB: Drug-specific characteristics of thrombocytopenia caused by non-cytotoxic drugs, *Eur J Clin Pharmacol* 54:701–706, 1998; and Pedersen-Bjergaard U, Andersen M, Hansen PB: Drug-induced thrombocytopenia: clinical data on 309 cases and the effect of corticosteroid therapy, *Eur J Clin Pharmacol* 52:183–189, 1997.

- Paraproteinemias may cause destruction or dysfunction of platelets
- Myeloproliferative disorders may be associated with thrombocytopenia or thrombocytosis; one third of these patients have bleeding complications, and one third have thrombosis
- Myelodysplasia may result in decreased platelet production or in production of abnormal platelets
- Post-transfusion purpura develops when alloantibodies are produced against platelet surface antigens, resulting in a decline in platelet count 7 to 10 days after RBC transfusion; treatment is with intravenous immune globulin (IVIG)
- Immune thrombocytopenic purpura (ITP), thrombotic thrombocytopenic purpura (TTP), hemolysis/elevated liver enzymes/low platelet count (HELLP syndrome), and disseminated intravascular coagulation (DIC) are described in Table 47-5
- **HIV and hepatitis C can cause thrombocytopenia directly**
  - HIV can infect the stromal cells of the bone marrow, leading to decreased platelet production
  - HIV can also be associated with ITP
  - Hepatitis C appears also to have a direct effect on platelets that is not well understood. Recent literature suggests that clearance of hepatitis C virus infection can result in resolution of thrombocytopenia.

TABLE 47-4	*Medical Disease–Related Platelet Disorders*	
Medical Disease	**Mechanism**	**Notes**
Uremia	Multifactorial, with uremic toxins causing defect in platelet aggregation	Treatment options include dialysis, DDAVP, cryoprecipitate, or estrogen DDAVP increases release of factor VIII:von Willebrand factor from endothelial cells Cryoprecipitate includes factor VIII:von Willebrand factor Mechanism of estrogen not understood; given IV, it can be efficacious in 24 hr Erythropoietin or transfusions should be given to maintain a hematocrit of 30% Dialysis improves platelet adhesion to the vessel wall and can decrease bleeding
Liver disease	Dysfibrinogenemia, not thrombocytopenia, leads to bleeding risk	Sequestered platelets will be available should need arise Platelet transfusion, DDAVP, and cryoprecipitate may be used
Cardiopulmonary bypass	Destruction of platelets in bypass circuit as well as platelet dysfunction from activation of platelets	50% drop in platelets common postoperatively Platelet dysfunction a minor cause of postoperative bleeding Prophylactic administration of platelets preoperatively not indicated
Sepsis	Increased platelet phagocytosis mediated by increased concentration of macrophage colony-stimulating factor	Sepsis can also precipitate DIC
HIV	ITP is a major cause, also direct infection of marrow stromal cells contributing to hematopoiesis	1.7% of patients with HIV and 8.7% of patients with AIDS will be asymptomatically thrombocytopenic Increased risk associated with IVDA, anemia, lower CD4 Treatment is the same as for conventional ITP but with the addition of HAART AZT seems to improve platelet count and so should be considered in selecting a regimen Response to prednisone is 80–90%
Hepatitis C	Unknown mechanism	Recent research has demonstrated a correlation between clearance of viremia and platelet count recovery

AIDS, acquired immunodeficiency syndrome; AZT, zidovudine; DDAVP, desmopressin; DIC, disseminated intravascular coagulation; HAART, highly active antiretroviral therapy; HIV, human immunodeficiency virus; ITP, idiopathic thrombocytopenic purpura; IV, intravenously; IVDA, intravenous drug abuse.

Disease	Basic Information	Diagnosis	Treatment
TABLE 47-5		*Selected Hematologic or Immunologic Disease–Related Platelet Disorders*	
ITP	Most commonly affects women in second and third decade of life Mechanism is autoantibodies against platelet membrane glycoproteins	Diagnosis of exclusion Antiplatelet antibodies demonstrated in 80% of cases Bone marrow shows normal or increased megakaryocytes May be secondary to HIV, SLE, thyroid disease, CLL, lymphoma, and solid tumors	Corticosteroids 1–2 mg/kg/day IVIG in refractory cases or if active bleeding Splenectomy rarely needed Transfuse platelets only if severe thrombocytopenia (platelet count <20,000/mm³) and bleeding
TTP	More common in women, typically in their fourth decade of life 10–40% report viral URI in 2 wk before onset Due to autoantibodies against ADAMTS 13: Metalloproteinase that cleaves ultralarge vWF multimers	Pentad of symptoms: Microangiopathic hemolytic anemia, thrombocytopenia, neurologic symptoms, fever, renal dysfunction Most have hemolytic anemia, thrombocytopenia, and neurologic symptoms; only 40% have complete pentad Neurologic symptoms may range from headache to coma Renal symptoms may include hematuria or proteinuria, with or without renal insufficiency	Plasmapheresis is treatment of choice; done daily until neurologic symptoms, platelet count, and LDH have been normal for 3 consecutive days 30% will relapse Corticosteroids have a questionable role in treatment Splenectomy reserved for refractory cases
HELLP syndrome	One of several causes of thrombocytopenia in pregnant women Normal pregnancy associated with mild thrombocytopenia (100,000–150,000/mm³) ITP, TTP, and DIC also may be associated with pregnancy	Patient typically presents with right upper quadrant pain Often associated with eclampsia/preeclampsia Hematologic findings include hemolysis and low platelet count	Delivery of fetus is definitive treatment, although abnormalities may persist Some evidence that corticosteroids are effective if delay of delivery desired
DIC	Process may be initiated by infection (especially gram-negative bacteria), obstetric complications, tissue injury, burns, or certain malignancies Generation of thrombin is central to pathogenesis; this allows consumption of fibrinogen, factor V, and factor VIII	Coagulopathy usually overshadowed by symptoms of illness that initiated DIC, but bleeding is major clinical manifestation, with thrombosis less common Common laboratory markers include elevated D-dimer, elevated fibrin degradation products, prolongation of PT and PTT, low fibrinogen and low platelet counts	Treat underlying disorder while initiating aggressive supportive measures Platelet transfusions, cryoprecipitate, and FFP may be used if bleeding predominates, especially if associated with very low fibrinogen or platelet counts Heparin indicated if thrombotic complications predominate

CLL, chronic lymphocytic leukemia; DIC, disseminated intravascular coagulation; FFP, fresh-frozen plasma; HELLP, hemolysis, elevated liver enzymes, and low platelet count; ITP, idiopathic thrombocytopenic purpura; IVIG, intravenous immune globulin; LDH, lactate dehydrogenase; PT, prothrombin time; PTT, partial thromboplastin time; SLE, systemic lupus erythematosus; TTP, thrombotic thrombocytopenic purpura; URI, upper respiratory infection; vWF, von Willebrand factor.

Diagnosis

- **This group of disorders is distinguished by onset of a new platelet-related bleeding disorder in a patient without a preexisting platelet-related bleeding disorder**
- Diagnosis requires a thorough review of all medications that affect either platelet function or production because medications are a common cause of acquired platelet disorders
  - Because the life of a platelet is 7 to 10 days, exposure to a medication that affects platelet function would have to occur within this time
  - Medications (and toxins) that affect platelet production may have a longer interval between exposure and clinical presentation
- **Evaluation of the peripheral blood smear remains essential in this group of disorders to exclude TTP in any patient with an acquired platelet disorder (Fig. 47-4)**

FIGURE 47-4 Thrombocytopenia due to disseminated intravascular coagulation. Note that platelets are nearly absent. *(From Forbes CD, Jackson WF: Color atlas and text of clinical medicine, ed 3, St. Louis, Mosby, 2003, Fig. 10.115.)*

47

- Antibodies
  - Antiplatelet antibodies are seen in 80% of individuals with ITP
  - Anti–heparin:platelet factor 4 complex antibodies are seen in HIT type 2 and mediate platelet activation, which results in increased thrombosis
- Evaluation of the bone marrow may be needed in ITP in elderly patients to exclude myeloproliferative, lymphoproliferative, or myelodysplastic disorders

Treatment

- Treatment is based in part on the presence or absence of immediate complications, including either bleeding or thrombosis. If life-threatening bleeding is present, platelet transfusion should be considered.
  - An exception is patients with thrombocytopenia resulting from TTP. **Patients with TTP should not receive platelet transfusions; treatment is plasmapheresis.**
    - **If plasmapheresis is not immediately available, patients should receive fresh-frozen plasma**
- At times, correction of the underlying disorder (e.g., dialysis in a patient with uremia and dysfunctional platelets) may be all that is needed to correct the bleeding disorder
- Medications that are used to treat platelet disorders include the following:
  - DDAVP: A synthetic form of arginine vasopressin that increases plasma levels of vWF factor and factor VIII
  - Corticosteroids are used in disorders in which an immune component predominates; they are the initial treatment of choice for ITP
  - $Rh_o(D)$ immune globulin (RhoGAM) can also be used effectively in Rh-positive patients with ITP and bleeding, inducing splenic sequestration of Rh-positive antibody–coated RBCs, thereby sparing platelets. Caution should be taken in using $Rh_o(D)$ as it can cause significant, even life-threatening hemolysis.
  - Thrombopoietin (TPO) mimetics: Drugs that mimic the effect of TPO available to treat thrombocytopenia; increase the platelet count in more than 80% of patients with ITP
- Plasmapheresis separates plasma from RBCs via centrifugation, allowing preservation of RBCs while plasma can be discarded
  - Plasmapheresis is essential treatment for TTP but is also used for some paraproteinemias
- Cryoprecipitate is a fraction of plasma that is frozen and then thawed (hence the name); the freeze-thaw process results in high concentrations of factor VIII, vWF, and fibrinogen
  - Cryoprecipitate can be used in patients who have depleted fibrinogen as a result of DIC and can be useful in patients with bleeding from uremia

Thrombocytosis

Basic Information

- **Thrombocytosis is most commonly diagnosed when the platelet count is greater than 600,000/mm³**
- Thrombocytosis may occur either in response to medical illness (i.e., reactive thrombocytosis) or as a clonal disorder

FIGURE 47-5 Thrombocytosis causing vessel occlusion and gangrene. *(From Haslett C, Chilvers ER, Boon NA, et al: Davidson's principles and practice of medicine, ed 19, New York, Churchill Livingstone, 2002, Fig. 19.15.)*

- **Reactive thrombocytosis is much more common than clonal disorders**

Clinical Presentation

- Reactive thrombocytosis may occur in response to infections (e.g., pneumonia, osteomyelitis, tuberculosis) or chronic inflammatory conditions (e.g., vasculitis, rheumatoid arthritis)
  - Other causes of reactive thrombocytosis include iron deficiency, acute hemorrhage, hemolysis, and splenectomy; some nonhematologic malignancies may also be accompanied by thrombocytosis
  - Clinical manifestations of reactive thrombocytosis are rarely seen, and symptoms of the underlying illness predominate
- Clonal thrombocytosis may be caused by an isolated clonal overproduction of platelets (i.e., essential thrombocytosis, Fig. 47-5), but is also commonly seen in polycythemia vera. Other clonal disorders include idiopathic myelofibrosis, myelodysplastic syndromes, and chronic granulocytic leukemia.
  - Hemorrhagic complications, although mild, are seen in up to 20% of individuals with essential thrombocytosis or polycythemia vera but rarely unless the platelet count exceeds 1,000,000/mm³
  - **Thrombotic complications may be venous or arterial and are not predicted by the platelet count (see Fig. 47-5)**
    - Advanced age and previous thrombosis are the greatest predictors of increased risk of thrombosis

Diagnosis

- **As reactive thrombocytosis is by far more common, efforts should be made to exclude infection, chronic inflammation, and iron deficiency (among others) in any patient with thrombocytosis**
- Clonal thrombocytosis is confirmed by associated clinical features and often with cytogenetic markers, including the presence of *JAK2* mutations. Rarely, bone marrow aspirate and biopsy are needed. Clonal thrombocytosis may be associated with the phenomenon of erythromelalgia (painful erythema, typically of the feet and hands), mediated by platelet thrombi in the peripheral vasculature.
  - Aspirin is the treatment of choice for this symptom

Treatment

- Reactive thrombocytosis is treated by treating the underlying illness
- Clonal thrombosis treatment is dictated by the type of clonal disorder
  - Aspirin therapy reduces risk of thrombosis and may be used prophylactically in patients with essential thrombocytosis or polycythemia vera, provided they do not have acquired von Willebrand disease
- Cytotoxic agents, including hydroxyurea, may be used short term to reduce platelet counts, even when cure is not possible
  - Anagrelide is an agent that prevents the maturation of megakaryocytes into platelets. This is used to decrease the platelet count in those with essential thrombocytosis. Caution is recommended with use in elderly patients because side effects can include heart failure, myocardial infarction, and pulmonary hypertension.

REVIEW QUESTIONS

For review questions, please go to www.expertconsult.com.

SUGGESTED READINGS

George JN: Platelets, *Lancet* 355:1531–1539, 2000.

George JN, Woolf SH, Rashkob GE, et al: Idiopathic thrombocytopenic purpura: a practice guideline developed by explicit methods for the American Society of Hematology, *Blood* 88:3–40, 1996.

Pedersen-Bjergaard U, Andersen M, Hansen PB: Drug-induced thrombocytopenia: clinical data on 309 cases and the effect of corticosteroid therapy, *Eur J Clin Pharmacol* 52:183–189, 1997.

Pedersen-Bjergaard U, Andersen M, Hansen PB: Drug-specific characteristics of thrombocytopenia caused by non-cytotoxic drugs, *Eur J Clin Pharmacol* 54:701–706, 1998.

Peterson P, Hayes TE, Arkin CF, et al: The preoperative bleeding time test lacks clinical benefit: College of American Pathologists and American Society of Clinical Pathologists position article, *Arch Surg* 133:134–139, 1998.

Warkentin TE, Kelton JG: A 14-year study of heparin-induced thrombocytopenia, *Am J Med* 101:502–507, 1996.

Williams WJ: *Hematology*, New York, 1995, McGraw-Hill.

47

CHAPTER 48

Coagulation Disorders

MICHAEL B. STREIFF, MD

Normal hemostasis is achieved by the cooperative function of coagulation proteins, platelets, and the vessel wall. Qualitative or quantitative abnormalities in any one of these components can precipitate excessive bleeding or thrombosis. Coagulation disorders are fairly common; therefore, internists should be familiar with the components of the hemostatic system, the tests used to evaluate their function, and the most common diseases that affect hemostasis. This chapter focuses on the coagulation system. Platelet disorders are covered in Chapter 47.

Bleeding Disorders

Basic Information

- Bleeding disorders vary in frequency and severity
- Can be categorized as congenital or acquired
- To understand and diagnose these conditions, one needs an understanding of the coagulation cascade (Fig. 48-1)
    - Intrinsic pathway: Factors XII, XI, IX, and VIII, prekallikrein, and high-molecular-weight kininogen
    - Extrinsic pathway: Factor VII, tissue factor
- **Common congenital coagulation disorders include factor deficiencies such as hemophilia A (factor VIII deficiency), hemophilia B (factor IX deficiency), and hemophilia C (factor XI deficiency), as well as von Willebrand disease (vWD; Table 48-1)**
    - **vWD, the most common inherited bleeding disorder, may affect as many as 0.1% of the population**
        - von Willebrand factor (vWF) serves two functions in hemostasis:
            - It mediates the adhesion of platelets to damaged vessel walls
            - It binds to and protects factor VIII from degradation by activated protein C, thus prolonging factor VIII half-life in the plasma
        - Several types of vWD exist:
            - Type I vWD (75% of all vWD) is caused by mutations that result in a quantitative deficiency of functional vWF
            - Type II vWD subtypes (20–25%) are due to mutations that result in the production of a dysfunctional vWF protein
            - Type III vWD (<5%) is rare and results in a severe quantitative deficiency of vWF
    - **Bleeding symptoms in vWD patients tend to be in mucosal sites (epistaxis, gum bleeding, menorrhagia, etc.) and mild to moderate in severity;** the exception is patients with type III

disease, who can develop severe bleeding similar to hemophilia (hemarthroses, etc.)
- **Acquired coagulation disorders include the following:**
    - **Liver disease**
        - **Results in decreased synthesis of all coagulation factors except for factor VIII**
        - Laboratory tests typically show prolongation of the prothrombin time (PT), the activated partial thromboplastin time (aPTT), and the thrombin time (TT) (the last one caused by decreased or dysfunctional fibrinogen)
        - Treatment
            - Fresh-frozen plasma (FFP) for bleeding
            - Recombinant human factor VIIa (rhFVIIa or Novo Seven [Novo Nordisk, Princeton, NJ]) has been used off-label for life-threatening bleeding refractory to FFP, but it may be associated with an increased risk of thrombotic complications
            - Liver transplantation for long-term management
    - **Disseminated intravascular coagulation (DIC; Box 48-1)**
    - **Vitamin K deficiency**
        - Vitamin K is required for the synthesis of active forms of factors II, VII, IX, and X, as well as the natural anticoagulant proteins C and S

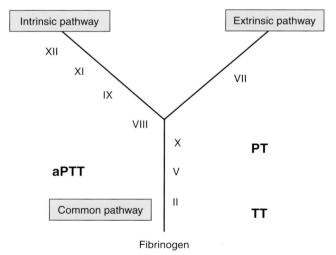

FIGURE 48-1 A simplified view of the coagulation cascade. (aPTT, activated partial thromboplastin time; PT, prothrombin time; TT, thrombin time.)

- Vitamin K deficiency is common with the following conditions:
  - Poor nutrition (especially diets deficient in green, leafy vegetables)
  - Broad-spectrum antibiotics (which kill intestinal bacteria, a significant source of vitamin K)
  - Antibiotics with an *N*-methylthio-tetrazole (MTT) side chain (e.g., moxalactam, cefamandole, cefoperazone), which can interfere with vitamin K metabolism and potentiate the deficiency state
  - Malabsorption (e.g., biliary disease, which interferes with delivery of bile necessary for absorption of fat-soluble vitamins)
- Vitamin K deficiency is characterized by a prolonged PT initially (factor VII has the shortest half-life of the coagulation factors; factors X and II also influence the PT), then prolonged aPTT (reflects factors IX, X, and II deficiency)
- Coagulation factor inhibitors: Antibodies directed against specific coagulation factors
  - Factor VIII inhibitors are the most common inhibitors that result in bleeding
    - Develop in 10% to 15% of hemophilia A patients because of chronic exposure to exogenous factor VIII
    - Rarely occur in nonhemophiliacs (1:1,000,000); most common associations are with tumors, pregnancy, drugs, and rheumatologic conditions
    - Inhibitor titer (concentration of the antibody) measured by the Bethesda assay
      - Low-titer inhibitors (<5 Bethesda units) can be transiently overcome with large doses of factor VIII

TABLE 48-1 *Selected Congenital Bleeding Disorders*

Disorder	Deficiency	Inheritance	aPTT	Laboratory Findings	Clinical Issues	Treatment
Hemophilia A	Factor VIII	X-linked recessive (1:10,000 male births)	↑	Reduced factor VIII level	Mild: Factor VIII >5%; bleed after significant trauma Moderate: Factor VIII = 1–5%; bleed after minor trauma Severe: Factor VIII <1%; spontaneous bleeding	Factor VIII concentrate
Hemophilia B (Christmas disease)	Factor IX	X-linked recessive (1:50,000 male births)	↑	Reduced factor IX level	Clinically similar to hemophilia A Same severity scale as hemophilia A	Factor IX concentrate
Hemophilia C (Rosenthal disease)	Factor XI	Autosomal-recessive; rare except among Ashkenazi Jews	↑	Reduced factor XI level	Variable severity, but usually mild; bleeding usually in response to trauma	FFP
von Willebrand disease (vWD)	Quantitative or qualitative defect in von Willebrand factor (vWF)	Autosomal dominant or recessive (1:1000 live births)	Normal or ↑	vWF antigen detects the quantity of vWF protein Ristocetin cofactor activity measures vWF function Factor VIII activity may be low or normal Tests of platelet function (e.g., bleeding time) may also be abnormal	Function of vWF: Aids in platelet adhesion and protection of factor VIII from inactivation Types of vWD: Type I: Partial deficiency of vWF; 75% of vWD Type II: Qualitative defect in vWF Type III: Complete deficiency of vWF	DDAVP, which causes the release of preformed vWF multimers from endothelium Factor VIII concentrates that contain vWF (e.g., Humate P)
Factor XIII deficiency	Factor XIII	Autosomal recessive (rare: <1:1,000,000 live births)	Normal	Factor XIII screen Tests for clot solubility in 5 M urea (clot will dissolve because of lack of fibrin cross-links)	Factor XIII is important for cross-linking fibrin strands to make a clot more resistant to fibrinolysis Clinical symptoms include delayed bleeding after trauma or surgery, poor wound healing	FFP

aPTT, activated partial thromboplastin time; DDAVP, 1-deamino-8-D-arginine vasopressin; FFP, fresh-frozen plasma.

BOX 48-1 *Disseminated Intravascular Coagulation*

Unbridled activation of the coagulation and fibrinolytic cascades due to excessive tissue factor expression

Exuberant thrombin generation results in excess fibrin clot formation, platelet activation, and secondary fibrinolysis

Results in bleeding due to consumption of coagulation factors (including fibrinogen) as well as platelets

If fibrinolysis is inadequate or inhibited, thrombosis may predominate

Causes: Infections, neoplasms, snake venom, endothelial disruption and abnormalities, tissue factor release (from trauma, obstetric complications)

Clinical presentation
    May see bleeding from wounds and venipuncture sites, petechiae, ecchymoses, hematuria, hematemesis, and diffuse bleeding
    Thromboembolic phenomena may include pulmonary emboli, necrotic skin lesions, and stroke

Lab diagnosis (suggestive but not diagnostic)
    Prolonged aPTT, PT
    Low fibrinogen concentration
    Elevated D-dimer or fibrin degradation products are most sensitive tests
    Thrombocytopenia and schistocytes on the peripheral blood smear are supportive but nonspecific

Treatment: Treat underlying disorder; supportive care (FFP, platelets); heparin may be worthwhile if thrombosis predominates (contraindicated if CNS lesions present)

Mortality rate: 50–80% in severe cases

---

aPTT, activated partial thromboplastin time; CNS, central nervous system; FFP, fresh-frozen plasma; PT, prothrombin time.

FIGURE 48-2 Regulation of the fibrinolytic system. (FDP, fibrin degradation products; tPA, tissue plasminogen activator; UK, urokinase.)

FIGURE 48-3 Massive hematomas in the absence of major trauma suggest hemophilia, Christmas disease, von Willebrand disease, or supratherapeutic anticoagulant therapy. *(From Forbes CD, Jackson WF: Color atlas and text of clinical medicine, ed 3, St. Louis, Mosby, 2003, Fig. 10.104.)*

- High-titer inhibitors (>5 Bethesda units) require alternative plasma products, such as factor VIII inhibitor bypassing activity (FEIBA VH; Baxter, Westlake Village, CA) or rhFVIIa, which can activate the coagulation cascade in the presence of a factor VIII inhibitor
- Hemophilia B patients have a lower incidence of inhibitor formation (2–4%)
- **Vessel wall disorders**
  - Immune complex–mediated destruction (cryoglobulinemia)
  - Inflammation (infection, vasculitis)
  - Destructive infiltration with proteins (amyloidosis)
  - Defective connective tissue structure (Ehlers-Danlos syndrome, vitamin C deficiency)
- **Fibrinolytic disorders can also result in bleeding**
  - Fibrinolytic system is responsible for clot digestion and remodeling (Fig. 48-2)
  - Excessive amounts of plasmin (the primary fibrinolytic enzyme) or its activators (tissue plasminogen activator, urokinase), or deficiency of inhibitors (plasminogen activator inhibitor-1, α_2-antiplasmin), can result in bleeding
  - These are rare disorders characterized by delayed bleeding

Clinical Presentation

- **Bleeding history**
  - Easy bruisability is very common and not always pathologic
  - More specific indications of a bleeding disorder are excessive bleeding with surgical procedures, an excessive transfusion requirement, a history of reoperation for bleeding, a positive family history of bleeding, and chronic iron deficiency anemia
  - Hemarthroses and soft tissue bleeds suggest a coagulation factor deficiency (Fig. 48-3)
  - Skin (petechiae) and mucosal (epistaxis, gingival bleeding, menorrhagia) bleeding are more suggestive of vWD or platelet disorders (Fig. 48-4)
  - Delayed bleeding is typical of factor XIII deficiency or fibrinolytic defects; factor XIII deficiency is also associated with poor wound healing
- Physical examination findings for bleeding
  - Ecchymoses at inaccessible sites suggest a coagulation disorder (Fig. 48-5)
  - **Palpable purpura indicates vessel wall inflammation (e.g., vasculitis)**

FIGURE 48-4 Hemorrhage after dental extraction is a common presentation of von Willebrand disease. *(From Forbes CD, Jackson WF: Color atlas and text of clinical medicine, ed 3, St. Louis, Mosby, 2003, Fig. 10.105.)*

FIGURE 48-5 Ecchymoses and petechiae on the lateral thigh of a patient with septicemic plague complicated by disseminated intravascular coagulation. *(From Mandell GL, Bennett JE, Dolin R: Principles and practice of infectious diseases, ed 6, Philadelphia, Churchill Livingstone, 2005, Fig. 226-7.)*

FIGURE 48-6 A mixing study. *Blue* denotes normal clotting activity; *white* denotes abnormal clotting activity.

- Nonpalpable purpura suggests vessel wall disorders, such as scurvy (vitamin C deficiency) or connective tissue disorders (e.g., Ehlers-Danlos syndrome)

Diagnosis and Evaluation

- Basic laboratory evaluation
  - PT: Measures factors in the extrinsic and common pathways (see Fig. 48-1)
  - **International normalized ratio (INR): A method for reporting PT results in patients on vitamin K antagonists (e.g., warfarin) that helps to normalize interlaboratory differences in reagent sensitivity**
  - aPTT: Measures factors in the intrinsic and common pathways
  - TT: Measures fibrinogen function
- Basic coagulation test scenarios
  - Isolated prolonged PT: Extrinsic pathway defect (e.g., factor VII deficiency; see Fig. 48-1)

- Isolated prolonged aPTT: Intrinsic pathway defect (e.g., in order of frequency, factor VIII, factor IX, factor XI, factor XII, prekallikrein, or high-molecular-weight kininogen deficiency—the latter two accelerate factor XII activation)
  - Isolated prolonged aPTT (usually markedly prolonged) in the absence of clinical bleeding suggests factor XII, prekallikrein, or high-molecular-weight kininogen deficiency
- Both PT and aPTT prolonged: Common pathway defect (e.g., factor X, factor V, or prothrombin deficiency)
- Isolated prolonged TT: Fibrinogen deficiency or dysfunction, heparin or presence of a heparin-like factor (e.g., monoclonal proteins, fibrin degradation products), thrombin inhibitor
- Prolonged PT, aPTT, TT: Generally the same considerations as isolated prolonged TT except heparins do not consistently prolong the PT
- Normal PT and aPTT: Think of platelet disorders, vWD, factor XIII deficiency, fibrinolytic disorders, and vessel wall disorders
- **Distinguishing between a factor deficiency and a factor inhibitor**
  - **Factor deficiency: The clotting time will correct when 1 part patient plasma is mixed with 1 part normal pooled plasma (NPP; 1:1 mix; Fig. 48-6)**
  - **Factor inhibitor: The clotting time fails to correct when 1 part patient plasma is mixed with 1 part normal pooled plasma (see Fig. 48-6)**
    - Weak inhibitors may only be identified in a mix of 3 parts patient plasma with 1 part NPP

Treatment

- Goal is to stop bleeding
- Treatment of individual factor deficiencies (see Table 48-1)
- Recombinant products (e.g., recombinant factor VIII concentrate) are preferred because they are less likely to transmit blood-borne infectious agents (e.g., HIV, hepatitis B and C)
- **DDAVP (1-deamino-8-D-arginine vasopressin)**
  - An analogue of arginine vasopressin that may be administered intravenously or nasally
  - **Induces factor VIII and vWF release from liver and endothelial cells**

48

- **Useful in type I vWD, mild hemophilia A (minor bleeds), and acquired and congenital platelet disorders**
- Side effects may include flushing, headache, hyponatremia, hypertension, and mild hypotension
- Doses may be repeated every 12 to 24 hours up to three or four doses, after which tachyphylaxis develops
- Acquired coagulation disorders: Usually treat the underlying cause
  - **Vitamin K deficiency: Administer FFP for rapid correction; oral or IV vitamin K (correction begins in 8–12 hours) for more gradual but definitive correction**
  - Liver disease: FFP for bleeding; rhFVIIa has been used for life-threatening bleeding unresponsive to FFP; eventual liver transplantation

Thrombotic Disorders

Basic Information

- The procoagulant function of the coagulation proteins is opposed by natural anticoagulants and the fibrinolytic system
- Defects or deficiencies in anticoagulant proteins or excessive function of coagulation proteins predisposes patients to thrombosis (thrombophilia; Table 48-2)
- **Extravascular risk factors for venous thromboembolism: Surgery, trauma, cancer, limb paresis or immobility, pregnancy/postpartum, obesity, smoking, estrogen use (including oral contraceptives; see Chapter 21)**

Clinical Presentation

- Patients generally have symptoms suggestive of venous thromboembolism
  - Pain, erythema, swelling of an extremity
  - Dyspnea, pleuritic chest pain
- Headache and mental status changes (suggesting cerebral vein sinus thrombosis) and abdominal pain, hepatomegaly, and ascites (suggesting Budd-Chiari syndrome or mesenteric vein thrombosis) are less common presentations

Diagnosis and Evaluation

- **Whom do you test for thrombophilia?**
  - Not all patients with thrombosis require a work-up
  - Consider work-up in patients with
    - Age younger than 50 years
    - Recurrent thrombosis
    - Positive family history
    - Thrombosis in unusual sites
    - Thrombosis with minimal provocation
    - Unexplained, recurrent pregnancy loss
- PT and aPTT will most often be normal
- Initial work-up should include factor V Leiden, prothrombin gene (20210) mutation, antiphospholipid antibody testing, antithrombin III activity, protein C activity, protein S activity
- Thrombophilia evaluation: Factor V Leiden, prothrombin gene mutation, antiphospholipid antibody testing, antithrombin III, protein C, and protein S may be tested in the acute setting
  - Antithrombin III activity may be affected by acute thrombosis and heparin therapy
  - Protein C and S activity and antigen levels may be affected by acute thrombosis and warfarin therapy
  - Protein S levels are also reduced by estrogens
  - The dilute Russell viper venom time may be affected by warfarin therapy
  - Homocysteine levels should be measured after fasting

Treatment

- General principles
  - Modify risk factors
  - Treat symptomatic patients (with thrombosis) with anticoagulation
- Treat underlying disorder, if one is found (see Table 48-2), often with anticoagulation
  - **If patient is asymptomatic, may defer treatment (because some will never develop thrombosis)**
  - **If patient develops thrombosis, indefinite anticoagulation may be necessary (for combined thrombophilic defects; antiphospholipid antibody syndrome; homozygous factor V Leiden; antithrombin III, protein C, and protein S deficiencies)**
  - For asymptomatic patients with thrombophilia, it is reasonable to provide aggressive deep venous thrombosis (DVT) prophylaxis during periods of increased risk
  - For hyperhomocysteinemia, vitamin supplementation (with folate, vitamins B_{12} and B_6) can lower homocysteine levels, but does not reduce the risk of clinical events
- Anticoagulation options
  - **Unfractionated heparin**
    - Binds to antithrombin III and potentiates its inhibition of thrombin (factor IIa), factor Xa, factor IXa, and factor XIa
    - Quick onset of action (within minutes to hours)
    - Delivered intravenously to treat thromboembolism; may be used subcutaneously (5000 units subcutaneously two or three times daily) for prophylaxis
    - **Monitor aPTT (goal is 1.5–2.5 times control): Therapeutic range should be established using heparin (anti-Xa) levels**
    - Safe during pregnancy
    - Side effects include bleeding, osteoporosis with prolonged use, thrombocytopenia (see Chapter 47)
    - Reversal with IV protamine infusion (1 mg/100 units of heparin)
  - **Low-molecular-weight heparin (LMWH)**
    - Enzymatically/chemically fractionated form of heparin that can be administered subcutaneously in fixed weight-based doses
    - Useful for prophylaxis or treatment
    - Examples: Dalteparin, enoxaparin, tinzaparin
    - **Laboratory monitoring of therapy is usually not necessary; aPTT is not useful for monitoring, must use LMWH (anti-Xa) assay**
    - Lower risk of heparin-induced thrombocytopenia
    - Partially reversible (60–80%) with protamine (1 mg/100 units or 1 mg)

TABLE 48-2   *Selected Disorders Leading to Hypercoagulability*

Disorder	Pathogenesis	Importance	Increase in Relative Risk of Thrombosis	Laboratory Findings
Factor V Leiden (activated protein C resistance)	Mutation in the first protein C cleavage site in factor V Prevents down-regulation of factor V activity	Common: 5% of white U.S. population Less common in African Americans and Asians Is synergistic with other thrombophilic states (e.g., prothrombin 20210 mutations)	Heterozygotes: 8× Homozygotes: 50×	Screening test: Activated protein C resistance assay DNA-based test for confirmation
Prothrombin 20210 gene mutation	Mutation beyond the coding region of the prothrombin gene Results in a 25% increase in prothrombin levels	Common: 1–2% of white U.S. population Less common in African Americans and Asians	2–3×	DNA-based test for mutation
Hyperhomocysteinemia	Homocysteine is a sulfur-containing amino acid produced during methionine metabolism Elevated in folate or vitamin B_{12} deficiency, homocysteinuria (autosomal recessive inherited enzyme deficiency state associated with dislocated lenses, mental retardation, vascular thrombosis), renal failure Pathophysiology of thrombosis is unclear	Mild hyperhomocysteinemia (15–30 μmol/L) is present in 5–10% of the general population	2×	Serum fasting homocysteine level >15 μmol/L is considered abnormal
Antiphospholipid antibody syndrome	Antibodies directed at phospholipid-binding proteins Associated with rheumatic disease (SLE, rheumatoid arthritis), neoplasms, drugs (procainamide, phenothiazines), viral infections (HIV), or idiopathic Pathophysiology of thrombosis is unclear	Predisposes to venous *and* arterial thrombosis Recurrence rate off therapy as high as 50% May also see thrombocytopenia and recurrent fetal loss	10×	Prolonged aPTT; no correction with 1:1 mix with normal plasma Prolonged dilute Russell viper venom time (dRVVT) Elevated anticardiolipin or β_2-glycoprotein 1 antibodies
Antithrombin (AT) III deficiency	In the presence of endogenous or exogenous heparins, AT III binds and inactivates thrombin, factors Xa, IXa, and XIa	Heterozygous deficiency present in 1:2000 to 1:5000	15–20×	Can measure AT III activity in the absence of heparin and acute thrombosis Family studies can be diagnostically useful
Protein C deficiency	In complex with protein S, it inactivates the activated forms of factors V and VIII	Heterozygous deficiency present in 1:250 to 1:500	5–10×	Protein C activity can be measured in the absence of warfarin, vitamin K deficiency, and acute thrombosis Family studies may be helpful
Protein S deficiency	Cofactor of protein C in the inactivation of activated forms of factors V and VIII	Heterozygous deficiency in 1:1000	5–10×	Protein S activity can be measured in the absence of warfarin, acute thrombosis, vitamin K deficiency, inflammation, pregnancy, and estrogen therapy

aPTT, activated partial thromboplastin time; HIV, human immunodeficiency virus; SLE, systemic lupus erythematosus.

48

- **Use with caution in patients with severe renal insufficiency (creatinine clearance <30 mL/min)**
- Use actual body weight for dosing as dose capping may increase the risk of recurrent thrombosis (e.g., enoxaparin 150 mg subcutaneously every 12 hours for 150-kg patient)
- **Warfarin**
  - A vitamin K antagonist that interferes with synthesis of vitamin K–dependent coagulation factors (II, VII, IX, and X), protein C, and protein S
  - Oral bioavailability
  - **Requires at least 96 to 120 hours for onset of antithrombotic effects (reduction in thrombin and factor X levels)**
  - Overlap initiation of warfarin with heparin to prevent initial depletion of protein C (before factors II, IX, and X) and theoretical risk of temporary hypercoagulability
  - **Monitor with INR**
    - **Standard therapeutic range for venous thromboembolism (VTE), aortic bileaflet mechanical heart valves, atrial fibrillation (INR 2–3)**
    - **Mitral bileaflet mechanical valves, recurrent VTE (INR 2.5–3.5); antiphospholipid syndrome with recurrent thromboembolism (INR 3–4)**
  - Contraindicated in pregnancy
  - Many drug interactions (Box 48-2)
  - Avoid use with nonsteroidal anti-inflammatory drugs, aspirin, or platelet inhibitors (increase bleeding risk)
  - **Warfarin reversal**
    - INR less than 5, no bleeding: Hold dose, monitor INR closely; restart at lower dose when approaching therapeutic range
    - INR 5 to 9, no bleeding: Hold dose, monitor INR closely; may give 1 to 2.5 mg oral vitamin K if at high risk for bleeding, restart at lower dose when approaching therapeutic range
    - INR greater than 9, no bleeding: Hold dose, monitor INR closely; may give 2.5 to 5 mg oral vitamin K if at high risk for bleeding; restart at lower dose when approaching therapeutic range
    - Any INR, life-threatening bleeding: Reverse warfarin with 10 mg vitamin K IV; use prothrombin complex concentrate (e.g., Bebulin [Baxter Healthcare, Westlake, CA]; or Profilnine [Grifols USA, LLC, Los Angeles, CA]) or rhFVIIa or FFP for rapid INR reversal; monitor INR closely
  - Warfarin skin necrosis (Fig. 48-7)
    - A rare hypercoagulable state most commonly seen in association with the use of large loading doses of warfarin (10 mg or more daily) in the absence of concomitant heparin anticoagulation
    - Results from rapid decrease in protein C levels (plasma half-life, 6–8 hours) preceding the decline of procoagulant factors II (prothrombin half-life, 72 hours) and X (half-life, 42 hours), which tips the hemostatic balance toward thrombosis

BOX 48-2   Selected Drug Interactions with Warfarin*

Drugs That Potentiate Warfarin Effects
Acetaminophen
Allopurinol
Amiodarone
Azole antifungals
Broad-spectrum antibiotics
Cimetidine
Ciprofloxacin
Clarithromycin
Disulfiram
Erythromycin
Isoniazid
Metronidazole
Norfloxacin
Omeprazole
Phenylbutazone
Propafenone
Quinidine
Sulfa-containing medications (e.g., trimethoprim-sulfamethoxazole)

Drugs That Decrease Absorption of Warfarin
Cholestyramine and other bile acid resins

Drugs That Increase the Hepatic Metabolism of Warfarin
Azathioprine
Barbiturates
Carbamazepine
Phenytoin
Rifampin

*This list is not all-inclusive. The international normalized ratio should be monitored whenever a patient's medical regimen is modified.

FIGURE 48-7 Warfarin-induced skin necrosis. *(From Hoffman R, Benz EJ Jr, Shattil SJ, et al: Hematology: basic principles and practice, ed 4, Philadelphia, Churchill Livingstone, 2005, Fig. 112-19.)*

- Timing: Usually within 1 to 10 days of warfarin initiation
- Histopathology: Dermal microvascular thrombosis typically involving the breast, buttocks, or thighs

- Hypercoagulable states such as factor V Leiden, prothrombin gene mutation, antiphospholipid antibody syndrome, antithrombin III, protein C, and protein S deficiencies increase the risk of warfarin skin necrosis
- Treatment: Heparin anticoagulation, protein C concentrate (Ceprotin), or FFP; skin grafting in severe cases

REVIEW QUESTIONS

For review questions, please go to www.expertconsult.com.

SUGGESTED READINGS

Ansell J, Hirsh J, Hylek E, et al: The pharmacology and managment of vitamin K antagonists: the American College of Chest Physicians Evidence-Based Clinical Practice Guidelines ed 8, *Chest* 133:160S–198S, 2008.

Kearon C, Kahn S, Agnelli G, et al: Antithrombotic therapy for venous thromboembolic disease: the American College of Chest Physicians Evidence-Based Clinical Practice Guidelines ed 8, *Chest* 133:454S–545S, 2008.

Hirsh J, Bauer K, Donati MB, et al: Parenteral anticoagulants: the American College of Chest Physicians Evidence-Based Clinical Practice Guidelines ed 8, *Chest* 133:141S–159S, 2008.

Hoffman R, Benz EJ Jr, Shattil SJ, et al editors: *Hematology: basic principles and practice*, ed 4, Philadelphia, 2005, Churchill Livingstone.

Kitchens CS, Alving BA, Kessler CM, editors: *Consultative hemostasis and thrombosis*, Philadelphia, 2002, WB Saunders.

Levine MN, Raskob G, Beyth RJ, et al: Hemorrhagic complications of anticoagulant and thrombolytic therapy: the American College of Chest Physicians Evidence-Based Clinical Practice Guidelines ed 8, *Chest* 133:257S–298S, 2008.

Seligsohn U, Lubetsky A: Genetic susceptibility to venous thrombosis, *N Engl J Med* 344:1222–1231, 2001.

48

Acute and Chronic Leukemias

TARA LIN, MD; and B. DOUGLAS SMITH, MD

Leukemias arise from the malignant transformation of hematopoietic cells and proliferate primarily in the bone marrow. In general, leukemias are classified as "acute" based on the rapidity of presentation and progression as compared to "chronic," which generally have a more insidious nature. In addition, leukemic cells in acute leukemias are often morphologically poorly differentiated (blasts), while chronic leukemias show a more normal differentiation pattern. Finally, leukemias are further classified by the cell of origin being either myeloid or lymphoid. A comparison of the clinical features of the broad leukemia subtypes is seen in Table 49-1. This chapter focuses on three of these types: acute myelogenous leukemia (AML), acute lymphocytic leukemia (ALL), and chronic myeloid leukemia (CML). Chronic lymphocytic leukemia (CLL) is discussed in Chapter 55.

Acute Myelogenous Leukemia

Basic Information

- Definition: AML is a clonal disorder of a primitive hematopoietic stem cell resulting in excess proliferation of immature cells and suppression of normal hematopoiesis
- Classification of AML was traditionally based on morphology according to the French-American-British (FAB) classification system (Table 49-2). This system has been largely replaced by the WHO classification (Table 49-3) based on molecular features of the various AML subtypes.
- Epidemiology
  - Median age at diagnosis: 62 to 65 years
  - Approximately 13,000 new cases annually in the United States
- Risk factors
  - Preceding myelodysplastic syndrome
  - Exposure to ionizing radiation
  - Exposure to chemicals (i.e., benzene)
  - Exposure to drugs: Alkylating agents (cyclophosphamide, chlorambucil, melphalan) and topoisomerase II inhibitors (etoposide, anthracyclines)
  - Genetic factors: Identical twins of leukemic patients have higher rates of leukemia; there is an increased rate of leukemia in patients with Down syndrome, Bloom syndrome, Fanconi anemia, ataxia-telangiectasia, and Klinefelter syndrome

Clinical Presentation

- Leukemic cells infiltrate the marrow and other organs (e.g., gums, skin, central nervous system [CNS]) and suppress normal hematopoiesis, resulting in cytopenias

- Most common presenting signs and symptoms caused by decreased production of normal cells:
  - Anemia: pallor, fatigue, and dyspnea
  - Thrombocytopenia: petechiae, hematoma, and bleeding (oral, GI)
  - Neutropenia: recurrent infections (sepsis, cellulitis, pneumonia)
- **Splenomegaly is uncommon**
- Individual subtypes of AML may have unique features (see Table 49-2)
- **Leptomeningeal involvement is more common with elevated white blood cell (WBC) count at diagnosis or M4/M5 morphology**
  - **Headache and altered mental status are common symptoms**
  - **Cranial nerve palsies are the most common sign**
- Hyperleukocytosis due to increased WBC count (may be seen with WBC 35,000–50,000/mL, more common with WBC >100,000/mL) results in obstruction of capillaries and small blood vessels, causing widespread ischemic changes such as stroke and/or mental status changes, congestive heart failure and/or myocardial ischemia, pulmonary congestion and/or hypoxia, and renal failure
- Tumor lysis syndrome (see Chapter 57)
- Disseminated intravascular coagulopathy is seen most commonly with acute promyelocytic leukemia (APL, or M3) and is an oncologic emergency

Diagnostic Evaluation

- Diagnosis depends on identification of myeloblasts in peripheral blood smear or bone marrow preparations
- Peripheral smear may vary from pancytopenia without circulating blasts to marked leukocytosis and leukostasis (Fig. 49-1)
- **Auer rods, which can be present and are considered pathognomonic for AML, are cytoplasmic inclusions of aggregated lysosomes (Fig. 49-2)**
- Morphology and immunologic/cytologic markers define the AML subtypes
- Other laboratory features
  - WBC count can be low or high (low WBC count raises suspicion of M3/APL)
  - Blast count may be low or high
  - Hematocrit usually low
  - Platelet count usually low
  - Increased cell turnover can increase serum potassium, phosphate, and uric acid
  - Spurious abnormalities are related to utilization (oxygen, glucose) by the high WBC count or excessive cell death (potassium) in the phlebotomy tube

TABLE 49-1	Comparison of the Different Types of Leukemia			
	AML	**ALL**	**CML**	**CLL**
Median age at diagnosis (yr)	60	4	50	60
Median survival (yr)	1–2 yr	Adults: 2 yr Children: >10 yr	5 yr	5 yr
Initial remission rate	60–70%	90%	90%	90%
WBC count at presentation	High or low	High or low	Elevated with ↑ myeloid cells	Elevated with ↑ lymphocytes
Hemoglobin at presentation	Low	Low	Low or normal	Low or normal
Platelet count at presentation	Low	Low	High or normal	Low or normal
Splenomegaly	Rarely	Common	Common	Common
Adenopathy	Rarely	Common	Rarely	Common
Infection risk	Elevated	Elevated	Normal	Elevated

ALL, acute lymphocytic leukemia; AML, acute myelogenous leukemia; CLL, chronic lymphocytic leukemia CML, chronic myeloid leukemia; WBC, white blood cell.

TABLE 49-2	French-American-British (FAB) Classification for Acute Myeloid Leukemias	
FAB Classification	**Degree of Myeloid Differentiation**	**Associated Cytogenetic Abnormalities**
M0	Minimal differentiation	
M1	Without maturation	
M2	With granulocytic maturation	t(8;21)
M3	Acute promyelocytic leukemia (APL)	t(15;17)
M4	Myelomonocytic	inv(16), del(16q)
M4Eo	Myelomonocytic with eosinophilia	inv(16), t(16;16)
M5	Monocytic	del(11q), t(9;11)
M6	Erythroblastic leukemia	
M7	Megaryoblastic leukemia	t(1;22)

FIGURE 49-1 Acute myelocytic leukemia (FAB AML M4) bone marrow. This category is typified by nearly equal numbers of myeloblasts and monoblasts plus promonocytes. *(From Henderson ES, Lister A, Greaves MF: Leukemia, ed 7, Philadelphia, WB Saunders, 2002, Fig. 11-14.)*

TABLE 49-3	World Health Organization (WHO) Classification for Acute Myeloid Leukemias	
WHO Classification	**Description**	
AML w/characteristic genetic abnormalities	AML with t(8;21) AML with inv(16) APL with t(15;17)	
AML w/multilineage dysplasia	Includes patients with preceding MDS or MPD that transforms into AML	
AML and MDS, therapy-related	Prior history of chemotherapy ± radiation therapy Often characterized by 11q23 or whole chromosome losses	
AML not otherwise categorized		

AML, acute myeloid leukemia; APL, acute promyelocytic leukemia; MDS, myelodysplastic syndrome; MPD, myeloproliferative disease.

FIGURE 49-2 Bone marrow showing promyelocytes with azurophilic granules. The cell in the center of the field reveals numerous needle-like Auer rods. *(From Kumar V, Fausto N, Abbas A: Robbins & Cotran: pathologic basis of disease, ed 7, Philadelphia, WB Saunders, 2004, Fig. 14-29.)*

49

TABLE 49-4	Acute Myeloid Leukemia Cytogenetic Risk Groups	
Risk Status	**Karyotype**	
Favorable	inv 16 or t(16;16) t(8;21) t(15;17)	
Intermediate	Normal cytogenetics +8 t(9;11) Other nondefined	
Poor	Complex (≥3 abnormal clones) −5, −5q, −7, −7q 11q23 inv 3 or t(3;3) t(6;9) t(9;22)—very rare	

TABLE 49-5	FAB Classification of Acute Lymphocytic Leukemia (ALL)
FAB Classification	**Morphology**
ALL L1	Fine to slightly condensed chromatin
ALL L2	Variable nuclear size, moderate cytoplasm
ALL L3 (Burkitt leukemia/ lymphoma)	Homogeneous, round nucleus, deeply basophilic, highly vacuolated

TABLE 49-6	WHO Classification of Acute Lymphocytic Leukemia (ALL)
WHO Classification	**Description**
Precursor B-cell ALL	t(12;21)(p12,q22) TEL/AML-1 t(1;19)(q23;p13) PBX/E2A t(9;22)(q34;q11) ABL/BCR t(V,11)(V;q23) V/MLL
Precursor T-cell ALL	
Burkitt leukemia/lymphoma	t(8;14), t(2;8), t(8;22)

Prognosis

- Cytogenetic abnormalities are most predictive of prognosis (Table 49-4). Emerging data suggest that there are other important molecular markers of prognosis such as *FLT3*-ITD mutations (poor prognosis) or mutations in *NPM1* (better prognosis)
- **Clinical features associated with a worse prognosis include age over 60 years, poor performance status, therapy-related AML (secondary to prior chemotherapy) or AML arising from another marrow disorder (i.e., myelodysplastic syndrome or myeloproliferative disease), WBC count greater than 100,000/mL.**

Treatment

- Chemotherapy is the mainstay of AML treatment and consists of two parts: induction and consolidation
  - Induction therapy is based on a combination of cytarabine (felt to be the most important and active agent for AML) and an anthracycline (daunomycin/idarubicin). It has the goal of stabilizing the sick patient and restoring bone marrow function to state of morphologic remission. **Hyperleukocytosis at diagnosis is often treated with leukophoresis (temporizing measure) and emergent lowering of counts with chemotherapy (more longitudinal measure) prior to full induction.**
    - APL (M3) induction includes the use of all-*trans* retinoic acid (ATRA) and has resulted in the highest cure rates of the AML subtypes
    - "Retinoic acid syndrome" or "differentiation syndrome" is an important side effect of ATRA (as well as arsenic trioxide) and is associated with increasing leukocyte counts, capillary leak, cytokine release resulting in weight gain, respiratory distress, serous effusions (pulmonary/pericardial), and potentially respiratory, cardiac and/or renal failure. Differentiation syndrome can occur in up to 15% of patients receiving ATRA, is more common with high-WBC-count presentations of APL, and may be fatal.
  - Consolidation: Consists of typically of several additional cycles of intensive cytarabine-based chemotherapy or stem cell transplantation. The goal of consolidation is to *cure* the patient by eradicating remaining microscopic disease.

- Allogeneic stem cell transplantation (SCT) is potentially curative but is associated with an increased treatment-related mortality compared to traditional chemotherapy. It often reserved for younger patients (<60–65 years) or those considered incurable by routine chemotherapy (i.e., those patients with poor-risk cytogenetics or leukemias related to previous therapy or arising from previous bone marrow disorders)
- Expected that 35% to 40% of the patients will be alive and free of disease at 5 years; relapse rate declines sharply after 3 to 4 years

Acute Lymphocytic Leukemia

Basic Information

- Definition: ALL is a clonal disorder of a malignant hematopoietic stem cell resulting in excess blasts and suppression of normal bone marrow function
- Epidemiology
  - Most common malignancy in children, but occurs in all ages
  - Median age at diagnosis (adults): 39 years
  - Approximately 5200 new cases annually
  - Traditional classification system (Table 49-5) and WHO classification system (Table 49-6) are used

Clinical Presentation

- Usually acute onset of symptoms (less than 2 weeks) and patients present with fatigue, pallor, bleeding or bruising, or infection
- **Up to 50% will present with fever due to either pyrogenic cytokine release or true concurrent infection**
- Approximately 50% have lymphadenopathy and splenomegaly
- Anterior mediastinal mass is common, especially with T-cell infiltration of the thymus
- CNS involvement is common in all types of ALL

FIGURE 49-3 Acute lymphoblastic leukemia/lymphoma. Lymphoblasts with condensed nuclear chromatin, small nucleoli, and scant agranular cytoplasm. *(From Kumar V, Fausto N, Abbas A: Robbins & Cotran: pathologic basis of disease, ed 7, Philadelphia, WB Saunders, 2004, Fig. 14-5.)*

Diagnostic Evaluation

- Lymphoblasts are seen on peripheral smear and bone marrow preparations (Fig. 49-3) but may be difficult to differentiate from myeloblasts on morphology alone
- Flow cytometry is helpful in distinguishing ALL and AML
- **Evaluation always includes analysis of cerebrospinal fluid for CNS involvement**

Prognosis

- Generally worsens with increasing age
  - Nearly 90% of children ages 2 to 10 are long-term survivors, with decreased survival rate as age increases
  - Elderly patients with ALL are rarely, if ever, cured. Overall survival for adults is 35% to 40% at 5 years
- Cytogenetics provide invaluable information on prognosis
- **Clinical features that affect prognosis include age, initial WBC count, and time to treatment response**

Treatment

- Standard treatment consists of multiple cycles of multiagent chemotherapy plus maintenance therapy for at least 2 years
- Salvage chemotherapy for relapsed ALL is rarely effective, and clinical trials are recommended
- Emerging treatment strategies include risk stratification to intensify chemotherapy for patients at highest risk of disease relapse
- Allogeneic SCT is recommended for adults with standard or poor risk features
- CNS chemoprophylaxis with intrathecal chemotherapy with or without CNS radiation is critical to reduce the chance of CNS relapse

Chronic Myeloid Leukemia

Basic Information

- Definition: CML is a malignant stem cell disorder characterized by a reciprocal translocation between chromosomes 9 and 22 [t(9;22), the Philadelphia chromosome]

FIGURE 49-4 The Philadelphia chromosome. A reciprocal translocation involving the long arms of chromosomes 9 and 22 results in the production of the Philadelphia chromosome. The t(9;22) translocation results in the fusion of the c-*abl* oncogene on chromosome 9 with the *bcr* gene on chromosome 22. *(From Rakel RE: Conn's current therapy, ed 57, Philadelphia, WB Saunders, 2005, Fig. 1.)*

that results in a *bcr/abl* gene fusion and a constitutively active tyrosine kinase causing uncontrolled cell proliferation and blocked apoptosis (Fig. 49-4)
- Epidemiology
  - There are three distinct phases of CML: Chronic, accelerated, or blast crisis depending on the degree of leukemic blasts versus mature cells
  - **Median age at diagnosis about 60 years**
  - Incidence: 1 to 2 cases/100,000 with slight male predominance

Clinical Presentation

- Chronic-phase patients often present with asymptomatic elevation of peripheral blood counts. When symptomatic, common features include early satiety, left upper quadrant fullness, and fatigue.
- **Splenomegaly on examination present in more than 50% of patients**
- Complete blood count typically shows WBC count greater than 100,000/mL with left-shifted differential, anemia, and thrombocytosis. In CML, the mature WBCs are functional and there does not appear to be an increased risk of infection in patients with chronic-phase presentations.
- **Anemia, thrombocytopenia, and monocytosis are red flags that you may *not* be dealing with chronic-phase CML**
- Blast crisis may present with constitutional symptoms such as fever, night sweats, bone pain, and symptoms resulting from suppression of normal hematopoiesis and resulting anemia and thrombocytopenia

Diagnostic Evaluation

- Peripheral smear typically shows the presence of virtually all cells of the neutrophilic series, from myeloblasts to bands and mature neutrophils (Fig. 49-5).
- **Diagnosis is established by demonstration of the Philadelphia chromosome by traditional marrow karyotyping or detection by peripheral blood**

49

FIGURE 49-5 Chronic myeloid leukemia. Note the abundance of granulocytes at all stages of maturation. *(From Forbes CD, Jackson WF: Color atlas and text of clinical medicine, ed 3, St. Louis, Mosby, 2003, Fig. 10.77.)*

fluorescent *in situ* hybridization (FISH) testing; molecular testing for the *bcr/abl* fusion by polymerase chain reaction is the most sensitive test and is used in diagnosis and monitoring response to treatment

Prognosis

- Better for patients younger than age 40, those diagnosed in chronic phase versus accelerated or blast crisis, normal or elevated platelet counts, and mild splenomegaly
- Natural progression of untreated disease moves from a relatively benign chronic phase to fatal blast crisis in 3 to 5 years. Blast crisis is typically myeloid (70%), but can be lymphoblastic (20%) or undifferentiated and carries a very poor median survival of a few months.

Treatment

- Allogeneic SCT remains only known curative therapy, with cure rates as high as 70% reported with human leukocyte antigen–matched donors, and is generally more successful early in the course of disease and/or during chronic phase
- Graft-versus-leukemia effects are critical for success in CML and are weighed against the potential risks of graft-versus-host disease, which remains the most critical component of morbidity and mortality
- **Medical management: The development of effective tyrosine kinase inhibitors (TKIs) for CML has significantly altered outcomes for patients with CML, so much so that allogeneic SCT is now reserved for patients who have failed medical management or present in blast crisis**

- Imatinib mesylate (IM; Gleevec) is a TKI that blocks the activity of *bcr/abl*
- Durable, complete hematologic remissions achieved in over 90% of patients
- Durable complete cytogenetic remissions achieved in over 80% of patients
- TKIs also effective in treating patients with advanced CML (accelerated, blast crisis) as well as Ph+ ALL; however, remissions in these advanced diseases are often short without additional therapy (i.e., allogeneic SCT)
- Second-generation TKIs dasatinib (Sprycel) and nilotinib (Tasigna) were originally developed for IM-resistant CML. More recently they have each shown efficacy and improved time to remission when compared to imatinib for newly diagnosed patients with CML and are now both Food and Drug Administration approved for use as first-line treatment. Long-term outcomes data are emerging; however, there are no convincing data that any of the three agents is best in the first-line setting.

REVIEW QUESTIONS

For review questions, please go to www.expertconsult.com.

SUGGESTED READINGS

Burns CP, Armitage JO, Frey AL, et al: Analysis of the presenting features of adult acute leukemia: The French-American-British classification, *Cancer* 47:2460–2469, 1981.

Cassileth PA, Harrington D, Appelbaum F, et al: Chemotherapy compared with autologous or allogeneic bone marrow transplantation in the management of acute myeloid leukemia in first remission, *N Engl J Med* 339:1649–1656, 1998.

Estey E, Dohner H: Acute myeloid leukaemia, *Lancet* 368:1894–1907, 2006.

Hoelzer D, Thiel E, Loffler H, et al: Prognostic factors in a multicenter study for treatment of acute lymphoblastic leukemia in adults, *Blood* 71:123–131, 1988.

National Comprehensive Cancer Network (NCCN) Guidelines: Available at, www.NCCN.org.

Pui CH, Robinson LL, Look AT: Acute lymphoblastic leukemia, *Lancet* 37:1030–1043, 2008.

Schiffer CA: BCR-ABL tyrosine kinase inhibitors for chronic myeloid leukemia, *N Engl J Med* 357:258–265, 2007.

CHAPTER 50

Myelodysplastic Syndrome

TARA LIN, MD; and B. DOUGLAS SMITH, MD

Myelodysplastic syndromes (MDS) are a complex and heterogeneous group of disorders characterized by ineffective hematopoiesis (in the absence of nutritional deficiencies), dysplasia, cytopenias, and increased risk of infection. In the general population, the incidence is approximately 2 to 10 cases per 100,000 people; however, as age increases the incidence rises to approximately 50 cases per 100,000 people over age 70.

Basic Information

- Etiology
  - Idiopathic: no known or explained cause of MDS development
  - Secondary: accounts for 20% to 30% of cases. Risk factors include
    - Benzene
    - Ionizing radiation
    - Tobacco/ethanol (ETOH)
    - Immunosuppressive therapy
    - Viral infections
    - Treatment-related or chemotherapy-related MDS:
      - Topoisomerase II inhibitors (e.g., etoposide, topotecan): Associated with 11q23 cytogenetic abnormality; typical onset between 1 and 3 years after chemotherapy
      - Alkylating agents (e.g., cyclophosphamide): Associated with unbalanced cytogenetic changes, including abnormalities of chromosome 5 or 7; typical onset is 5 to 7 years after chemotherapy
- Pathophysiology
  - Complete understanding of the MDS pathophysiology has not yet been achieved
  - Inciting genetic event occurs within an early hematopoetic progenitor in a milieu of inflammation with increased levels of the cytokines tumor necrosis factor-α and interferon-γ
    - **Detectable cytogenetic abnormalities are evident in approximately 40% to 70% of patients with primary MDS and greater than 90% of treatment-related MDS. The cytogenetic abnormality predicts outcome.**
  - Early MDS: Increased levels of apoptosis + increased proliferation → hypercellular bone marrow with peripheral cytopenias
  - Later MDS: Apoptosis decreases and proliferation increases → more aggressive disease and possible transformation to acute myelogenous leukemia
- Classifications
  - Subtle differences exist between a number of classification systems that have been developed

- Staging systems follow the natural progression of the disease by describing the number of cell lines affected, cellularity of the bone marrow, and percentage of blasts within the bone marrow and blood
  - The French-American-British (FAB) classification system (Table 50-1) mainly focuses on morphologic descriptions and is less accurate for predicting prognosis for an individual patient
  - The World Health Organization (WHO) classification system (see Table 50-1) focuses more specifically on the biology of MDS and takes into account blast percentage, estimation of degree of dysplasia, and establishment of genetic subclassifications

Clinical Presentation

- Symptoms derive from the bone marrow cell line or lines most affected
  - Anemia can present with fatigue, pallor, dyspnea, or weakness
  - Thrombocytopenia can present with bruising or bleeding
  - Neutropenia can present with infection
- **Red blood cells are typically the first cell line affected, followed by white blood cells and then platelets**
- Splenomegaly can be seen in some cases, usually in chronic myelomonocytic leukemia

Diagnosis

- Anemia or pancytopenia is typically seen
- The mean corpuscular volume is usually increased, indicating macrocytosis
- Differential diagnosis
  - Vitamin B_{12} or folate deficiency
  - Viral infections (e.g., HIV)
  - Alcohol abuse
  - Benzene exposure
  - Chemotherapy
  - Aplastic anemia or paroxysmal nocturnal hemoglobinuria (PNH) (in settings of a hypoplastic marrow)
- Peripheral blood smear
  - Hypersegmented (5–6 lobes) neutrophils (Fig. 50-1)
  - Macrocytosis of red blood cells
  - **Presence of pseudo Pelger-Huët cells: Hyposegmented "dumbbell"-shaped nuclei of neutrophils (Fig. 50-2)**
- Bone marrow biopsy
  - Required for diagnosis
  - Cellularity: Typically normocellular to hypercellular

TABLE 50-1	Classification Systems for Myelodysplastic Syndromes (MDS)
FAB Classification (Morphologic Classification)	**WHO Classification (Biologic Classification)**
Refractory Anemia (RA) • Cytopenia of one PB lineage • Normocellular or hypocellular BM • <1% PB blasts • <5% BM blasts	1) Refractory Anemia (RA) 2) Refractory Cytopenias with Multilineage Dysplasia (RCMD)
Refractory Anemia w/ Ringed Sideroblasts (RARS) • Cytopenia, dysplasia, and same blast percentage as RA *but* • >15% ringed sideroblasts	3) Refractory Anemia with Ringed Sideroblasts (RARS) 4) RCMD RS
Refractory Anemia with Excess Blasts (RAEB) • Cytopenia of two or more lineages • Dysplasia in all three lineages • <5% PB blasts or • 5–20% BM blasts	5) RAEB-1: 5–10% blasts 6) RAEB-2: 11–20% blasts 7) 5q– syndrome 8) MDS unclassified
Refractory Anemia with Excess Blasts in Transformation (RAEB-t) • Same hematologic parameters as RAEB • >5% PB blasts *or* • 21–30% BM blasts	Acute Myelogenous Leukemia (AML): >20% BM blasts 1) AML with recurrent genetic abnormalities 2) AML with multilineage dysplasia 3) AML and MDS 4) AML NOS
Chronic Myelomonocytic Leukemia (CMML) • Monocytosis in PB • <5% PB blasts *and* • Up to 20% BM blasts	

BM, bone marrow; NOS, not otherwise specified; PB, peripheral blood.
Adapted from Catenacci DV, Schiller GJ: Myelodysplasic syndromes: a comprehensive review, *Blood Rev* 19:301–319, 2005.

FIGURE 50-1 Hypersegmented neutrophils. *(From ASH Image Bank.)*

FIGURE 50-2 Pseudo Pelger-Huët cells. *(From ASH Image Bank.)*

- ▪ **Hypocellular MDS (<20% of cases) can occur and can be difficult to distinguish from aplastic anemia or PNH. However, because cytogenetic abnormalities are typically seen in MDS and not in aplastic anemia or PNH, chromosome analysis can assist in defining the disorders.**
  - ▪ Dysplasia: 1+ cell lines
    - ▪ White blood cells: Hypogranular, poor maturation, abnormal segmentation of nuclei
    - ▪ Red blood cells: Binucleate or multinucleate forms, megaloblastic changes, nuclear-cytoplasmic asynchrony
    - ▪ Platelets: Small, monolobated
  - ▪ Cytogenetic abnormalities: Helpful in determining prognosis
    - ▪ **Good prognosis: 20q–, 5q– syndrome, normal, –Y**
    - ▪ Intermediate prognosis: trisomy 8, other
    - ▪ Poor prognosis: abnormality of chromosome 7, complex cytogenetics
- ▪ Prognosis
  - ▪ The International Prognostic Staging System (IPSS) (Table 50-2)
    - ▪ Scoring system that assigns a point scale for three categories:
      - ▪ Number of cell lines affected
      - ▪ Percentage of blasts within the bone marrow (blasts are usually distinguished by an increase in CD34-positive cells)
      - ▪ Cytogenetic abnormalities
    - ▪ Calculations based on these categories risk-stratify patients into low-risk, intermediate-1, intermediate-2, and high-risk categories
  - ▪ Recently, a revised prognostic scoring system, the Global MD Anderson MDS Score, was developed that includes additional clinical factors in order to more precisely predict outcomes and risk of transformation to acute leukemia (see Table 50-2)

Treatment

- ▪ Regardless of stage of disease of MDS patients, there are four major generalizable goals of medical treatment

TABLE 50-2	*Prognostic Scoring Systems for Myelodysplastic Syndrome (MDS)*			
	IPSS	**Assigned Points**	**Global MD Anderson MDS Score**	**Assigned Points**
Percentage marrow blasts	<5	0	<5	0
	5–10	0.5	5–10	1
	11–20	1	11–29	2
	21–30	2		
Cytogenetics	*Good:* normal, –Y, 20q–, 5q–	0	–7, del(7)q or complex	3
	Intermediate: trisomy 8	0.5	All others	0
	Poor: abnormal 7, complex	1		
Cytopenias (number of lineages)	0–1	0		
	2–3	0.5		
Performance status (Zubrod)			0 or 1	0
			≥2	2
Age			<60	0
			60–64	1
			≥65	2
Platelets (K/µL)			<30	3
			30–49	2
			50–199	1
			≥200	0
Hemoglobin			<12.0	2
			≥12.0	0
WBC (K/µL)			≤20	0
			>20	2
Prior transfusion (RBC or PLT)			No	0
			Yes	1
MDS Risk Category				
Low		0		0–4
Intermediate-1		0.5–1		5–6
Intermediate-2		1.5–2		7–8
High		>2.5		>9

IPSS, International Prognostic Staging System; PLT, platelet; RBC, red blood cell; WBC, white blood cell.

- Control the symptoms caused by cytopenias and minimize transfusion needs
- Improve overall quality of life
- Decrease risk of progression to acute myelogenous leukemia (AML)
- Improve overall survival
- Supportive care
  - Careful blood count monitoring with transfusion support
    - Iron overload can occur with repeated transfusions
    - Iron chelation recommended for patients who have had greater than 20 to 30 transfusions: monitor ferritin levels with goal ferritin less than 1000 ng/mL
  - Growth factor support
    - **Erythropoietin (EPO) effective only when EPO levels are low; response seen in less than 20% of patients**
    - Granulocyte colony-stimulating factor only indicated in setting of repeated infections or in combination with EPO to boost red blood cell response (the combination is especially important for refractory anemia with ringed sideroblasts)

- Allogeneic stem cell transplantation
  - **Only curative approach to treatment**
  - Best outcome generally seen in younger patients with a matched donor (either sibling or unrelated) and with good performance status
    - Numerous studies now confirm that nonmyeloablative, or "mini," transplants are feasible in elderly MDS patients with decreased treatment-related mortality (15–20%) but at the expense of slightly increased relapse rates
  - Approximately 30% to 50% disease-free survival at 3 years
  - Treatment-related mortality can be as high as 30+% with standard myeloablative transplants
- Medical management
  - Numerous new agents approved by the Food and Drug Administration for the treatment of MDS over the last 5 years
  - Hypomethylating agents (azacitidine or decitabine): traditionally studied in higher risk patients (intermediate-1, intermediate-2, and high IPSS risk score)
    - Overall response rate is approximately 40% to 60% (includes complete response, partial response, and hematologic improvement)

- Trilineage responses are common and expected, with transfusion independence rates ranging from 40% to 60%
- Azacitidine shown to delay time to AML and prolong overall survival in Phase III studies
- Lenalidomide is a new thalidomide analogue with immunomodulatory effects recently found to have significant activity in MDS patients with 5q− syndrome
  - **5q− syndrome: A syndrome that typically occurs in older women characterized by anemia, bone marrow findings of small hyposegmented megakaryocytes, and less than 5% blasts.** Treatment is typically supportive care only as transformation to acute leukemia rarely occurs. This is a separate entity from deletions of 5q.
  - Best responses seen in those patients with anemia only, 5q− abnormality, and low or intermediate-1 IPSS risk score
    - Response aim is to decrease or eliminate transfusion requirements
- Conventional chemotherapy (cytarabine based)
  - High-dose chemotherapy targets the abnormal clonal cells
  - Results often short lived and toxicity is high
  - Overall survival not improved by intense chemotherapy but this is sometimes needed for those patients with high blast percentage

REVIEW QUESTIONS

For review questions, please go to www.expertconsult.com.

SUGGESTED READINGS

Aul C, Giagounidis U, Germing U: Epidemiological features of myelodysplastic syndrome: real or factitious? *Int J Hematol* 73:405–410, 2001.

Bennett JM, Catovsky D, Daniel MT, et al: Proposals for the classification of the myelodysplastic syndromes, *Br J Haematol* 51:189–199, 1982.

Catenacci DV, Schiller GJ: Myelodysplasic syndromes: a comprehensive review, *Blood Rev* 19:301–319, 2005.

Fenaux P, Mufti GJ, Hellstrom-Lindberg E, et al: Efficacy of azacitidine compared with that of conventional care regimens in the treatment of higher-risk myelodysplastic syndromes: a randomized, open-label, phase III study, *Lancet Oncol* 10:223–232, 2009.

Kantarjian H, O'Brien S, Ravandi F, et al: Proposal for a new risk model in myelodysplastic syndrome that accounts for events not considered in the original International Prognostic Scoring System, *Cancer* 113:1351–1361, 2008.

Mufti GJ: Pathobiology, classification, and diagnosis of myelodysplatic syndromes, *Best Pract Res Clin Haematol* 17:543–557, 2004.

National Comprehensive Cancer Network Guidelines for Myelodysplastic Syndromes: Available at www.NCCN.org.

CHAPTER 51

Blood Smear and Bone Marrow Review

JONATHAN M. GERBER, MD

An internist should be familiar with the key components of a peripheral blood smear (PBS). Findings on a PBS, coupled with information obtained from the complete blood count (CBC), can help to narrow the differential diagnosis. Uncertainties not answered by the PBS and CBC may necessitate an examination of the bone marrow.

Peripheral Blood Smear

- Role of PBS in the evaluation of a patient
  - Part of the initial evaluation for any abnormality in the CBC
  - Useful in narrowing the differential diagnosis
    - Sometimes what is not seen on the PBS can be of great value in ruling in or out a specific diagnosis
- Two components of evaluation of a PBS are the descriptive report and the prepared slide
  - In describing the PBS, terms often used to describe red blood cells (RBCs) include the following (Figs. 51-1 and 51-2):
    - Anisocytosis: Differently sized RBCs (see Fig. 51-1B and C)
    - Poikilocytosis: Differently shaped RBCs (see Figs. 51-1A and 51-2B, D, and F)
    - Polychromasia: Indicating an increase in young RBCs (see Fig. 51-2E)
    - Microcytosis: Small RBCs (see Figs. 51-1C and 51-2A)
    - Macrocytosis: Large RBCs (see Fig. 51-1B)
    - Schistocytes: Fragmented RBC forms (see Fig. 51-1A)
- The prepared slide may provide the diagnosis or narrow the differential diagnosis (Figs. 51-3 and 51-4; Tables 51-1 and 51-2; see also Figs. 51-1 and 51-2)
  - Poor slide preparation may result in artifacts such as rouleaux (stacked RBCs), which may be caused by an overly thick smear but also may be a sign of inflammation, infection (e.g., hepatitis or HIV), or myeloma
- The normal PBS
  - **RBCs should be round and the size of a lymphocyte nucleus, with one-third central pallor**
  - Lymphocytes should have small, compact nuclei
  - **Polymorphonuclear neutrophils (PMNs) should have three to four lobes**
  - Platelets should number 15 to 20 per high-power field (1 platelet on PBS at high power equals ~10,000 in CBC)

- In addition to a microscopic examination, peripheral blood may also be sent for the following:
  - **Flow cytometry: Quantitates cell surface markers and can also establish clonality**
  - Fluorescent *in situ* hybridization (FISH): A sensitive method of determining specific cytogenetic abnormalities. It does not require proliferating cells and can thus be performed on peripheral blood, but limited to specific probes for known abnormalities.
  - Polymerase chain reaction (PCR): A highly sensitive method for looking at mutations; can be qualitative or quantitative, but limited to known mutations for which there are primers

Bone Marrow Analysis

- A bone marrow examination consists of two components: (1) a bone marrow aspirate and (2) a bone marrow biopsy
  - **The aspirate is a smear of the marrow elements;** it is stained and examined for cell morphology, such as when considering myelodysplastic syndrome, vitamin deficiency, and other conditions
  - Tests performed on a bone marrow aspirate include the following:
    - Iron staining: The gold standard for diagnosis of iron deficiency
    - Culture: Note that the sensitivities of bone marrow culture and blood culture are similar
    - Flow cytometry, FISH, and PCR (as previously stated with peripheral blood)
    - Cytogenetics: Often used in the evaluation of leukemias; used to detect chromosomal aberrations, including translocations (such as 9;22 in chronic myeloid leukemia or 15;17 in acute promyelocytic leukemia [the M3 variant of acute myelogenous leukemia]). *Note:* Cytogenetic analysis requires dividing cells, which are usually found only in the marrow (as opposed to peripheral blood); it is less sensitive than FISH or PCR but not limited by specific probes.
  - The bone marrow biopsy is a core biopsy that is then decalcified
    - **The bone marrow biopsy is most helpful in determining cellularity** (e.g., hypocellular, as in aplastic anemia, or hypercellular, as in

FIGURE 51-1 **A**, Schistocytes. **B**, Macrocytes. **C**, Spherocytes. **D**, Teardrops, bizarre shapes.

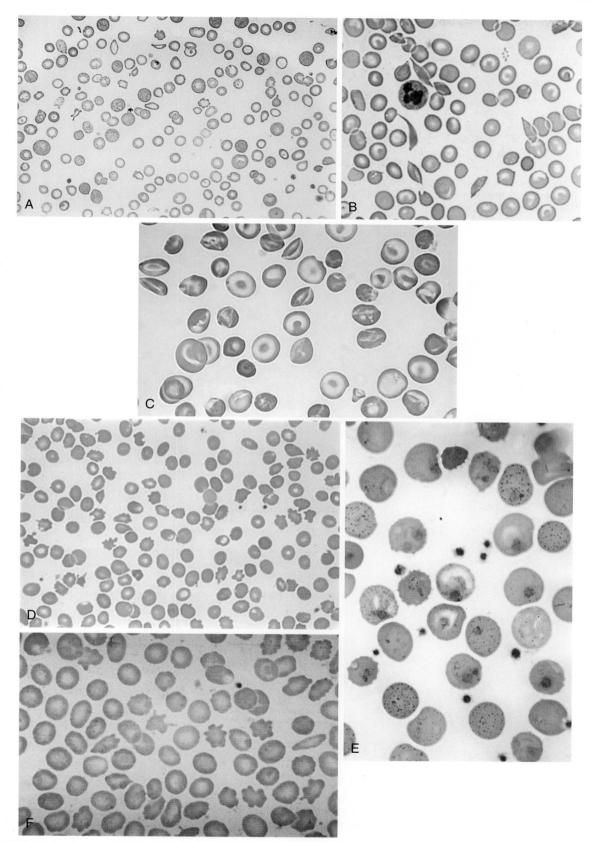

FIGURE 51-2   **A,** Hypochromic, microcytic. **B,** Sickle cells. **C,** Target cells. **D,** Burr cells. **E,** Basophilic stippling. **F,** Acanthocytes.

FIGURE 51-3   Leukopenia with nucleated red blood cells (RBCs) (**A**) and hyposegmented polymorphonuclear neutrophils (PMNs) (**B**). **C**, Parasite inclusions. **D**, Leukopenia with hypersegmented PMNs. **E**, Microangiopathic hemolytic anemia with schistocytes and thrombocytopenia. **F**, Lymphocytosis with normal-appearing lymphocytes.

FIGURE 51-4 **A,** Lymphocytosis with cell membrane projections. **B** and **C,** Leukocytosis with wide range of immature forms, including blasts. (Note the large nuclei with open chromatin and prominent nuclei, seen well in part **B.**)

TABLE 51-1	*Abnormalities on Peripheral Blood Smear (PBS): Red Blood Cells*		
Findings on PBS	**Appearance**	**Differential Diagnosis**	**Further Testing***
Hypochromic, microcytic		Iron deficiency Thalassemia Anemia of chronic disease	Iron studies; Hgb electrophoresis
Target cells		Hemoglobin C Liver disease Thalassemia	Hgb electrophoresis; studies of liver function
Basophilic stippling		Hemolysis Lead poisoning Thalassemia	Coombs' test; lead levels; Hgb electrophoresis; reticulocyte count
Sickle cells		Sickle cell syndromes	Hgb electrophoresis

Continued on following page

51

TABLE 51-1   *Abnormalities on Peripheral Blood Smear (PBS): Red Blood Cells* (Continued)

Findings on PBS	Appearance	Differential Diagnosis	Further Testing*
Burr cells		Renal disease	Studies of renal function
Acanthocytes		Liver disease Abetalipoproteinemia	Studies of liver function; lipid profile
Schistocytes		Microangiopathic hemolytic anemia (e.g., TTP, DIC) Malignant hypertension Prosthetic heart valve	See Chapter 46
Spherocytes		Autoimmune hemolytic anemia Hereditary spherocytosis	See Chapter 46
Macrocytes		Vitamin B_{12} deficiency Folate deficiency Myelodysplastic syndrome Liver disease Hypothyroidism	Serum vitamin B_{12} and RBC folate levels; TSH; liver function tests; bone marrow examination
Teardrops, nucleated RBCs, bizarre forms		Myelofibrosis Marrow infiltration (e.g., tumor, tuberculosis)	Bone marrow examination; splenomegaly suggests extramedullary hematopoiesis
Bite cells		G6PD deficiency Unstable hemoglobinopathy	Enzyme assays; drug history; Heinz body preparation; heat stability test
Parasite inclusions		Malaria (shown) Babesiosis	Thick and thin blood smear remains gold standard for diagnosis of malaria; polymerase chain reaction and antibody testing now available for babesiosis

DIC, disseminated intravascular coagulopathy; G6PD, glucose-6-phosphate dehydrogenase; Hgb, hemoglobin; RBC, red blood cell; TSH, thyroid-stimulating hormone; TTP, thrombotic thrombocytopenic purpura.
*See also Chapter 46.

TABLE 51-2 *Abnormalities on Peripheral Blood Smear (PBS): Platelet and Leukocyte Disorders*

Findings on PBS	Appearance	Differential Diagnosis	Further Testing
Thrombocytopenia		Idiopathic thrombocytopenic purpura (if RBC fragments present, suspect microangiopathic hemolytic anemia)	Bone marrow examination if patient >50 yr old, other cytopenias present, or any other abnormality seen on the PBS; immature platelet fraction (typically high if destructive cause)
Leukopenia with hyposegmented PMNs		Myelodysplastic syndrome Stress, infection Pelger-Huët anomaly	Bone marrow examination with cytogenetics/FISH if myelodysplastic syndrome suspected
Leukopenia with hypersegmented PMNs		Vitamin B_{12} deficiency Folate deficiency	Serum B_{12} and RBC folate levels
Lymphocytosis with normal-appearing lymphocytes		Chronic lymphocytic leukemia	Flow cytometry
Lymphocytosis with cell membrane projections		Hairy cell leukemia	Flow cytometry
Lymphocytosis with open nuclei/nucleoli		Activated lymphocytes (e.g., seen in viral infection)	Clinical correlation and viral serologies as appropriate; flow cytometry to rule out leukemia/lymphoma
Leukocytosis with wide range of immature forms		Reactive bone marrow (i.e., leukemoid reaction) Chronic myelogenous leukemia Myeloproliferative neoplasm	Clinical correlation and bone marrow examination (with additional studies) as appropriate
Immature cells (blasts)		Leukemia	Bone marrow examination with flow cytometry; cytogenetics/FISH/PCR (see also Chapter 56)
Blasts with Auer rods		Acute myeloid leukemia	Bone marrow examination with flow cytometry; cytogenetics/FISH/PCR (see also Chapter 56)

FISH, fluorescent in situ hybridization; PCR, polymerase chain reaction; PMNs, polymorphonuclear neutrophils; RBC, red blood cell.

51

myelodysplastic syndrome), in assessing fibrosis or marrow replacement by tumor (metastatic or hematologic), and in determining the relative quantities of cell populations in a marrow (e.g., increased number of plasma cells in myeloma)

- Tests performed on the biopsy include the following:
    - Immunohistochemical stains for specific cell populations (such as κ or λ)
    - Special stains for fibrosis (reticulin) or amyloid (Congo red)
    - Stains for infections (fungal, acid-fast bacilli, some viral antigens)
- Indications for bone marrow analysis
    - **Bone marrow aspirate** is used for evaluation of:
        - Pancytopenia
        - Unexplained anemias (especially with teardrops or bizarre forms on PBS)
        - Isolated thrombocytopenia (if patient >50 years, if there are any other abnormalities in the CBC or in the PBS, or if there are other concerns for myelodysplasia)
        - Suspected hematologic malignancy
        - **Bone marrow aspirate has a relatively low yield for evaluation of fever of unknown origin or aggressive lymphoma (excisional biopsy of an affected lymph node is preferred)**
    - Bone marrow biopsy is used for evaluation of:
        - Overall cellularity of bone marrow (normal overall cellularity can be approximated by 100 minus the patient's age; so for a 70-year-old patient, the bone marrow should be 30% cellular)

- Diagnosis (and staging) of a suspected clonal process: The biopsy can be stained for cell markers (e.g., if most plasma cells stain positive for κ rather than λ, a monoclonal process such as myeloma is suggested). Bone marrow biopsy is part of the staging work-up for lymphoma.
- Bone marrow biopsy can also be examined for fungus, acid-fast bacilli, or granuloma, which may greatly facilitate the diagnosis of some infectious disorders

Acknowledgment

This chapter was adapted from a chapter written by Lawrence Gardner, MD, for the second edition of the *Johns Hopkins Internal Medicine Board Review*.

REVIEW QUESTIONS

For review questions, please go to www.expertconsult.com.

SUGGESTED READINGS

Hoffbrand AV, Pettit JE: *Clinical haematology*, London, 1988, Gower Medical Publishing.

Hoffbrand AV, Pettit JE: *Color atlas of clinical hematology*, ed 4, London, 2010, Mosby.

Tkachuk DC, Hirschmann JV: *Wintrobe's atlas of clinical hematology*, Philadelphia, Lippincott, 2007, Williams & Wilkins.

Zucker-Franklin D: *Atlas of blood cells: function and pathology*, ed 2, Philadelphia, 1988, Lea & Febiger.

SECTION NINE

Oncology

Colorectal Cancer

DAVID COSGROVE, MD

Colorectal cancer (CRC) is the third most common malignancy seen in both men and women. Over 140,000 cases of colon cancer are diagnosed each year, making it a disease that ultimately affects 8% of the population in the United States.

Basic Information

- Epidemiology
  - Starting at age 40 years, CRC incidence increases with age, with a mean presentation between ages 60 and 65 years
  - Incidence higher in developed countries
  - Third leading cause of cancer deaths
    - 52,000 deaths each year in the United States
  - African Americans have a higher incidence and mortality from CRC than any other ethnic group
- Etiology
  - CRC development proceeds in stepwise fashion from adenoma to invasive carcinoma, with accumulation of oncogenic mutations (Fig. 52-1)
- Classification by location
  - Rectal cancers are those arising below the peritoneal reflection or less than 12 to 15 cm from the anal verge
  - Cancers arising proximal to this area are designated as colon cancers
  - Incidence of CRC by anatomic location: see Table 52-1
- Risk factors
  - Polyposis syndromes are associated with a higher risk of CRC (Table 52-2)
  - **Familial adenomatous polyposis (FAP) increases risk to almost 100% unless prophylactic total colectomy is performed (Fig. 52-2)**
  - Hereditary nonpolyposis colon cancer (HNPCC)—also known as the Lynch syndromes (Table 52-3)—can increase risk as much as seven times that of the general population
    - Lynch syndromes are associated with *mutHLS* gene complex leading to genetic instability; 4% of CRC cases
      - Usually right-sided lesions
      - Median age 44 years
      - Prognosis not worse than in sporadic tumors
      - Caused by germline mutations of DNA mismatch repair genes (*MLH1, MSH2, PMS1, PMS2*)
      - Total colectomy recommended by some authorities after diagnosis of this syndrome; most recommend total colectomy after a recurrence
  - Risk increases in patients with personal or family history of sporadic CRC or adenoma
  - **Sporadic CRC occurs in 80% of the cases, with mutations of adenomatous polyposis coli (APC) gene found in 70% of sporadic tumors**
- There is also a higher incidence of CRC in patients with inflammatory bowel disease (IBD), either ulcerative colitis or Crohn disease
  - Risk is associated with duration of IBD, extent of disease, and development of mucosal dysplasia
- Weaker risk factors include environmental, nutritional, and lifestyle factors
  - Increased risk of CRC is associated with higher total calories, animal fat, and protein in diet
  - Lower risk is associated with increased calcium; vitamins A, C, D; folate; and selenium
  - Dietary fiber is currently an area of controversy
- ***Streptococcus bovis* bacteremia: Patients who develop this condition have a high incidence of occult CRC**

Clinical Presentation

- Clinical presentations may differ depending on the tumor location
- Right-sided lesions commonly produce the following:
  - Vague abdominal aching
  - Abdominal mass
  - Anemia from chronic blood loss (Fig. 52-3)
  - Fatigue
- Left-sided tumors more commonly produce the following:
  - Obstructive symptoms
  - Colicky abdominal pain
  - Changes in bowel habits, with or without rectal bleeding
- Rectal tumors commonly present with the following:
  - Change in caliber of stools
  - Sensation of rectal fullness
  - Urgency
  - Hematochezia, tenesmus
- **Pelvic pain usually indicates local extension into pelvic nerves (later stage of disease)**

Diagnosis and Evaluation

- Screening
  - Because the only definitive cure is via surgical resection, detection at an early stage is imperative
  - The American Cancer Society (ACS) recommends the following tests and precautions:
    - Fecal occult blood test (FOBT) or fecal immunochemical test (FIT) annually beginning at age 50 years
    - Plus flexible sigmoidoscopy every 5 years, colonoscopy every 10 years, double-contrast barium enema every 5 years, or computed tomographic colonography (virtual colonoscopy) every 5 years.

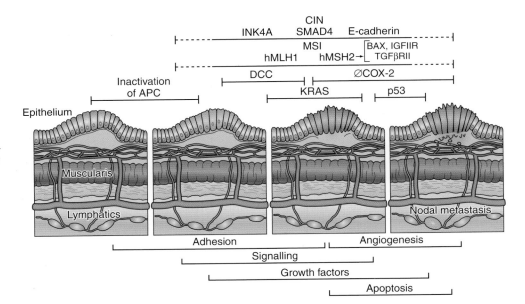

FIGURE 52-1 Adenoma-to-carcinoma sequence and the associated molecular alterations involved in colon cancer development. *(From Abeloff MD, Armitage JO, Niederhuber JE, et al: Clinical oncology, ed 3, Philadelphia, Churchill Livingstone, 2004, Fig. 80-3.)*

TABLE 52-1	Location of Colorectal Cancers
Location	**Incidence (%)**
Cecum	12.5
Ascending colon	9
Transverse colon	11
Descending colon	6.1
Sigmoid colon	23.6
Rectosigmoid junction	8.6
Rectum	22.1

- Although there are no proven screening recommendations for high-risk patients, it is reasonable to begin screening at an earlier age and conduct it with increased frequency in these populations. Colonoscopy is the test of choice in high-risk populations.
- The U.S. Preventive Services Task Force (USPSTF) recommends:
  - Annual high-sensitivity FOBT or sigmoidoscopy every 5 years combined with high-sensitivity FOBT every 3 years or screening colonoscopy at intervals of 10 years
  - **Against routine screening in patients older than age 75 years**
- Initial diagnostic evaluation for suggested CRC
  - Complete history and physical examination are warranted
  - Preoperative staging includes the following:
    - Complete blood count
    - Liver function tests
    - Renal function studies
    - Urinalysis
    - Serum carcinoembryonic antigen (CEA)
    - Computed tomography (CT) scans of the chest, abdomen and pelvis
    - Tumor-node-metastasis (TNM) staging (Table 52-4)

TABLE 52-2	Polyposis Syndromes	
Syndrome	**Inheritance Pattern**	**Clinical Features**
Familial adenomatous polyposis: 1% of colorectal cancer (CRC) cases	Autosomal dominant	Pancolonic adenomatous polyposis by late adolescence; almost all patients will develop CRC unless prophylactic colectomy is performed
Gardner syndrome	Autosomal dominant	Small and large bowel adenomas, extracolonic tumors of soft tissue (desmoid tumors, fibromas, lipomas), bone (osteomas), and ampulla; epidermoid and sebaceous cysts also associated; almost all patients will develop CRC
Turcot syndrome	Autosomal recessive	Bowel polyposis associated with malignant CNS tumors; CRC commonly develops
Peutz-Jeghers syndrome	Autosomal dominant	Hamartomas of the small intestine and colon; also associated with mucocutaneous pigmented lesions of the hands, feet, and mouth; tumors of ovary, breast, pancreas, and endometrium can be seen; rarely transforms to malignancy
Juvenile polyposis	Autosomal dominant	Hamartomas may be limited to the stomach or colon or may be distributed throughout the GI tract; low malignant potential

CNS, central nervous system; GI, gastrointestinal.

FIGURE 52-2 A segment of a large intestine covered with adenomatous polyps in a patient with familial adenomatous polyposis. The entire colon is covered with hundreds of polyps. *(From Skarin AT, Shaffer K, Wieczorek T [eds]: Atlas of diagnostic oncology, ed 3, St. Louis, Mosby, 2003, p 152. In Abeloff MD, Armitage JO, Niederhuber JE, et al: Clinical oncology, ed 3, Philadelphia, Churchill Livingstone, 2004, Fig. 80-7.)*

TABLE 52-3	*Lynch Syndromes (HNPCC)*
Lynch I	Autosomal dominant trait, early-onset trait; early development of primarily proximal colon cancers; colon specific
Lynch II	Associated with colonic and extracolonic adenocarcinomas of the ovary, breast, stomach, small bowel, endometrium, pancreas, bile duct, kidney, and urinary tract

Treatment

- Surgical treatment
  - The primary goal of surgery is resection for cure
  - In the setting of known metastatic disease, the need for surgery depends on the presence or risk of obstruction or bleeding
  - Types of surgical resections performed also depend on location and extent of tumor. Right, transverse, or left hemicolectomy; wide sigmoid resection; or a low anterior resection with end-to-end anastomosis for proximal rectal cancers may be performed.
  - For distal rectal tumors, when unable to spare the sphincter, abdominoperineal resection with permanent colostomy is often necessary
  - An alternative procedure for tumors 2 to 5 cm from the anal verge is a coloanal anastomosis
  - In selected rectal cancer cases with tumors smaller than 3 to 4 cm, T1, well to moderately differentiated, and without lymphovascular involvement, local excision alone may be performed with a full-thickness negative margin
  - Preoperative endorectal ultrasound is an extremely useful tool in defining rectal lesions that are amenable to local excision alone
- Postoperative adjuvant therapy
  - Offered to those at high risk for recurrence because approximately 50% of CRC patients die secondary to metastatic disease
  - For colon cancer
    - The current standard adjuvant chemotherapy regimen in the United States is 5-fluorouracil (5-FU) and leucovorin, with oxaliplatin

52

FIGURE 52-3 Colonoscopic view of bleeding carcinomas of the sigmoid colon (**A**) and cecum (**B**). Carcinomas of the colon often bleed intermittently. Patients may present with evidence of microcytic anemia or with red blood per rectum (hematochezia), depending on tumor site and amount of blood loss. *(From Feldman M: Sleisenger and Fordtran's gastrointestinal and liver disease, ed 7, Philadelphia, WB Saunders, 2002, Fig. 115-22.)*

TABLE 52-4 *Tumor-Node-Metastasis (TNM) Staging for Colorectal Cancer*

TNM Stage	Primary Tumor	Lymph Node Classification	Distant Metastasis	Duke's Stage
0	Tis (carcinoma *in situ*)	N0 (no regional lymph node metastasis)	M0 (no distant metastasis)	—
I	T1 (tumor invades the submucosa)	N0	M0	A
	T2 (tumor invades the muscularis propria)			A
IIA	T3 (tumor invades through the muscularis propria)	N0	M0	B
IIB/C	T4a/b (tumor invades visceral peritoneum/ other organs)	N0	M0	B
IIIA/B/C	T1–T4 (stage III tumors encompass any T stage with N1 or N2 disease)	N1/2 (metastasis in 1–3/≥4 pericolic or perirectal lymph nodes along the course of a named vascular trunk)	M0	C
IV	Any T	Any N	M1 (distant metastasis)	D

- **Adjuvant chemotherapy has been demonstrated to significantly improve survival in stage III disease**
  - Benefit of chemotherapy in stage II patients is currently unclear, but is typically offered to patients with high-risk features (T4 lesions, perforation, bowel obstruction, high-grade tumors)
  - Radiation therapy is not routinely used adjuvantly; however, it may be useful in achieving better local control in T4 tumors
- For rectal cancer
  - The combination of radiation therapy and 5-FU does increase locoregional control, disease-free survival, and overall survival for stages II and III
  - With the preoperative use of combined-modality treatment, locally advanced (T3 or T4) or unresectable cancer may be rendered resectable and sphincter preservation can be achieved
- Recurrence patterns
  - Sites of colon cancer recurrence
    - Liver
    - Peritoneum
    - Other distant sites
  - Rectal cancer commonly associated with locoregional recurrences; in these cases, radiation therapy is important for local control
  - Recurrence evaluation
    - If a patient is found to have only an elevated CEA, colonoscopy and CT scans of chest, abdomen, and pelvis should be performed
    - If imaging is negative, repeat CT scans should be ordered every 3 months
    - If imaging is positive, patients should undergo salvage therapy
- Treatment of local recurrence and metastatic disease
  - Local recurrences
    - Whenever possible, resection is recommended
    - Recurrence to regional or retroperitoneal lymph nodes is associated with poor prognosis
    - Pelvic recurrences may be cured by pelvic exenteration in some patients

TABLE 52-5 *Surveillance of Patients After Treatment for Colon Cancer*

Surveillance Method	Frequency/Comment
Colonoscopy	At 1 yr after surgery, then every 3 yr if no polyps on previous endoscopy
Physical examination, including rectal examination	Every 3 mo for 2 yr, then every 6 mo until 5 yr post-therapy (for stage II and III disease)
Fecal occult blood testing	Every 3 mo for 2 yr, then every 6 mo until 5 yr post-therapy (for stage II and III disease)
CBC and chemistries	Every 3 mo for 2 yr, then every 6 mo until 5 yr post-therapy (for stage II and III disease)
Carcinoembryonic antigen	Every 6 mo for 2 yr, then annually for 5 yr
Chest and abdominal CT	Every 6 mo for 2 yr, then annually for 3 yr in patients who have undergone resection or completed other therapy

CBC, complete blood count; CT, computed tomography.

- Recurrences in the liver
  - **If the liver is the only site of recurrence, resection of liver metastases is a viable, and potentially curative, treatment option in selected patients**
- In the setting of metastatic disease
  - 5-FU–based chemotherapy (preceded by leucovorin) is still the standard systemic palliative treatment, with other cytotoxic agents such as irinotecan and oxaliplatin available. Targeted chemotherapy with epidermal growth factor receptor monoclonal antibodies (cetuximab, panitumumab) or vascular endothelial growth factor monoclonal antibodies (bevacizumab) can be used in conjunction with chemotherapy in select cases.

- Palliative radiation therapy for regionally recurrent rectal cancer
  - Can decrease pain and bleeding in 70% to 80% of patients
- Prognosis
  - At diagnosis, 25% of colon cancers have extended through the bowel wall. Of all rectal cancers, up to 60% have extended through the bowel wall or to regional lymph nodes.
  - **The most common site of distant metastasis is the liver**
  - The most commonly affected extra-abdominal organ is the lung
  - Stage of disease is the single most significant prognostic factor
  - Other unfavorable clinical prognostic factors include the following:
    - Long duration of symptoms
    - Bowel obstruction or perforation
    - Elevated preoperative CEA level
  - Surveillance after therapy: see Table 52-5

Acknowledgment

This chapter is based on the chapter written by Mark Levis, MD, PhD, for the 3rd edition.

REVIEW QUESTIONS

For review questions, please go to www.expertconsult.com.

SUGGESTED READINGS

Andre T, Boni C, Navarro M, et al: Improved overall survival with oxaliplatin, fluorouracil and leucovorin as adjuvant treatment in stage II or III colon cancer in the MOSAIC trial, *J Clin Oncol* 27:3109, 2009.

Engstrom PF, Arnoletti JP, Benson AB, et al: Clinical practice guidelines in oncology: colon cancer, *J Natl Compr Canc Netw* 7:778–831, 2009.

Kemeny N: The management of resectable and unresectable liver metastases from colorectal cancer, *Curr Opin Oncol* 22:364–373, 2010.

Nelson H, Petrelli N, Carlin A, et al: Guidelines 2000 for colon and rectal cancer surgery, *J Natl Cancer Inst* 93:583, 2001.

Vasen HF, Moslein G, Alonso A, et al: Guidelines for the clinical management of familial adenomatous polyposis (FAP), *Gut* 57:704–713, 2008.

52

Breast and Ovarian Cancer

DEBORAH K. ARMSTRONG, MD

Breast cancer is the most commonly diagnosed malignancy in women, affecting 1 out of every 8 women in the United States. It is the second most common cause of cancer deaths in women. Ovarian cancer is less prevalent, affecting 1 out of every 50 to 70 women, but it is associated with high mortality rates because of difficulties in diagnosing early-stage disease. This chapter provides an overview of these two very important malignancies.

Breast Cancer

Basic Information

- Affects 12% of the female population in the United States
  - Less than 1% of breast cancer cases occur in men
- There are significant variations in breast cancer incidence and mortality between countries. This is thought to be due to variations in genetic, reproductive, environmental, dietary, and social factors.
  - Japan and other Asian countries have the lowest death rates
  - England and Wales have the highest death rates
- A number of breast cancer risk factors have been identified (Box 53-1)
- Genetics of breast cancer
  - **More than 90% of breast cancer cases appear to be sporadic without an apparent familial or genetic predisposition**
  - Factors suggestive of a familial or genetic inheritance of breast cancer
    - Multiple affected family members
    - Multiple generations involved
    - Early age of onset (before age 50)
    - Bilateral disease
    - Presence of ovarian cancer within the family
    - Male breast cancer
  - Approximately 10% of breast cancers appear to be familial (Table 53-1)
    - The causative gene(s) have not been identified in approximately half of familial breast cancers
    - Less than 1% of familial breast cancer is ascribed to rare frequency genes such as *TP53*, *PTEN*, and *CDH1*
  - *BRCA* mutations
    - The two *BRCA* genes account for about 50% of familial breast cancer and the vast majority of identified genetic mutations associated with breast cancer
    - Lifetime breast cancer risk in women with a deleterious *BRCA* mutation is 40% to 85%

- Lifetime risk of male breast cancer is 6% for *BRCA2* carriers
- The inheritance pattern is autosomal dominant
- The *BRCA* genes are not sex-linked, but they are silent in most males
- There is a high penetrance of disease in female carriers
- Certain *BRCA* mutations are seen more often in specific populations (i.e., three founder mutations in people of Ashkenazi Jewish descent)
- Hormonal prevention with tamoxifen or raloxifene, oophorectomy, and mastectomy are all potential prophylactic measures in *BRCA*-positive patients (see Breast Cancer Prevention section below)
- Breast cancer screening recommendations are controversial. The American Cancer Society suggests more aggressive screening (Table 53-2) than the U.S. Preventive Services Task Force (USPSTF), which suggests mammography every 2 years for average-risk women ages 50 to 74.
- Pathology
  - Generally classified by the anatomic area of the breast that is affected (ducts versus lobules), by the level of tumor invasion (carcinoma *in situ* versus invasive carcinoma) and grade of the tumor cells
    - Ductal carcinoma *in situ* (DCIS) is a marker for development of subsequent invasive disease at the same site
    - **Lobular carcinoma *in situ* (LCIS) is a marker for development of invasive cancer in either breast, so close surveillance of both breasts is required**
    - Infiltrating (invasive) ductal carcinoma is the most common histologic type of breast cancer

Clinical Presentation and Diagnosis

- Most cases manifest as a palpable breast mass or abnormality on mammogram
  - Palpable breast mass
    - **A mammogram should be obtained after discovering a mass; however, the absence of a mammographic abnormality does not eliminate the need for tissue diagnosis of a new palpable mass**
  - Tissue diagnosis
    - Fine-needle aspiration does not preserve tissue architecture and is most appropriate for likely benign cystic lesions
    - **Incisional (core) biopsy maintains tissue architecture of the sample and is the best approach for diagnosis, but the lesion is not completely removed**

53

BOX 53-1 *Risk Factors Associated with Breast Cancer*

Known carrier of a deleterious *BRCA1* or *BRCA2* mutation

Personal history of prior breast, endometrial, or ovarian cancer

Family history of breast or ovarian cancer

Increasing age

Nulliparity or late age at first pregnancy (age 30 yr or older)

Absence of breast-feeding

Early menarche

Late menopause

Hormone replacement therapy

Prior breast biopsy, especially with documented hyperplasia

Prior radiation to breast area (e.g., mantle radiation for lymphoma)

TABLE 53-1 *Causes of Hereditary Susceptibility of Breast Cancer*

Gene	Contribution to Hereditary Breast Cancer
BRCA1	~30%
BRCA2	~20%
TP53, PTEN, CDH1*	<1%
Undiscovered genes	~50%

*TP53, Li-Fraumeni syndrome; PTEN, Cowden syndrome; CDH1, hereditary diffuse gastric cancer syndrome.

TABLE 53-2 *American Cancer Society Breast Cancer Screening Recommendations**

Age (yr)	Examination	Frequency
20–39	Breast self-examination	Optional
	Clinical breast examination	Every 3 yr
≥40	Breast self-examination	Optional
	Clinical breast examination	Yearly
	Mammography	Yearly

*Women at increased risk due to family history, genetic risk, or prior breast cancer should have individualized recommendations that may include starting mammography earlier, additional screening tests such as breast ultrasound or magnetic resonance imaging, or having more frequent exams.

- Excisional biopsy involves complete removal of the lesion
- Mammographic abnormality
  - Risk of the abnormality is stratified based on patient history, exam findings, and imaging characteristics
  - A core biopsy of a mammographic abnormality is frequently done by the radiologist with the assistance of imaging

Treatment

- DCIS
  - Requires complete excision (goal of attaining negative margins)
  - May be treated with lumpectomy and radiation therapy (RT) or mastectomy
  - Lymph node evaluation not required for pure DCIS without invasion
    - Sentinel node evaluation sometimes done with mastectomy for DCIS in case invasion is ultimately found
  - **Tamoxifen decreases risk of a contralateral cancer and decreases in-breast recurrence after lumpectomy and RT**
- LCIS
  - The optimal treatment strategy is unknown at this time and may involve careful surveillance of both breasts, with or without tamoxifen therapy, or bilateral prophylactic mastectomies
    - Excision of the lesion is recommended to rule out invasion, but negative margins are not required
    - Lymph node evaluation not required for pure LCIS without invasion
- Invasive breast cancer
  - Local control of disease in the breast
    - Removal of the tumor
      - Modified radical mastectomy (MRM) involves removal of the breast and draining axillary lymph nodes, sparing the musculature of the chest wall
      - Lumpectomy involves removal of tumor with the goal of attaining pathologically negative margins and requires RT for optimal control; contraindicated in patients who are pregnant, have a history of prior radiation to the breast, have evidence of diffuse breast calcifications, have certain connective tissue disorders, or have more than one distinct tumor
    - Pathologic evaluation of the regional lymph nodes can be done by sentinel lymph node biopsy. Complete axillary lymph node dissection for a positive sentinel node is now not always required, but is done if the information will affect chemotherapy or RT recommendations.
    - RT is used after lumpectomy and for selected node-positive patients after mastectomy
    - Choosing between lumpectomy plus RT and MRM
      - **Survival is equivalent**
      - Most patients (>80%) are good candidates for lumpectomy plus RT; patient preference is a critical element
      - In patients with large tumors, large breast size, or tumors under the nipple, mastectomy may be preferable because of poor cosmetic outcome with lumpectomy
      - Approximately 9% risk of local recurrence in the conserved breast with lumpectomy plus RT (0.5–1% per year)
      - Local recurrences after lumpectomy can be salvaged with MRM
  - Staging (Box 53-2)
  - Poor prognostic factors
    - Larger tumor size
    - Axillary lymph node metastases
    - Absent estrogen/progesterone receptor (ER/PR)

- Poor nuclear grade
- Elevated measures of proliferation (S-phase fraction, Ki67)
- Molecular markers such as *Her-2/neu* are increasingly used to aid in prognosis and to direct treatment
  - **Tumors that have negative ER, PR, and *Her-2/neu* carry an especially poor prognosis and are referred to as "triple-negative" breast cancer**
- Adjuvant systemic therapy
  - Even though 90% of women present with apparently localized disease (i.e., breast and regional lymph nodes), only about 70% will be free of disease 5 years later, despite adequate local therapy
  - **Adjuvant therapy is given when no disease is apparent, with the goal of eradicating potential micrometastatic disease and thereby reducing the risk of relapse**
  - Important factors to keep in mind with regard to adjuvant therapy:
    - The higher the risk of relapse, the greater the absolute reduction in the risk of relapse with adjuvant therapy
    - The choice of the type of adjuvant therapy is based on patient factors (age, comorbidities, and menopausal status) and on disease factors (nodal status, hormone receptor status [ER/PR], and *Her-2/neu* status) (Table 53-3)

- In certain clinical situations a genetic profile of the tumor (e.g., oncotype DX) can aid in predicting relapse risk and determining the benefit of adding chemotherapy
- Types of adjuvant therapy (hormone therapy, chemotherapy, antibody therapy)
  - Hormonal therapy
    - Used when the tumor expresses ER, PR, or both
    - The highest response rates seen when both receptors expressed
    - Response rate negligible when neither receptor expressed
    - Generally recommended for 5 years; sequential use of different agents may extend duration of therapy
  - Postmenopausal patients
    - Aromatase inhibitors (e.g., anastrozole, letrozole, exemestane)—prevent conversion of androgens to estrogen, thereby suppressing plasma estrogen levels
    - Tamoxifen: Mixed ER antagonist/agonist (Box 53-3)
  - Premenopausal patients
    - Tamoxifen: Mixed ER antagonist/agonist (see Box 53-3)
    - Inhibition of the pituitary-hypothalamic-gonadal axis with gonadotropin-releasing hormone analogues (goserelin, leuprolide acetate)
    - Surgical removal of the ovaries
    - Radiation of the ovaries (rarely used in the United States)

BOX 53-2 | *Simplified Staging Schema for Invasive Breast Cancer*

Stage I: Small primary tumor (≤2 cm), negative nodes, no distant metastases

Stage II: Involved axillary lymph nodes *or* large primary tumor (>2 cm), no distant metastases

Stage III: Locally advanced disease
Large tumor and involved nodes
Matted or fixed axillary nodes
Tumor with direct extension to the skin or chest wall
Inflammatory breast cancer: Redness, warmth, peau d'orange skin changes

Stage IV: Distant metastases; common sites (in order of frequency) are bone, lung, liver, adrenals, and brain/cerebrospinal fluid

---

BOX 53-3 | *Tamoxifen Therapy for Breast Disease*

It is a nonsteroidal antiestrogen when acting on breast tissue

It binds to the estrogen receptor protein and competitively inhibits estrogen action in breast and breast tumors

In some tissues, it acts as a partial estrogen agonist
Uterus: Estrogenic activity of tamoxifen increases endometrial cancer risk (increase of 1–2:1000)
Bone: Increases bone density and delays bone loss
Cardiovascular: Lowers low-density lipoprotein and total cholesterol

Side effects
Hot flashes and other vasomotor symptoms
Weight gain
Thromboembolic disease (rare)
Increased risk of endometrial cancer (rare)
Keratopathy and optic neuritis (very rare)

TABLE 53-3 | *Adjuvant Therapy Options for Breast Cancer*

	Node-Negative	Node-Positive	Node-Positive and *Her-2* Positive
Premenopausal			
Estrogen receptor–positive	Hormone therapy ± chemotherapy	Chemotherapy + hormone therapy	Chemotherapy + trastuzumab + hormone therapy
Estrogen receptor–negative	Chemotherapy	Chemotherapy	Chemotherapy + trastuzumab
Postmenopausal			
Estrogen receptor–positive	Hormone therapy	Hormone therapy ± chemotherapy	Chemotherapy + trastuzumab + hormone therapy
Estrogen receptor–negative	Chemotherapy	Chemotherapy	Chemotherapy + trastuzumab

- The toxic effect of chemotherapy drugs on ovarian follicular cells frequently results in cessation of menses. The closer a woman is to natural menopause, the more likely that amenorrhea will be permanent.
- Chemotherapy
  - Considered for tumors that are more than 1 cm in size and occasionally for smaller, aggressive tumors
  - **Shown to increase survival for women younger than 70 years regardless of node or receptor status**
  - The effects of chemotherapy are additive with hormonal therapy when used sequentially. However, they may have antagonistic effects when used together.
  - Breast cancer is responsive to a variety of cytotoxic chemotherapeutic agents, including anthracyclines (doxorubicin, epirubicin), microtubule inhibitors (taxanes [paclitaxel, docetaxel], ixabepilone), alkylating agents (cyclophosphamide), antimetabolites (5-fluorouracil, capecitabine, gemcitabine), and mitotic inhibitors (eribulin, vinorelbine)
  - Combination multiagent chemotherapy for 3 to 6 months standard
- Trastuzumab (Herceptin)
  - *HER-2/neu* proto-oncogene is overexpressed in 20% to 30% of human breast cancers
  - Cell surface localization of *HER-2/neu* allows for immunotherapeutic targeting
  - Trastuzumab: Recombinant humanized anti–*HER-2* monoclonal antibody
    - Synergistic cardiac toxicity when used with doxorubicin
    - Single-agent activity in *HER-2/neu* overexpressing breast cancer
    - At least additive effects in combination with chemotherapeutic agents
    - **Significantly improves survival when used with adjuvant chemotherapy in patients with *Her-2*–overexpressing tumors**
- Follow-up after diagnosis and treatment of localized breast cancer
  - Regular history and physical examination
  - Standard blood work: complete blood count, calcium, and liver function testing
  - Yearly mammography; every 6 months for 3 years in involved breast after lumpectomy plus RT
  - Computed tomography (CT), nuclear scanning, and tumor markers should not be routinely employed unless specific symptoms or exam findings dictate their use
- Advanced or recurrent disease
  - Treatment goals for the patient with disseminated breast cancer are to prolong life, improve the quality of life, and palliate symptoms
  - Treatment of advanced disease depends on several factors, including prior therapy, time from diagnosis, sites of metastases, hormone receptor status, and *Her-2/neu* status
  - Two thirds of metastatic breast cancer patients respond to chemotherapy
  - Quality of life is improved for some advanced breast cancer patients receiving chemotherapy

- Response rates are higher for patients who have received no prior chemotherapy or who have had a long treatment-free interval since prior chemotherapy
- Patients with lytic bone metastases have decreased skeletal morbidity (pain and fractures) with the use of IV bisphosphonate therapy

Breast Cancer Prevention

- Bilateral mastectomy prevents greater than 95% of breast cancers. Some breast tissue remains on the chest wall, which is why prevention is not 100%. Preventive mastectomy has significant cosmetic, psychological, social, and sexual impact and is usually reserved for those at highest risk.
- Hormonal chemoprevention
  - Tamoxifen, raloxifene, and the aromatase inhibitor exemestane have each been shown to reduce the risk of breast cancer in women at increased risk
  - These drugs all have side effects that may be relative contraindications to treatment or may not be tolerated in the prevention setting
  - Raloxifene and exemestane can only be used in postmenopausal women

Epithelial Ovarian Cancer

Basic Information

- Cancers that arise from the epithelium of the ovary (not germ cell or stromal tumors)
- Fourth leading cause of cancer deaths in American women
- **High mortality because of difficulty in diagnosing localized (early-stage) disease**
- Risk factors
  - Clear-cut cause has not been established for most cases of ovarian cancer
  - Family history
    - Risk of ovarian cancer significantly increased in patients with a familial predisposition (Table 53-4)
    - Patients with *BRCA1* mutations appear to have ovarian cancer onset about 10 years earlier (median age 54 years) than patients with *BRCA2* mutations or sporadic ovarian cancer (64 years)
    - Three inherited genetic mutations currently are associated with an increased risk of ovarian cancer
      - *BRCA1* is associated with a lifetime risk of 14% to 45%
      - *BRCA2* is associated with a lifetime risk of 10% to 20%

TABLE 53-4	*Familial Risk of Ovarian Cancer**	
Relationship	**Risk**
One second-degree relative	1:25 (4%)
One first-degree relative (any age)	1:20 (5%)
Age <55 yr	1:10 (10%)
Age <45 yr	1:5 (20%)
Two first-degree relatives	1:2 (50%)

*Familial ovarian cancer accounts for only 5–10% of all cases.

53

- Lynch syndrome (aka hereditary nonpolyposis colorectal cancer, or familial cancer syndrome) associated with increased risk of GI, ovarian, and endometrial cancers (see Chapter 52)
- Direct relationship between number of lifetime ovulations and the risk of ovarian cancer
  - Ovulation causes injury to the epithelial surface of the ovary
  - Repeated injury or the process of repairing injury may contribute to malignant transformation
  - **Conditions that cause a relative increase in the number of ovulations (e.g., early menarche, late menopause, and infertility) associated with an increased risk of ovarian cancer**
  - Conditions that cause a relative decrease in the number of ovulations (e.g., oral contraceptive use, multiple pregnancies, early pregnancy, and breast-feeding for more than a year) associated with a decreased risk of ovarian cancer
  - Recent studies have implicated fallopian tube cells as the cells of origin for many ovarian and peritoneal cancers
- Risk reduction for high-risk patients
  - Oral contraceptives can reduce the risk by more than 50% when used for over 5 years
  - Bilateral salpingo-oophorectomy
    - The degree of risk reduction is estimated to be 90% to 95%
    - Risk of peritoneal cancer remains and is not reduced by removal of the ovaries
    - Oophorectomy results in premature menopause for menstruating women and reduces the risk of breast cancer in these women, but may result in vasomotor symptoms and an increased risk of heart disease and osteoporosis
    - Premenopausal *BRCA* mutation carriers who have undergone prophylactic oophorectomy frequently receive low-dose, short-term hormone replacement therapy to manage hormone withdrawal symptoms without apparent excess risk of breast cancer
  - Close surveillance and screening
- Screening
  - **No ovarian cancer screening techniques have sufficient sensitivity, specificity, or cost-effectiveness to routinely recommend their use for the general population**
  - Screening (with transvaginal ultrasound or cancer antigen 125 [CA 125]) is commonly used in women at high risk for ovarian cancer based on personal or family history

Clinical Presentation

- Specific symptoms are uncommon when disease localized to the ovary
- Symptoms of advanced disease are vague and are nonspecific for ovarian cancer but are usually present
  - Abdominal fullness or bloating
  - Pelvic heaviness or pressure
  - Pain with intercourse
  - Vaginal bleeding or discharge
  - GI symptoms such as lack of appetite, nausea, vomiting, constipation

- Tumor spread can occur by a number of different mechanisms (in order of decreasing frequency):
  - Local shedding of tumor cells into the peritoneal cavity followed by implantation on the peritoneal surfaces
  - Lymphatic spread to local or distant lymph nodes
  - Hematogenous spread to distant sites (parenchyma of liver, lungs, pleura)
  - Local invasion of bowel or bladder

Diagnosis

- Not commonly diagnosed by pelvic examination
- Can be found incidentally on ultrasound or CT scan
- Surgical laparotomy necessary for diagnosis, staging, and tumor debulking but laparoscopy and robotic surgery are increasing in use
- CA 125 tumor marker
  - CA 125 common to most ovarian tumors
  - **82% of advanced ovarian cancer patients have an elevated CA 125, but less than 50% with stage I disease show an elevation**
  - Rising or falling titers correlate with disease in 93% of patients, making it a useful tool for monitoring disease
  - Persistent elevation of CA 125 after treatment strongly associated with residual disease
  - Doubling or an absolute value greater than 100 usually indicates recurrence
  - Even though an elevation of CA 125 may antedate appearance of disease or recurrence, it is not a useful screening tool in unaffected women because of its lack of sensitivity and specificity

Treatment

- Surgery
  - **Aggressive tumor debulking is usually indicated even in advanced disease**
  - Volume of tumor after surgery and before chemotherapy is a major prognostic factor for survival
    - After surgical debulking, patients categorized as
      - Optimally debulked (≤1 cm postoperative residual disease)
      - Suboptimally debulked (>1 cm postoperative residual disease)
- Staging: see Box 53-4
- Chemotherapy
  - Chemotherapy is not used in borderline, low malignant potential, or atypical proliferating tumors
  - Use of chemotherapy for stage I invasive ovarian cancer based on risk

BOX 53-4	*Simplified Staging Schema for Ovarian Cancer*

Stage I: Disease limited to the ovaries: 5-year survival, 80–90%

Stage II: Disease confined to the pelvis: 5-year survival, 60–70%

Stage III: Disease spread to upper abdomen or regional lymph nodes: 5-year survival, 15–30%

Stage IV: Distant metastases (liver parenchyma, lung, pleura): 5-year survival, 5–10%

- Patients with well-differentiated stage I tumors have a 5-year disease-free survival rate of over 90% and do not benefit from chemotherapy
- Chemotherapy justified for patients with high-grade stage I tumors, tumors involving the surface of the ovary, or when there is ascites or positive peritoneal washings
  - Postoperative, platinum-based chemotherapy, usually in combination with a taxane
  - Three to six courses standard
- Stage II, III, or IV disease
  - All patients receive systemic, platinum-based chemotherapy
  - Usually receive six courses of treatment
  - Combination of a taxane (paclitaxel or docetaxel) plus platinum (carboplatin or cisplatin) standard
  - Intraperitoneal administration of chemotherapy improves survival in selected low-volume patients
  - Small percentage of patients (10–15%) will be cured
  - The addition of bevacizumab (antibody to vascular endothelial growth factor) to chemotherapy improves progression-free survival (prolongs time to recurrence) but does not improve overall survival

- Recurrent ovarian cancer
  - High rate of response to therapy but is generally not curable
  - Noncurative treatment can prolong life
  - Number of chemotherapeutic options available

REVIEW QUESTIONS

For review questions, please go to www.expertconsult.com.

SUGGESTED READINGS

Clarke-Pearson DL: Screening for ovarian cancer, *N Engl J Med* 361:170–177, 2009.

Goss PE, Ingle JN, Alés-Martínez JE, et al: Exemestane for breast-cancer prevention in postmenopausal women, *N Engl J Med* 364:2381–2391, 2011.

Gradishar WJ: Safety considerations of adjuvant therapy in early breast cancer in postmenopausal women, *Oncology* 69:1–9, 2005.

Jelovac D, Armstrong DK: Recent progress in the diagnosis and treatment of ovarian cancer, *CA Cancer J Clin* 61:183–203, 2011.

Kuhl CK, Schrading S, Leutner CC, et al: Mammography, breast ultrasound, and magnetic resonance imaging for surveillance of women at high familial risk for breast cancer, *J Clin Oncol* 23:8469–8476, 2005.

Perez EA, Romond EH, Suman VJ, et al: Four-year follow-up of trastuzumab plus adjuvant chemotherapy for operable human epidermal growth factor receptor 2-positive breast cancer: joint analysis of data from NCCTG N9831 and NSABP B-31, *J Clin Oncol* 29:3366–3373, 2011.

53

Genitourinary Cancer

MICHAEL A. CARDUCCI, MD; and HANS HAMMERS, MD, PhD

Cancers of the genitourinary system are commonly seen in the United States and result in significant morbidity and mortality. Neoplasms of the prostate and testicle are the leading causes of cancer in elderly and young men, respectively. This chapter describes the clinical features of these two cancers, as well as cancers of the bladder and kidney.

Prostate Cancer

Incidence

- Most common cancer for men in the United States
- **One in 6 lifetime risk for a man to develop invasive prostate cancer**
- For 2010, it is estimated that 217,730 new cases were diagnosed, and 32,050 deaths were attributed to this disease. Second most common cause of cancer death in men after lung cancer.

Epidemiology

- The Japanese and mainland Chinese have the lowest rates of invasive prostate cancer
- Incidence of prostate cancer is highest in Scandinavian countries
- Socioeconomic status appears unrelated to risk
- Risk may be inversely related to ultraviolet light exposure (vitamin D) because the incidence increases the farther one lives from the equator

Etiology and Risk Factors

- **Age: Autopsy studies suggest that nearly 60% of men will have prostate cancer by age 80**
- Family history: Men with a first-degree relative with prostate cancer have a twofold increased risk; an individual with two first-degree relatives with prostate cancer has a ninefold increased risk; hereditary prostate cancer may account for 5% to 10% of all prostate cancers and tends to develop at a very early age (<55 years)
- Race: African Americans have a 9.8% lifetime risk
- Intake of dietary fat may increase the risk of prostate cancer
- Vasectomy, sexual activity, and sexually transmitted disease are not associated with an increased risk of prostate cancer. Some studies have shown a lower risk of prostate cancer with a higher frequency of ejaculation.

Signs and Symptoms

- Early-stage disease
  - **Most are asymptomatic**
  - Some present with bladder outlet obstruction

- Locally advanced disease
  - Bladder outlet obstruction causing urinary frequency, urgency, irritative voiding symptoms, hematuria, or urinary tract infections most commonly seen
  - Extension to seminal vesicles may manifest with hematospermia
  - Extension to the periphery of the gland and involvement of the neurovascular bundles may manifest as impotence or erectile dysfunction
- Advanced disease
  - Bulky lymph node metastasis can manifest with bilateral lower extremity edema
  - **Men with bony metastasis may have bone pain or lower extremity weakness or paralysis from spinal cord compression**

Screening and Diagnosis

- If prostate cancer is detected early, treatment can be effective and result in minimal morbidity
- No universally agreed-on strategic plan for its diagnosis and management
- Digital rectal examination (DRE)
  - 7% to 15% of men older than 50 years will have suggestive results on DRE
  - Positive predictive value of DRE for prostate cancer is 15% to 30%, and varies little with age
  - DRE has 1% to 2% detection rate when used alone
  - **A normal DRE does not reduce the odds of clinically significant prostate cancer**
- Prostate-specific antigen (PSA)
  - Serine protease specific to prostate tissue, not just cancer
  - **Can be elevated from benign prostatic hypertrophy, acute prostatitis, transrectal needle biopsy, acute urinary retention, prostate surgery, and ejaculation**
  - In general, DRE does not increase serum PSA
  - PSA doubles the detection rate of DRE
  - It detects nearly 70% of prostate cancer cases
  - PSA and DRE are complementary as screening tests for prostate cancer
  - PSA levels greater than 4 ng/mL are seen in 15% of men older than 50 years; the probability that this PSA level indicates cancer is 20% to 30%
  - In recent Prostate Cancer Prevention Study, 16% of men diagnosed with prostate cancer had a PSA below 1 ng/mL
  - **Most men with PSA greater than 10 ng/mL, and Gleason grade 7 or greater, are found to have extracapsular disease that is much less likely to be curable**

- PSA rise of more than 2 ng/mL in year prior to diagnosis is associated with high-risk disease
- American Cancer Society screening recommendations
  - Annual examination with DRE and PSA beginning at age 50 years in patients with an anticipated survival of 10 years
  - Begin earlier (age 40 years) in high-risk groups (e.g., African American men, those men with a positive family history)
- American College of Physicians recommends that the decision to screen be individualized after discussion with the patient
- The U.S. Preventive Services Task Force (USPSTF) recently concluded that current evidence is insufficient to assess the balance of benefits and harms of prostate cancer screening in men younger than age 75 years. The USPSTF recommends against screening for prostate cancer in men age 75 years or older.
- Transrectal biopsy
  - Should be done only in those patients who would require therapy, either definitive or palliative
  - Men with PSA values greater than 4 ng/mL or an abnormal DRE suggestive of prostate cancer should consider prostate biopsy. Age-specific thresholds and rate of rise within the normal range may be reason to consider biopsy in younger or high-risk men.
  - Side effects of the transrectal biopsy include hematuria, hematochezia, and hematospermia
  - **If the biopsy specimen is negative, the patient should be followed conservatively with serial PSAs and DREs.** Consideration for an earlier repeat biopsy depends on the number of cores taken initially and the pretest likelihood of finding cancer.

Pathology

- Adenocarcinomas make up the vast majority of tumors, although ductal adenocarcinoma, transitional cell carcinoma, and small-cell neuroendocrine tumors can occur
- Most (70%) occur in the peripheral zone of the gland; only 10% occur in the area surrounding the prostatic urethra
- Histologic grade is summarized using the Gleason system
  - Based on architectural patterns of the tumor
  - A score for each cancer based on the sum of the grade assigned to the most predominant (1–5) and secondary (1–5) architectural patterns (Fig. 54-1)
  - Gleason grades 2 to 6 are associated with a better prognosis
  - **The risk of developing metastatic disease with a Gleason grade of 8 to 10 is about 43% (17–81%)**
- Adenocarcinoma may spread locally to periprostatic fat, seminal vesicles, and regional lymph nodes; hematogenous spread is predominantly to bone, particularly the lumbosacral spine and the axial skeleton

Staging and Prognosis

- Prognosis depends on tumor stage, Gleason score, and pretreatment PSA value
- Table 54-1 summarizes the basic staging for prostate cancer

- **In general, cure is anticipated for men with organ-confined disease and local treatments.** Men with recurrence despite local treatment can have a long survival. Median survival for men with PSA recurrence after local therapy is 13 to 15 years. Median survival for men presenting with metastatic disease approaches 7 years.

Treatment

- Needs to be individualized; decisions are based on the disease stage and grade, on pretreatment PSA, and on the patient's age and life expectancy
- Physiologic age is of greater importance than chronologic age
- **Patients with short life expectancy (<10 years) should probably be observed because there is little evidence to support a prolonged life expectancy with interventions**
- Localized disease (stages A and B): Radical prostatectomy and radiation therapy are clearly effective forms of treatment in the attempt to cure tumors limited to the prostate for appropriately selected patients; comparisons across studies suggest comparable 10-year survival rates with either form of management
- Locally advanced disease (stage C): Improved survival may be seen with androgen deprivation (see following discussion) plus radiation
- Advanced disease: First-line therapies include surgical or medical castration (androgen deprivation)
  - Advanced symptomatic or metastatic disease requires medical or surgical castration. Men with PSA recurrence after local therapy have a high likelihood of micrometastatic disease. Use of androgen ablation in the absence of clinically evident or radiographically evident metastasis is commonplace, although this approach has not been clearly shown to improve survival.
  - Androgen ablation is effective in 80% to 90% of patients, with an average duration of response of 18 to 24 months
  - Surgical castration (bilateral orchiectomy) removes testicular androgens. It is a safe and inexpensive procedure that ensures patient compliance; however, the psychological impact can be severe.
  - Medical castration is primarily in the form of luteinizing hormone–releasing hormone agonists. These regulate the release of luteinizing hormone, thereby producing chemical castration by ultimately decreasing testosterone levels.
  - **Androgen ablation is associated with significant hot flashes, sexual dysfunction (e.g., loss of libido, erectile dysfunction, and microgenitalia), decreases in bone and muscle mass, gynecomastia, fatigue, anemia, and metabolic syndrome, as well as neurocognitive effects. Use of early androgen ablation for men with PSA recurrence and no radiographic metastasis potentially exposes men to these negative aspects of hormonal therapy without known survival benefit.**
  - Second-line hormonal therapies include the addition and subtraction of antiandrogens, ketoconazole, or estrogens such as diethylstilbestrol. Antiandrogens (e.g., flutamide, nilutamide, bicalutamide) block the

54

FIGURE 54-1 Gleason scoring system for grading of adenocarcinoma of the prostate. **A,** Schematic of the system. **B** to **F,** Histologic sections showing Gleason patterns 1 through 5, respectively. *(From Walsh PC: Campbell's urology, ed 8, Philadelphia, WB Saunders, 2002, Fig. 86.2.)*

TABLE 54-1	Simplified Staging System for Prostate Cancer
Stage	**Description**
A	Incidental finding of localized tumor
B	Tumor confined within the prostate capsule
C	Extracapsular disease
D	Disseminated disease to lymph nodes or distant sites

effects of androgens at the prostate tissue level by interfering with receptor binding of active androgens. Some experts suggest the addition of antiandrogens to either medical or surgical castration. 17-Lyase inhibitors such as abiraterone, which are similar in their action to ketoconazole, either are in clinical development or are awaiting Food and Drug Administration (FDA) approval.

- Antiandrogens are reported to act as agonists in up to 25% of treated men. In these cases, the removal of the antiandrogen may be associated with a clinical response and is recommended for men with a rising PSA or progressive disease while on an antiandrogen.
- Disease progression (rising PSA, new lesions, or new symptoms) while on androgen ablation (castrate levels of testosterone) defines castration-resistant disease
- Docetaxel and predisone in combination is FDA-approved for men with metastatic castration-resistant prostate cancer based on randomized, Phase III clinical trials demonstrating an improvement in overall survival. Median survival for men receiving docetaxel approximates 19 months.
- Cabazitaxel in combination with prednisone has recently been approved for patients with metastatic castration-resistant prostate cancer who progressed after prior treatment with docetaxel. Cabazitaxel/prednisone improved median survival by 2.5 months (15.1) when compared to mitoxantrone/prednisone.
- Sipuleucel-T has been approved by the FDA as an autologous cellular immunotherapy for the treatment of asymptomatic or minimally symptomatic metastatic castration-resistant prostate cancer. Sipuleucel-T improved median survival by 4 months (25.8) when compared to placebo.
- Radiopharmaceuticals (strontium-89 and samarium) may be beneficial for men with symptomatic metastatic hormone-refractory cancer. External beam radiation remains an important method to improve pain and reduce fracture at isolated painful bone metastasis.
- Abiraterone in combination with prednisone has shown a median 4.5 month improvement in survival over prednisone alone in men with castration-resistant prostate cancer and prior treatment with chemotherapy, primarily docetaxel-based.
- The bisphosphonate zolendronic acid is FDA-approved to reduce skeletal-related events (fractures, cord compression) in men with metastatic hormone-refractory prostate cancer. Increases in creatinine and osteonecrosis of the jaw are concerns associated with long-term use of this bisphosphonate. Denosumab, an antibody against RANK ligand (RANKL, an osteoclast survival factor), has recently been shown to improve time to the first skeletal-related event when compared to zoledronic acid in prostate cancer patients and has been FDA approved. Like zoledronic acid, it can cause osteonecrosis of the jaw.

Urothelial (Bladder, Ureteral, and Renal Pelvis) Cancer

Incidence

- In 2010, an estimated 70,530 cases were diagnosed and 14,680 deaths were attributed to cancer of the bladder
- Bladder cancer is much more common than ureteral cancer or cancer of the renal pelvis
- When cancer of the upper urinary tract is diagnosed, there is a 30% to 50% chance of cancer of the bladder developing
- When bladder cancer is diagnosed, there is a 2% to 3% chance of developing cancer of upper urinary tract

Epidemiology

- More common in men (3:1); incidence in women increasing secondary to tobacco use
- Peak incidence in the seventh decade of life
- More common in whites than in African Americans

Etiology and Risk Factors

- **Cigarette smoking**
- Analgesic abuse, phenacetin use
- Chronic urinary tract inflammation (stones in upper tract, recurrent infections)
- Occupational exposures (exposure to aryl amines in organic chemicals, rubber, paint, and dyes)
- Balkan nephropathy: A familial nephropathy of unknown cause that results in progressive inflammation of the renal parenchyma, leading to renal failure and multifocal, superficial, low-grade cancers of the renal pelvis and ureters
- *Schistosoma haematobium* infection usually associated with squamous cell carcinoma of the bladder

Signs and Symptoms

- Hematuria: Often painless
- Urinary voiding symptoms (e.g., frequency, urgency, or dysuria)
- Vesical irritation without hematuria: Common in carcinoma *in situ* of bladder
- Symptoms of advanced disease: Pain from metastatic sites, edema of lower extremities, cough or dyspnea from lung metastases

Diagnosis

- **Excretory urography/intravenous pyelogram (Fig. 54-2) followed by cystoscopy**
- Retrograde pyelography is best for detecting upper tract lesions
- Urine cytology may be helpful; brush biopsies may increase the diagnostic yield

FIGURE 54-2 **A** and **B**, Excretory urography in a patient with a bladder tumor. Note the filling defect in the right inferior portion of the bladder. *(From Bragg DG, Rubin P, Hricak H: Oncologic imaging, ed 2, Philadelphia, WB Saunders, 2002, Fig. 30-1.)*

- Biopsies of any lesion must be of adequate size to include bladder wall muscle
- Computed tomography (CT) scan of abdomen: Evaluate for local extension and nodal involvement
- Obtain bone scan if bony symptoms are present
- Chest radiograph completes staging evaluation

Pathology

- Transitional cell carcinoma: 90% to 95% of all urothelial cancers
  - Superficial lesions most commonly low-grade papillary lesions that rarely become invasive
  - Carcinoma *in situ* (CIS)
    - Often accompanies higher stages of disease
    - Has high likelihood of progressing to muscle-invasive disease
- Squamous cell carcinoma: 3% to 7% of urothelial cancers, mostly renal pelvis and ureters
- Adenocarcinomas: Less than 3% of urothelial cancers; those arising from the dome of the bladder are urachal in origin

Staging and Prognosis

- Most important prognostic factors are T stage (Table 54-2) and differentiation pattern
- Superficial bladder cancer: Papillary tumors that involve only the mucosa (Ta) or submucosa (T1) and flat carcinoma *in situ* (Tis) (Note: This is different from CIS)
  - Natural history is unpredictable; recurrences are very common
  - Most superficial tumors recur within 6 to 12 months and are the same stage and grade
  - 10% to 15% of superficial cancers develop into invasive or metastatic disease
  - Well-differentiated lesions have a 95% survival rate, whereas high-grade (less differentiated) T1 lesions have a 10-year survival of 50%
- Muscle invasive carcinoma (T2) carries a 5-year survival of 20% to 50%; with regional node involvement and metastatic disease (stage IV), the 5-year survival is 0% to 20%

Treatment

- Localized disease
  - Superficial bladder cancer

TABLE 54-2	*Simplified Staging System for Bladder Cancer*
Stage	**Description**
Tis, Ta	Noninvasive (superficial) carcinoma
T1	Tumor invades lamina propria
T2	Tumor invades muscle
T3	Tumor invades through muscle into perivesicular fat
T4	Invasion of other structures/organs

  - Surgical approaches
    - Transurethral resection: Removes existing tumor; patients require close follow-up
    - Laser: Not adopted for general use because of limitations of obtaining stage and grade
    - Partial cystectomy: If tumor not accessible or amenable to transurethral resection
    - **Radical cystectomy: Generally not used for superficial bladder cancer; indications are unusually large tumors, some high-grade tumors, multiple tumors or frequent recurrences, symptomatic diffuse CIS, prostatic stromal involvement**
  - Intravesical therapy
    - Indications are: Stage T1 tumors, multifocal papillary Ta lesions, rapidly recurring superficial disease
    - Agents used: Bacille Calmette-Guérin (BCG), thiotepa, or mitomycin; BCG has the greatest efficacy
- Invasive bladder cancer
  - Surgical approaches
    - Radical cystectomy is the gold standard; indicated in patients with muscle-invasive tumors (regardless of grade), diffuse CIS, or recurrent superficial cancers not responding to intravesical therapy
    - Patients can undergo urinary reconstruction with intestinal conduits, continent cutaneous diversions, or orthotopic reconstruction

- Surgical approaches to ureteral and renal pelvic tumors: Nephroureterectomy with resection of cuff of bladder
- Role of radiation therapy
  - Therapy of choice for patients with clinical condition precluding surgery
  - Addition of chemotherapy as radiosensitizing agent of benefit if patient can tolerate chemotherapy
  - Palliative radiation therapy is quite effective in controlling pain from local or metastatic disease
- Treatment of advanced disease is palliative; cisplatin-based regimens are commonly used; gemcitabine and paclitaxel appear most active as single agents and in combination with cisplatin/carboplatin. Median survival is 14 to 20 months depending on prognostic factors, such as performance status, sites of metastasis, and laboratory measures.

Renal Cell Carcinoma

Incidence

- Estimated new cases in 2010 were 58,240 (increasing in incidence)
- Estimated deaths in 2010 were 13,040

Epidemiology

- Twice as common in men as in women
- **Most cases diagnosed in fourth to sixth decades of life**
- More common in persons of northern European ancestry

Etiology and Risk Factors

- Sporadic form
  - Etiology unclear
  - Associated with smoking, obesity, and renal dialysis
  - Sporadic renal cell carcinomas of the clear cell type are associated with deletions or hypermethylation on chromosome 3 (location of Von Hippel-Lindau gene)
- Familial form
  - **Von Hippel-Lindau disease: Autosomal dominant disease, deletions of short arm on chromosome 3; associated with retinal angiomas, central nervous system hemangioblastomas, and renal cell carcinomas (sometimes bilateral); carries the same prognosis as sporadic disease**
- Signs and symptoms
  - Classic triad of hematuria, flank mass, and flank pain occurs in only 10% of patients and is associated with a poor prognosis
  - Hematuria: More than 50% of patients describe hematuria
  - Normocytic, normochromic anemia, fever, and weight loss are other common manifestations
  - Less common manifestations: Paraneoplastic syndromes (polycythemia from excess erythropoietin production, thrombocytosis from increased interleukin [IL]-6, hypercalcemia from release of parathyroid hormone–related peptide), hepatic dysfunction not associated with metastases (Stauffer syndrome)
  - **Varicocele: If acute in onset, right sided, or does not decrease in size in the supine position, consider renal cell carcinoma with obstruction of the venous system**

TABLE 54-3	Simplified Staging System for Renal Cell Carcinoma

Stage	Description
I	Tumor ≤7 cm and limited to kidney
II	Tumor >7 cm and limited to kidney
III	Tumor extension outside of kidney but within Gerota's fascia or one regional lymph node involved
IV	Tumor extends beyond Gerota's fascia or more than one regional lymph node involved or distant metastasis

- With wide use of CT and ultrasound, renal cell cancer is being diagnosed more commonly as an incidental finding

Diagnosis

- **Standard evaluation includes CT scan of abdomen and pelvis, chest radiograph, urinalysis, urine cytology**
- Contrast-enhanced CT scan differentiates solid from cystic masses; supplies information on nodal or renal vein or inferior vena cava (IVC) involvement
- Venography or magnetic resonance imaging: Best test to look at IVC involvement
- Evaluation of extra-abdominal disease: Bone scan if symptoms suggestive; CT of chest if plain film suggestive of metastasis

Pathology

- Tumor cells arise from proximal renal tubular epithelium
- Histologic cell types include clear cell, papillary, and chromophobe
- **Clear cell carcinomas are the most common**
- Sarcomatoid variants are more aggressive and associated with a worse prognosis

Staging and Prognosis

- Staging based on tumor size and extension from the kidney (Table 54-3)
- Approximately 30% of patients have metastatic disease at diagnosis
- Five-year survival rates for tumors confined to the kidney are greater than 80%; renal vein involvement does not affect survival
- Prior to the introduction of approved targeted therapies, patients with metastatic disease had a median 1-year survival rate of 0% to 20%. Survival is improving for patients with metastatic disease.

Treatment

- Surgery
  - Radical nephrectomy is the established therapy for localized disease. Partial, nephron-sparing nephrectomy should be performed when possible
  - **In the presence of metastatic disease, nephrectomy should be considered to debulk the primary tumor and is associated with a 4-month improvement in survival.** Not all patients are surgical

54

candidates, or the burden of metastatic disease may be too great and the nephrectomy may delay other systemic therapies.
- Radiation therapy to metastatic sites may provide benefit
  - Most commonly used for palliation of bony metastasis
- Systemic therapy of advanced disease
  - Metastatic renal cell carcinoma is relatively resistant to chemotherapeutic agents, although chemotherapy agents such as gemcitabine and capecitabine are used rarely in select patients
  - Immunotherapy and tyrosine kinase inhibitors are the most common approach to therapy
  - Patients with best response to immunotherapy are those with excellent performance status, lung-only disease, history of nephrectomy, nephrectomy longer than 1 year from treatment, and a long interval history from diagnosis to recurrence and need for treatment
  - IL-2 is FDA-approved treatment for metastatic renal cell carcinoma
    - Response rates range from 15% to 30% (8% are complete, durable responses)
    - Major toxicity is sepsis-like syndrome
  - Interferon-alfa had been used commonly in the past, but has been surpassed by newer targeted agents
    - Response rate as a single agent ranges from 15% to 20%
    - Responses are often short lived, but there is some suggestion of improved survival in interferon-treated patients
    - The combination of interferon and bevacizumab improves progression-free survival over interferon alone by approximately 6 months. The combination of bevacizumab and interferon has been approved by the FDA for previously untreated patients but is used infrequently in the United States.
  - Targeting vascular endothelial growth factor and its tyrosine kinase receptors has demonstrated clinical benefit. Sunitinib, pazopanib, and sorafenib are FDA-approved for advanced renal cancer.
    - Sorafenib, a multitargeted tyrosine kinase, has been approved for advanced metastatic disease based on randomized data demonstrating a 12-week improvement in time to disease progression for sorafenib over placebo in cytokine-pretreated patients. The overall response rate for sorafenib is reported at 2%.
    - Sunitinib, a multitargeted kinase inhibitor, has been approved for advanced metastatic disease. Survival of patients receiving sunitinib for first-line metastatic disease approaches 28 months.
    - Pazopanib, another multitargeted kinase inhibitor, has been approved for metastatic disease, with response rates reported as 30%. Progression-free survival for cytokine-naïve patients was approximately 11 months.
    - Common side effects of these agents include hypertension, hand-foot syndrome, and fatigue. Other potential side effects are a decrease in the cardiac ejection fraction (sunitinib), liver toxicity, and hypothyroidism.

- Temsirolimus and everolimus are mammalian target of rapamycin (mTOR) inhibitors, and both are FDA-approved. Temsirolimus demonstrated a 3-month improvement in survival over interferon alone in patients with metastatic renal cell cancer and poor risk features. Everolimus demonstrated a 3-month improvement in progression-free survival over best supportive care in patients who had disease progression after sunitinib, sorafenib, or both.
- At this time, the most effective sequence or combinations of agents have not been defined. Clinical trials remain an appropriate first step for patients with metastatic disease.

Testicular Cancer

Incidence
- Estimated new cases in 2010 were 8480 (increasing in incidence)
- Estimated deaths in 2010 were 350

Epidemiology
- **Most common cancer in men in the 20- to 34-year age group**
- There is a secondary peak after age 60 years (mostly seminoma)
- Incidence is rare in African Americans

Etiology and Risk Factors
- Prior testicular cancer (500-fold increase in risk)
- Cryptorchidism (20- to 40-fold increase in risk)
- High prevalence (90%) have isochromosome 12p
- Association of extragonadal germ cell tumors with Klinefelter and possibly Marfan syndromes
- Association of extragonadal germ cell tumors with hematologic malignancy
- Prior trauma, elevated scrotal temperature, wearing briefs instead of boxer shorts, sleeping with electric blankets, and activities such as horseback and motorcycle riding are not related to development of testicular cancer

Pathology
- **Vast majority are germ cell tumors: Seminomas and nonseminomas**
- Seminoma: 30% of all germ cell tumors
- Nonseminoma cell types: Embryonal, endodermal sinus, teratoma, choriocarcinoma
- Other non–germ cell tumors are rare: Leydig cell tumors, Sertoli cell tumors

Presentation
- Most germ cell tumors manifest in the testis (90%)
- Extragonadal (10%) tumors typically manifest in the retroperitoneum, mediastinum, or pineal gland; primary tumor in the testis may be occult
- Classically manifests as an enlargement or mass within testicle
  - Pain and swelling commonly occur
  - An associated hydrocele may be present in 20% of patients

- Gynecomastia (usually bilateral) caused by excess β-human chorionic gonadotropin (β-hCG) production can be seen
- **Inguinal lymphadenopathy is usually not a presenting feature because the regional lymph nodes for the testis are in the retroperitoneum**
- Metastatic spread may present with low back pain (retroperitoneal adenopathy), chest pain, cough, dyspnea, or hemoptysis (mediastinal adenopathy or lung metastases)

Diagnosis

- Testicular ultrasound can easily distinguish extratesticular from testicular abnormalities, and solid from cystic lesions
- **All solid intratesticular lesions should be removed by an inguinal orchiectomy. Biopsy or scrotal orchiectomy is contraindicated because it is associated with local spread of tumor cells.**

Staging

- Tumor marker studies should be obtained pre- and postorchiectomy
  - Elevation of β-hCG or α-fetoprotein (AFP) is seen in 80% to 90% of nonseminomatous germ cell tumors
  - Pure seminoma may have elevated β-hCG, but not AFP
  - **Elevated AFP indicates presence of nonseminomatous elements**
  - False-positive β-hCG elevations can be seen with hypogonadism and use of marijuana. AFP may be elevated in patients with liver disease.
  - Lactate dehydrogenase levels may also be elevated in patients with bulky disease and can serve as a useful tumor marker
- CT scan of chest, abdomen, and pelvis should be obtained to search for metastatic sites
- CT of head and bone scan unnecessary unless symptoms or signs are suggestive of spread to those areas
- Overall staging is based on extent of spread (Table 54-4)

Treatment

- Seminomas
  - Very sensitive to radiation therapy (RT), so very low doses (25 Gy) should be used; acute side effects include nausea, vomiting, diarrhea; late side effects include peptic ulcers, infertility, and second malignancies
  - Stage I disease: In compliant patients, observation is preferred. Adjuvant RT has been the primary adjuvant approach, with single-dose carboplatin as an alternative.
  - Stage II disease: Treat with RT after inguinal orchiectomy for nonbulky disease and with chemotherapy for bulky disease
  - Stage III disease: Chemotherapy with bleomycin/etoposide/cisplatin (BEP)
- Nonseminomas
  - Stage I: Inguinal orchiectomy with or without retroperitoneal lymph node dissection (RPLND); adjuvant BEP can be considered for patients whose risk for relapse exceeds 50% (e.g., embryonal carcinoma with vascular invasion)

TABLE 54-4	*Simplified Staging System for Testicular Cancer*
Stage	**Description**
I	Tumor limited to testis, epididymis, or spermatic cord
II	Tumor extends to but not beyond the regional (retroperitoneal) lymph nodes
III	Disseminated disease

- Stage II: Inguinal orchiectomy followed by RPLND with or without adjuvant chemotherapy (BEP)
- Stage III: Chemotherapy with BEP
- Recurrent disease: Treat with salvage chemotherapy

Prognosis

- **Five-year survival of all patients is approximately 95%**
- Cure rates high for disease with minimal-to-moderate spread
- Infertility is common in all stages of testicular cancer, but risk of permanent infertility increases with therapy and stage; sperm banking must be considered in all patients undergoing therapy for testis cancer

REVIEW QUESTIONS

For review questions, please go to www.expertconsult.com.

SUGGESTED READINGS

Chee KG, Cambio A, Lara PN Jr: Recent developments in advanced urothelial cancer, *Curr Opin Urol* 15:342–349, 2005.
De Bono JS, Oudard S, Ozguroglu M, et al: for the TROPIC Investigators: Prednisone plus cabazitaxel or mitoxantrone for metastatic castration-resistant prostate cancer progressing after docetaxel treatment: a randomised open-label trial, *Lancet* 376:1147–1154, 2010.
International Germ Cell Cancer Collaborative Group: International germ cell consensus classification: a prognostic factor-based staging system for metastatic germ cell cancers, *J Clin Oncol* 15:594–603, 1997.
Kanda S, Miyata Y, Kanetake H: Current status and perspective of antiangiogenesis therapy for cancer: urinary cancer, *Int J Clin Oncol* 11:90–107, 2006.
Kantoff PW, Higano CS, Shore ND, et al: for the IMPACT Study Investigators:Sipuleucel-T immunotherapy for castration-resistant prostate cancer, *N Engl J Med* 363:411–422, 2010.
Motzer RJ, Escudier B, Oudard S, et al: for the RECORD-1 Study Group:Efficacy of everolimus in advanced renal cell carcinoma: a double-blind, randomised, placebo-controlled phase III trial, *Lancet* 372:449–456, 2008.
Nelson WG, DeMarzo AM, Isaacs WB: Prostate cancer, *N Engl J Med* 349:366–381, 2003.
Pienta KJ, Smith DC: Advances in prostate cancer chemotherapy: a new era begins, *CA Cancer J Clin* 55:300–318, 2005.
Rini BI, Campbell SC, Escudier B: Renal cell carcinoma, *Lancet* 373:1119–1132, 2009.
Sarvis JA, Thompson IM: Prostate cancer chemoprevention: update of the prostate cancer prevention trial findings and implications for clinical practice, *Curr Oncol Rep* 10:529–532, 2008.
Sternberg CN, Davis ID, Mardiak J, et al: Pazopanib in locally advanced or metastatic renal cell carcinoma: results of a randomized phase III trial, *J Clin Oncol* 28:1061–1068, 2010.

54

Lymphoma and Chronic Lymphocytic Leukemia

YVETTE L. KASAMON, MD

Leukemia and lymphoma are both hematologic malignancies. Whereas leukemias proliferate primarily in the blood and bone marrow, lymphomas are characterized by uncontrolled proliferation of cells residing in the lymphoid tissues. Some diseases, like chronic lymphocytic leukemia (CLL), can have features of both.

Classic Hodgkin Lymphoma

Basic Information

- Usually arises from B cells
- Bimodal age distribution (third and seventh decades)
- Subset associated with Epstein-Barr virus infection

Clinical Presentation

- **Patients commonly present with "B symptoms" (fever, weight loss, night sweats) and pruritus**
- Most present with an asymptomatic enlarged lymph node or a mass found on chest radiograph (Fig. 55-1A and B)
  - Nodes are usually painless and rubbery
  - Most common sites are neck and mediastinum
  - Hodgkin lymphoma starts at a single site within the lymphatic system, then progresses to adjacent lymph nodes
  - Alcohol-induced pain is a rare symptom of Hodgkin lymphoma
- **A mediastinal mass in a young person is most often Hodgkin lymphoma,** followed in frequency by non-Hodgkin lymphoma
  - Mediastinal masses may be incidental findings or cause chest pain, cough, dyspnea, or superior vena cava syndrome
- Common laboratory findings include
  - Elevated white blood cell (WBC) count
  - Lymphopenia
  - Thrombocytosis
  - Elevated erythrocyte sedimentation rate

Diagnosis

- Usually diagnosed by lymph node biopsy
  - **Reed-Sternberg cells (giant "owl's-eye" cells) are characteristic and are surrounded by a dense inflammatory infiltrate** (see Fig. 55-1C)
  - Fine-needle aspiration is usually insufficient because of limited architecture
  - Mediastinoscopy may be performed to sample a mediastinal tumor

- Most common subtypes: nodular sclerosis, followed by mixed cellularity
- Lymphocyte-predominant Hodgkin (a rare variant) is not classic Hodgkin
- Staging (Table 55-1) requires computed tomography (CT) of chest, abdomen, and pelvis, preferably with positron emission tomography (PET)
  - Exploratory laparotomy is now rarely performed for staging
  - Bone marrow biopsy is not always necessary; consider especially with B symptoms, cytopenias, or advanced disease
  - PET is a useful adjunct to CT

Prognosis

- Majority are curable
- Adverse prognostic factors include
  - Age older than 45 years
  - Male gender
  - Stage IV disease
  - Abnormal complete blood count (CBC): WBC ≥15,000/μL, lymphopenia, anemia
  - Albumin less than 4 g/dL
  - Large mediastinal mass

Treatment

- Treatment is based on staging
  - Stages I and II are usually treated with combination chemotherapy followed by radiation. Some cases may be treated with chemotherapy alone.
  - Stages III and IV are treated with full-course chemotherapy. Radiation may be added afterward to areas of bulky tumor.
  - Combination therapy with doxorubicin, bleomycin, vinblastine, and dacarbazine (ABVD) is standard; full-course is six to eight cycles
- Scans are followed during and after treatment to assess remission
- Autologous stem cell transplant is considered for most patients who relapse after first-line treatment
- Sequelae from treatment are common. Treatment toxicities are leading considerations because most Hodgkin lymphoma patients are cured.
  - Pulmonary toxicity from bleomycin can occur, usually during treatment. Patient may be asymptomatic, or bleomycin may cause cough, fever, dyspnea, and infiltrates.
  - Anthracyclines can cause late cardiomyopathy

FIGURE 55-1 Hodgkin's lymphoma. Most patients present with asymptomatic lymphadenopathy (**A**) or a mediastinal mass (**B**). Multinucleated Reed-Sternberg cells are characteristic pathologic findings (**C**). *(A and B, From Shah B, Laude T: Atlas of pediatric clinical diagnosis, Philadelphia, Saunders, 2000, Fig. 7-32. C, From Hoffman R, Benz EJ Jr, Shattil SJ, et al: Hematology: basic principles and practice, ed 4, Philadelphia, Churchill Livingstone, 2005, Fig. 74-36.)*

55

TABLE 55-1	*Staging of Lymphoma**
Stage I	Disease in one nodal or one extralymphatic site
Stage II	Two or more nodal areas on same side of diaphragm
Stage III	Nodes on both sides of diaphragm
Stage IV	Disseminated extralymphatic spread

*Stages are designated as: A, absence of constitutional symptoms (unexplained fever >38°C, drenching night sweats, or unexplained >10% weight loss in preceding 6 months), or B, presence of these constitutional symptoms.

- Radiation significantly increases the risk of solid tumors (including lung, breast, thyroid)
- **Mediastinal radiation can also cause cardiac complications, including premature coronary artery disease, constrictive pericarditis, restrictive cardiomyopathy, and valve disease**

- Thyroid function tests should be monitored for hypothyroidism after radiation
- Chemotherapy increases the risk of myelodysplastic syndrome and acute leukemia

Non-Hodgkin Lymphoma

Basic Information

- Incidence
  - **Diffuse large B-cell lymphoma (DLBCL) is the most common non-Hodgkin lymphoma (NHL), followed by follicular lymphoma**
  - Incidence of lymphoma rises with age
- Histology
  - Most lymphomas arise from B cells
  - Broadly divided into "low-grade" (indolent) or "high-grade" (aggressive) lymphomas (Box 55-1)

BOX 55-1 *Examples of Non-Hodgkin Lymphomas*

Indolent
Follicular lymphoma, grade 1 or 2
Marginal zone lymphoma, including mucosa-associated lymphoid tissue lymphoma
CLL/SLL
Most skin lymphomas

Aggressive
Follicular lymphoma, grade 3B
Diffuse large B-cell lymphoma
Mediastinal large B-cell lymphoma
Peripheral T-cell lymphoma
Mantle cell lymphoma
Burkitt lymphoma*
Acute lymphoblastic lymphoma/leukemia (ALL) *

CLL, chronic lymphocytic leukemia; SLL, small lymphocytic leukemia.
*These are highly aggressive.

- Risk factors
  - Altered immunity (HIV infection, organ transplantation, autoimmune diseases, congenital immunodeficiency)
    - Aggressive B-cell lymphoma is an AIDS-defining illness
  - Infections
    - Epstein-Barr virus (especially in African Burkitt lymphoma and AIDS-related lymphomas)
    - HTLV-1 in adult T-cell leukemia/lymphoma
    - Hepatitis C virus in some low-grade lymphomas
    - *Helicobacter pylori* in gastric mucosa–associated lymphoid tissue (MALT) lymphoma **(H. pylori treatment can eradicate the lymphoma)**
    - Consider antibiotics as first line for low-grade, localized gastric lymphoma that is positive for *H. pylori*, with radiation as second-line
  - Chemical exposure (pesticides)

Clinical Presentation

- Low-grade lymphomas (e.g., follicular lymphomas) manifest subtly
  - Lymph nodes can wax and wane, possibly for years
  - May be discovered incidentally
- More aggressive lymphomas (e.g., DLBCL) usually manifest with firm, enlarging lymph nodes or widespread lymphadenopathy, with or without B symptoms
- **Very high-grade lymphomas (e.g., Burkitt, lymphoblastic) can grow extremely rapidly, usually manifesting as a single large mass or widespread disease and a markedly elevated lactate dehydrogenase (LDH)**

Diagnosis

- Incisional lymph node biopsy is generally preferable to needle biopsy
- Staging (see Table 55-1) includes chest/abdomen/pelvis CT, preferably with PET, and a bone marrow biopsy
- Consider HIV antibody in most patients with aggressive NHL

Prognosis

- Stage is relatively poor indicator of outcome, because spread is hematogenous
  - Adverse prognostic features in aggressive lymphomas include
    - Age older than 60 years
    - Elevated LDH
    - Stage III or IV disease
    - More than one extranodal site
    - Poor performance status
- In AIDS-related lymphomas
  - CD4 count is most important prognostic feature
  - Addition of highly active antiretroviral therapy (HAART) improves survival

Treatment

- Low-grade lymphomas are treatable but usually incurable
  - Many treatment options (e.g., watchful waiting, chemotherapy, monoclonal antibodies such as rituximab, radiation)
  - **No benefit to early or aggressive treatment if patient is asymptomatic; consider observation**
  - Transformation to high-grade lymphoma may occur
  - In low-grade follicular lymphoma
    - Median survival is 8 to 10 years
    - Radiation may cure limited-stage disease
    - Most have disseminated disease at diagnosis
    - Transformation occurs in ~40% and is treated like high-grade lymphoma
- Aggressive lymphomas are treated promptly with combination chemotherapy, with or without radiation, and are potentially curable (~60% cure rate in DLBCL)
  - Cyclophosphamide, doxorubicin, vincristine, and prednisone (CHOP) is a widely used regimen
  - Addition of rituximab (monoclonal anti-CD20 antibody) to chemotherapy (e.g., rituximab-CHOP) improves outcomes in B-cell lymphomas
  - **Monitor for tumor lysis syndrome due to rapid cell breakdown**
    - Hyperuricemia
    - Hyperkalemia
    - Hyperphosphatemia
    - Hypocalcemia
    - Acute renal failure
  - Spread to the central nervous system (CNS) may occur
    - Usually leptomeningeal disease, rather than a brain mass
    - May be diagnosed by lumbar puncture
    - Risk factors include
      - HIV infection
      - Extranodal sites, such as bone marrow, sinuses, or testicles
      - High LDH
      - Burkitt lymphoma or lymphoblastic histology
    - CNS lymphoma requires directed therapy
      - Intrathecal chemotherapy, with or without radiation, is the mainstay
      - Most systemic chemotherapies are ineffective
  - Autologous stem cell transplant is considered for most patients with relapsed aggressive lymphoma

FIGURE 55-2 **A,** Peripheral blood smear showing "smudge cells" in chronic lymphocytic leukemia. **B,** Lymphocytes with fine surface projections or "hairs" (*arrow*) in hairy cell leukemia. *(A, From Hoffman R, Benz EJ Jr, Shattil SJ, et al: Hematology: basic principles and practice, ed 4, Philadelphia, Churchill Livingstone, 2005, Fig. 79-5. B, From Rodak BF: Diagnostic hematology, Philadelphia, Saunders, 1995.)*

Chronic Lymphocytic Leukemia

Basic Information

- Most common leukemia in the United States
- Median age of diagnosis is 65 years, with male predominance
- Arises from B cells
- Leading cause of death is infection

Clinical Presentation

- Often asymptomatic at diagnosis
  - About 25% present with **lymphocytosis** found on routine labs
  - **WBC greater than 100,000/μL can be asymptomatic and not require therapy**
- May also present with lymphadenopathy (usually painless), splenomegaly, anemia, thrombocytopenia, or B symptoms
- **Hypogammaglobulinemia increases infection risk**
- Autoimmune complications may occur, including hemolytic anemia and immune-mediated thrombocytopenia

Diagnosis

- Lymphocytosis in blood
  - At least 5000/μL circulating B cells, with characteristic phenotype
  - **Peripheral smear shows small, mature lymphocytes, some appearing as "smudge cells" (an artifact) (Fig. 55-2A)**
- Lymphocytosis in bone marrow is common (often >30% lymphocytes)
- Staging (Table 55-2) based on CBC and presence of enlarged lymph nodes, spleen, or liver

TABLE 55-2	Rai Staging of Chronic Lymphocytic Leukemia	
Risk Group	**Stage**	**Features**
Low	0	Lymphocytosis only (blood or marrow)
Intermediate	I	Lymphocytosis + lymphadenopathy
	II	Lymphocytosis + hepatomegaly or splenomegaly
High	III	Lymphocytosis + anemia (hemoglobin <11 g/dL)
	IV	Lymphocytosis + thrombocytopenia (platelets <100,000/μL)

- Small lymphocytic lymphoma (SLL) is the same disease as CLL, but with more lymphadenopathy than leukemia

Prognosis

- Virtually incurable
- Variable natural history
  - Median survival ranges from less than 4 years to more than 20 years, depending on risk factors
- Adverse features include
  - Rapid lymphocyte doubling time (12 months)
  - Advanced stage at diagnosis
  - Cytogenetics (17p deletion, 11q deletion are unfavorable; isolated 13q deletion is most favorable)
  - Immunoglobulin gene mutation status (unmutated immunoglobulin heavy-chain variable region [*IgVH*] gene is unfavorable)
- **Richter syndrome** (transformation to aggressive lymphoma) occurs in ~5% and is difficult to treat
  - Suspect if rapid growth in one or more lymph nodes or worsening B symptoms

Treatment

- **Observation is appropriate for early-stage or asymptomatic CLL**
  - No proven advantage to early treatment if asymptomatic
- Indications for treatment
  - Bulky lymphadenopathy or organomegaly
  - Constitutional symptoms (weakness, B symptoms)
  - Bone marrow failure (anemia or thrombocytopenia) from progressive CLL
  - Autoimmune hemolysis or autoimmune thrombocytopenia failing usual therapy
  - Rapidly progressive disease or Richter transformation
- Active drugs include
  - Purine analogues: fludarabine
  - Antibodies: rituximab, alemtuzumab (Campathanti-CD52 antibody)
  - Alkylating agents: chlorambucil (commonly used as single agent), cyclophosphamide
  - Other: bendamustine, biologic agents
- **Intravenous immune globulin may be given for hypogammaglobulinemia and frequent infection**

55

Hairy Cell Leukemia

Basic Information
- Rare B-cell leukemia
- Median age of onset 55 years, with strong male predominance
- Indolent course, but progressive

Clinical Presentation
- **Manifests with pancytopenia and massive splenomegaly**
- A **"dry" bone marrow tap** despite marrow hypercellularity is characteristic

Diagnosis
- Peripheral smear may show small- to medium-sized lymphocytes with hair-like projections (see Fig. 55-2B)
- Cells have a specific phenotype

Treatment
- Cladribine (2-CdA) or pentostatin (both purine analogues) usually induces complete remission

REVIEW QUESTIONS
For review questions, please go to www.expertconsult.com.

SUGGESTED READINGS

Armitage JO: Early stage Hodgkin's lymphoma, *N Engl J Med* 363:653–662, 2010.
Armitage JO: How I treat patients with diffuse large B-cell lymphoma, *Blood* 110:29–36, 2007.
Dighiero G, Hamblin TJ: Chronic lymphocytic leukaemia, *Lancet* 371:1017–1029, 2008.
Hasenclever D, Diehl VA: A prognostic score for advanced Hodgkin's disease. International Prognostic Factors Project on Advanced Hodgkin's Disease, *N Engl J Med* 339:1506–1514, 1998.
Ng AK, Lacasce A, Travis LB: Long-term complications of lymphoma and its treatment, *J Clin Oncol* 29:1885–1892, 2011.
The International Non-Hodgkin's Lymphoma Prognostic Factors Project: a predictive model for aggressive non-Hodgkin's lymphoma, *N Engl J Med* 329:987–994, 1993.

Plasma Cell Dyscrasias

CAROL ANN HUFF, MD

Plasma cell dyscrasias are **clonal B-cell disorders characterized by the overproduction of monoclonal immunoglobulins.** Patients with plasma cell dyscrasias may present with any of a number of symptoms, but many patients are asymptomatic at the time of diagnosis.

Basic Information

- Definition
  - There are seven categories of plasma cell dyscrasias (Table 56-1)
  - Each has an immunohistochemically identical production of antibody
  - Autoimmune disorders and chronic inflammatory conditions may lead to the production of monoclonal immunoglobulins; this is not malignant and is separate from plasma cell dyscrasias; examples include
    - Systemic lupus erythematosus, Sjögren syndrome, and cold agglutinin disease
    - Infections such as tuberculosis, endocarditis, hepatitis; carcinoid tumors, polycythemia rubra vera, and pyoderma gangrenosum
  - **Monoclonal immunoglobulins (Igs) seen in 1% of adults;** prevalence increases with increasing age
    - Prevalence: IgG > IgM > IgA
- Evaluation of the patient with possible monoclonal immunoglobulin production (Figs. 56-1 and 56-2)
  - Diagnostic clues to initiate evaluation
    - Asymptomatic individual: Elevated total protein; elevated globulin fraction of protein; normochromic, normocytic anemia
    - Symptomatic individual: Normochromic, normocytic anemia; recurrent bacterial infections; renal insufficiency; bone pain; pathologic fracture or osteolytic lesion on radiograph; osteoporosis; sensorimotor neuropathy; pyoderma gangrenosum

Multiple Myeloma

Basic Information

- **Second most common hematologic malignancy** (after non-Hodgkin lymphoma [NHL]), resulting in 1% of cancer deaths each year
- Male predominance
- Twice as common in African Americans as whites
- Median age at diagnosis: 68 years
- Median survival after diagnosis is 5 years and improving

- Poor prognostic indicators include renal insufficiency, hypercalcemia, anemia, elevated β_2-microglobulin, hypoalbuminemia; cytogenetic abnormalities including hypodiploidy, 13q deletion, or complex karyotype, or t[4;14], t[14;16], or p53 deletions detected with fluorescent *in situ* hybridization (FISH) or cytogenetics

Clinical Presentation

- Most common presenting features are calcium elevation, renal insufficiency, anemia, and bone pain (group of findings referred to as CRAB)

TABLE 56-1	*Plasma Cell Dyscrasias*
Disorders	**Disease Definition**
Monoclonal gammopathy of undetermined significance (MGUS)	Overproduction of monoclonal immunoglobulin (<3 g/dL) with <10% clonal plasma cells on bone marrow aspiration and biopsy and absence of end-organ damage (hypercalcemia, renal insufficiency, anemia, bone lesions).
Multiple myeloma	Clonal plasma cells ≥10% in the bone marrow and/or presence of serum and/or urinary monoclonal protein; when associated evidence of lytic bone lesions, anemia, hypercalcemia, or renal insufficiency, it is active myeloma. In the absence of associated symptoms, termed smoldering or asymptomatic.
Plasmacytoma	Biopsy-proven solitary lesion with clonal plasma cells and insufficient criteria to diagnose multiple myeloma (see above).
POEMS syndrome	Presence of monoclonal plasma cells; **p**olyneuropathy, **o**rganomegaly, **e**ndocrinopathy, **M** protein, and **s**kin changes.
AL amyloidosis	Presence of monoclonal plasma cells creating a syndrome where insoluble proteins deposit in tissues and cause end-organ damage.
Waldenström macroglobulinemia	Immunoglobulin M monoclonal gammopathy with >10% bone marrow lymphoplasmacytic infiltration.
Cryoglobulinemia	Group of disorders associated with overproduction of monoclonal or polyclonal protein production: defining characteristic is that proteins precipitate when cooled and dissolve when heated.

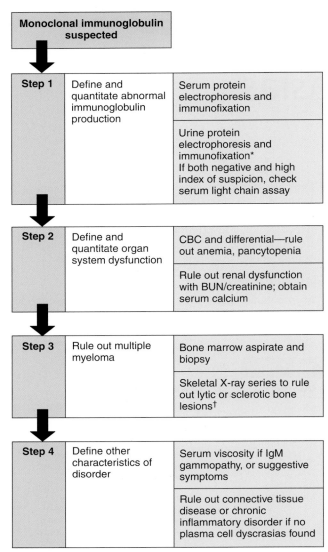

FIGURE 56-1   Evaluation of a monoclonal immunoglobulin. *Spot urine for qualitative assessment: 24-hour collection for quantitative assessment. †Bone scan evaluates for blastic lesions and will be normal in multiple myeloma. (BUN, blood urea nitrogen; CBC, complete blood count; IgM, immunoglobulin M.)

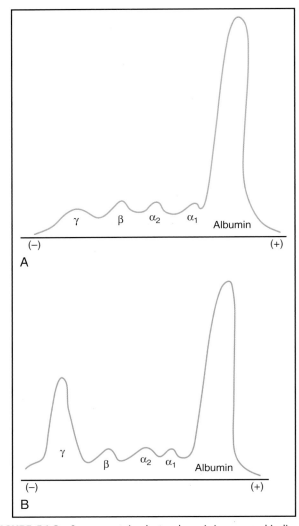

FIGURE 56-2   Serum protein electrophoresis in a normal individual (**A**) and in an individual with a monoclonal gammopathy (**B**). *(From Waldman SD: Interventional pain management, ed 2, Philadelphia, WB Saunders, 2001, Fig. 9-1A, C.)*

- Figure 56-3 illustrates the clinical manifestations of multiple myeloma

Diagnosis and Evaluation

- Diagnostic criteria for multiple myeloma
  - Smoldering/asymptomatic (Box 56-1)
    - Clonal bone marrow plasma cells greater than or equal to 10% *or*
    - Presence of serum and/or urinary monoclonal protein greater than or equal to 3 g/dL
  - Active
    - Above criteria with the addition of end-organ damage that can be attributed to the underlying plasma cell proliferative disorder, specifically the CRAB criteria
      - **C**alcium greater than 11.5 g/dL
      - **R**enal insufficiency (creatinine >2 mg/dL)

- **A**nemia (hemoglobin [Hbg] <10 g/100mL or 2 g/100 mL < normal)
- **B**one disease (osteopenia or lytic lesions)
- Common complications include the following:
  - Hypercalcemia: Present in 25% of patients; results from lytic bone disease; treated with saline hydration, loop diuretics, and bisphosphonates
  - Anemia: Normochromic, normocytic with an Hbg value of greater than 2 g/100 mL below the lower limit of normal or an Hbg value less than 10 g/100 mL
  - Renal insufficiency: Occurs in 50% of patients; usually progresses insidiously, but acute renal failure may be present
    - **Bence Jones proteinuria** (may be missed on routine urine dipstick, which detects albumin; sulfosalicylic acid effectively precipitates light chains), tubular casts, glomerular lesions
  - Hyperviscosity syndrome: Results from elevated serum proteins; symptoms usually not seen until serum viscosity greater than 4 cP (centiPoises; Box 56-2)

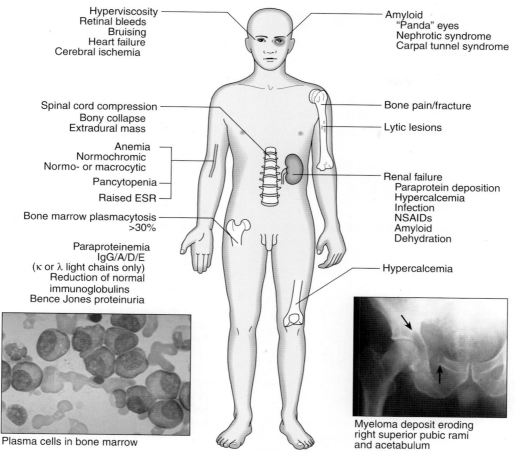

Hyperviscosity
Retinal bleeds
Bruising
Heart failure
Cerebral ischemia

Amyloid
"Panda" eyes
Nephrotic syndrome
Carpal tunnel syndrome

Spinal cord compression
Bony collapse
Extradural mass

Bone pain/fracture

Lytic lesions

Anemia
Normochromic
Normo- or macrocytic

Pancytopenia

Raised ESR

Bone marrow plasmacytosis
>30%

Renal failure
Paraprotein deposition
Hypercalcemia
Infection
NSAIDs
Amyloid
Dehydration

Paraproteinemia
IgG/A/D/E
(κ or λ light chains only)
Reduction of normal
immunoglobulins
Bence Jones proteinuria

Hypercalcemia

Plasma cells in bone marrow

Myeloma deposit eroding
right superior pubic rami
and acetabulum

56

FIGURE 56-3 Clinical manifestations of multiple myeloma. (ESR, erythrocyte sedimentation rate; Ig, immunoglobulin; NSAIDs, nonsteroidal anti-inflammatory drugs.) *(From Haslett C, Chilvers ER, Boon NA, et al: Davidson's principles and practice of medicine, ed 19, New York, Churchill Livingstone, 2002, Fig. 19.33.)*

BOX 56-1 | *Diagnostic Criteria for Multiple Myeloma*

Smoldering

M protein ≥3 g/dL and/or clonal plasma cells on bone marrow ≥10%

No evidence of end-organ impairment and asymptomatic

Active

Requires one or more of the following in addition to the criteria for smoldering disease:
    Calcium >11.5 g/dL
    Renal insufficiency (creatinine >2 mg/dL)
    Anemia (hemoglobin <10 g/100mL or 2 g/100 mL < normal)
    Bone disease (osteopenia or lytic lesions)

- Neurologic: Sensory or sensorimotor neuropathy
- Immunodeficiency: Increased risk of recurrent bacterial infections due to suppression of normal immunoglobulins
- Bone lesions: Lytic lesions, severe osteopenia or pathologic fractures (most commonly vertebral compression fractures)

- To diagnose: Obtain skeletal survey to identify high-risk areas and consider prophylactic radiotherapy or surgical pinning of areas at high risk
- Positron emission tomography (PET) scans and spine magnetic resonance imaging (MRI) are not routinely recommended at this point but are useful in certain situations
- **Bone scan is typically normal in myeloma patients because it only shows blastic lesions**
- Spinal cord compression serious complication that could present with pain, lower extremity paresthesias or weakness, and urinary retention or fecal incontinence; treatment with IV dexamethasone and radiation therapy and, sometimes, with urgent surgical decompression

Treatment

- **Chemotherapy: Not curative; should be instituted when patients are symptomatic or demonstrate end-organ dysfunction as described earlier**
  - Melphalan and prednisone; inferior results when compared to melphalan/prednisone combinations listed below
  - Melphalan, prednisone, and thalidomide
  - Melphalan, prednisone, and bortezomib

FIGURE 56-4   Bone marrow replaced with plasma cells. *(From Stevens A, Lowe J: Pathology, ed 2, St. Louis, Mosby, 2000, Fig. 15.16.)*

- Thalidomide and dexamethasone
- Lenaldiomide and dexamethasone
- Bortezomib and dexamethasone
- Bortezomib, liposomal adriamycin, and dexamethasone
- Lenalidomide, bortezomib, and dexamethasone
- Cyclophosphamide, bortezomib, and dexamethasone
- Bone marrow transplantation
  - Autologous: Increases survival by 12 to 18 months on average; all patients eventually relapse
  - Allogeneic: Potentially curative (25–30%) but with greatest toxicities
- Symptomatic management
  - **Bone lesions: Bisphosphonates decrease risk of fracture and improve quality of life;** surgical intervention for pathologic fractures; vertebroplasty or kyphoplasty for symptomatic vertebral lesions
  - Anemia: Erythropoietin in symptomatic patients who are not hyperviscous
  - Infectious: Vaccinate against *Pneumococcus, Haemophilus influenzae,* and influenza; consider prophylactic antibiotics if on long-term corticosteroids, varicella-zoster prophylaxis if on bortezomib

Plasmacytomas

Basic Information

- **Plasmacytomas are proliferations of monoclonal plasma cells forming a mass at extramedullary or osseous sites**
- No evidence of multiple myeloma or end-organ dysfunction (hypercalcemia, renal insufficiency, anemia, or other bone lesions, and no evidence of plasmacytosis on bone marrow biopsy)
- 50% of osseous plasmacytomas develop into overt myeloma; only 15% of extraosseous lesions develop overt myeloma

Clinical Presentation

- Solitary plasmacytoma: Single tumor of plasma cells resulting in localized complaints (bone pain, pathologic fracture); no evidence of diffuse plasma cell overgrowth throughout remainder of bone marrow (Fig. 56-4); most common sites are vertebrae, ribs, skull, and pelvis
- Extramedullary plasmacytoma: Tumor of plasma cells arising outside of the bone marrow; most commonly found in the upper respiratory tract (nasal passages, sinuses, nasopharynx, larynx); occasionally described in the lower extremity, GI tract, lung, lymph nodes; can be associated with HIV infection

Diagnosis and Evaluation

- Diagnosis made by biopsy, typically when mass or structural abnormality noted on imaging study
- Serum protein electrophoresis (SPEP), urine protein electrophoresis (UPEP), bone marrow aspiration, and biopsy, as well as skeletal survey should be done at diagnosis to rule out extramedullary spread of multiple myeloma; if negative, consider spine MRI and PET scan to exclude occult lesions elsewhere; if truly isolated, follow serially in case of progression to myeloma

Treatment

- Radiation therapy to the involved area; 15% to 25% are disease-free at 10 years

Monoclonal Gammopathy of Undetermined Significance

Basic Information

- Most common plasma cell dyscrasia (3% of population older than age 50 years)
- Asymptomatic premalignant disorder
- Rate of progression of monoclonal gammopathy of unknown significance (MGUS) to myeloma or related malignancy is 1% per year
- **Characterized by overproduction of a monoclonal immunoglobulin without other abnormalities;** diagnosis of exclusion, usually made retrospectively, when one demonstrates stability over time in the quantity of M protein and the absence of other findings

Clinical Presentation

- **No symptoms associated with MGUS; diagnosed entirely on laboratory criteria**
- Evaluation: SPEP and immunofixation electrophoresis (IFE); 24-hour UPEP and IFE; complete blood count (CBC) and differential, creatinine, calcium, albumin, serum light-chain assay, skeletal survey, bone marrow aspiration, and **biopsy recommended for all patients with M protein greater than 1 g/dL and in those with non-IgG paraprotein, regardless of quantification of M protein**

Diagnostic Criteria

- **M protein less than 3 g/dL** (as determined by SPEP)
- **Less than 10% plasma cells on bone marrow**
- Normal Hgb, creatinine, calcium
- Absence of lytic bone disease
- Asymptomatic

Treatment/Follow-up

- **Observation alone, without therapy**
- No formal guideline for follow-up: Serial laboratories including SPEP, UPEP, CBC, and metabolic panel for creatinine and calcium at least yearly
- Increased risk of progression to myeloma: High monoclonal protein concentration; high percentage of plasma cells in the bone marrow, a non-IgG paraprotein, an abnormal serum-free κ/λ light-chain ratio

POEMS Syndrome

Basic Information

- **Syndrome resulting from overproduction of light chains, usually λ, without significant overgrowth of plasma cells in the bone marrow; many organ systems involved, with characteristic abnormalities**
- Also called osteosclerotic myeloma

Clinical Presentation

Table 56-2 summarizes the clinical presentation of POEMS syndrome.

- Polyneuropathy is an inflammatory demyelinating process with predominantly sensory symptoms
- Organomegaly most common in spleen and liver
- Endocrinopathies seen include hypogonadism and hyperprolactinemia
- M protein is usually λ light chains
- Skin changes include hypertrichosis and thickening of the dermis
- Sclerotic bone lesions
- Elevated vascular endothelial growth factor
- Papilledema
- Thrombocytosis or polycythemia

Diagnosis

- Based on clinical suspicion and constellation of findings (see Table 56-2); neuropathy is typically the most prominent symptom; SPEP/immunofixation/serum-free light-chain assay demonstrating λ light chains

TABLE 56-2	*Criteria for the Diagnosis of POEMS Syndrome*
Major criteria	Polyneuropathy* Monoclonal plasma cell–proliferative disorder (95% are λ)* Sclerotic bone lesions Castleman disease Vascular endothelial growth factor elevation
Minor criteria	Organomegaly (splenomegaly, hepatomegaly, or lymphadenopathy) Extravascular volume overload (edema, pleural effusion, or ascites) Endocrinopathy (adrenal, thyroid,† pituitary, gonadal, parathyroid, pancreatic†) Skin changes (hyperpigmentation, hypertrichosis, white nails) Papilledema Thrombocytosis, polycythemia
Other signs and symptoms	Clubbing, weight loss, hyperhidrosis, pulmonary hypertension, restrictive lung disease, low vitamin B_{12}, diarrhea, thrombotic diatheses
Possible associations	Arthralgias, cardiomyopathy, fever

*Polyneuropathy and monoclonal plasma cell disorder must be present in all patients; to make diagnosis, at least one other major criterion and one minor criterion are required.

†Endocrinopathy other than isolated thyroid disease or diabetes mellitus is required to meet this criterion (due to the relative frequency of these in the general population).

Treatment

- Includes radiation therapy to bone lesion if isolated; if diffuse changes, then systemic therapy with corticosteroids, low-dose alkylator therapy, and high-dose chemotherapy followed by consideration of stem cell transplantation

Waldenström Macroglobulinemia

Basic Information

- Also known as lymphoplasmacytic lymphoma
- **A rare lymphoma characterized by bone marrow infiltration by clonal B cells with production of M protein (IgM)**

Clinical Presentation

- **Signs and symptoms commonly related to both tumor infiltration of the marrow and elevated monoclonal IgM**
- Most dangerous: Hyperviscosity (Fig. 56-5; see Box 56-2) because of high production of IgM
- Polyneuropathy and cryoglobulinemia (with digital infarcts) also may be seen because of high production of IgM
- Tumor infiltration causing organomegaly, lymphadenopathy, B symptoms (fevers, night sweats, weight loss)
- Only 25% of patients with IgM monoclonal gammopathy have Waldenström macroglobulinemia; others have MGUS, multiple myeloma, chronic lymphocytic leukemia, NHL, or cold agglutinin disease

Diagnosis

- **Based on presence of IgM and evidence of B-cell lymphoma by pathology**

Treatment

- Plasmapheresis is performed to treat hyperviscosity and its related symptoms
- Chemotherapy: Use monoclonal antibody therapy, such as rituximab (anti-CD20) or nucleoside analogues (e.g., fludarabine) or oral alkylating agents (e.g., melphalan or cyclophosphamide)
- Some patients develop aggressive lymphoma (Richter transformation)

Cryoglobulinemia

Basic Information

- Group of disorders characterized by the production of soluble proteins that precipitate on cooling, typically associated with symptoms; often evidence of an

FIGURE 56-5 Waldenström macroglobulinemia (hyperviscosity syndrome). The retina of a patient who presented with blurred vision, headache, and dizziness exhibits gross distention of vessels, particularly the veins, which show bulging and constriction (the "linked sausage" effect), as well as areas of hemorrhage. *(From Skarin AT [ed]: Atlas of diagnostic oncology, ed 3, Philadelphia, WB Saunders, 2003, Fig. 15.56.)*

underlying clonal disorder; divided into three subtypes (Table 56-3)

Clinical Presentation

- Varies by subtype (see Table 56-3)

Diagnosis

- **Key to detection is proper transport of sample—must be taken to lab at body temperature—(ideally in a warm-water bath); diagnosis requires the demonstration of protein precipitation on cooling of blood**

Treatment

- Focused on correcting underlying disease
- Plasmapheresis for those symptomatic patients in whom underlying disease is not treatable

Amyloidosis

Basic Information

- Relatively rare
- **Characterized by deposition of insoluble protein in organs and tissues, resulting in organ dysfunction**
- Disease classified by which protein precursor forms the fibril deposits
  - AL amyloidosis: Amyloid protein is primarily the variable region of Ig light chains ($\lambda > \kappa$)
    - AL amyloidosis is a plasma cell dyscrasia related to myeloma
  - AA amyloidosis: Secondary amyloidosis in which the amyloid protein is serum amyloid protein A (an acute-phase reactant produced in response to inflammation)
    - Protein A is not related to a known immunoglobulin
    - AA amyloidosis is associated with chronic infections (e.g., tuberculosis, osteomyelitis, bronchiectasis), chronic inflammatory disorders (e.g., rheumatoid arthritis, inflammatory bowel disease, and familial Mediterranean fever)
  - Familial amyloidosis: Autosomal dominant disorder in which mutant protein (most commonly transthyretin) forms amyloid fibrils

TABLE 56-3	The Cryoglobulinemias		
Subtype	Immunoglobulin	Disease Association	Features
I	Presence of isolated monoclonal immunoglobulin (usually IgG or IgM, less commonly IgA or free light chains)	Waldenström macroglobulinemia, multiple myeloma	Many patients are asymptomatic; classic symptoms related to hyperviscosity: digital ischemia, Raynaud's phenomenon, purpura, livedo reticularis
II	"Essential mixed CG" is a mixture of polyclonal immunoglobulin with a monoclonal immunoglobulin (usually IgM or IgA); can also have RF activity	Persistent viral infectious—most often hepatitis C or HIV	Membranoproliferative glomerulonephritis, mononeuritis muliplex, vasculitis; classic Meltzer's triad of purpura, arthralgias, and weakness
III	Polyclonal immunoglobulins	Most often secondary to connective tissue disorders or chronic inflammatory conditions	Treatment directed at primary disorder

CG, cryoglobulinemia; HIV, human immunodeficiency virus; Ig, immunoglobulin; RF, rheumatoid factor.

TABLE 56-4		*Clinical Presentation of Amyloidosis*		
Amyloid Subtype	**Dominant Protein**	**Organ Deposit**	**Symptoms**	
AL	Immuno-globulin light chains	Heart	Low-voltage ECG Right-sided heart failure with volume overload Echocardiogram shows classic myocardium speckled pattern; orthostatic hypotension	
		Kidney	Nephrotic-range proteinuria	
		Tongue	Macroglossia	
		GI tract	Infiltration of gut with malabsorptive process	
		CNS	Peripheral neuropathy, carpal tunnel syndrome	
AA	Serum amyloid protein A	Kidney	Most commonly involved with nephrotic-range proteinuria	
		Liver, spleen	Organomegaly	
Familial	Transthyretin	CNS	Neuropathy with sensory or autonomic insufficiency	
		Heart	Conduction abnormalities (see also symptoms of cardiac deposit of AL above)	

CNS, central nervous system; ECG, electrocardiogram; GI, gastrointestinal.

Clinical Presentation

- Determined by the organs predominantly affected by protein deposition and differs according to amyloid subtype (Table 56-4)

Diagnosis

- **Requires demonstration of deposition of amyloid fibers, typically with a fat pad aspirate; staining with Congo red demonstrates apple green birefringence under polarized light (Fig. 56-6)**
- Underlying plasma cell dyscrasias should be ruled out with SPEP/UPEP/serum IFE/urine IFE, bone marrow aspirate/biopsy, CBC and differential diagnosis, chemistry panel, and serum light-chain assay
- Variant transthyretin (familial amyloidosis) should also be ruled out by DNA testing

FIGURE 56-6 Amyloidosis. Congo red stain of a glomerulus that is largely replaced by amyloid demonstrates the characteristic birefringence under polarized light. *(From Goldman L: Cecil textbook of medicine, ed 23, Philadelphia, Elsevier Saunders, 2007, Fig. 115-14.)*

- If no plasma cell dyscrasias, transthyretin normal, consider AA amyloidosis

Treatment

- Directed at the underlying disease, with goal to prevent further deposition of amyloid (resorption of amyloid fibers usually does not occur); management must also focus on control of symptoms from organ dysfunction
- AL: Systemic chemotherapy shown to prolong survival—melphalan and prednisone
  - Small studies suggest that autologous bone marrow transplantation may further improve survival in selected patients
  - Prognosis: Median survival is 1 to 2 years, depending on degree of organ involvement; median survival is 6 months if symptomatic cardiac involvement, 21 months with renal involvement
- AA amyloidosis: Treat underlying infection or inflammatory disease
- Familial amyloidosis: Liver transplantation is curative; often does not reverse the damage

REVIEW QUESTIONS

For review questions, please go to www.expertconsult.com.

SUGGESTED READINGS

Blade J: Clinical practice: monoclonal gammopathy of undetermined significance, *N Engl J Med* 355:2765–2770, 2006.
Comenzo RL: Amyloidosis, *Curr Treat Options Oncol* 7:225–231, 2006.
Dispenzieri A: POEMS syndrome, *Blood Rev* 21:285–299, 2007.
Kyle R, Rajkumar S: Monoclonal gammopathy of undetermined significance and smouldering multiple myeloma: emphasis on risk factors for progression, *Br J Haematol* 139:730–743, 2007.
Kyle R, Rajkumar V: Multiple myeloma, *Blood* 15:2962–2972, 2008.
Rajkumar S, Kyle R, Buadi FK: Advances in the diagnosis, classification, risk stratification, and management of monoclonal gammopathy of undetermined significance: implications for recategorizing disease entities in the presence of evolving scientific evidence, *Mayo Clin Proc* 85:945–948, 2010.

56

Selected Topics in Oncology

DAVID COSGROVE, MD

Previous chapters in this section have focused on the diagnosis and treatment of specific types of cancers. This chapter emphasizes other important aspects in the identification and care of oncologic patients. Specifically, the evaluation of patients with cancer of unknown primary, as well as the identification of oncologic emergencies and paraneoplastic syndromes, is emphasized. Although specific chemotherapeutic regimens are generally left to oncologists, basic toxicities and complications of chemotherapeutic agents should be recognized by all internists.

Cancer of Unknown Primary

Basic Information

- 3% to 5% of all patients with newly diagnosed cancers present with primary tumors of unknown origin
- Equal incidence in men and women
- Median age 60 years
- Most common site: Lymph nodes
- Only 20% to 30% of patients have a primary site identified after work-up
- Cytopathology
  - Helpful in determining the primary tumor site
  - Histology
    - Adenocarcinoma **is the most commonly identified tumor type (60% of cases)**
      - Prostate-specific antigen stain may be helpful in identifying prostate cancer
    - Poorly or undifferentiated carcinoma is seen in about 30% of cases
    - Squamous cell carcinoma is seen in 5% to 10% of cases
    - Specific immunoperoxidase stains may be helpful in suggesting specific causes (Table 57-1)
  - Genetic studies may be helpful in identifying non-Hodgkin lymphomas and sarcomas

Clinical Presentation

- Depends on site of organ involvement
- Weight loss, fatigue, and malaise are common systemic symptoms
- Lymphadenopathy (cervical, supraclavicular, mediastinal, axillary, retroperitoneal) may be the only clinical abnormality

Diagnosis

- **Avoid the impulse to randomly order tumor markers and imaging studies**

- Start with a thorough history and physical (including gynecologic examination or prostate examination) to guide your evaluation
- Make sure appropriate cancer screening is up to date
- Complete blood count (CBC), chemistry profile, liver function tests
- Computed tomography (CT) scan of the chest, abdomen, and pelvis should be ordered routinely. A positron emission tomography/CT scan should be considered.
- Colonoscopy should be considered if clinical symptoms dictate or if screening measures are not up to date
- Mammography for women should be considered if indicated by symptoms or initial work-up, or if screening measures are not up to date
- Order biopsy of mass and special studies (as described previously)
- Specific evaluation measures dictated by location of discovered tumor (Table 57-2)

Treatment

- Directed at the primary site of origin, if discovered
- In cases in which the primary tumor is not identified, treatment is based on tumor histology, location, and most likely primary site (see Table 57-2)
- In cases in which the histology and location do not suggest a specific primary site (most cases), empirical chemotherapy can extend median survival by a few months in select cases

Oncologic Emergencies

SPINAL CORD COMPRESSION

Basic Information

- More than 5% of patients who die from cancer have evidence of spinal cord compression
- The most common primary malignancies include lung cancer, breast cancer, prostate cancer, renal cell cancer, and multiple myeloma
- Compression most commonly caused by extradural metastases involving the spinal cord
- **Any delay in diagnosis and treatment may result in paralysis and incontinence of bowel and bladder that may be irreversible**
- Spinal cord compression may be the initial manifestation of a malignancy
- Most cases (60%) involve the thoracic spine, but compression can occur at the lumbosacral (20%) and cervical (10%) regions as well

Clinical Presentation

- Back pain that continues to increase in intensity is the most common initial finding (90% of cases)
  - Pain can be worsened by movement, coughing, sneezing
  - Radicular symptoms can develop (more common with lumbosacral lesions)
- Progressive motor weakness leading to instability of gait and paralysis is also common
- Sensory loss is seen in over half of patients
- Change in deep tendon reflexes (hyper- or hyporeflexia) and extensor plantar responses may be seen
- Incontinence of stool or urine is usually a late finding

Diagnosis

- History and physical examination should focus on neurologic abnormalities
- **Radiologic imaging should be immediately done in all cancer patients who present with persistent back pain with or without radicular symptoms**
  - Plain spinal radiographs may detect vertebral compression fractures or collapse or erosive spinal lesions, but there is a high false-negative rate

TABLE 57-1 — *Immunoperoxidase Stains*

Tumor Type	Immunoperoxidase Stain
Carcinoma	Cytokeratin, chromogranin
Melanoma	S100, HMB45
Sarcoma	Vimentin, desmin
Lymphoma	Leukocyte common antigen
Neuroendocrine	Cytokeratin, synaptophysin, chromogranin

- Magnetic resonance imaging (MRI) is now the test of choice given its widespread availability
  - The entire vertebral column should be imaged, even if symptoms suggest involvement at a specific level, as multiple metastatic deposits are common, and should all be treated
  - CT myelogram is an alternative for patients who cannot lie still for an MRI or who have a contraindication to MRI

Treatment

- Goal is to control pain and preserve neurologic function
- Options are surgical resection or decompression, radiation therapy, and, in some cases, systemic chemotherapy. Urgent surgical, radiation, and medical oncology consults should be obtained.
  - **Surgery, when feasible, has been shown to result in better neurologic outcomes and possibly a survival benefit compared with radiation alone**
- Steroids should be given promptly
  - Initially, high-dose steroid therapy (dexamethasone 96 mg/day) may be given for palliation of pain and improvement of neurologic status, but this regimen may be associated with a higher treatment complication rate than a lower-dose regimen (16 mg/day)
- Surgery
  - Consider in patients who
    - Have tumors that are not sensitive to radiation
    - Have received prior radiation therapy to the affected area
    - Have a predicted survival of greater than 6 months
    - Need a tissue diagnosis
    - Need spinal stabilization

57

TABLE 57-2 — *Evaluation and Treatment of Specific Carcinomas*

Clinical Finding	Histology/Treatment*	Evaluation
Isolated axillary adenopathy in women	Adenocarcinoma	Breast examination Stage II breast cancer Mammogram/breast MRI Estrogen/progesterone receptor studies
Cervical adenopathy and neck mass	Squamous cell carcinoma	Head and neck examination Panendoscopy of the aerodigestive tract CT scan of head and neck area
Inguinal adenopathy	Squamous cell carcinoma	Full gynecologic examination in women Evaluation of prostate and penis in males Rectal examinations Tumor markers (PSA, CA 125)
Bone metastases	Adenocarcinoma or poorly differentiated carcinoma	Physical examination Stage IV prostate cancer or breast cancer X-rays of spine/weight-bearing joints to rule out fracture PSA in men
Mediastinal/retroperitoneal adenopathy in young males	Poorly differentiated carcinoma	Extragonadal germ cell tumor Tumor markers (hCG, AFP, LDH)
Peritoneal carcinomatosis	Adenocarcinoma	Full gynecologic examination in women Colonoscopy

AFP, α-fetoprotein; CA 125, cancer antigen 125; CT, computed tomography; hCG, human chorionic gonadotropin; LDH, lactate dehydrogenase; MRI, magnetic resonance imaging; PSA, prostate-specific antigen.
*Empirical treatment if the evaluation failed to confirm the primary site.

- Chemotherapy should be considered as a primary treatment option only in patients with exquisitely chemosensitive tumors
- Radiation therapy is the mainstay of treatment to control spinal cord compression
- Overall, prognosis is poor; median survival after diagnosis is 6 months

SUPERIOR VENA CAVA SYNDROME

- **Defined as obstruction of blood return to the heart by invasion, compression, or thrombosis of the superior vena cava**
- Most cases are associated with lung cancer (small cell), lymphoma, thymoma, testicular or breast cancer
- Can also result from venous thrombosis caused by indwelling venous access devices or fibrosing mediastinitis from infections (e.g., histoplasmosis, tuberculosis)
- Signs and symptoms include shortness of breath, facial swelling, fullness of face, cough, arm swelling, and prominent neck and chest veins (Fig. 57-1)
- CT scanning of the chest with contrast or MRI with gadolinium enhancement are the diagnostic modalities of choice
- If the cause is unknown, an evaluation that may include CT-guided biopsy, bronchoscopy, mediastinoscopy, or thoracotomy should be considered
- Treatment with radiation or chemotherapy may be indicated once the tumor type has been identified
- Intraluminal metal stents may provide palliation when cancer is refractory to chemotherapy or radiation
- Thrombolytics and anticoagulation may be necessary for patients with thrombosis

PERICARDIAL TAMPONADE

See also Chapter 8.
- Rarely occurs as the initial manifestation of a cancer
- Seen most commonly in patients with lung or breast cancer, lymphoma, or leukemia
- Cannot assume that all pericardial effusions in cancer patients are caused by metastasis

FIGURE 57-1 Superior vena caval obstruction in bronchial carcinoma. Note the swelling of the face and neck and the development of a collateral circulation in the veins of the chest wall. *(From Goldman L, Bennett JC, Ausiello D: Cecil textbook of medicine, ed 22, Philadelphia, WB Saunders, 2004, Fig. 95-6.)*

- Treatment options in symptomatic patients include prolonged catheter drainage, substernal pericardiotomy, pericardiectomy, or injection of a sclerosing agent
- **No need to treat asymptomatic pericardial effusions**

VENOUS THROMBOSIS

- Thromboembolism is the second leading cause of death in patients with malignancy
- Venous thrombosis is seen most commonly with visceral cancers from pancreas, lung, stomach, colon, breast, and ovary
- **Trousseau syndrome refers to migratory thrombophlebitis in the setting of visceral cancers**
- The risk of thrombosis is increased because of release of procoagulants by tumor cells, immobility of patients because of weakness, or obstruction of blood vessels by tumors
- Patients should be treated initially with heparin, then warfarin
- Sometimes the thromboembolism is resistant to warfarin and requires low-molecular-weight heparin therapy or inferior vena cava filter placement
- See Chapter 21 for detailed information regarding deep venous thrombosis and thromboembolism

METABOLIC EMERGENCIES

- Hypercalcemia of malignancy (see Chapter 39)
- Hyponatremia (see Chapter 32)

Paraneoplastic Syndromes

Basic Information

- Defined as conditions that arise as a result of factors produced by cancer cells
- **In some cases, the symptoms of these syndromes may precede the actual diagnosis of malignancy**
- Presence does not necessarily imply a poor prognosis
- Long-term treatment is geared toward the underlying malignancy

NEUROLOGIC SYNDROMES

- A number of specific syndromes have been described that may affect all parts of the nervous system (Table 57-3)
- Antineuronal antibodies may be helpful in diagnosis and in searching for particular neoplasms; however, they may not always be present

RHEUMATOLOGIC SYNDROMES

- Hypertrophic osteoarthropathy (Fig. 57-2)
  - Abnormal proliferation of bone and skin in the extremities
  - Most commonly associated with adenocarcinoma of the lung but sometimes seen with other lung cancers, lung infections, or conditions that result in right-to-left shunting of blood
  - Symptoms include joint pain with or without effusions
  - Examination may reveal new digital clubbing
  - Radiographs show periosteal new bone formation
  - **If the diagnosis is made, the thorax should be imaged to search for lung cancer**

TABLE 57-3	*Selected Neurologic Paraneoplastic Syndromes*		
Syndrome	**Description**	**Most Commonly Associated Tumors**	**Antibody**
Encephalomyelitis	Precedes discovery of the tumor in most patients Symptoms vary because it can involve a number of different areas of the nervous system Subacute sensory neuronopathy causing asymmetrical paresthesias is the most common early symptom	SCLC	Anti-Hu (also called antineuronal nuclear antibodies or ANNA-1)
Cerebellar degeneration	Abrupt onset of dysarthria and ataxia Nystagmus and oculomotor dysfunction can occur	SCLC Ovarian cancer Breast cancer Uterine cancer Hodgkin lymphoma	Anti-Yo Anti-Tr (in Hodgkin lymphoma only)
Limbic encephalitis	Presents with memory loss, mood changes, emotional lability Hallucinations and seizures may occur	SCLC Testicular germ cell tumors Thymoma Hodgkin lymphoma	Anti-Hu Anti-Ta (testicular or breast)
Stiff-person syndrome	Muscle stiffness or rigidity Usually begins asymmetrically Can cause significant pain EMG shows abnormal continuous firing of motor units	SCLC Breast cancer Thymoma Hodgkin lymphoma	Anti-amphiphysin Anti-GAD (breast)
Lambert-Eaton myasthenic syndrome (LEMS)	Presents with proximal weakness that improves with exercise Bulbar weakness not seen (as opposed to myasthenia gravis) EMG shows motor unit potentials whose amplitude increases with exercise Treatment is geared to malignancy but plasmapheresis or immunosuppressives may be helpful	SCLC	LEMS antibody

EMG, electromyography; GAD, glutamic acid decarboxylase; SCLC, small cell lung cancer.

FIGURE 57-2 **A,** Dorsal view of the hand shows clubbing, with widening of the fingertips replacing the normally tapered appearance of the digits. **B,** A lateral view of the index finger demonstrates clubbing with loss of the normal 15-degree angle between the nail and the cuticle due to accentuated convexity of the nail. There is also enlargement of the distal finger pad and shininess of the nail and adjacent skin. *(From Harris ED, Budd RC, Genovese MC, et al [ed]: Kelley's textbook of rheumatology, ed 7, Philadelphia, WB Saunders, 2005, Figs. 110-2 and 110-3.)*

FIGURE 57-3 Dermatomyositis. **A,** Gottron papules of the hands. **B,** Facial rash with periorbital and malar distribution. *(From Albert RK, Spiro SG, Jett JR [ed]: Clinical respiratory medicine, ed 2, St. Louis, Mosby, 2004, Fig. 48.6.)*

- Dermatomyositis/polymyositis (see Chapter 45)
  - Presents with proximal muscle weakness with or without pain (polymyositis)
  - Dermatomyositis is diagnosed if skin involvement is also present (Fig. 57-3)
  - Associated primarily with ovarian, breast, and lung cancers
  - Tumors usually present within 5 years of the diagnosis
  - Laboratory data reveal increased sedimentation rate and creatine phosphokinase level, and abnormal electromyogram
  - Muscle biopsy confirms the diagnosis

ENDOCRINOLOGIC SYNDROMES

- Carcinoid syndrome
  - Associated with carcinoid tumors of the small intestine, cervix, stomach, rectum, and lung
  - **Usually presents when there is metastasis to the liver**
  - Clinical symptoms include episodic flushing, diarrhea, abdominal pain, and wheezing
  - Fibrosis of the endocardium (predominantly tricuspid valve) is a late complication
  - Diagnose with 24-hour urine for 5-hydroxyindole-acetic acid, or elevated serum or platelet serotonin levels
  - Treat with surgical resection whenever possible
  - Somatostatin analogues may help control symptoms
- Cushing syndrome
  - Seen predominantly with small cell lung cancer, pancreatic islet cell tumors, thymic cancer, and bronchial carcinoid
  - Usually caused by ectopic secretion of adrenocorticotropic hormones from cancer cells but can rarely occur secondary to ectopic secretion of corticotropin-releasing hormone
  - Signs and symptoms include truncal obesity, fatigue, weakness, hypertension, abdominal striae, hyperpigmentation, hirsutism, polyuria, polydipsia
  - Laboratory evaluation (see Chapter 41)
  - Treatment is geared toward the underlying malignancy
  - Ketoconazole, metyrapone, or aminoglutethamide may be used to inhibit steroid production and provide symptomatic relief
- Acromegaly
  - Usually caused by ectopic release of growth hormone–releasing hormone (GH-RH)
  - Associated with bronchial carcinoids, pancreatic islet cell tumors, lung cancer, breast cancer, and colon cancer
  - Signs and symptoms include increasing glove and shoe size, impotence, hypertension, amenorrhea, diabetes
  - Elevated insulin-like growth factor-1, GH-RH, and glucose-suppressed growth hormone levels establish the diagnosis (see Chapter 41)
  - Treat the underlying malignancy
  - Bromocriptine and octreotide may be used to suppress growth hormone secretion from the pituitary
- Hypercalcemia (see Chapter 39)
  - Can be caused by parathyroid hormone–related protein, osteolytic metastases, and tumor production of calcitriol (seen mainly with lymphomas)
  - Most commonly occurs with lung cancer, breast cancer, and multiple myeloma
- Syndrome of inappropriate antidiuresis (see Chapter 32)
  - Caused by ectopic secretion of antidiuretic hormone
  - Most commonly seen with small cell lung cancer

NONBACTERIAL THROMBOTIC ENDOCARDITIS

- Caused by clotting and platelet activation by procoagulants released by tumors
- Associated primarily with adenocarcinomas (e.g., lung, GI tract)
- Sterile, verrucous lesions are seen, usually on left-sided heart valves
- Clinically may present as embolic stroke, seizure, confusion
- Can be associated with disseminated intravascular coagulation
- Diagnose with echocardiogram and/or cerebral angiogram with negative blood cultures
- Treatment is geared to the underlying malignancy

TABLE 57-4	*Delayed Toxicity of Selected Chemotherapeutic Agents*
Drug	**Toxicity**
Bleomycin	Pneumonitis and pulmonary fibrosis
Cisplatin	Hearing loss, nephrotoxicity, peripheral neuropathy
Cyclophosphamide	Hemorrhagic cystitis
Daunorubicin	Cardiomyopathy
Doxorubicin	Cardiomyopathy
Fluorouracil	Severe diarrhea, oral or GI ulcers, palmar or plantar rash
Methotrexate	Oral/GI ulcers, pulmonary infiltrates and fibrosis, cirrhosis
Paclitaxel	Peripheral neuropathy
Vincristine	Peripheral neuropathy

CUTANEOUS SYNDROMES

See Chapter 65.

Cancer Chemotherapy

Basic Information

- Most drugs are designed to impair cell division
- Selectivity stems from the effect on cells that are more rapidly dividing (i.e., tumor cells)
- Normal cells that rapidly divide are also affected, causing common toxicities (e.g., bone marrow suppression, hair loss, mucosal sloughing)
- Chemotherapy toxicity may be acute or chronic, dose dependent, or idiosyncratic

CHEMOTHERAPY TOXICITY

- Acute toxicities are common and include nausea, vomiting, diarrhea, headache, and fatigue
- Delayed toxicities
  - Bone marrow suppression is a common side effect of many agents
  - Some selective toxicities are listed in Table 57-4

TUMOR LYSIS SYNDROME

- Caused by rapid destruction of a large number of cancer cells
- **Results in hyperuricemia, hyperkalemia, hyperphosphatemia, lactic acidosis, hypocalcemia, and acute renal failure**
- Seen most commonly after treatment of leukemias and lymphomas
- Prevention of renal failure with fluid administration, allopurinol, and sodium bicarbonate should be attempted in high-risk patients (i.e., patients with high tumor burdens, baseline renal dysfunction, baseline hyperuricemia)
- Treatment with IV fluids, loop diuretics, alkalinization of the urine, and allopurinol can by tried initially in patients developing acute renal failure

- Treatment with rasburicase can lower the serum uric acid level rapidly, helping to prevent renal failure
- Hemodialysis may be necessary if the response is inadequate

FEBRILE NEUTROPENIA

Basic Information and Clinical Presentation

- Neutropenia is defined as absolute neutrophil count (ANC) less than 500/mL
- Fever usually defined as one temperature greater than 38.5°C or three temperatures above 38°C within 24 hours
- Usually occurs as a result of chemotherapy
- Patients may or may not have any localizing symptoms to suggest a source for infection
- Typical etiology is bacterial translocation from the GI tract
- Infectious agents to consider include *Staphylococcus aureus, Staphylococcus epidermidis, Escherichia coli, Klebsiella pneumoniae, Pseudomonas aeruginosa,* and fungi

Diagnosis

- History and physical examination
- Inspect rectal area but avoid digital rectal examination because it may introduce infection
- Obtain CBC and calculate ANC
- Obtain chest radiograph or CT chest
- Panculture (i.e., blood, urine, sputum, throat, stool [including *Clostridium difficile*])

Treatment

- **Empirical antibiotics should be administered immediately**
- Evaluation usually identifies a primary source of infection in only 20% of patients
- Antibiotic choice depends on hospital practice, but in general should be broad-spectrum unless causal organism is clear
- Possible antibiotic regimens
  - Single-agent therapy: Cefipime, cefotetan, imipenem-cilastin, meropenem, ceftazidime
  - Combination therapy: β-Lactam (e.g., piperacillin, ticarcillin) plus an aminoglycoside (e.g., gentamicin, tobramycin) or ciprofloxacin
- In patients with persistent fever, the addition of vancomycin or antifungal drugs (e.g., amphotericin or fluconazole) should be considered

TYPHLITIS

- Necrotizing infection of the cecum and colon
- Symptoms include fever, diarrhea, and right lower quadrant abdominal pain (mimics appendicitis)
- Seen predominantly after treatment for acute leukemia
- Treat with broad-spectrum antibiotics
- Surgery may be necessary

Acknowledgment

This chapter was based on the chapter by Mark Levis, MD, PhD, written for the third edition of the Johns Hopkins Internal Medicine Board Review.

57

REVIEW QUESTIONS

For review questions, please go to www.expertconsult.com.

SUGGESTED READINGS

Dropcho EJ: Update on paraneoplastic syndromes, *Curr Opin Neurol* 18:331–336, 2005.

Ettinger DS, Aqulnik M, Cristea M, et al: Occult primary, *J Natl Compr Canc Netw* 6:1026–1060, 2008.

Morris GJ, Greco FA, Hainsworth JD, et al: Cancer of unknown primary site, *Semin Oncol* 37:71–79, 2010.

Picazo JJ: Management of the febrile neutropenic patient: a consensus conference, *Clin Infect Dis* 39(Suppl 1):S1–S6, 2004.

Rice TW, Rodriguez RM, Light RW: The superior vena cava syndrome: clinical characteristics and evolving etiology,, *Medicine (Baltimore)* 85:37–42, 2006.

Schmidt MH, Klimo P Jr, Vrionis FD: Metastatic spinal cord compression, *J Natl Compr Canc Netw* 3:711–719, 2005.

Walji N, Chan AK, Peake DR: Common acute oncologic emergencies: diagnosis, investigation, and management, *Postgrad Med J* 84:418–427, 2008.

CHAPTER 58

Lung Cancer and Head and Neck Cancer

DAVID COSGROVE, MD

Lung cancer is now the most common cause of death due to cancer in both men and women in the United States, claiming 160,000 lives per year, about 28% of all cancer-related deaths. Given the well-established relationship between smoking and most types of lung cancer, it also remains the most preventable neoplastic disorder. Although head and neck cancer is less common than lung cancer, its relationship to tobacco use is similar, making it a highly preventable disease. This chapter will serve to highlight the features of these two smoking-related diseases.

Lung Cancer

Basic Information

- **Most common cause of death due to cancer in both genders**
- Incidence over the past decade has been declining in men but slowly increasing in women
- African American males have highest incidence rates for lung cancer
- Risk factors
  - Tobacco
    - **80% to 90% of lung cancer cases result from cigarette smoking**
    - Risk is dependent upon total lifetime consumption of cigarettes
    - Risk of lung cancer begins to decrease 5 years after smoking has ceased, although the risk always remains higher than that for a nonsmoker
    - Passive or secondhand smoke associated with increased risk (3–5% of all lung cancer cases)
    - Smoking of cigars may also increase risk, although the association is highly variable
  - Asbestos
    - Increases risk of bronchogenic carcinoma and mesothelioma
    - A potential hazard for a number of occupations, including plumbers, pipefitters, carpenters, electricians, welders, and insulation workers
  - Radon
  - Uranium
  - Ionizing radiation
  - Nickel, chromium
- Screening
  - Prospective studies of lung cancer screening do not support use of chest radiograph or sputum cytology

- Spiral computed tomography (CT) scan of chest is more sensitive than chest film and is being evaluated in multiple clinical studies in high-risk populations
- Initial studies suggest a lung cancer specific and overall survival benefit with CT screening in high risk groups, those with high lifetime tobacco exposure
- Pathology
  - Non–small cell lung cancer (60–80% of cases)
    - Adenocarcinoma
      - **Most common type in nonsmokers**
      - Peripheral location
      - Bronchoalveolar carcinoma is a subtype that presents diffusely within the lungs
    - Squamous cell
      - Can be associated with hypercalcemia as a paraneoplastic syndrome (see Chapters 39 and 57)
      - Central location
      - 10% undergo cavitation
    - Large cell lung cancer—usually peripheral location
  - Small cell lung cancer (15–20% of cases)
    - Small primary tumors, but adenopathy may be bulky
    - Associated with a number of paraneoplastic syndromes, most commonly syndrome of inappropriate antidiuretic hormone (SIADH)
  - Mesothelioma (Box 58-1)

Clinical Presentation

- Cough, dyspnea, and chest pain are the most common presenting symptoms
- Hemoptysis is seen more commonly with central lesions
- Recurrent or unresolving pneumonia caused by obstruction
- Hoarseness: Caused by recurrent laryngeal nerve compression
- **Horner syndrome: Ptosis, miosis, ipsilateral anhydrosis from sympathetic chain involvement of tumor**
- Paraneoplastic syndromes (see Chapter 57)
- **Shoulder pain: Pancoast tumors—apical tumors locally invading the lower brachial plexus (C8-T2) and chest wall, resulting in shoulder pain and plexopathy—may be missed on chest radiograph**
- Poor prognostic factors
  - Weight loss of more than 5% body weight
  - Advanced stage (see following discussion)
  - Poor performance status
  - *K-ras* oncogene mutation (non–small cell)

BOX 58-1	*Malignant Mesothelioma*

Most common risk factor is asbestos exposure

Male predominance

Disease manifests 20–30 yr after initial exposure; usually around age 60 yr

Presenting symptoms include dyspnea and chest pain

Chest imaging typically reveals pleural abnormality with a large pleural effusion

Diagnosis is made by thoracentesis and pleural biopsy

Treatment options are limited

    Extrapleural pneumonectomy with or without chemotherapy and radiation is one treatment strategy

Prognosis (even with treatment) is currently poor

FIGURE 58-1 **A** and **C,** Positron emission tomography/computed tomography (PET/CT) scans demonstrate right adrenal mass (*arrow*). **B,** Less well-delineated mass on CT scan (*arrow*). (*From Abeloff MD, Armitage JO, Niederhuber JE, et al [eds]: Clinical oncology, ed 3, Philadelphia, Churchill Livingstone, 2004, Fig. 75-9.*)

Diagnosis

- All patients should have a history and physical examination, complete blood count, chemistry profile, liver function tests, and CT scan of chest and abdomen
- Bronchoscopy
  - 80% to 85% effective in establishing a diagnosis for centrally located tumors
  - Not as effective for peripheral lesions
- CT-guided biopsy is about 90% effective for establishing a diagnosis for peripherally located tumors
- Mediastinoscopy may be used for diagnosis or staging (especially for anterior mediastinal lymph nodes)
- Positron emission tomography (PET) scan
  - Hypermetabolic tumors enhance on scanning
  - Considered more sensitive than CT for mediastinal disease (Fig. 58-1)
  - Currently recommended to confirm the presence of resectable non–small cell cancer
- Bone scan and head CT
  - For non–small cell cancers: Obtain if symptoms are suggestive of bony metastasis or neurologic disease

TABLE 58-1	*Staging for Non–Small Cell Lung Cancer*	
Stage	**Description**	**5-Year Survival Rate (%)**
I	Any size tumor with or without extension into visceral pleura, at least 2 cm from carina, no nodal involvement	60–80
II	Any size, extension into intrabronchial lymph nodes	40–50
IIIa	Any size, extension into parietal pleura, chest wall, or mediastinal pleura, or into hilar or ipsilateral mediastinal lymph nodes	20–30
IIIb	Any size, extension into mediastinal structures, contralateral hilar, mediastinal, or supraclavicular lymph nodes	10–20
IV	Evidence of distant metastasis	<5

- For small cell cancers: Obtain routinely as part of the staging work-up
- Staging
  - Non–small cell lung cancer: tumor-node-metastasis (TNM) staging criteria (Table 58-1)
  - Small cell lung cancer
    - Limited stage: Disease confined to one hemithorax and can be encompassed within a single radiation therapy port
    - Extensive stage: Disease spread outside of the preceding area

Treatment

- Non–small cell lung cancer (NSCLC)
  - Stages I to IIIa
    - **Surgery is the treatment of choice if performance status is good and postresection pulmonary reserve is deemed to be adequate (forced expiratory volume in 1 second [FEV$_1$] >0.8 L)**
    - Adjuvant chemotherapy or radiation may be beneficial for stage II and IIIa disease, but not for stage I disease
  - Stage IIIb: Definitive radiation therapy with or without chemotherapy
  - Stage IV
    - Goal is palliation
    - Chemotherapy prolongs survival
    - Erlotinib, a small molecule inhibitor of epidermal growth factor receptor (EGFR), is indicated as first-line treatment for patients with nonsquamous NSCLC with known activating mutations in EGFR
    - Bevacizumab, a monoclonal antibody targeting vascular endothelial growth factor, is indicated in conjunction with chemotherapy for patients with nonsquamous NSCLC, as long as no contraindication exists
- Small cell lung cancer
  - Limited stage
    - Combined chemotherapy (platinum-/etoposide-based regimen) plus concurrent radiation

- Consider prophylactic cranial irradiation
  - Decreases risk of brain metastases
  - No effect on survival in individual studies, but trend toward improved survival in meta-analysis
- Surgical resection may be an option in a small subset of patients after chemoradiation
- Median survival is 18 months
- Extensive stage
  - Chemotherapy with platinum/etoposide or irinotecan/etoposide
  - Median survival is 9 months

Head and Neck Cancer

Basic Information

- Responsible for as many as 11,000 cancer deaths per year, out of 48,000 cases diagnosed in the United States
- More common in men
- Median age is 60 years
- Can affect the oral cavity, larynx, pharynx, or nasopharynx
- Risk factors
  - Tobacco
    - Dose-response relationship between the occurrence of cancer and duration and amount of cigarette use
    - Secondhand smoke and cigars may also be risk factors
  - Alcohol
    - Increased risk with heavy use (>50 g/day)
    - No increased risk with moderate use (<19 g/day)
    - Risk is greatly increased in people who drink and smoke cigarettes heavily
  - Prior radiation therapy: Increased risk of salivary gland tumors
  - Plummer-Vinson syndrome
    - Characterized by dysphagia, iron deficiency anemia, and esophageal webs in women
    - Increased incidence of cancer of the hypopharynx and esophagus
  - **Epstein-Barr virus (EBV)**
    - **Strong association with nasopharyngeal carcinoma, which has a high incidence in southern China**
    - Pathology is usually undifferentiated rather than squamous cell type
  - Human papillomavirus (HPV)
    - Type 16 most strongly associated with invasive tumors of the oral cavity and oropharynx
    - Presence of HPV may confer a better prognosis
- Pathology
  - Most cancers in the United States are squamous cell carcinomas
  - Precancerous lesions
    - Leukoplakia (Fig. 58-2): Hyperkeratosis associated with a low malignant potential (<5% of cases)
    - Erythroplakia
      - Red, superficial patches adjacent to normal mucosa
      - Associated with dysplasia
      - Significant malignant potential (40% of cases)
    - Dysplasia
      - Presence of mitoses and prominent nucleoli
      - Can involve entire mucosa (carcinoma *in situ*)
      - Commonly progresses to invasive cancer

FIGURE 58-2 Leukoplakia of the hard palate. *(From Cummings CW, Flint PW, Harker LA, et al: Otolaryngology: head and neck surgery, ed 4, Philadelphia, Mosby, 2005, Fig. 64-5B.)*

- Lymphoepithelial: Undifferentiated tumors predominantly seen in nasopharyngeal carcinoma because of EBV (see preceding discussion)

Clinical Presentation

- Symptoms vary by the site of the tumor
  - Nasal cavity: Epistaxis, ulceration, nasal obstruction
  - Paranasal sinuses: Recurrent or persistent sinusitis
  - Nasopharyngeal: Mass, eustachian tube dysfunction, serous otitis media
  - Oral cavity, tongue, lips: Mass with or without ulceration
  - Laryngeal/glottic: Hoarseness, dysphagia, odynophagia, hemoptysis
- Cervical lymphadenopathy may sometimes be the only finding on presentation

Diagnosis

- History and physical examination with emphasis on risk factors and direct visualization of tumor
- **Fiberoptic endoscopy is necessary to assess the extent of the tumor as well as vocal cord mobility**
- Diagnosis is usually made by direct biopsy of tumor or fine-needle aspiration of a metastatic lymph node
- CT scan of the head and neck aids in the staging process
- Chest CT and panendoscopy (e.g., laryngoscopy, esophagoscopy, bronchoscopy) are helpful for detecting distant metastases and second primary lesions
- PET scan is useful for detecting recurrent tumors in patients who have had surgery and may be useful in detecting occult head and neck cancers

Treatment

- Staging system and treatments vary depending on the primary tumor site
- Primary therapy of squamous cell carcinoma usually includes surgery (possibly neck dissection; Fig. 58-3) and radiation therapy, although the role of chemotherapy continues to expand
  - Early (stages I and II)
    - Goal is for cure with either radiation or surgery
  - Advanced resectable (stages III and IV, without distant metastases)

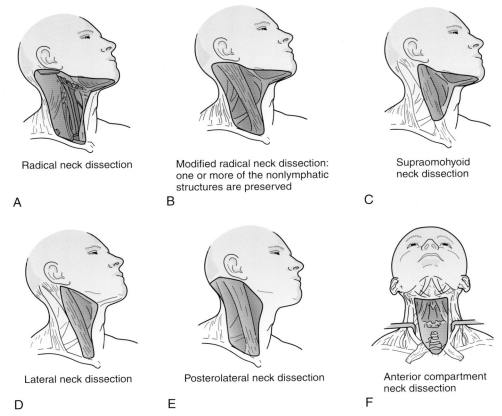

FIGURE 58-3   Types of neck dissection. **A,** Radical. **B,** Modified radical: One or more of the nonlymphatic structures are preserved. **C,** Supraomohyoid. **D,** Lateral. **E,** Posterolateral. **F,** Anterior compartment. *(From Abeloff MD, Armitage JO, Niederhuber JE, et al [eds]: Clinical oncology, ed 3, Philadelphia, Churchill Livingstone, 2004, Fig. 71-6.)*

- Oral cavity: Surgery and postoperative radiation plus chemotherapy
  - Pharynx: Definitive concurrent chemoradiation
- Advanced unresectable
  - Treat with chemoradiotherapy
  - Prognosis is poor
- Metastatic disease (typically remains localized to head and neck or thorax)
  - Radiation with or without chemotherapy
- Nasopharyngeal cancer is primarily treated with radiation therapy and chemotherapy
- Significant morbidity can be associated with treatment
  - Physical disfiguration
  - Loss of voice or hoarseness
  - Dysphagia or odynophagia leading to malnutrition
  - Xerostomia
    - Artificial saliva can provide temporary relief of symptoms
    - Oral pilocarpine is effective as a treatment and for prophylaxis
  - Osteoradionecrosis of the mandible
  - Fibrosis of neck, pharynx, temporomandibular joint, esophagus
  - Hypothyroidism
- Most tumor recurrences occur within 2 years of the initial treatment
- After 2 years, second primary aerodigestive tumors occur at 3% to 7% per year (field cancerization)

- **Recurrence risk higher in patients who continue to smoke**

Acknowledgment

This chapter was based on the chapter by Mark Levis, MD, PhD, written for the third edition of the Johns Hopkins Internal Medicine Board Review.

REVIEW QUESTIONS

For review questions, please go to www.expertconsult.com.

SUGGESTED READINGS

Cappuzzo F, Ciuleanu T, Stelmakh L, et al: Erlotinib as maintenance treatment in advanced non-small-cell lung cancer: a multicentre, randomized, placebo-controlled phase 3 study, *Lancet Oncol* 11:521–529, 2010.

Cognetti DM, Weber RS, Lai SY: Head and neck cancer: an evolving treatment paradigm, *Cancer* 113:S1911–S1932, 2008.

Hann CL, Rudin CM: Management of small-cell lung cancer: incremental changes but hope for the future, *Oncology* 22:1486–1492, 2008.

Jemal A, Siegel R, Ward E, et al: Cancer statistics, 2008, *CA Cancer J Clin* 58:71–96, 2008.

Molina JR, Yang P, Cassivi SD, et al: Non-small cell lung cancer: epidemiology, risk factors, treatment, and survivorship, *Mayo Clin Proc* 83:584–594, 2008.

Schiller JH, Adak S, Cella D, et al: Topotecan versus observation after cisplatin plus etoposide in extensive-stage small-cell lung cancer: E7593—a phase III trial of the Eastern Cooperative Oncology Group, *J Clin Oncol* 15:2114–2122, 2001.

Suzuki K, Nagai K, Yoshida J, et al: Prognostic factors in clinical stage I non-small cell lung cancer, *Ann Thorac Surg* 67:927–932, 1999.

SECTION TEN

Neurology

Headaches

APRIL S. FITZGERALD, MD

It has been estimated that as many as 90% of individuals experience at least one headache per year. The presentation in an outpatient setting is usually of benign origin, but headaches may also be the hallmark of a more ominous illness. Certain characteristics of the headache pattern will help guide the clinician in assessing the cause.

Primary Headache Syndromes

Basic Information

- A primary headache syndrome means the headache is the disease
  - More common in clinical practice than secondary headaches
  - No obvious structural or metabolic cause
- Common primary headache disorders
  - **Migraine** (see following section)
  - **Tension-type**
    - Episodic, occur less than 15 days a month
    - Chronic, occur more than 15 days a month
  - **Trigeminal autonomic cephalalgias (TACs)**
    - Short-lived attacks; unilateral pain in V1 distribution of trigeminal nerve (around eye) with autonomic features
    - **Cluster headache is most common subtype of TACs**
- Complete headache history is helpful in delineating headache type
- Complete physical exam should be done for a headache evaluation, with the focus on
  - Blood pressure
  - Optic exam: Papilledema may suggest increased intracranial pressure
  - Visual fields: Field cut warrants imaging
  - Facial tenderness (sinuses, temporal artery): Structural etiology versus giant-cell arteritis
  - Complete neurologic exam: Focal changes are more worrisome for a secondary headache etiology and warrant neuroimaging

Clinical Presentation

- Important features in the history that are helpful to categorize the headache type are listed in Table 59-1
- Also consider comorbid medical diseases in a patient with a headache
  - Hypertension, pregnancy, depression, infection, etc.

Diagnosis and Evaluation

- Diagnosis is based on history and physical
- If history is consistent with a primary headache syndrome and the physical exam is unrevealing, then central nervous system (CNS) imaging is usually unnecessary

Treatment

- Migraine (see following section)
- Tension-type headache
  - Nonsteroidal anti-inflammatory drugs (NSAIDs) or acetaminophen
  - Antianxiety medications or antidepressants if concomitant disorder exists
  - Biofeedback techniques to manage stress and tension (especially in chronic tension-type headache)
  - Avoid medication overuse as this may trigger a headache cycle
- Cluster headache
  - Abortive therapy
    - 100% oxygen inhalation (7 L/min) at onset of attack
    - Subcutaneous sumaptriptan
    - Dihydroergotamine (D.H.E. 45) IV or IM
    - Intranasal lidocaine for anesthesia during attack
  - Preventive therapy (during cluster phase)
    - Calcium channel blockers (verapamil)
    - Lithium
    - Prednisone taper
    - Valproate

Migraine Headache

Basic Information

- Pathophysiology is complex, starting in the brainstem and ultimately involving the trigeminal vascular system; abnormal signals cause release of neurotransmitters and dilation of blood vessels, leading to pain and further neural activation
- In migraine with aura subtype, familial hemiplegic migraine, there is an association with mutations in at least three genes that encode for neuron transmembrane channels (i.e., P/Q-type calcium channel, Na^+-K^+ pump)

Clinical Presentation

See Table 59-1 for clinical characteristics
- International Headache Society (IHS) classification scheme for migraine headache

TABLE 59-1	*Clinical Presentations of Primary Headache Syndromes*		
Characteristic	**Migraine Headache**	**Tension-Type Headache**	**Cluster Headache**
Onset (age/sex)	Peak incidence in adolescence More common in females Family history	Variable age of onset More common in females	Age 20–50 yr Male to female ratio 5:1
Frequency	1–2 attacks/mo, may be more frequent Often near menses	Episodic type: <15 days/mo Chronic type: >15 days/mo	*Nightly* or daily for 6–12 wk Circadian association Periods of headache freedom may last months to years
Potential triggers	Stress Too much or too little sleep Hormonal changes Variations in caffeine Red wine Foods: chocolate, cheese, MSG, nitrates	Fatigue Stress	Alcohol (in some or during a period of attacks)
Location	Unilateral > bilateral Bifrontal in 40%	Bilateral, neck, occipital	100% unilateral Temporal or orbital
Pain characteristics	Crescendo pattern Pulsating Moderate to severe pain Patient retreats to dark, quiet room	Pressure or squeezing Waxing/waning severity Patient may remain active	Quick onset of excruciating pain "Suicide headache" Deep and continuous (nonpulsating) Patient may pace or rock from severity of pain
Duration	4–72 hr	Minutes to days	30 min to 3 hr Average is 45–90 min
Associated symptoms	Nausea, vomiting, photophobia, phonophobia ± aura (visual, speech, or motor deficits)	None	*Ipsilateral* parasympathetic overactivity Ptosis, miosis, lacrimation, conjunctival injection Rhinorrhea, nasal congestion Cheek flushing, facial swelling

MSG, monosodium glutamate.

BOX 59-1	*Diagnostic Criteria for Migraine Without Aura*

At least five attacks fulfilling the following criteria:
Untreated headache lasting 4–72 hr
Group A (2 of 4):
1. Unilateral headache
2. Throbbing or pulsating pain
3. Moderate to severe pain that inhibits ability to function
4. Pain aggravated by routine physical activity
Group B (1 of 2):
1. Presence of nausea or vomiting
2. Presence of photophobia and phonophobia
Underlying disorders that may cause secondary headaches must be ruled out

- **Migraine without aura. Account for nearly 80% of migranes.** Diagnostic criteria outlined in Box 59-1.
- Migraine with aura
  - Requires three of four criteria with at least two attacks
  - One or more aura symptoms are fully reversible
  - Aura symptoms develop over more than 4 minutes, or two or more auras in succession
  - No aura lasts more than 60 minutes
  - Onset of headache within 60 minutes of aura termination
  - Underlying cranial disorder must be ruled out

- Retinal migraine
  - Monocular blindness with disk edema
  - Peripapillary hemorrhage and slow resolution of the vision loss
- Complications of migraine
  - Progression to chronic migraine
    - Migraines on more than 15 days a month
  - Infarction risk is increased in migraine with aura. Oral contraceptives significantly increases risk.

Diagnosis and Evaluation

- Based on history, physical examination, and classification scheme
- CNS imaging may be warranted for atypical presentations

Treatment

- Therapy for acute migraine attack
  - Treat attacks rapidly and consistently
  - Restore patient's ability to function
  - **Choose drug based on severity of headaches (stratified care approach)**
  - May need to use different approaches for different headaches in same patient
  - Analgesics
    - NSAIDs (e.g., aspirin, ibuprofen, naproxen sodium); combination agent of acetaminophen + aspirin + caffeine
      - Best for mild to moderate headaches but may be effective for severe attacks

- Decreased gastric motility may limit effectiveness
- Metoclopramide (Reglan)
  - Increases gastrointestinal motility and may help as antiemetic
  - Dopamine antagonist and may be used as monotherapy for treatment by IV route
- Serotonin$_{1B/1D}$ receptor agonists ("triptans")
  - **Drugs of choice for moderate or severe migraines or if no response to analgesics**
  - Contraindications: Ischemic cardiac or cerebrovascular disease, uncontrolled hypertension, basilar or hemiplegic migraines, ergotamine use
  - Use in pregnancy is Category C drugs: Inadequate data exist
  - Sumatriptan: Subcutaneous form with rapid onset of action
    - Inhaled and oral forms also available: Vary in half-life, onset time, tolerability, efficacy, return of headache
- Ergotamine with or without caffeine
  - Nonspecific serotonin agonist and vasoconstrictor
  - Frequent adverse effects including medication overuse headache
  - Contraindications: Vascular disease, liver disease, pregnancy (potent vasoconstrictor)
- Dihydroergotamine
  - Available in intranasal form with evidence for efficacy and safety
  - Less vasoactive than ergotamine
- Combination agents (acetaminophen/dichloralphenazone/isometheptene)
- Preventive therapy for migraine
  - Behavioral modification
    - Avoid "triggers" (e.g., foods, alcohol, caffeine, nicotine, nitrates)
    - Regular sleeping patterns
    - Minimize stress
  - Migraine diary to record patterns of headache and identify possible triggers
  - Consider prophylactic medication if
    - **Two or more attacks a month with 3 or more days of disability**
    - Failure or contraindication of acute therapy
    - Abortive medications required more than twice a week
  - Recommendations for use of prophylactic migraine medication
    - Start with low dose and titrate slowly
    - Decrease in headache frequency may be imperceptible the first month
      - First month, 10% decrease in frequency is considered successful
      - Improvement is cumulative, may take 6 months to reach efficacy
    - After a 6-month period of headache stability, consider taper
  - Migraine headache prevention medications
    - Antihypertensives
      - β-Blockers (propranolol, timolol, nadolol) demonstrate best evidence
      - Verapamil
      - Candesartan
      - Lisinopril (small trial showing efficacy)

BOX 59-2	"Red Flags" of Secondary Headache Syndromes

New-onset headache in absence of headache history
Onset age older than 40 yr
Unusually severe headache ("worst of life")
Headaches with progressive course
Significant change in headache pattern over prior 3 mo
Precipitation with exercise, Valsalva maneuver, head turning, supine position
Association with seizure or focal neurologic signs
Systemic symptoms (fever, weight loss, jaw pain)

- Antidepressants
  - **Tricyclics (amitriptyline); effect is unrelated to antidepressant activity**
  - Venlafaxine, selective serotonin reuptake inhibitors may also be effective
- Neuromodulators
  - Divalproex sodium (teratogenic)
  - Topiramate (may cause weight loss)
- NSAIDs (especially useful for menstrually related migraine)
- Botulinum toxin injection is being evaluated for those with muscular stress as migraine trigger
- Acupuncture
  - No more effective than "sham acupuncture" for migraine prevention, but both groups had fewer headaches than the untreated group so may have a role in acute treatment and prophylaxis
- Riboflavin (vitamin B$_2$)

Secondary Headaches

Basic Information

- A secondary headache syndrome means the headache is caused by an underlying pathologic or metabolic condition
  - Less common in clinical practice than primary headaches
  - Often abnormal neurologic exam
  - **Consider secondary headache even when a patient has a history of primary headaches but the headache pattern changes**

Clinical Presentation

- "Red flags" of secondary headache syndromes (Box 59-2)
- Secondary headache types
  - Subarachnoid hemorrhage (SAH)
    - **Classic "worst headache of life" caused by ruptured intracranial aneurysm**
    - Warning or "thunderclap" headache in 20% to 50% of patients with SAH (severe headache lasting minutes in the days to weeks prior to major bleed)
    - Headache is severe and develops in seconds
    - Diagnosis
      - Noncontrast computed tomography (CT) scan is first choice (Fig. 59-1)
      - If CT done within 24 hours, blood seen in subarachnoid space in 92% of cases

59

FIGURE 59-1 Computed tomography scan of the brain showing a subarachnoid bleed due to a middle cerebral artery aneurysm (*arrow*). *(From Townsend CM, Beauchamp RD, Evers BM, Mattox K: Sabiston textbook of surgery, ed 17, Philadelphia, WB Saunders, 2004, Fig. 71-1A.)*

- Sensitivity begins to decline after 24 hours after bleed
- Lumbar puncture if head CT negative
    - Xanthochromia is criterion for SAH (red blood cells break down, releasing hemoglobin, which is metabolized to reveal xanthochromia)
    - May be negative if bleed less than 12 hours or more than 2 weeks old
- Meningeal irritation or meningitis
    - Systemic symptoms, stiff neck, fever
    - Diagnosis made by lumbar puncture
- Brain tumor
    - Usually other neurologic findings present (seizures, vomiting, papilledema)
    - Worse in morning or if supine
    - Diagnosis made by CNS imaging
- Temporal arteritis (giant-cell arteritis)
    - Vasculitis of large and medium blood vessels
    - **Two thirds of patients with giant-cell arteritis have headache with localized temporal pain or jaw claudication**
    - Patients are typically older than 50 years
    - Other systemic features present (fever, fatigue, weight loss)
    - Diagnosis made by temporal artery biopsy
    - Other autoimmune illnesses (lupus, vasculitis) may present with headache
- Low-pressure headaches
    - Occur from contraction of subarachnoid space from a cerebrospinal fluid leak or lumbar puncture (Marfan and Ehler-Danlos syndromes predispose to spontaneous leak)
    - Pain is worse with standing and relieved when supine

- Bed rest, hydration, and analgesics are mainstay of therapy
- Caffeine (PO or IV) may help relieve the pain
- Subdural hematoma
    - Gradual onset of headache often associated with fall
    - Often seen with elderly patients presenting with headache
    - Diagnosis made with CNS imaging
- Idiopathic intracranial hypertension (previously known as pseudotumor cerebri)
    - Increased intracranial pressure without mass
    - **More commonly presents in overweight young women**
    - Associated with isotretinoin (Accutane), tetracycline, hypervitaminosis A, oral contraceptives
    - Headache pattern similar to tension-type headache
    - **Neurologic exam is normal except for papilledema. Can have sixth nerve palsy and possible vision loss.**
    - Diagnosis
        - Patient has normal head CT but elevated opening pressure on lumbar puncture without other cause for increased pressure
- Cerebral venous thrombosis
    - Rare cause of headache with increased intracranial pressure
    - CT scan may be normal in 30% of cases
    - Magnetic resonance venogram is gold standard

Chronic Daily Headache

Basic Information

- Category of headaches that represent primary and secondary types
- Headache frequency more than 15 days of the month and duration longer than 3 months
- Chronic migraine and medication overuse headaches are two of the more common types of chronic daily headache

Clinical Presentation

- Chronic migraine and medication overuse headache patients are more frequently women and have history of episodic migraines
- Medications implicated in causing medication overuse headache
    - Overuse of any headache medication for more than 3 months
    - Simple analgesic use more often than 15 days a month
    - Combination analgesics, narcotics, ergotamine, triptans more than 10 days a month

Treatment (Medication Overuse Headache)

- Lifestyle modification (discontinue caffeine; exercise, regular sleep patterns, etc.)
- Stop all medications (taper opioids)
- If severe headache, try NSAIDs or dihydroergotamine (parenteral route)
- Consider preventive migraine therapy
- A short course of steroids can reduce headache severity during withdrawal

Acknowledgment

This chapter was based on the chapter by Dr. Kimberly Peairs written for the third edition of the Johns Hopkins Internal Medicine Board Review.

REVIEW QUESTIONS

For review questions, please go to www.expertconsult.com.

SUGGESTED READINGS

Buse D, Rupnow M, Lipton R: Assessing and managing all aspects of migraine: migraine attacks, migraine-related functional impairment, common comorbidities, and quality of life, *Mayo Clin Proc* 84:422–435, 2009.

Detsky M, McDonald D, Baerlocher M, et al: Does this patient with headache have a migraine or need neuroimaging? *JAMA* 296:1274–1283, 2006.

Edlow JA, Caplan LR: Avoiding pitfalls in the diagnosis of subarachnoid hemorrhage, *N Engl J Med* 342:29–36, 2000.

Halker RB, Hastriter EV, Dodick DW: Chronic daily headache: an evidence-based and systematic approach to a challenging problem, *Neurology* 76:S37–S43, 2011.

Kaniecki R: Headache assessment and management, *JAMA* 289:1430–1433, 2003.

Lipton RB, Loder EW: Migraine: primary care challenges in diagnosis and treatment, *Am J Med* 118(Suppl 1):28S–35S, 2005.

Marks DR, Rapoport AM: Practical evaluation and diagnosis of headache, *Semin Neurol* 17:307–312, 1997.

Olesen J, Bousser MG, Diener H, et al: The International Classification of Headache Disorders, ed 2, *Cephalalgia* 23(Suppl 1):1–160, 2004.

Wilson JF: In the clinic. Migraine, *Ann Intern Med* 147, 2007. ITC11-1–ITC11-16.

59

Cerebrovascular Disease and Seizure Disorders

RAFAEL H. LLINÁS, MD; and ROBERT J. WITYK, MD

Cerebrovascular disease is a common disorder in the United States, occurring at a rate of 1 per 1000 population. It is the third leading cause of medical deaths in developed countries. Stroke can be classified into ischemic disease (80%) and hemorrhagic disease (20%). Mortality from ischemic stroke has been declining in the United States because of an increased awareness and attention to modification of risk factors.

Seizures are electrical events of the brain, with varied clinical manifestations, that can be a cause of significant morbidity. Epilepsy is the chronic recurrence of seizures with a usual onset before age 20 years. Often, the underlying cause of epilepsy is unknown.

Cerebrovascular Disease

Basic Information

- Definitions
  - **Ischemic stroke: Focal neurologic deficit lasting more than 24 hours because of loss of blood flow to a portion of the brain that results in irreversible cell death (Fig. 60-1)**
    - Mechanisms
      - Large-vessel atherosclerosis
      - Embolic disease
  - **Transient ischemic attack (TIA): Transient focal neurologic deficit caused by loss of regional blood flow; lasts less than 24 hours, but typically only 10 to 60 minutes**
  - **Intracerebral hemorrhage: Bleeding into the brain parenchyma (Fig. 60-2)**
  - **Subarachnoid hemorrhage (SAH): Bleeding into the subarachnoid space around the brain**
- Classification of ischemic cerebrovascular disease (Table 60-1)

Clinical Presentation

- **Ischemic atherosclerotic stroke risk factors are similar to those of coronary artery disease (CAD)**
  - Increasing age
  - Male sex
  - African American
  - Hypertension, diabetes, high cholesterol
  - Smoking
  - Drug abuse (cocaine, amphetamines)
  - Sedentary lifestyle, obesity

- Family history
- **Embolic stroke risk factors**
  - Cardiac arrhythmias: Atrial fibrillation, sick sinus syndrome
  - Dilated cardiomyopathy, including left ventricular aneurysm
  - Valvular disorders, including prosthetic valves, rheumatic heart disease
  - Infective and nonbacterial endocarditis
  - Left ventricular or left atrial thrombus
  - Cardiac myxoma
  - Atrial and ventricular septal defects, patent foramen ovale
- TIAs
  - Usually last 10 to 15 minutes; most resolve within 1 hour
  - High correlation with future stroke (lifetime risk is 33%)
  - Predictor of vascular death, especially myocardial infarction
  - Amaurosis fugax is a common presentation
    - Temporary monocular blindness ("shade falling over vision")
    - Secondary to carotid artery atherosclerosis with embolization
- Classic (common) ischemic stroke presentations (see Table 60-1)
- Hemorrhagic stroke (Table 60-2)
  - **Subarachnoid hemorrhage**
    - **Bleeding in the space between the brain and the pia arachnoid**
    - **Mortality 50%; prognosis particularly poor for patients who present in coma**
    - Often seen in younger patients (age 35–65 years)
    - Causes, presentation, treatment (see Table 60-2)
    - Berry aneurysm is common cause (Fig. 60-3)
    - May occur with exertion, during rest, or even in sleep
    - **Complications of SAH**
      - **Rebleeding: Most common in first 2 weeks; 50% mortality**
      - **Hydrocephalus**
      - **Vasospasm: Cause of late ischemic infarctions**
      - **Hyponatremia (caused by atrial natriuretic factor)**
      - **Autonomic dysfunction**

FIGURE 60-1 Magnetic resonance angiogram demonstrating occlusion of the left middle cerebral artery (*arrow*), consistent with a thromboembolic event. *(From Forbes CD, Jackson WF: Color atlas and text of clinical medicine, ed 3, St. Louis, Mosby, 2003, Fig. 11.34.)*

FIGURE 60-2 Hemorrhagic cerebral infarction demonstrated by a noncontrast computed tomography scan. *(From Forbes CD, Jackson WF: Color atlas and text of clinical medicine, ed 3, St. Louis, Mosby, 2003, Fig. 11.66.)*

TABLE 60-1	*Classification of Ischemic Cerebrovascular Disease*		
	Examples	**Clinical Presentation**	**Treatment**
Large artery atherosclerosis	Carotid stenosis (extra- or intracranial) Vertebrobasilar disease	Carotid stenosis Ipsilateral face and hand numbness/weakness Aphasia or dysarthria Amaurosis fugax Vertebrobasilar disease Dizziness Vertigo Ataxia "Drop attack"	For intracranial carotid disease: antiplatelet agent or anticoagulation For extracranial carotid disease: <30%: Antiplatelet agent 50–70%: Modest benefit of carotid endarterectomy (CAE) >70% and symptomatic: CEA For vertebrobasilar disease: Antiplatelet agent or anticoagulation
Lacune (small-vessel disease)	Atherosclerosis of small, penetrating vessels Associated with hypertension and diabetes	Pure motor ipsilateral hemiparesis (caused by internal capsule or pons lesion) Pure ipsilateral hemisensory stroke (caused by thalamic lesion)	Antiplatelet agents
Cardiac embolism	Atrial fibrillation Dilated cardiomyopathy Endocarditis	Presentation depends on site of embolization Often occurs at gray-white junction	Anticoagulation for primary or secondary prevention (except for endocarditis—bleeding risk too high) Acute anticoagulation not advised because of bleeding risk
Nonatherosclerotic vasculopathy	Fibromuscular dysplasia (FMD) Arterial dissection Vasculitis	Depends on location FMD more common in women May have systemic symptoms with vasculitis May have neck pain with arterial dissection	Treat underlying cause (i.e., vasculitis) Antiplatelet agent for FMD Antiplatelet agent for anticoagulation for arterial dissection
Hematologic disorders/coagulopathy	Antiphospholipid antibody Sickle cell disease	Depends on location	Treat underlying cause Consider anticoagulation for antiphospholipid antibodies
Watershed infarction	Caused by hypotension from various causes (e.g., shock)	Bilateral proximal weakness of arms and legs	Volume repletion Treat underlying cause
Other Drug abuse Migraine Venous infarction	Cocaine Sagittal sinus thrombosis	Depends on location	Individualize treatment Consider anticoagulation for cerebral vein thrombosis

60

TABLE 60-2	*Hemorrhagic Cerebrovascular Disease*			
	Etiology	**Clinical Presentation**	**Diagnosis**	**Treatment**
Subarachnoid hemorrhage	Berry aneurysm (at bifurcation of vessels in circle of Willis) Trauma (dissecting aneurysm) Atherosclerosis (fusiform aneurysm) Infection (mycotic aneurysm) Arteriovenous malformation (AVM)	Sudden, severe headache—"worst of life" Meningismus Often decreased consciousness Focal neurologic deficits possible Oculomotor palsy (CN III) is clue to posterior communicating artery aneurysm (common location)	CT is most sensitive to blood; >90% accuracy If CT is negative but suspicion high, must perform LP with RBC counts in tubes 1 and 4, as well as spin for xanthochromia MRI relatively insensitive Cerebral angiography to detect underlying aneurysm	Supportive care Nimodipine for associated vasospasm Early surgical clipping of aneurysms in patients with minor deficits Endovascular therapy (coiling of aneurysms)
Intracranial hemorrhage (ICH)	Chronic hypertension (50–80% of ICH) Cerebral amyloid angiopathy (older patients with Alzheimer disease) AVM (young patients) Tumor (renal cell, melanoma, glioma, choriocarcinoma) Drugs (cocaine, amphetamines, phenylpropanolamine) Other: vasculitis, coagulopathy, endocarditis, thrombocytopenia	Headache Vomiting Coma Seizures May be sudden onset or gradual progression of symptoms Lobar most common, followed by basal ganglia, thalamus, cerebellum, pons	CT most sensitive to blood MRI with gadolinium to detect underlying AVM, tumor Cerebral angiography if AVM suggested Avoid LP if mass effect from bleed	Control extreme hypertension Ventilation; airway protection Intracranial pressure management: Elevate head of bed, avoid hypotonic fluids, possibly mannitol and hyperventilation Surgical evacuation if possible
Subdural hemorrhage	Trauma (often minor in elderly)	Headache Confusion Seizures	CT: Concave-shaped bleed, may have mass effect	Supportive care Consider surgical evacuation
Epidural hemorrhage	Trauma	Headache Decreased level of consciousness	CT: Lens-shaped bleed between dura and skull, pushing on parenchyma	Often requires urgent surgical evacuation

CN, cranial nerve; CT, computed tomography; LP, lumbar puncture; MRI, magnetic resonance imaging; RBC, red blood cell.

FIGURE 60-3 Proximal left middle cerebral artery aneurysm. Comparison of computed tomographic angiography (CTA) with conventional catheter angiography. **A,** Maximum-intensity projection image from CTA of the circle of Willis shows a berry aneurysm of the M1 segment. **B,** Catheter angiography, submentovertex view following left internal carotid artery injection, shows excellent correlation. *(From Bradley WG, Daroff RB, Fenichel GM, Jankovic J: Neurology in clinical practice, ed 4, Philadelphia, Butterworth-Heinemann, 2004, Fig. 37B.16.)*

- Intracerebral hemorrhage
  - Numerous causes
  - Presentation and treatment (see Table 60-2)
- **Subdural hematoma**
  - **Classic "crescent" shape on computed tomography (CT) underlying inner table of the skull (Fig. 60-4)**
  - Often seen in elderly after trauma, particularly if on anticoagulants
- Epidural hematoma
  - Often seen with trauma associated with skull fracture
  - Classic "lens" shape pushing on parenchyma by CT

Diagnosis and Evaluation

- **General diagnostic evaluation: Tailor to individual presentation**
  - Brain imaging
    - CT (high sensitivity for blood)
    - Magnetic resonance imaging (MRI) (better for brainstem visualization or lacunar strokes)
  - Vascular imaging
    - Carotid duplex ultrasound
    - CT angiography
    - Transcranial Doppler (ultrasound of intracranial vessels)

FIGURE 60-4 Head computed tomography scan demonstrating an acute subdural hematoma. *(From Ferrera PC, Couciello SA, Marx J, Verdile V: Trauma management: an emergency medicine approach, St. Louis, Mosby, 2001, Fig. 11-2.)*

- Magnetic resonance angiography
- **Cerebral angiography (gold standard)**
  - **Better anatomic localization of disease**
  - **Involves dye load**
  - **1% risk of stroke with procedure**
- Cardiac evaluation
  - Electrocardiogram (examine rhythm, evidence of old CAD)
  - **Echocardiogram: Transesophageal preferred over transthoracic for better visualization of atria and aorta**
  - Holter monitor: Often low yield for arrhythmia
- Other
  - **Hypercoagulable evaluation (especially in young stroke patients; consider antiphospholipid antibodies and lupus anticoagulant)**
  - Toxicology
  - Blood cultures
- Differential diagnosis of stroke or TIA
  - Focal seizure with Todd paralysis (see following discussion)
  - Complicated migraine
  - Brain mass
  - Peripheral vestibular disorder
  - Cardiac arrhythmia

Treatment

- General treatment of ischemic stroke
  - Supportive medical care: Prevent aspiration, deep venous thromboembolism, pressure sores
  - **Recommend against aggressive blood pressure control in the acute setting because this may lower cerebral perfusion**
  - **Aggressively control fever and hyperglycemia (may worsen stroke outcome)**
  - Observe for cerebral edema (peaks typically at 48 hours)

- **Antiplatelet therapy: Reduction of future events by roughly 25%**
  - Aspirin: 81 to 325 mg/day
  - Clopidogrel: 75 mg/day
    - Rare cases of thrombotic thrombocytopenic purpura reported
  - Dipyridamole 200 mg plus aspirin 25 mg sustained-release orally twice daily
- Anticoagulants
  - **Heparin: No proven benefit and acutely increases bleeding risk**
  - Low-molecular-weight heparinoids: No proven benefit but alternative to IV heparin
  - **Warfarin for secondary prevention of cardioembolic stroke in atrial fibrillation**
  - **New thrombin inhibitors such as dabigatran have been shown to prevent stroke in atrial fibrillation to same degree as warfarin**
    - **It is important to remember that the thrombin inhibitors cannot be reversed with fresh-frozen plasma**
- **Thrombolytic therapy**
  - Food and Drug Administration approval for tissue plasminogen activator (tPA) in 1996
  - For use in acute ischemic stroke
  - **Criteria for use**
    - **Suggested acute ischemic stroke**
    - **Administration of tPA within 3 hours from onset of symptoms**
    - New data suggest that patients who received within 4.5 hour window have benefit also, but less so
    - **No contraindications for thrombolytic therapy (i.e., active GI bleeding and others as with thrombolysis for myocardial infarction)**
  - **Exclusions for use of tPA**
    - Time of onset uncertain or more than 3 hours
    - Minor stroke or resolving symptoms
    - Suggested or witnessed seizure
    - Blood pressure greater than 185/110 mm Hg or requiring aggressive treatment
    - Early hypodensity or other lesion on CT that would increase risk of bleeding (e.g., tumor)
  - Protocol
    - tPA dose 0.9 mg/kg, maximum dose of 90 mg (10% bolus followed by 60-minute infusion)
    - No invasive procedures for 24 hours
    - Strict blood pressure control to keep less than 185/110 mm Hg
- Carotid endarterectomy (CEA)
  - Useful for extracranial carotid stenosis
  - Helpful for long-term management and prevention of future events
  - **Indications (based on large trials)**
    - **50% to 70% symptomatic stenosis: Modest benefit from CEA; individualize treatment**
    - **Greater than 70% symptomatic stenosis: CEA superior to medical therapy in patients who are good surgical candidates**
    - **Greater than 60% asymptomatic stenosis: Modest benefit from CEA over medical therapy; individualize treatment**

60

- Carotid stenting
  - Useful for those patients who are not surgical candidates
  - Head-to-head trials versus CEA still pending
  - Surgery still preferred treatment for patients who are good surgical candidates

Seizure Disorders

Basic Information

- **Seizures do not necessarily imply epilepsy; they may be caused by a temporary underlying disorder**
- In adults, the most common type of seizure is complex partial (40%), followed by generalized and simple partial seizures
- **The most common cause of epilepsy is "idiopathic" or "cryptogenic"**
- Up to 70% of patients can achieve remission; about half of these (35%) can remain seizure-free without medication

Clinical Presentation

- Classification of seizures (Table 60-3)
  - **Partial seizures: Onset is limited to one cerebral hemisphere**
    - May be motor, sensory, or psychoillusory ("déjà vu")
    - May generalize secondarily
    - "Jacksonian march": Focal seizure that begins in motor cortex and spreads to rest of motor area; clinically, clonic movements that spread proximally (usually up a limb)
  - **Primary generalized seizures (grand mal): Involve the cerebral cortex diffusely from the beginning**
- Each class of seizures can have varied clinical presentations (see Table 60-3)
- Todd paralysis: A transient (not longer than 48 hours) neurologic deficit (e.g., motor weakness) after a seizure that reflects postictal depression of the involved area
- Tongue biting and incontinence can be hallmarks

Diagnosis and Evaluation

- **Diagnosis depends on the clinical presentation and setting; electroencephalogram (EEG) findings are helpful but not definitive**
- Goals of diagnosis
  - Classify the type of seizure
  - Determine if epilepsy is truly present
  - Identify the underlying cause if possible
- Seizures may have underlying structural causes (e.g., hippocampal sclerosis, glial tumors, cavernous malformations, encephalitis, trauma, hemorrhage)
- **Consider metabolic and other causes of seizure (secondary seizure) in the right clinical setting**
  - Hyperglycemia (often focal seizures)
  - Hypoglycemia
  - Hyponatremia
  - Hypoxia
  - Uremia
  - Meningitis, encephalitis
  - Head trauma
- Drugs that can precipitate seizures
  - Antibiotics such as metronidazole, ciprofloxacin, acyclovir, high-dose penicillin and its derivatives

TABLE 60-3	Classification of Seizures	
Class	**Definition**	**Examples**
Simple partial seizure	Normal consciousness	Simple motor (limb jerking) Simple sensory (paresthesias)
Complex partial seizure	Alteration of consciousness	"Temporal lobe epilepsy" Aura (strange odor, déjà vu, automatisms, lip smacking, agitation, nondirected violence) May be associated with frontal or temporal lobe tumors, herpes encephalitis, hippocampal sclerosis
Generalized seizure	Complete impairment of consciousness	Primary generalized tonic-clonic (grand mal) Secondary generalized tonic-clonic (focal seizure that spreads) Absence (petit mal) Myoclonic (juvenile myoclonic epilepsy) Atonic (Lennox-Gastaut syndrome; "drop attack")

- Bupropion
- Methylphenidate
- Rapid withdrawal of barbiturates, alcohol, benzodiazepines
- Differential diagnosis of seizures
  - Convulsive syncope
  - **Pseudoseizures**
    - **Also known as psychogenic seizures**
    - **Change in behavior not associated with abnormal brain electrical activity**
    - Often helpful to check prolactin 15 to 45 minutes after the event (will be normal in pseudoseizures, elevated in true seizure disorder)
  - Anoxic myoclonus
- Evaluation of new-onset seizures
  - History: Focality of onset, aura, family history (may need to talk with witnesses)
  - Brain imaging: MRI with gadolinium enhancement is best to rule out structural abnormalities
  - EEG (Fig. 60-5)
    - **"Spikes" or "sharp waves" help localize seizure focus and classify seizure type**
    - **Most useful if obtained during a clinical attack to avoid false negatives**
    - EEG in the setting of sleep deprivation enhances seizure detection
    - Video EEG for unusual symptoms or suggested pseudoseizures
  - **Serum prolactin may be elevated at 45 minutes with partial complex or generalized seizures**
  - Increased recurrent seizure risk: Focal neurologic deficit, brain lesion, abnormal EEG
  - **First isolated seizure: Recurrence rate is 50% within 2 years if untreated (25% if treated); risk drops to about 20% if physical examination, MRI, and EEG are all normal**

FIGURE 60-5   Electroencephalogram recorded at the onset of a generalized tonic-clonic seizure. *(From Goetz B: Textbook of clinical neurology, ed 2, Philadelphia, WB Saunders, 2003, Fig. 24-7.)*

Treatment

- General principles
  - New seizure onset
    - **Work-up as in preceding section; hospitalization is usually not necessary**
    - **Initiation of drug treatment for first seizure is controversial; must tailor to individual; assessing risk of further seizures is helpful**
      - Low risk: Normal physical examination, MRI, EEG, no history of brain trauma, and no family history of epilepsy
      - Higher risk (consider drug therapy): Two or more of preceding risk factors
  - Seizures that do not need long-term treatment: Drug- or alcohol-related, seizures immediately associated with head injury, convulsive syncope
  - Seizures from metabolic causes: Treat the underlying metabolic abnormality
- Common antiepileptic drugs (Table 60-4)
- Antiepileptic drugs of choice by diagnosis (Table 60-5)
- **Adverse effects common to most antiepileptic drugs**
  - **Dose-related side effects: Ataxia, nausea, sedation, diplopia**
  - "Allergic" effects (all except phenobarbital): Neutropenia, thrombocytopenia, aplastic anemia
  - **Drug interactions: Can be complex, but most antiepileptics induce cytochrome P450 and increase metabolism of other drugs (e.g., warfarin, other anticonvulsant drugs, folate, oral contraceptives)**
- Birth defects
  - All antiepileptics increase birth defects twofold (3% increased to 6%)
  - Valproate felt to be worst offender
  - Patient should be on folic acid supplements at time of conception
- Surgical treatment

- Consider when drug therapy fails (usually defined as two trials of high-dose monotherapy and one trial of combination therapy)
- Most common procedure: Focal cortical resection
  - Must be able to identify focal epileptogenic region
  - Surgery must not leave patient with significant neurologic deficits
  - Most commonly used for refractory temporal lobe epilepsy
- **Treatment of status epilepticus**
  - Medical emergency
  - Untreated, a variety of complications may occur, including aspiration, hypertension, cardiac dysrhythmias, lactic acidosis, rhabdomyolysis, hyperpyrexia, and, ultimately, death
  - Assess: Give oxygen; obtain IV access; send stat chemistry (glucose, calcium, magnesium)
  - Give IV normal saline, thiamine 100 mg, and 1 ampule of D50 empirically
  - Seizure-specific therapy (in usual order of preference)
    - Lorazepam 2 to 4 mg IV at 2 mg/min (0.05–0.2 mg/kg), maximum 8 mg for adults
    - Phenytoin 20 mg/kg IV in 50 mL normal saline at maximum rate of 50 mg/min (e.g., 1000 mg over 20 minutes for an adult), or fosphenytoin 20 "phenytoin equivalents" (PE)/kg IV at maximum rate of 150 PE/min (1 g IV over 10 minutes)
      - Monitor for hypotension, arrhythmia
    - Phenobarbital 20 mg/kg IV at 100 mg/min (5–10 mg/kg)
      - Monitor for respiratory depression
    - Pentobarbital coma
      - Last resort
      - Potential complications: Hypotension, hypothermia, decreased cardiac output

60

TABLE 60-4	Common Antiepileptic Drugs		
Drug	**Indication**	**Typical Dose**	**Side Effect**
Lorazepam	Rapid treatment of acute seizures Not useful for long-term prophylaxis	0.5–1 mg PO every 6–8 hr	Sedation Respiratory compromise
Phenytoin	Partial seizures Generalized seizures	300 mg PO daily	IV dose may cause cardiac arrhythmias Nausea, ataxia, sedation Rash Hypersensitivity (mononucleosis-like) syndrome with rash, fever, lymphadenopathy Gingival hyperplasia Peripheral neuropathy Cerebellar degeneration Osteoporosis Fosphenytoin may be safer but is more costly
Carbamazepine	Partial seizures Generalized seizures Temporal lobe epilepsy	200 mg PO bid–tid	Nausea, ataxia, sedation Rash Leukopenia Aplastic anemia Hyponatremia Osteoporosis
Phenobarbital	Generalized seizures	30–120 mg PO daily	Sedation Respiratory depression with IV dosing
Valproic acid (valproate)	Partial seizures Generalized seizures Myoclonic seizures Lennox-Gastaut seizures	500–1000 mg PO bid–tid	Nausea Weight gain Birth defects Tremor Thrombocytopenia and platelet dysfunction Hair loss Pancreatitis
Gabapentin	Add-on to other therapy	300–900 mg tid	Sedation Ataxia
Levetiracetam	Add on therapy	500 mg bid	Agitation, exacerbation of psychiatric symptoms

bid, twice daily; IV, intravenous; PO, orally; tid, three times daily.

TABLE 60-5	Antiepileptic Drugs of Choice by Diagnosis
Type of Seizure	**Drug of Choice**
Generalized seizure	Phenytoin Carbamazepine Valproate Phenobarbital Levetiracetam
Partial complex seizure	Carbamazepine
Absence seizure	Ethosuxomide
Myoclonic seizure	Valproate
Add-on therapy	Gabapentin Lamotrigine Topiramate Levetiracetam

REVIEW QUESTIONS

For review questions, please go to www.expertconsult.com.

SUGGESTED READINGS

Brodie MJ, Dichter MA: Antiepileptic drugs, *N Engl J Med* 334:168–175, 1996.

International Stroke Trial Collaborative Group: The International Stroke Trial (IST): a randomized trial of aspirin, subcutaneous heparin, both, or neither among 19,435 patients with acute ischemic stroke, *Lancet* 349:1569–1581, 1997.

Moore WS, Barnett HJ, Beebe HG, et al: Guidelines for carotid endarterectomy: a multidisciplinary consensus statement from the Ad Hoc Committee, American Heart Association, *Circulation* 91:566–579, 1995.

The National Institute of Neurological Disorders and Stroke rt-PA Stroke Study Group: Tissue plasminogen activator for acute ischemic stroke, *N Engl J Med* 333:1581–1587, 1995.

Wityk RJ, Caplan LR: Hypertensive intracerebral hemorrhage: epidemiology and clinical pathology, *Neurosurg Clin North Am* 3:521–532, 1992.

Movement Disorders

SHAWN F. SMYTH, MD; RAINER von COELLN, MD, PhD; and JOSEPH M. SAVITT, MD, PhD

The primary motor pathways from the cerebral cortex to the brainstem and spinal cord (upper motor neuron) and from the brainstem and spinal cord to the muscle (lower motor neuron) control the basics of voluntary muscle contraction. The term *movement disorders* refers to disorders at a higher level of control over movement, such as the speed, timing, gain, accuracy, planning, feedback, and integration of directed movement. While ancillary testing can help in the diagnosis of disorders of higher level movement control, the diagnosis predominantly depends on the recognition of clinical patterns of movement. Thus, understanding the nature and types of abnormal movements is crucial to the diagnosis of these disorders.

- Initial questions regarding movement disorders:
  - Are abnormal movements present?
  - Are there impairments in normal movements?
  - What is the nature of the abnormality (i.e. what is it called)?
  - What is the cause?
  - Are there treatments to address the underlying cause of the disorder and/or to control the abnormal movement?

There are two categories of abnormal movements based on whether excessive movement (hyperkinesis) or not enough movement (hypokinesis) is seen. Also addressed in this chapter are other topics in movement disorders that do not neatly fit this distinction.

- **Hyperkinesis = too much movement:**
  - Tremor
  - Chorea, athetosis, and ballism
  - Dystonia
  - Myoclonus
  - Urge to move: Tics, restless legs syndrome, akathisia
- **Hypokinesis = too little movement:**
  - Parkinsonism
  - Parkinson disease
  - Catatonia (often classified as a psychiatric disorder)
  - Apraxia (often classified as a cognitive disorder)
- Other topics in movement disorders:
  - Ataxia
  - Drug-induced movement disorders
  - Psychogenic movement disorders

Hyperkinesis

TREMOR

Basic Information

- Definition: Rhythmic oscillations of any body part
- **Three types of tremor:**
  - **Rest:** Present when a body part is completely relaxed

- **Postural:** Present when a body part is held, not moving, against gravity (arms extended, or holding a cup or newspaper)
- **Kinetic:** Present during motion of a body part (reaching, pouring)
- Intention tremor is a subtype of kinetic tremor that increases in amplitude/intensity at the end of movement (close to target)
- Etiologies
  - Physiologic tremor: Normal, very small oscillations usually unnoticed in most people
  - Enhanced physiologic tremor: An increase in physiologic tremor triggered by a substance or condition
    - Medications/toxins: Caffeine, antidepressants, β-agonists, others
    - Metabolic: Hyperthyroidism, liver disease
    - Anxiety
  - Essential tremor (ET)
    - This condition is influenced by genetic factors. Roughly **50% have a first-degree relative with ET**
    - **Gradual onset** (average = fourth decade of life but can be any age) and slow progression of a postural > kinetic limb tremor, but can have tremor in the head and voice. Worsens with anxiety, caffeine, lack of sleep, some medications, and **may improve with relatively small amounts of alcohol consumption.**
  - **Cerebellar tremor: intention/kinetic > postural tremors,** often with coincident ataxia. Can result from degenerative disorders, masses, strokes, multiple sclerosis, etc.
  - Dystonic tremor: See section on Dystonia
  - Parkinsonian tremor: See section on Parkinsonism
  - Psychogenic tremor: See section on Psychogenic Movement Disorders

Diagnosis and Evaluation of Tremor

- History and examination: Define the pattern of tremor
- Determination of etiology: Assess for underlying metabolic and toxic conditions, medications, anatomical lesions, and other identifiable etiologies. Often the determination revolves around distinguishing ET from parkinsonian tremor (Table 61-1).

Treatment

- Treatment of tremor dependent on cause
- Enhanced physiologic tremor: **Remove the triggering cause** if known

TABLE 61-1	Essential Tremor versus Parkinson Disease–Associated Tremor	
Clinical Feature	**Essential Tremor**	**Parkinson Disease**
Family history	Positive in 50%	Usually negative
Response to alcohol	Tremor attenuates	No obvious effect
When does it occur?	With action	At rest
Speed	Fast (6–10 Hz)	Slow (4–6 Hz)
Appearance	Flexion-extension of wrists	Pill-rolling movement of fingers with pronation-supination of wrist
Location	Hands/arms (bilateral), head/neck, voice	Hands/arms (unilateral), jaw/chin
Associated features	Mild imbalance	Masked face, cogwheel rigidity, bradykinesia, gait impairment

Hz, Hertz (cycles per second).

- Essential tremor (ET)
  - Pharmacotherapy: see Box 61-1
  - Surgical treatment: For medically refractory and functionally disabling tremors
    - Thalamotomy: A small lesion is made in the thalamus (rarely done now)
    - Deep brain stimulation: Implanted brain electrodes connected to a battery pack/pulse generator in the chest, to electrically stimulate the thalamus
- Cerebellar tremor: Sometimes responds to benzodiazepines, carbamazepine, and more traditional ET treatments
- Dystonic tremor: See discussion under Dystonia
- Parkinsonian tremor: See discussion under Parkinson Disease
- Psychogenic tremor: See discussion under Psychogenic Movement Disorders

DYSTONIA
Basic Information

- Definition: **Involuntary excessive muscle contractions that tend to be sustained and patterned,** causing abnormal postures (often twisting of limbs) or movement
- Most often associated with dysfunction of the neural circuits of the basal ganglia, cerebellum, as well as cerebral cortex
- Etiologies
  - Inherited diseases: Wilson disease (dysfunction of copper metabolism), DYT1 gene–associated dystonia, and others
  - Ischemia or stroke: Putamen
  - Toxic/metabolic: Carbon monoxide poisoning
  - Medications: Antipsychotics and antiemetics
  - Infections: Viral encephalitis

BOX 61-1	Pharmacotherapy for Essential Tremor

First Line:
Propranolol (both short- and long-acting formulations)
Primidone (with or without propranolol)

Second Line:
Other β-blockers (e.g., metoprolol, atenolol)
Anticonvulsants (e.g., gabapentin, topiramate)
Benzodiazepines (e.g., clonazepam, lorazepam)

TABLE 61-2	Subtypes of Dystonia Based on Involved Area	
Dystonia Subtype	**Affected Region**	
Focal	Limited body region	
Torticollis	Neck muscles	
Blepharospasm	Periocular muscles	
Spasmodic dysphonia	Vocal cords	
Writer's cramp	Hand muscles	
Segmental	Two contiguous regions	
Meige syndrome	Periocular and perioral muscles	
Oromandibular	Mouth, jaw, tongue	
Hemidystonia	Half of the body	
Generalized	Majority of the body	

- Parkinson disease: Often affects the foot, with dystonia first
- Idiopathic: In many cases the cause remains undetermined

Clinical Presentation

- Dystonias may develop at any age
  - **Childhood**-onset cases are more likely to be **genetic,** with progression from focal/segmental to generalized involvement
  - **Adult**-onset cases are more likely to be **idiopathic,** with progression in a focal/segmental pattern over weeks or months followed by stabilization (not generalized usually)
- **Dystonias are often categorized according to the body part affected,** with several well-recognized syndromes such as cervical dystonia (neck), blepharospasm (eyelids), spasmodic dysphonia (voice), and writer's cramp (Table 61-2)
- Dystonic head tremor may often mimic ET
- Severity can range from mildly exaggerated normal movements to intermittent contractions and twisting postures, to sustained postures with fixed deformities, severe incapacitation, and death

Diagnosis and Evaluation

- History and exam: age of onset, manner of progression, family history, region affected, and associated clinical features

TABLE 61-3	*Drug-Induced Movement Disorders**			
Tremor	**Parkinsonism**	**Choreoathetosis**	**Acute Dystonia**	**Tardive Dyskinesia**

Stimulants
  Amphetamine
  Pemoline
  Cocaine
  Caffeine
  Adrenergics
    Ephedrine
    β-Agonists
Anticonvulsants
  Valproic acid
  Lamotrigine
  Phenytoin
Others
  Cyclosporine
  Amiodarone
  Thyroxine
  Lithium
	Dopamine antagonists
	  Classical
	  Atypical
	Antiemetics
	  Metoclopramide
	  Prochlorperazine
	Cardiovascular
	  Reserpine
	  α-Methyldopa
	  Calcium channel blockers
	  Amiodarone
	Antidepressants
	  SSRIs
	  Lithium
		Stimulants
		  Amphetamine
		  Pemoline
		  Cocaine
		  Theophylline
		  Adrenergics
		    Ephedrine
		    β-Agonists
		Anticonvulsants
		  Carbamazepine
		  Phenytoin
		Others
		  Lithium
		  Oral contraceptives
		  Levodopa
			Dopamine antagonists
			  Classical
			  Atypical[†]
			Antiemetics
			  Metoclopramide
			  Prochlorperazine
			Antihistamines
			  Cimetidine
			  Ranitidine
			Antitussives
				Dopamine antagonists
				  Classical
				  Atypical[†]
				Antiemetics
				  Metoclopramide
				  Prochlorperazine
				Antidepressants
				  SSRIs

SSRI, selective serotonin reuptake inhibitor.
*This is a partial list of the most common offenders.
[†]Exceptions: It is less likely for quetiapine, and extremely rare for clozapine, to cause these movement disorders, compared with the other atypical neuroleptics.

- Brain and/or spine magnetic resonance imaging (MRI) is indicated in many cases
- **Test for reversible/treatable causes,** especially in early-onset cases
  - **Wilson disease:** Check for increased 24-hour urinary copper excretion, low serum ceruloplasmin, liver biopsy, and Kayser-Fleischer rings by ophthalmologic exam
  - **Dopa-responsive dystonia** (DRD): Give diagnostic or therapeutic trial of levodopa/carbidopa (Sinemet)
  - *DYT1* **gene–associated dystonia:** The most common heritable form of generalized dystonia (autosomal dominant but reduced penetrance, so family history may be negative). Send this gene test for generalized and atypical focal dystonia.
  - Consider Parkinson disease or parkinsonian syndrome

Treatment

- **Always treat the underlying cause,** if found and if possible
- Symptomatic treatment
  - **For focal dystonias: The most effective treatment is injected botulinum toxin** every 3 to 6 months. When larger regions are involved (hemi- or generalized dystonia), this often is not feasible.
  - For more generalized dystonia
    - First: **Carbidopa/levodopa** to rule out DRD
    - If unresponsive, then try **anticholinergics, benzodiazepines, or baclofen**
    - Surgical procedures are used for medically refractory cases: Selective denervation (cutting nerves), intrathecal baclofen pump, or deep brain stimulation of the globus pallidus

CHOREA, ATHETOSIS, AND BALLISM
Basic Information

- These three terms refer to a group of movements that exist on a spectrum
  - Definitions

- **Chorea: Involuntary, irregular, unpatterned, and unsustained movements** with variable timing and distribution
- **Athetosis: Involuntary slow and irregular writhing movements** most often affecting the distal limbs
- **Ballism: Involuntary, large-amplitude, flinging movements,** typically involving proximal muscles that move an entire limb
- These three movements often blend together, with distinctions being the speed and location of movements. The term *choreoathetosis* acknowledges the frequent co-occurrence of chorea and athetosis.
- Anatomy: These movements are most often associated with dysfunction of neural circuits of the basal ganglia
- Etiology
  - **Inherited diseases:** Usually gradual onset
    - **Huntington disease:** Autosomal dominant inheritance with gene test for triplet nucleotide repeat. Chorea, psychiatric symptoms, and cognitive dysfunction progress over 10 to 20 years until death.
    - Inborn errors of metabolism (mainly in children)
  - Stroke: Often to the subthalamic nucleus or another nucleus of the basal ganglia
  - Toxic or metabolic: Cocaine intoxication, hyperthyroidism
  - Medications (Table 61-3)
  - Infections
  - Autoimmune disorders: Lupus, anticardiolipin syndrome, or Sydenham chorea (after rheumatic fever/strep infection)
  - Pregnancy (chorea gravidarum): Occurs just during pregnancy

Clinical Presentation

- The mildest forms of chorea are **easily overlooked as occasional fidgeting movements**
- Affected individuals often try to mask the abnormal movements by blending them into more purposeful-appearing movements

61

Diagnosis and Evaluation

- History and exam
- Possible ancillary testing: thyroid-stimulating hormone; antinuclear antibodies, antistreptolysin O, and other antibodies
- Huntingtin gene testing
- Brain MRI

Treatment

- Consider if the movement interferes with daily activities or is significantly embarrassing
  - **Antipsychotic medications:** Used with caution since they can cause tardive dyskinesias (that look like chorea) and can cause parkinsonism
  - Tetrabenazine (Xenazine): A newer Food and Drug Administration–approved medication with less tardive dyskinesia or parkinsonism but risk of depression and suicide
  - Chorea from stroke often improves on its own. Chorea from some autoimmune disorders, medications, hormonal imbalance, and other causes may improve with correction of the underlying disorder or withdrawal of the medication.

MYOCLONUS

Basic Information

- Definition: **Involuntary, abrupt, brief and jerky movement of a body part. Often described as "lightning fast."**
- Anatomy: The origin ("generator") of this movement can be the cerebral cortex, subcortical structures (basal ganglia, thalamus, brainstem), or spinal cord
- Classification of myoclonus by etiology
  - Physiologic myoclonus (e.g., when falling asleep; startle reaction; hiccups)
  - Essential myoclonus
  - Myoclonic epilepsies (Unverricht-Lundborg disease, myoclonic epilepsy with ragged red fibers, neuronal ceroid lipofuscinoses, sialidosis, and Lafora body disease)
  - **Symptomatic myoclonus** (the most common form) from a variety of **underlying conditions:**
    - **Metabolic encephalopathies** (most commonly hepatic or renal encephalopathy), typically with asterixis (wrist flapping)
    - **Toxic encephalopathies** (cocaine, marijuana, tricyclic antidepressants, levodopa, penicillin, others)
    - **Neurodegenerative diseases** (Wilson disease, Creutzfeldt-Jakob disease, Huntington disease, etc.)
    - **Viral encephalitis**
    - **Posthypoxic myoclonus** (Lance-Adams syndrome)
- Classification of myoclonus by distribution
  - Focal, segmental, multifocal, or generalized
- Classification of myoclonus by character
  - Arrhythmic (random), rhythmic (regular pattern), or oscillatory (resembling a tremor)

Clinical Presentation

- **These jerks can be spontaneous, stimulus-induced, or associated with action**
- Etiology determines the onset, progression, distribution, and character

Diagnosis and Evaluation

- History and exam: **Characterize the myoclonus regarding the distribution, spontaneity, triggering factors,** and accompanying symptoms
- Routine laboratories, MRI of the brain and/or spine, lumbar puncture, and/or electrophysiology (electroencephalography [EEG], somatosensory evoked potentials, electromyography)

Treatment

- **Treatment is difficult,** and in many cases therapeutic response is incomplete
- **The most common treatments include valproic acid, levetiracetam, and benzodiazepines** (i.e., clonazepam)

Disorders with the "Urge to Move"

TICS AND TOURETTE SYNDROME

Basic Information

- Definitions
  - **Tics: Brief stereotyped movements, preceded by an urge, followed by a sense of relief,** that are usually temporarily suppressible (thus are not truly "involuntary," but are classified as "unvoluntary")
  - **Tourette syndrome: Multiple motor and vocal tics beginning before age 18** and lasting for at least 6 months
- Etiology
  - **Idiopathic:** In most cases; may be developmental in the neurocircuity and neurochemistry of the basal ganglia, forebrain, and other regions
  - Medication-induced
  - Neurodegenerative

Clinical Presentation

- Varied, with onset at any age, but more commonly in childhood
- Symptoms may be chronic or have a waxing/waning course, which may remit for years
- **Common simple tics include eye squinting or shoulder shrugging, while complex ones may include neck rolling, brief ritualized sequences, utterances of phrases**
- Coprolalia (blurting out of obscenities) only occurs in a minority of patients
- Suppression of a tic is accompanied by a buildup of tension that is released when the tic is expressed
- Tics can closely resemble other movement disorders such as chorea, dystonia, or myoclonus
- **Tics and Tourette syndrome are frequently associated with obsessive-compulsive disorder or attention-deficit/hyperactivity disorder**

Diagnosis and Evaluation

- History and exam
- Not much is needed with regard to ancillary tests except for adult-onset tics (without any previous childhood history), as the movement may be a sign of a neurodegenerative disorder and further investigation may be needed (if medications are excluded)

Treatment

- **Only treat if functionally limiting or significantly embarrassing**
- Antipsychotics (low doses): Haloperidol, pimozide, risperidol, atypical antipsychotics. Risk of long-term side effects.
- Other medications include clonidine, guanfacine, gabapentin, baclofen

RESTLESS LEGS SYNDROME

Basic Information

- Definition: **Discomforting sensations in the legs, most prominent at rest and in the evening/nighttime, causing an urge to move.** Leg movement usually temporarily relieves the discomfort.
- Epidemiology: Approximately 10% of the adult population will have restless legs syndrome (RLS); it is **more common in women who have been pregnant**
- Etiology
  - **Primary RLS (~67%): About 50% of these patients have a first-degree relative with RLS**
  - **Secondary RLS (~33%): Iron deficiency anemia, end-stage renal disease, pregnancy, peripheral neuropathy, lumbar radiculopathy, autoimmune disorders, vitamin B$_{12}$, folate, or magnesium deficiencies,** and medications/substances (antipsychotics, antidepressants, alcohol, caffeine, etc.)
  - Pathophysiology: Iron metabolism and dopaminergic transmission may be involved

Clinical Presentation

- Most commonly **begins in early adulthood with slow progression**
- It is often unrecognized or misdiagnosed
- Sometimes symptoms are described as vague discomfort, restlessness, irritation, creeping/tingling sensations, or less commonly pain
- Symptom relief by movement: stretching, cycling legs, walking, etc.
- Symptoms can disrupt sleep that can lead to daytime sleepiness
- In more serious cases, discomfort may appear during any period of rest (sitting to read), at any time of day, and can affect the arms and trunk

Diagnosis and Evaluation

- History and exam: The exam is usually normal in RLS
- Overnight polysomnogram can document coexisting periodic limb movements in sleep PLMS), which are usually asymptomatic and often present
- Other testing: Check for iron deficiency, renal dysfunction, diabetes, peripheral neuropathy
- Also, differentiate from akathisia (see below)

Treatment

- Usually dosed once in the evening
- **Dopaminergic agents:** Much lower doses than in Parkinson disease
  - Dopamine agonists: Primarily ropinirole (Requip) or pramipexole (Mirapex)
  - Carbidopa/levodopa (Sinemet)

- Two problems can occur with dopaminergic medications:
  - Rebound: Symptoms can worsen in the morning when the medication wears off
  - Augmentation: Symptoms occur earlier in the evening and eventually during the day the longer these medications are used
- **Nondopaminergic agents**
  - Antiepileptic medications: Gabapentin (Neurontin), pregabalin (Lyrica), carbamazepine (Tegretol), valproic acid (Depakote)
  - Benzodiazepines: These promote sleep if needed, but do not suppress RLS symptoms. Effective for PLMS.
  - Opioids: Effective in refractory cases

AKATHISIA

Basic Information

- Definition: **An inner sense of restlessness that temporarily improves upon voluntary movement, and can be temporarily suppressed by the patient, though anxiety/tension builds during that suppression**
- Etiology
  - Often medication induced: Antipsychotics, dopamine blocking antinausea medications (metoclopramide, prochlorperazine), antidepressants
  - Sometimes seen in degenerative parkinsonian disorders

Clinical Presentation and Characteristics

- **Restlessness or uneasiness is relieved by movement but does NOT predominate in the legs** and is NOT more common while resting or lying down (as in RLS)
- It is differentiated from anxiety since it is temporarily relieved by movement and is not typically associated with recurrent worry

Treatment

- Remove offending medication, or treat underlying disorder

Hypokinesis

PARKINSONISM

Basic Information

- Definition: A clinical syndrome defined by **bradykinesia** (slowness), **rest tremor**, **rigidity** (stiffness), and **postural instability** (balance and gait dysfunction)
  - Bradykinesia is best assessed by rapidly tapping the index finger on the thumb and rapidly opening and closing a fisted hand
  - *Parkinsonism* simply defines a collection of symptoms that can have many different etiologies, while *Parkinson disease* refers to a specific disorder that is the most common cause of parkinsonism
- Etiology
  - Primary: Parkinson disease (PD; see below)
  - **Secondary**

61

TABLE 61-4	Red Flags for the Parkinson Imitators*	
Parkinson Imitator	**Characteristic Clinical Features**	**Brain MRI**
Progressive supranuclear palsy	Parkinsonism, gaze palsies, slow saccades, imbalance with falls, dysarthria, or truncal dystonia	Normal or slight midbrain atrophy
Dementia with Lewy bodies	Parkinsonism, early dementia, fluctuating alertness, early visual hallucinations	Diffuse atrophy
Corticobasal degeneration	Parkinsonism, asymmetrical stiffness, apraxia, or dysfunction of one arm, dysarthria, or dementia	Normal or asymmetrical cortical atrophy
Multiple system atrophy	Parkinsonism, early autonomic dysfunction, sometimes cerebellar ataxia	Normal or brainstem and cerebellar atrophy
Normal-pressure hydrocephalus	Prominant gait dysfunction (imbalanced, slow, feet sliding on ground), dementia, urinary incontinence, possible parkinsonism	Enlarged lateral ventricles with normal cortical sulci
Vascular parkinsonism	Parkinsonism of the lower body more than upper body, prominent gait disability, cognitive dysfunction (or dementia)	Extensive patchy or diffuse white matter disease

*The Parkinson imitators are sometimes called Parkinson-plus syndromes or akinetic-rigid syndromes. The characteristic clinical features are combined with other features of parkinsonism.

- Parkinson-plus (atypical parkinsonian) disorders: Other neurodegenerative disorders with parkinsonism plus other atypical features (Table 61-4)
- Hereditary-degenerative disorders: **Huntington disease, Wilson disease,** and others
- **Vascular parkinsonism:** Accumulation of small or large strokes that may produce parkinsonism more centered in the lower half of the body
- Hydrocephalus: Enlarged ventricles (cerebrospinal fluid–filled spaces) in the brain. Most commonly **normal-pressure hydrocephalus,** which can be assessed by neuroimaging and high-volume lumbar puncture/drainage (see Table 61-4). The latter is to determine if the patient is a candidate for ventriculoperitoneal shunt as chronic treatment for this disorder.
- **Metabolic/toxic:** Hypothyroidism, methylphenyltetrahydropyridine (MPTP), manganese, carbon monoxide
- **Medication-induced** (Table 61-5)
- Traumatic brain injury
- Postencephalitis

TABLE 61-5	Medications Associated with Secondary Parkinsonism
Class of Medication	**Drug(s)**
Cardiovascular drugs	α-Methyldopa Reserpine
Dopamine antagonists for nausea	Prochlorperazine Metoclopramide
Dopamine antagonists for psychosis	**Typical Antipsychotics** Haloperidol Thioridazine Fluphenazine Pimozide Chlorpromazine Perphenazine **Atypical Antipsychotics** Risperidone Paliperidone Olanzapine Ziprasidone Aripiprazole (Quetiapine)*
Neurologic or psychiatric drugs	Valproic acid Lithium

*Much less so than the other atypical neuroleptics.

Diagnosis

- History and exam: Determine if the syndrome is consistent with PD or if there are atypical features that suggest a different etiology
- Ancillary testing: Brain MRI (if suspected vascular or hydrocephalic changes), TSH, etc.
- Medication trial: **PD also is characterized by a robust and sustained response to dopaminergic medications (especially carbidopa/levodopa), while other etiologies have only a partial or short-lived response**

Treatment

- Depends on the underlying etiology. If there is a concern for hydrocephalus, refer to a specialist. **Treat vascular risk factors if vascular parkinsonism is suspected.** Correct underlying metabolic changes and remove medications that may be contributing.
- **PD movement-related symptoms respond well to dopaminergic medications** (see below)
- Other forms of parkinsonism may also respond somewhat to dopaminergic medications and therefore may be considered

PARKINSON DISEASE

Basic Information

- Definition: A disorder characterized by **bradykinesia, rest tremor, rigidity,** and **postural instability** caused by the progressive degeneration of dopaminergic neurons within the **substantia nigra.** Also seen are the formation of cytoplasmic inclusions (Lewy bodies; Fig. 61-1) and neurodegeneration in other parts of the central nervous system.
- Secondary symptoms: Drooling, anxiety, constipation, poor olfactory function, executive cognitive dysfunction, depression, apathy, dysarthria, dysphagia, and dystonia

FIGURE 61-1 **A,** Substantia nigra in a patient with Parkinson disease, showing area of depigmentation due to neuronal loss. **B,** Normal substantia nigra showing typical pigmentation for comparison. **C,** A large neuron showing a typical irregularly shaped nucleus and rounded cytoplasmic Lewy body with surrounding halo. Surrounding the Lewy body are the typical pigmentary granules of substantia nigra neurons.

- Epidemiology
  - **Average age of diagnosis is 62 years, and increased age is a risk factor for developing PD,** though 4% to 10% of patients present younger than 40
  - **Most cases are idiopathic, but several rare monogenetic forms have been identified** (mutations in genes for parkin, alpha-synuclein, LRRK2, and others), as well as several "risk genes"

Clinical Presentation

- Onset is usually insidious, and progression is lifelong
- There are four cardinal motor (movement) symptoms: Bradykinesia (slowness), tremor at rest, rigidity (muscle resistance to movement), and postural instability (balance and gait dysfunction). **It is a common misconception that all PD patients must have a rest tremor.** This leads to a delay in diagnosis in those who lack tremor.
- **Initial manifestations may include a single isolated symptom, making early diagnosis more difficult.** Examples include rest tremor of one hand/arm, stiff or awkward movements of one limb, slow or labored gait, or the finding that daily tasks are taking longer to perform.
- **Asymmetry is a key feature distinguishing PD from many other causes of parkinsonism.** Thus it should start in one arm or side, prior to progressing to the other side and typically remaining worse on the initially affected side.
- Nonmotor symptoms
  - Psychiatric: Anxiety, depression, hallucinations
  - Cognitive: Executive or memory dysfunction, and often eventual dementia
  - Autonomic: Orthostatic hypotension, urinary urgency or retention, sexual dysfunction, and constipation

- Usually autonomic or cognitive symptoms are absent or mild initially and slowly worsen over time. Hallucinations are usually a late feature unless they are triggered by a dopaminergic medication. Anxiety and depression can occur early.

Diagnosis

- History and exam: **Look for asymmetrical motor features that must include bradykinesia plus one of the other three cardinal motor features of parkinsonism (does not have to include tremor)**
- Assess for any "red flags" that would suggest a different cause of the patient's parkinsonism (see Table 61-4)
  - *Early, prominent* dementia, imbalance with falls, autonomic findings, posturing of one limb, or eye movement changes may suggest another etiology
- Response to a dopaminergic agent: A medication trial of a dopaminergic agent that provides *significant* improvement in motor symptoms supports a diagnosis of PD
- Brain imaging (MRI, computed tomography) is helpful if vascular disease or hydrocephalus is suspected. Should be normal in PD.
- Functional imaging, including radioactive tracers (i.e., DaTscan), may offer additional evidence for disease

Treatment

- See Figure 61-2 for a treatment algorithm for PD.
- Symptomatic medication treatments
  - **Carbidopa/levodopa** (Sinemet) is still the most effective treatment. In later stages of the disease, levodopa therapy is typically complicated by fluctuation of effectiveness (wearing off) and dyskinesias (i.e., drug-induced choreoathetosis).

61

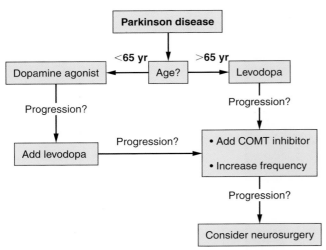

FIGURE 61-2 Algorithm for treatment of Parkinson disease. (COMT, catechol-O-methyltransferase.)

- **Dopamine agonists:** Pramipexole (Mirapex) and ropinirole (Requip). These have longer lasting effects than carbidopa/levodopa but usually more side effects, especially in the elderly (>70 years).
- **Monoamine oxidase (MAO)-B inhibitors:** Selegiline (Eldepryl, Zelapar) and rasagiline (Azilect). These provide mild symptomatic benefits but may prolong the per dose benefits of carbidopa/levodopa. May offer some neuroprotective effects.
- **Catechol-O-methyltransferase (COMT) inhibitors:** Entacapone (Comtan) can be packaged with carbidopa/levodopa (Stalevo). Entacopone given with carbidopa/levodopa prolongs the effect of each dose. Tolcapone (Tasmar) also may be used though hepatic monitoring is required.
- **Amantadine:** Has weak symptomatic benefits and may suppress levodopa-induced dyskinesias
- Symptomatic nonmedication treatments
  - Exercise: Three to four times weekly with aerobic and strength training improves overall function and might have mild protective effects
  - Yoga, tai chi, dancing, walking, and physical therapy: Focus on balance and likely reduce the risk of falling. Often improves overall function, independence, and quality of life.
  - Occupational therapy for manual dexterity, optimizing activities of daily living, and ensuring safe driving is important
  - Speech therapy aids with dysarthria and hypophonia should be used when needed
  - Swallowing evaluation and therapy are important to reduce choking hazards
- Possible disease-modifying (neuroprotective) therapies
  - These are being researched as interventions that may slow the progression of PD neurodegeneration
  - Currently, there is no conclusive evidence of disease-modifying effects of any agent
  - Data are suggestive of *possible* such effects for coenzyme Q-10 (1200–2400 mg/day), creatine (5–10 g/day), antioxidant vitamins, MAO-B inhibitors (selegeline and rasagiline), and exercise. Recent data suggests

that coenzyme Q-10 offers no protection, while that for rasagiline continues to be controversial.
- Surgical therapies
  - Treatment usually is reserved for medically refractory cases of PD (not shown to be helpful in other causes of parkinsonism)
  - **Deep brain stimulation: The most frequent surgical intervention;** it involves stimulation of the subthalamic nucleus or the globus pallidus

CATATONIA SYNDROMES

Basic Information

- Often considered a psychiatric disorder
- Definition: **A motor and behavioral dysregulation syndrome with the inability to move despite full physical capability, with difficulty initiating and terminating movement.** Postures become frozen or oddly positioned, and actions become contrary to intent.
- Epidemiology
  - Incidence not known
  - **It occurs most commonly in the setting of mood disorders and psychotic disorders** and also general medical conditions, and neurologic disorders
- Etiologies: Often more than one per patient
  - Psychiatric disorders: Mood disorders (especially bipolar mania), psychotic disorders
  - Neurologic disorders: Cerebral structural damage (stroke, mass, trauma to specific regions), encephalitis, seizures
  - Medical and toxic disorders: Liver dysfunction or post–liver transplantation; renal dysfunction; other metabolic dysfunction; hypothyroidism; lupus; HIV/AIDS; other infection; low iron, vitamin B_{12}, folate; and drug intoxications (phenylcyclidine, disulfiram, corticosteroids)

Clinical Presentation

- **"Hypokinetic"/"retarded" form is the most common:** Posturing, rigidity, mutism, staring, repetitive actions, negativism (resistance to commands or examination), waxy flexibility (can position the patient), and stupor
- **"Excited" form:** Similar to an agitated deilirum or mania
- **"Malignant" form:** Acute onset, fever, autonomic dysfunction, and with other similarities to neuroleptic malignant syndrome (see section on Drug-Induced Movement Disorders below)

Diagnosis

- History (from family/friends is helpful) and exam
- Brain MRI and EEG are typically recommended
- Additional testing for etiologies listed above should be employed as indicated

Treatment

- **Supportive care:** Intensive nursing care, artificial hydration or nutrition as needed, deep venous thrombosis prevention, urinary catheterization, and range of motion through physical therapy
- **Address the underlying etiology**

- **Benzodiazepines:** With a test dose of lorazepam 1 to 2 mg IV, often within minutes there is lessening of symptoms, but not in all cases. Repeating the same dose every 4 to 12 hours can be used symptomatically.
- **Electroconvulsive therapy:** Can be used under the supervision of a psychiatrist for cases that do not respond to benzodiazepines
- *N*-methyl-D-aspartate (NMDA) receptor antagonists: Amantadine and memantine have been used successfully when added to lorazepam and electroconvulsive therapy
- Atypical antipsychotics: Data for these agents are uncertain, and some patients will worsen or progress to neuroleptic malignant syndrome when these are used

APRAXIA
Basic Information

- Often considered a cognitive disorder
- Definition: **Dysfunction in performing learned, skilled movements that is not due to primary neurologic dysfunctions such as weakness, sensory loss, changes in posture or tone, incoordination, or impaired attention, comprehension of the task, or cooperation.** Apraxia is a higher order motor-cognitive symptom, where it is as if all the appropriate pieces were in place, but the patient cannot "put it all together."
- Examples
  - Difficulty using objects appropriately (picks up toothbrush not knowing what to do with it, or tries to eat with it)
  - Difficulty gesturing, interpreting gestures, or with imitation
  - Difficulty in orienting movements appropriately in relation to other body parts
  - Difficulty in imagining and planning complex movements
- Etiologies
  - Localizes best to the parietal lobes, frontal lobes, and their subcortical connections. Disorders that cause dysfunction in these regions can cause apraxia.
    - **Focal brain damage:** Stroke, trauma, masses
    - **Degenerative disorders:** Corticobasal degeneration, Alzheimer disease, progressive supranuclear palsy, and other dementias or parkinsonian conditions
    - Other causes of general cognitive dysfunction and/or delirium can cause apraxia within the setting of general brain dysfunction

Diagnosis

- History and exam: Verifying normal basic motor and sensory function on neurologic exam as well as comprehension of tasks is necessary
- Look for additional features of dementia (memory, language, executive function, visuospatial impairments) and signs of parkinsonism that may suggest a particular disorder. Assess for focal neurologic signs that may indicate focal brain damage.
- Have the patient demonstrate how to do specific tasks with imagined objects ("show me how you would brush your teeth as if you were holding a toothbrush"), or imitate complex hand postures (interlocking hands in various ways)

Treatment

- **Apraxia is difficult to treat.** Addressing any underlying conditions that can be modified is the first step.
- Strategies from occupational and speech/language therapists to augment each step in the sequence of actions to accomplish daily tasks can be helpful and implemented by patients
- Correctly identifying apraxia as the problem can remove the need to perform further testing or treatments

Other Movement Disorders

ATAXIA
Basic Information

- Definition: **Incoordination arising from dysfunction in timing, rhythm, accuracy (targeting), and smoothness of movement** (Fig. 61-3). This is usually due to abnormalities in the cerebellum or its motor and/or sensory pathways (cerebellar or spinocerebellar ataxia). Sensory ataxia may arise from neuropathy. Ataxic patients may appear drunk. The term *ataxia* is often incorrectly applied to movement abnormalities caused by weakness, dystonia, chorea, or poor attention.
  - **Dysmetria** ("poorly measured"): **Irregular timing or trajectory of targeted movements**
  - **Dysdiadochokinesis: Breakdown of the normal timing and sequencing of rapid alternating movements** (e.g., rapid succession of pronation and supination)
- Etiology
  - Vascular: **Stroke to cerebellum or brainstem**
  - Autoimmune: Includes **celiac disease, anti-GAD syndrome, Miller Fisher syndrome**
  - Inherited disorders: **Spinocerebellar ataxia** (autosomal dominant trinucleotide repeat diseases), Friedreich ataxia, ataxia-telangiectasia, and others
  - Metabolic/toxic: **Vitamin E deficiency,** hypothyroidism, chronic alcoholism (alcohol often causes midline/gait ataxia)
  - Medications (**antiepileptics**)
  - Infections
  - Tumor/mass, or **paraneoplastic/parainfectious disease**

Clinical Presentation

- May be rapid or slow in onset depending on etiology
- **Common symptoms include imbalance, wide-based gait, falls, dysarthria, eye movement abnormalities, intention tremor, and mistargeting with the limbs** (trouble pouring water, poor handwriting, knocking over objects, etc.)

Diagnosis

- History and exam supplemented with laboratory testing and brain imaging (lesions, atrophy)
- Genetic tests can be done if there is a family history or after other testing is unrevealing

61

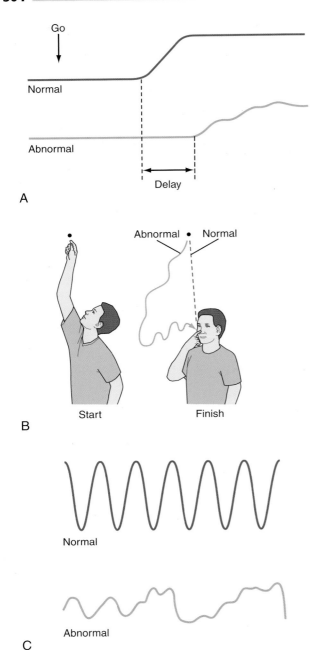

FIGURE 61-3 Typical defects in upper limb ataxia. **A,** Initiation of movement is delayed. **B,** Dysmetria (inaccuracy in range and direction) and kinetic tremor. **C,** Dysdiadochokinesis, an irregular pattern of alternating movements, can be seen in the abnormal position trace. *(From Kandel ER, Schwartz JH, Jessell TM [eds]: Principles of neural science, ed 3, Norwalk, CT, Appleton & Lange, 1991, Fig. 41-16, p 643. Adapted from Thach WT, Montgomery EB: Motor system. In Pearlman AL, Collins RC [eds]: Neurobiology of disease, ed. 3, New York, Oxford University Press, 1990, pp 168–196.)*

Treatment

- If found, treat the underlying cause
- No medication therapies have proven efficacy for ataxia, though several can be tried with possible mild benefits
- Physical, occupational, and speech therapies play an important role for maximizing function, preventing injury and aspiration, and optimizing an assistive walking device

DRUG-INDUCED MOVEMENT DISORDERS

Basic Information

- Medications can produce side effects that closely mimic "natural" movement disorders, including tremor, ataxia, chorea, dystonia, tics, and parkinsonism (see Table 61-3)
- Drug-induced movement disorders are important to recognize as many are "cured" by eliminating the offending agent

Clinical Presentation

- **Drug-induced tremor:** Can be **postural, kinetic and/or rest**
- Clinical features of drug-induced **ataxia, parkinsonism,** and **chorea** appear similar to the descriptions of these movements (listed above)
- Antidopaminergic agents: Antipsychotics (haloperidol, fluphenazine, and other typical antipsychotics more commonly than atypical antipsychotics), as well as some antinausea medications (metoclopramide and prochlorperazine), cause several types of movement disorders:
  - **Acute dystonic reaction: Sudden and forceful abnormal dystonic posturing; typically within hours of receiving an offending medication**
  - **Tardive dyskinesias:** Usually **choreoathetosis of the tongue, mouth, and/or face** more than other regions
  - **Parkinsonism:** More often **symmetrical rather than asymmetrical,** with or without tremor
  - **Neuroleptic malignant syndrome** (NMS): Characterized by **rigidity, fever, autonomic instability, decreased level of consciousness, and an elevated creatine kinase and white blood cell count**
    - Mortality may be as high as 50%
    - May follow chronic or acute exposure to an offending medication, often after an increase or decrease in dose
    - A partial syndrome may occur that is important to catch early

Diagnosis

- History and exam
- Reviewing the side effects and timing of medications

Treatment

- **Stop the offending medication,** if possible. Depending on why the patient is on the medication, it may need to be tapered.
- Resolution of the movement disorder may occur within hours or be delayed to weeks or months (often similar to the onset)
- **Acute dystonic reactions: Diphenhydramine (Benadryl) or benztropine (Cogentin)** can speed resolution
- Tardive dyskinesia can be permanent, but performing a very slow taper of the offending medication increases the chance of resolving the abnormal movements
- NMS: Hospitalization with supportive care is often required because the syndrome can be life-threatening. Intravenous fluids, benzodiazepines, dopamine agonists, dantrolene, and antipyretics have been used.

PSYCHOGENIC MOVEMENT DISORDERS

Basic Information

- Also known as "functional" or "nonorganic" disorders
- Definition: **Physical symptoms (resembling movement disorders listed above) that are brought on by psychological mechanisms.** Psychogenic movement disorders (PMDs) encompass a spectrum of mainly three types of psychological phenomena:
  - **Conversion disorder: A subconscious, nonwillful manifestation of a psychiatric disturbance that leads to physical symptoms**
  - **Factitious disorder: When a patient knowingly creates physical symptoms usually to gain the benfits of attention by assuming the sick role**
  - **Malingering: A deliberate production of symptoms for material gain or avoidance** (not strictly considered a psychiatric disorder)
- Epidemiology: About 2% to 3% of patients in a movement disorder clinic have PMDs, with a female-to-male ratio of 2:1
- Risk factors for PMDs: Sexual abuse, major emotionally stressful life events, and previous physical trauma (including surgery)

Clinical Presentation

- **Most common manifestations are tremor, dystonia, gait disorder, and myoclonus**
- Less common manifestations include parkinsonism, chorea, ataxia, and tics
- **Red flags** to suggest a PMD
  - **Acute onset and fast progression** to maximal severity
  - **Waxing and waning course;** temporary complete remissions
  - Symptoms are incongruent with any established organic disease
  - Symptoms are inconsistent over time and regarding involved body parts
  - Symptoms are distractible and increase with attention to the affected body part
  - Association with "false neurologic symptoms" (e.g., weakness only with certain tasks)

Diagnosis

- **History and careful examination** involving maneuvers to distract the patient, observe when the patient is not aware of being observed, and retest affected areas in similar or different ways to check for degree of variability
- Ancillary work-up, including imaging, electrophysiology, and lab tests, might be necessary depending on the presentation and the diagnostic certainty
- Evaluation by a psychiatrist and/or psychologist to evaluate for other psychiatric comorbidities and possible psychological factors underlying the movement disorder (though they may not be obvious)
- **Delivery of the diagnosis in an empathic and accurate manner is very important** for a patient to accept it and comply with treatment. Acknowledge symptoms as "real and serious," and emphasize that symptoms are not present 100% of the time and therefore normal function is possible and can be "tapped into" more and more over time. Give an unambiguous message that this is an established cause of movement disorders and that additional diagnostic tests are unnecessary.
- Avoid unnecessary work-up, including aggressive and costly procedures, or administration of potentially harmful drugs, solely based on reluctance of the physician and the patient alike to discuss or accept the diagnosis of PMD

Treatment

- **Treatment of psychiatric comorbidity** (i.e., anxiety, depression, etc.) and underlying psychological mechanisms, if identified. This may include antidepressants or psychotherapy.
- Stress management and relaxation techniques (e.g., biofeedback, yoga, meditation)
- Physical therapy and occupational therapy can help reestablish healthy patterns of movement
- Early and sustained treatment is important for recovery

REVIEW QUESTIONS

For review questions, please go to www.expertconsult.com.

SUGGESTED READINGS

Daniels J: Catatonia: clinical aspects and neurobiological correlates, *J Neuropsychiatry Clin Neurosci* 21:371–380, 2009.

Fahn S, Jankovic J, Hallett M: *Principles and practice of movement disorders*, Philadelphia, 2007, Churchill Livingstone Elsevier.

Fink M, Taylor MA: The catatonia syndrome, *Arch Gen Psychiatry* 66:1173–1177, 2009.

Janavs JL, Aminoff MJ: Involuntary movements in general medical disorders. In Aminoff MJ, editor: *Neurology and general medicine*, ed 3, New York, 2001, Churchill Livingstone, pp 983–1002.

Petreska B, Adriani M, Blanke O, et al: Apraxia: a review, *Prog Brain Res* 164:61–83, 2007.

Tolosa E, Koller WC, Gershanik OS: *Differential diagnosis and treatment of movement disorders*, Boston, 1998, Butterworth-Heinemann.

SUGGESTED WEB SITE

The following Web site provides useful basic information on many movement disorders for both practitioners and patients: *www.wemove.com.*

61

Selected Topics in Neurology

RAFAEL H. LLINÁS, MD

This chapter reviews a selection of central and peripheral neurologic disorders involving the spinal cord, peripheral nerves, and neuromuscular junction and toxic myopathies. Inflammatory myopathies are reviewed in Chapter 45. Localization of neurologic lesions, based on clinical evaluation or imaging studies, is the diagnostic theme.

Spinal Cord

Basic Information

- The spinal column is made up of vertebrae separated by intervertebral disks (Fig. 62-1)
- The spinal cord is found within the spinal canal, beginning at the end of the brainstem and extending to L1
- Below L1 is the "cauda equina," which consists of nerve roots
- Spinal cord circulation
  - The anterior spinal cord is dependent on a single anterior spinal artery
  - The posterior spinal cord is fed by numerous posterior spinal arteries
  - **Spinal stroke preferentially affects the anterior spinal cord**
- Table 62-1 lists the most common entities affecting the spinal cord

Clinical Presentation

- Spinal cord lesions may be categorized by presentation
  - Upper motor neuron signs (long tract signs): **Weakness, spasticity, hyperreflexia, and positive Babinski sign** (Fig. 62-2)
  - **Sensory signs** (anterior or posterior columns or both): **Sensory level or loss of single modality** (pinprick/temperature or light touch/proprioception)
  - **Bowel, bladder, and sexual dysfunction signs: Urinary overflow incontinence or bladder spasticity, and weak rectal tone with fecal incontinence**
  - **Local root dysfunction: Multimodal sensory and motor loss in a dermatomal distribution (Fig. 62-3)**
  - Caveats
    - No cranial nerve abnormalities should be present
    - In acute spinal cord trauma, weakness may be the only long tract sign present
    - The sensory level reveals only the lowest level possible for a lesion (e.g., a T10 sensory level may be caused by a cervical lesion)
- Spinal cord lesions may be categorized by location
  - **Anterior** spinal cord lesions

- Loss of **pain and temperature** sense (lateral spinothalamic tract)
- Fine touch, proprioception, and vibration sense are spared
- May occur with or without motor loss

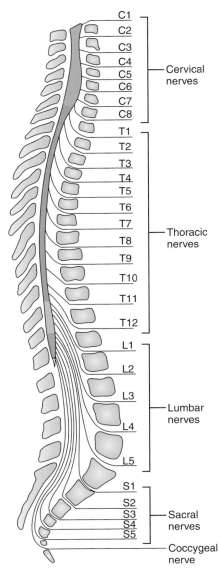

FIGURE 62-1 The spinal column, showing the relationships among the spinal cord, spinal nerves, and vertebral column. *(From Crossman AR, Neary D: Neuroanatomy, ed 3, Philadelphia, Churchill Livingstone, 2006, Fig. 8.3.)*

TABLE 62-1	*Diseases Affecting the Spinal Cord*				
	Multiple Sclerosis	**Vitamin B$_{12}$ Deficiency**	**Syringomyelia**	**Tabes Dorsalis**	**Epidural Abscess**
Basic information	Prototypical demyelinating disease "Transverse myelitis" when affects the spinal cord Most common presentation "optic neuritis"	Neurologic symptoms develop after prolonged B$_{12}$ deficiency (months to years) Neurologic symptoms occur in the majority of patients with pernicious anemia Anemia need not be present	Central cord cavitation, CSF accumulation and compression Often cervical cord Congenital (e.g., with Arnold-Chiari malformation) or post-traumatic	Onset many years after primary syphilitic infection	Often caused by *Staphylococcus aureus* May occur at any level
Clinical presentation	Two basic forms Chronic-progressive: Lesions develop, persist, and progress Relapsing-remitting: Lesions develop, resolve, and recur elsewhere	Loss of vibration and proprioception sense Loss of reflexes Mild weakness Mental status change Night blindness	Central cord syndrome (see Table 63-2) Atrophy, fasciculation, and lost reflexes	"Lightning shocks" in abdomen and legs Loss of vibration and proprioception sense Bladder dysfunction	Fever and chills Pain Cord or nerve root compression
Diagnosis and evaluation	Lesions "separated in time and space" Lhermitte's sign* MRI with contrast	Vitamin B$_{12}$ (low) Methylmalonic acid (high)	MRI	Argyll Robertson pupil† CSF VDRL (+)	Focal tenderness to percussion over spine Elevated WBC count
Treatment	Acute: Steroids Chronic: Immune modulators (e.g., interferon beta-1a or beta-1b, and glatiramer acetate)	Vitamin B$_{12}$ injections	Neurosurgical evaluation	IV penicillin	Antibiotics Urgent surgery for cord compression

CSF, cerebrospinal fluid; IV, intravenous; MRI, magnetic resonance imaging; VDRL, Venereal Disease Research Laboratory; WBC, white blood cell.
*Sensation of an electric shock radiating to the arms or legs and provoked by neck movement or cough.
†Pupils react to convergence but not to light.

62

FIGURE 62-2 Babinski sign. The normal adult response to stimulation of the lateral plantar surface of the foot (*top*). The abnormal adult response (*bottom*). (*From Goetz B: Textbook of clinical neurology, ed 2, Philadelphia, WB Saunders, 2003, Fig. 15-13.*)

FIGURE 62-3 Dermatome map. (*From FitzGerald MJT, Folan-Curran J: Clinical neuroanatomy and related neuroscience, ed 4, Philadelphia, WB Saunders, 2002, Fig. 11.10.*)

- **Posterior** spinal cord lesions
  - Loss of fine touch, proprioception, and vibration sense (posterior columns)
  - Pain and temperature sense are spared
  - May occur with or without motor loss
- **Central** spinal cord lesions (Fig. 62-4)
  - Lateral spinothalamic tract and local motor neurons disrupted
  - **Pain and temperature sense lost in "cape-like" distribution**
  - Fine touch, proprioception, and vibration sense spared
  - **Lower motor neuron weakness may be evident in the extremities**

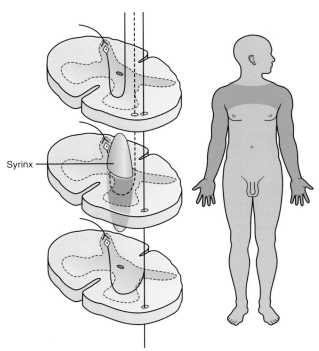

Syrinx

FIGURE 62-4 Central spinal cord lesion (in this case, syringomyelia), showing cape-like distribution of analgesia. *(From FitzGerald MJT, Folan-Curran J: Clinical neuroanatomy and related neuroscience, ed 4, Philadelphia, WB Saunders, 2002, Fig. 12.1.1.)*

Diagnosis and Evaluation

Table 62-2 provides a comparison of spinal cord syndromes.

- Anterior spinal cord syndromes are caused by the following:
  - Trauma
  - Rupture of disk, causing compression of the spinal cord (Fig. 62-5)
  - Occlusion of anterior spinal artery causing spinal stroke
  - Primary spinal cord tumors
  - Metastatic cancer
- Posterior spinal cord syndromes are caused by the following:
  - Cervical spondylosis (arthritis and ligamentous hypertrophy)
  - Epidural abscess
  - Vitamin B_{12} deficiency
  - Syphilis
  - Multiple sclerosis
  - Primary spinal cord tumors
  - Metastatic cancer
- Central spinal cord syndromes are caused by the following:
  - Syringomyelia (congenital or post-traumatic)
  - Primary spinal cord tumors
  - Hyperextension injuries that disrupt the central spinal cord gray matter
- Brown-Séquard syndrome
  - Caused by hemisection of the spinal cord
  - Findings depend on where each tract decussates
    - Motor tract lesions give ipsilateral weakness (**motor fibers cross in the brainstem**)
    - Sensory tract lesions give ipsilateral fine touch, proprioception, and vibration loss (**posterior columns cross in brainstem**); and contralateral pain and temperature sense loss (**spinothalamic tracts cross in the spinal cord** through the gray matter)

Treatment

See Table 62-1.

TABLE 62-2	**Comparison of Spinal Cord Syndromes**	
	Clinical Manifestations	**Possible Causes**
Anterior	Loss of pain and temperature sensation Motor weakness may or may not be present	Trauma Ruptured intervertebral disk Anterior spinal artery occlusion ("spinal stroke") Primary spinal cord tumors Metastatic cancer
Central	Loss of pain and temperature sensation Lower motor neuron weakness (in lower extremities)	Syringomyelia Primary spinal cord tumors Hyperextension injuries
Posterior	Loss of fine touch, vibratory sensation Loss of proprioception Motor weakness may or may not be present	Cervical spondylosis Epidural abscess Vitamin B_{12} deficiency Syphilis Multiple sclerosis Primary spinal cord tumors Metastatic cancer

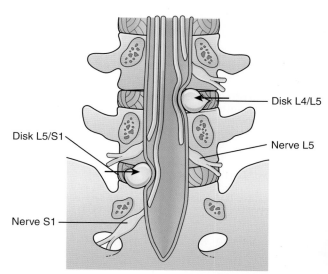

FIGURE 62-5 Nerve compression by rupture of intervertebral disks (*arrows*). *(From FitzGerald MJT, Folan-Curran J: Clinical neuroanatomy and related neuroscience, ed 4, Philadelphia, WB Saunders, 2002, Fig. 11.2.2.)*

Peripheral Nerves

Basic Information

- The peripheral nerves include the spinal roots, cauda equina, nerve plexus (brachial and lumbar), and named nerves

Clinical Presentations

- **Lower motor neuron signs (Box 62-1)**
  - Acute: **Weakness, multimodal sensory loss, lancinating pain, and loss of reflexes**
  - Chronic: **Atrophy and fasciculation**
  - Not all features need to be present
- Spinal roots (Table 62-3)
- Cauda equina syndrome: Bowel and bladder dysfunction, flaccid paralysis of bilateral lower extremities, and saddle anesthesia
- Plexus: Unilateral extremity affected without spinal cord signs; all sensory modalities are affected and upper motor neuron signs are absent
- Named nerves
  - **Compression neuropathies commonly present with pain** and are caused by repetitive or chronic external compression (Table 62-4)
  - **Inflammatory neuropathies present with motor more than sensory involvement** and are caused by demyelination (Table 62-5)
  - **Toxic neuropathies commonly present with lancinating pain** and are caused by axonal damage (Table 62-6)

Diagnosis and Evaluation

- Electromyography (EMG) and nerve conduction studies (NCS) are helpful in localizing peripheral nerve lesions
  - **EMG evaluates for myopathy and denervation**
  - **NCS can differentiate axonal from demyelinating neuropathy**
- Magnetic resonance imaging most useful imaging study

TABLE 62-3 *Cervical and Lumbar Root Lesion Presentation*

Root Level	Weakness	Sensory Loss Distribution	Reflex Dropped?
C5	Deltoid	Top of shoulder	None
C6	Biceps	Lateral upper and lower arm, including first finger and thumb	Biceps jerk
C7	Triceps	Medial arm and middle finger	Triceps jerk
C8	Grip strength	Lateral arm and little finger	Triceps jerk
L4	Knee extension	Posterolateral thigh	Knee jerk
L5	Foot dorsiflexion	Top of the foot	Hamstring jerk
S1	Foot plantar flexion	Sole of the foot and lateral foot	Ankle jerk

- Peripheral nerve lesions have the lengthiest differential diagnosis in neurology, being subject to acute trauma, chronic compression, inflammation, demyelination, and toxic and infectious injury
  - Spinal nerve roots: Most commonly caused by compression by intervertebral disk; consider mass lesion
  - Cauda equina syndrome: Most common causes are disk herniation, tumor, and epidural hemorrhage
  - Plexus: Pancoast tumors present with brachial plexus lesion and Horner syndrome

Treatment

- Eliminate or correct cause
- Symptomatic treatment with tricyclic antidepressants, gabapentin, and anticonvulsants
- See Tables 62-4 to 62-6

Neuromuscular Junction

Basic Information

- Myasthenia gravis is the prototypical disorder
- **Anti–acetylcholine receptor autoantibodies block the postsynaptic receptor and block effect of**

62

TABLE 62-4	Compressive Neuropathies		
	Carpal Tunnel Syndrome	**Ulnar Neuropathy**	**Peroneal Neuropathy**
Basic information	Caused by median nerve compression at wrist	Caused by ulnar nerve compression at elbow "funny bone"	Caused by peroneal compression at fibular head
Clinical presentation	Pain, numbness, and paresthesias in first through third fingers and radial half of fourth Weakness of thumb flexion, opposition, and abduction Nocturnal exacerbation	Pain, numbness, and paresthesias in fifth finger and ulnar half of fourth Weakness of finger abductors May resemble C8 radiculopathy	Footdrop Foot inversion spared
Diagnosis and evaluation	Positive median nerve "Tinel's sign"* and "Phalen's sign"† Abnormal EMG/NCS Rule out overuse, synovitis, hypothyroidism, amyloidosis, acromegaly, and pregnancy	Positive ulnar nerve "Tinel's sign" at the elbow‡ Rule out trauma caused by leaning on elbows or repetitive curls	May resemble L5 nerve root, but no sensory abnormalities Usually traumatic May be seen in diabetes
Treatment	Wrist splint, NSAIDs, steroid injection, and surgical release	Splinting, NSAIDs, and surgical transposition of the nerve	Splinting and physical therapy

EMG, electromyography; NCS, nerve conduction study; NSAIDs, nonsteroidal anti-inflammatory drugs.
*Provoke pain and paresthesias with percussion over nerve at the wrist.
†Provoke pain, paresthesias, or numbness with forced wrist flexion (reversed "prayer position").
‡Percussion between medial elbow epicondyle and olecranon process.

TABLE 62-5	Inflammatory Neuropathies	
	Acute Inflammatory Demyelinating Polyneuropathy (Guillain-Barré Syndrome)	**Chronic Inflammatory Demyelinating Polyneuropathy**
Basic information	Immune-mediated Onset 1–3 weeks after respiratory or GI illness, in two thirds of cases Herpesvirus (CMV and EBV) *Campylobacter jejuni* Nonseasonal, nonepidemic	Immune-mediated
Clinical presentation	Longest nerves affected first (presents with leg paresthesias and disordered gait) Motor > sensory Ascending pattern of progression Respiratory failure Bowel/bladder function preserved Dysautonomia Areflexia	Slowly progressive Atrophy and fasciculation Motor > sensory
Diagnosis and evaluation	Elevated CSF protein EMG/NCS normal early in course, except for loss of "F-waves"	EMG/NCS consistent with demyelination ↓ Conduction velocity Partial conduction block
Treatment	IVIG Plasmapheresis	Steroids IVIG Plasmapheresis

CMV, cytomegalovirus; CSF, cerebrospinal fluid; EBV, Epstein-Barr virus; EMG, electromyography; NCS, nerve conduction study; IVIG, intravenous immunoglobulins.

acetylcholine released from the presynaptic nerve ending to stimulate associated muscle cells

Clinical Presentation

- **Muscles fatigue and become weak with activity**
- **Presents with fatigue with chewing, swallowing disorder, and diplopia**
- **Often associated with other autoimmune disorders or thymoma**
- Can be precipitated or worsened by aminoglycosides, clindamycin, erythromycin, tetracycline, procainamide, quinine, quinidine, β-blockers, and calcium channel blockers (Box 62-2)

Diagnosis and Evaluation

- Neurologic examination is otherwise normal
- **Measure anti–acetylcholine receptor antibodies in serum**
- Deficits improve transiently with edrophonium (Tensilon) test
- **EMG/NCS repetitive stimulation shows fatigue, but is otherwise normal**

TABLE 62-6	Toxic Neuropathies			
	Diabetic Neuropathy	**Lead Neuropathy**	**Alcoholic Neuropathy**	**Critical Illness Neuropathy**
Basic information	Caused by hyperglycemia	Caused by lead toxicity	Caused by long-standing alcohol abuse	Associated with Prolonged stay in ICU Sepsis Exposure to steroids and paralytic agents
Clinical presentation	Distal symmetrical sensory or sensorimotor neuropathy Multimodal sensory loss	Unilateral or bilateral wristdrop (classic) Distal symmetrical sensorimotor neuropathy Abdominal pain	Pain Ataxia	Often difficult to wean from ventilator
Diagnosis and evaluation*	Host presentation	Host presentation Confirmed by serum and 24-hr urine lead measurement	Host presentation	Host presentation Nerve biopsy may be useful
Treatment	Glycemic control Symptomatic	Chelation therapy Symptomatic	Eliminate exposure Symptomatic	Remove offending agents Supportive care

ICU, intensive care unit.
*Axonal changes seen on electromyography/nerve conduction study.

BOX 62-2	Medications That Exacerbate Myasthenia Gravis

Aminoglycosides
Clindamycin
Erythromycin
Tetracycline
Procainamide
Quinine
Quinidine
β-Blockers
Calcium channel blocker

- Differential diagnosis includes: Lambert-Eaton myasthenic syndrome (see Chapter 57, Table 57-3), botulism, and drug toxicity

Treatment

- Prednisone, mestinon, IV immunoglobulin, and thymectomy

Toxic Myopathies

INFLAMMATORY MYOPATHIES

Basic Information

- Caused by a variety of agents, including **alcohol, cimetidine, colchicine, D-penicillamine, heroin, prednisone, and statins**

Clinical Presentation

- **Prolonged, high-dose steroid use is associated with chronic progressive proximal muscle weakness**
- Other agents present with a classic myopathic examination

Diagnosis and Evaluation

- **Prednisone myopathy is unique in that it has normal creatine phosphokinase (CPK) levels** and is diagnosed by myopathic changes on EMG
- The other agents cause elevated CPK levels, and the EMG shows myopathic changes

Treatment

- Tapering the steroid dose or changing to a steroid-sparing immunosuppressive is the only effective treatment for steroid myopathy
- Likewise, the other inciting agents must also be stopped

REVIEW QUESTIONS

For review questions, please go to www.expertconsult.com.

SUGGESTED READINGS

Bradley WG, Daroff RB, editors: *Neurology in clinical practice*, ed 2, Philadelphia, 1945, WB Saunders.
Canale ST, editor: *Campbell's operative orthopedics*, ed 9, St. Louis, 1998, Mosby.
Collins RD: *Illustrated manual of neurological diseases*, Philadelphia, 1962, JP Lippincott.

62

SECTION ELEVEN

Selected Topics in General and Internal Medicine

Selected Topics in Geriatric Medicine

COLLEEN CHRISTMAS, MD

The medical issues facing the elderly include those commonly seen in all adults, but also include issues that become increasingly prevalent with advancing age. With aging, people become increasingly less resilient and often suffer from several chronic diseases simultaneously. These issues call on special skills when approaching elderly patients. With the aging of the U.S. population, internists will need to be familiar with the diagnosis and management of health issues common among the elderly. In this chapter, we review four syndromes commonly seen in older adults: urinary incontinence, pressure ulcers, falls, and dementia.

Urinary Incontinence

Basic Information

- Definition: Involuntary loss of urine that causes a social, health, or hygiene problem
- Physiology of micturition involves the following:
  - Sympathetic innervation: Relaxes bladder and contracts bladder neck and urethra
  - Parasympathetic innervation: Contracts bladder (detrusor muscle) for emptying
  - Somatic innervation: Leads to voluntary contraction of external urethral sphincter
    - Helpful mnemonic: Sympathetics store, parasympathetics pee

Clinical Presentation

Table 63-1 summarizes the types of urinary incontinence.
- **Urge incontinence: The most common cause of incontinence (accounts for 40–70% of cases)**
  - **Results from detrusor overactivity, detrusor instability, or detrusor hyperreflexia**
  - **Characterized by a sudden urge and desire to void, a fear of leakage, and ultimately urine loss**
  - May lose small or large amounts of urine depending on sphincter function
  - May result from defects of neurologic inhibition of the bladder (e.g., stroke, cervical stenosis, central nervous system masses, multiple sclerosis, Parkinson disease, spinal cord injury, dementia) or local bladder irritants (e.g., infection, tumor, stone)
- **Stress incontinence: The second most common cause of incontinence in the elderly**

- **Characterized by small-volume losses of urine during times of increased intra-abdominal pressure (e.g., coughing, sneezing, laughing, exercising)**
- Usually seen in women who have lost pelvic support of the urethra, with resultant failure of the urinary sphincter mechanism during periods of increased intra-abdominal pressure
- If seen in men, typically seen in those who have undergone urologic procedures
- **Overflow incontinence: Accounts for 10% of urinary incontinence among elderly patients**
  - Typically associated with some form of urinary outflow obstruction (e.g., prostatic enlargement, urethral stricture, or cystocele)
    - Also seen in diabetes mellitus, in part because of neurogenic bladder and in part because of nerve damage to control of detrusor contractility
  - Patients complain of reduced urinary stream, incomplete voiding, frequent or continuous dribbling
  - Most commonly, leakage occurs without warning
- **Functional incontinence: Occurs when an individual is unable or unwilling to reach the toilet in time**
  - Associated factors include dementia, depression, physical impairments that impede mobility (e.g., degenerative arthritis, stroke, Parkinson disease), or physical restraints or inaccessible toilets

Diagnosis

- Important historical features in the incontinent patient
  - Frequency, timing, and situations associated with incontinent episodes
  - Volume of urine loss
  - Comorbid medical and psychiatric conditions
  - Medications (Box 63-1)
  - Bladder (or voiding) record: Patient or caregiver records continent and incontinent voids over 48 hours; used to diagnose cause, assess effect on daily life, and track response to therapy
- The physical examination in the incontinent patient
  - Abdominal examination for bladder distention
  - Rectal examination for rectal tone, fecal impaction, and, in males, prostatic enlargement

TABLE 63-1	Types of Urinary Incontinence		
Type	**Pathophysiology**	**Characteristic of Urine Lost**	**Common Causes**
Urge	Detrusor overactivity	Small to large with brief "warning"	UTI, fecal impaction, CVA, cord injury
Stress	Weak bladder outlet	Small, often with coughing or standing	Weakened pelvis from childbirth
Overflow	Bladder outlet obstruction	Small, frequently dribbling without "warning"	BPH, diabetes, cystocele
Functional	Can't or won't get to toilet	Can be small but usually large	Dementia, mobility problems, toilet inaccessible

BPH, benign prostatic hypertrophy; CVA, cerebrovascular accident; UTI, urinary tract infection.

BOX 63-1 *Medications That Exacerbate Incontinence*

Sedative/hypnotics
Diuretics
α-Adrenergic agonists
α-Adrenergic antagonists
Anticholinergics
Narcotics
Alcohol
Calcium channel blockers

TABLE 63-2	Treatment of Incontinence	
Type	**Nonpharmacologic**	**Pharmacologic**
Urge incontinence	Pelvic muscle exercises (Kegel exercises) Bladder retraining Scheduled or prompted voiding	Anticholinergics Oxybutinin Tolterodine Imipramine
Stress incontinence	Pelvic muscle exercises Biofeedback Surgery Colposuspension Sling procedure	α-Adrenergic agonists: Pseudoephedrine Anticholinergics: Imipramine Estrogen alone of no proven benefit; may be of use in combination with α-adrenergics
Overflow incontinence	Intermittent or chronic catheterization Surgical correction of obstruction	Discontinue medications that exacerbate overflow obstruction
Functional incontinence	Prompted or scheduled voiding Absorbent undergarments Remove barriers to bathroom Bedside commode when appropriate Optimize physical function	None

- In women, pelvic examination for cystocele, uterine prolapse, rectocele, atrophic vaginitis
- Full neurologic examination, including mental status and mobility assessment
- Laboratory examination in the incontinent patient should include measure of renal function as well as glucose and calcium (which cause osmotic diuresis)
  - Urinalysis as well as urine culture to exclude infection as cause of incontinence
- Postvoid residual: Patient voluntarily empties bladder completely, followed by bladder catheterization to measure residual volume in bladder
  - Normal is less than 50 to 100 mL
  - **Postvoid residual of more than 100 mL suggests overflow incontinence** either from impaired detrusor contractility (e.g., neurogenic bladder) or outlet obstruction
- Urodynamic testing: Used to assess lower urinary tract function; tests commonly include cystometry, urinary flow measurement, and measurement of urethral pressure (some would add intravenous pyelography and cystourethrography to this list)
  - In majority of cases of incontinence, diagnosis can be made without testing
  - No clear guidelines exist on when to refer for testing
  - May help in the following situations:
    - Failure of the initial treatment plan
    - Confusing or inconsistent history
    - To clarify need for surgery

Treatment

See Table 63-2.

Pressure Ulcers

Basic Information

- A pressure ulcer results when unrelieved pressure on skin and subcutaneous tissue results in infarction and necrosis
  - Moisture, friction, and body habitus may contribute to susceptibility and formation of ulcer
- Four stages of pressure ulcers (Table 63-3; Figs. 63-1 to 63-3)
  - Stage I: Damage to intact skin; apparent clinically as nonblanchable erythema of intact skin
  - Stage II: Partial-thickness skin loss involving epidermis or both epidermis and dermis; clinically apparent as a blister or superficial ulcer

TABLE 63-3	*Staging of Pressure Ulcers*
Stage I	Nonblanchable erythema of intact skin
Stage II	Superficial ulcer extending through the epidermis or dermis or both
Stage III	Full-thickness skin loss exposing fat or subcutaneous tissue
Stage IV	Full-thickness skin loss exposing bone, muscle, tendon, or joint capsule

- Stage III: Full-thickness skin loss exposing subcutaneous tissue, with damage to subcutaneous tissue as well; underlying fascia is not affected; clinically apparent as a deep ulcer but without exposure of bone, muscle, or joint capsule
- Stage IV: Full-thickness skin loss extending to and including underlying fascia, including muscle and bone; clinically apparent as a crater with visibly involved underlying structures

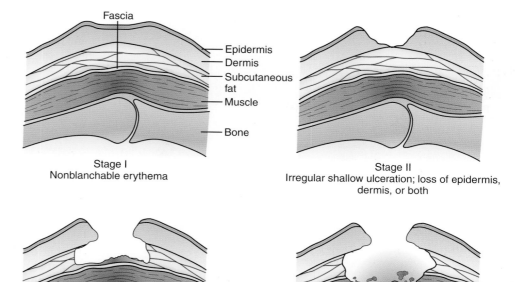

FIGURE 63-1 National Pressure Ulcer Advisory Panel classification of pressure ulcers. *(From Bolognia JL, Jorizzo JL, Rapini RP: Dermatology, St. Louis, Mosby, 2003, Fig. 106.20.)*

Stage I
Nonblanchable erythema

Stage II
Irregular shallow ulceration; loss of epidermis, dermis, or both

Stage III
Deep ulceration with necrotic base

Stage IV
Deep ulceration reaching underlying bone

FIGURE 63-2 Pressure ulcer demonstrating stages I, II, and III of ulceration.

FIGURE 63-3 Stage IV pressure ulcer on the sacrum.

TABLE 63-4	Principles of Pressure Ulcer Management
Ulcer Appearance	**Management**
Infected or necrotic	Sharp or chemical débridement Iodine product (e.g., Iodosorb) Bleach product (e.g., Chlorpactin)
Clean granulating	Supportive environment (e.g., Calginate, hydrogel)
Undermined	Fill tissue space with wick or vacuum device
Epithelializing	Petroleum gauze, collagen
Hypergranulating	Control granulation with salt foam (e.g., Mesalt) or silver nitrate

TABLE 63-5	Wound Care Products and Indications
Product	**Indication(s)**
Film covering (e.g., Opsite)	Stage I ulcer
Foam covering (e.g., Allevyn)	Noninfected stage II or III ulcer
Hydrocolloid covering (e.g., Duoderm)	Noninfected stage II ulcer; stage III ulcer with light exudate
Hydrogel (e.g., Carrington)	Stage II–IV ulcer with moderate drainage
Alginate (e.g., Sorbsan)	Stage II–IV ulcer with copious drainage

Clinical Presentation

- Risk factors have been quantified into clinical prediction rules for likelihood of developing a pressure ulcer
  - **Risk factors predictive of pressure ulcers include poor physical condition, decreased mental status, reduced activity, and incontinence**
  - Other clinical prediction rules add "poor nutritional status" (which is variably defined) and chronic skin moisture as risk factors for pressure ulcers
- Complications of pressure ulcers may accompany clinical presentation and include wound infection (manifesting as purulent drainage, often with foul odor, and surrounding erythema, warmth, and tenderness); osteomyelitis; and sinus tract formation
  - **Pressure ulcers are colonized with bacteria; a positive swab culture does not imply infection**
  - **Osteomyelitis is presumed if bone is grossly visible or can be reached with a probe**

Diagnosis

- Diagnosis based on preceding staging system
- If eschar overlies ulcer, staging cannot be performed

Treatment

Table 63-4 summarizes principles of management, and Table 63-5 provides information on wound care products.
- **Best treatment is identification of individuals at risk and prevention of ulcer development**

- **Pressure reduction: Turn and reposition immobile patients every 2 hours**
  - Specialized mattresses and beds may decrease risk of ulcer development, although it is unclear if they are superior to vigilant bedside care
  - Avoid friction: Use draw sheets to lift and turn patients; avoid any shearing forces to the skin
- Nutrition: It is unclear whether nutritional interventions improve pressure sore outcomes. Oral supplementation could play a role.
  - Despite this weak evidence, many authorities advise a diet providing 30 to 35 cal/kg/day and 1.25 to 1.5 g protein/kg/day in undernourished individuals with pressure ulcers
  - If tube feeding is used and causes increased immobility and diarrhea, pressure sore outcomes may be worsened
  - The role of zinc supplementation is unclear
  - Vitamin deficiencies should be corrected
- Optimize skin condition: avoid and treat maceration, fungal infection, or contact irritants
- Débridement: To remove necrotic material and promote healing
  - Mechanical débridement is achieved with scalpel or scissor or wet-to-moist dressings
  - Enzymatic débridement is achieved with collagenases
  - Autolytic débridement is achieved by covering ulcer with synthetic dressing, which allows enzymes in the wound to digest the necrotic but noninfected tissue
    - Should not be used in infected wounds
- **Infection: As noted previously, colonization is common and does not represent infection; swab cultures of the wound base have no clinical utility**
  - Use of topical antibiotics controversial; they may be toxic to fibroblasts
    - If used, topical antibiotics should be discontinued after 48 hours
  - **Systemic antibiotics are reserved for patients with signs of cellulitis, osteomyelitis, or systemic illness**
  - If a pocket of abscess is identified, culture of purulent contents may be useful in selecting antibiotics

Falls

Basic Information

- A fall represents an individual's unintentional coming to rest on the ground or other lower level without overwhelming intrinsic or extrinsic cause
- **Falls are distinct from syncope; with syncope, loss of consciousness occurs** (see Chapter 5)
- Incidence of falls increases with increasing age of patient
- Situational factors that predispose to falling include the type of activity and the environment
  - **70% of falls occur at home**
  - 10% of falls occur on the stairs
  - 50% of falls are associated with environmental hazards (e.g., wet surface, throw rugs)

BOX 63-2   *Risk Factors for Falling*

Medications
- Benzodiazepines
- Neuroleptics
- Tricyclic antidepressants
- Antihypertensives
- Diuretics
- Use of four or more medications simultaneously

Sensory impairment
- Visual loss
- Vestibular dysfunction
- Decreased proprioception

Central nervous system disease
- Stroke
- Parkinson disease
- Cognitive disorders

Musculoskeletal disorders
- Arthritis

Depression

Substance abuse

Past history of falling

BOX 63-3   *Home Environmental Modifications to Prevent Falls*

Stairs
Light switch at both ends
Clutter free
Tightly woven carpet or treads
Handrails

Kitchen
Avoid high shelves
Step stool with handrails
Keep floor dry

Living Area
Open pathway
No footstools, low tables, pets
Cords out of pathway
No throw rugs
Cordless phone

Bathroom
Night light
Nonskid rugs
Handrails in tub and toilet
Tub mat, chair

Bedroom
Clutter-free path
Night light
Sit on edge of bed before getting up

Footwear
Low heel, nonskid soles
Appropriate fit
Keep laces tied/Velcro

- In addition to risks associated with trauma, falls are associated with a decline in the ability to perform activities of daily living (ADLs) and an increasing likelihood of nursing home placement

Clinical Presentation

- Among the tasks of the clinician is to differentiate a fall from a syncopal event
  - Evidence of trauma should also raise concern for abuse or neglect
- Otherwise, the clinical presentation is straightforward

Diagnosis

- The events surrounding the fall and other fall history should be reviewed
  - The frequency of falling and the location of falling (e.g., in the home, on the stairs) should be reviewed
    - Look for patterns to falls, such as timing in relation to medications or meals or directions of falling (e.g., falling backward would suggest parkinsonism or falling to one side could suggest footdrop or a subtle weakness on that side)
- Risk factors for falling should be reviewed (Box 63-2)
  - More than one risk factor typically present in the patient who falls
  - **Medications such as sedatives, antidepressants, and neuroleptics are associated with the greatest risk for falling**
    - The more medications, the higher the risk of falling
  - Dementia increases the chances of falling fivefold
- Physical examination includes assessment of volume status (i.e., orthostatics), cognition, and the cardiovascular, musculoskeletal, and neurologic systems
  - Visual and auditory acuity should also be checked regularly
  - Many physicians informally evaluate fall risk with the "get up and go" test, in which they observe the patient rise from a chair and walk while paying attention to the speed and steadiness of the patient's gait

Treatment

- Prevention of falls for at-risk individuals
  - Exercise and balance training: Both have demonstrated effect at reducing falls
  - Home modification: Improve home lighting, maintain clutter-free passageways, install raised toilet seats, add grab bars in the bathroom, secure loose carpets, add stair rails (Box 63-3)
  - Adjust or avoid medications that increase risk of falling, **particularly sedating medications**
  - Emerging evidence suggest supplementation with vitamin D may reduce falls in older individuals. The ideal dose and formulation is not yet clear, however.
  - Evaluate for appropriate assistive devices, such as a cane or walker in those with imbalance or physical disability
  - Consider a referral to a physical therapist for assessment for assistive devices and for training to improve strength and balance
- Prevention of injury in those at risk of falling
  - Osteoporosis screening and treatment
  - Hip protectors
  - Lifeline or other contact strategy if fallen

63

Dementia

Basic Information

- **Dementia: A syndrome that results in a decline in memory and other cognitive abilities to the point that it interferes with ADLs**
  - Impairment of ADLs is an important distinction; age-related modest decline in intellectual function that does not impair physical function is normal and does not represent dementia
  - Mild cognitive impairment: A loss of cognition more significant than anticipated from age alone and a precursor to dementia; poorly understood
- At age 60 years, 1% of the population is demented
  - The age-related prevalence of dementia then doubles every 5 years
- Once diagnosed, estimates of average survival range from 5 to 9 years, but may be as short as 3 years
- Common causes of dementia
  - **Alzheimer disease is the most common cause of dementia (70% of cases)**
  - Vascular dementia is the second most common cause (10–20% of cases)
  - Dementia with Lewy bodies may be more common than previously thought
  - Alcohol-related causes are commonly associated with dementia; one out of five patients with dementia has a significant alcohol history
  - Often individuals will have clinical features of more than one type of dementia and will be labeled as having "mixed-type" dementia
- Uncommon causes of dementia include infectious causes (e.g., HIV, neurosyphilis); endocrine or metabolic causes (e.g., hypothyroidism, hypercalcemia, vitamin B_{12} deficiency); and neurologic disorders, including Parkinson disease, frontotemporal dementia (formerly known as Pick disease), Creutzfeldt-Jacob disease, subdural hematoma, and normal-pressure hydrocephalus
- **Only 2% of cases of dementia are caused by reversible causes; even when found and treated (e.g., hypothyroidism, syphilis), dementia may not resolve**
  - Depression may present with impairments of cognition ("pseudodementia") that improve significantly when the depression is adequately treated. Thus, depression is very important to consider in the differential diagnosis of someone with cognitive concerns.

Clinical Presentation

- With dementia, family members or caregivers are usually the ones who initially raise concern for dementia
  - **A patient who complains of memory problems is more likely to be depressed or under stress than demented**
  - **Consciousness is clear in the demented patient;** clouded consciousness (especially waxing and waning symptoms) suggests delirium
- Clinical features vary based on cause of dementia
  - **Alzheimer disease results in a gradual decline in cognitive function**

BOX 63-4 *Diagnostic Criteria for Dementia*

Part 1: The development of multiple cognitive defects, manifested by both
  Memory impairment *plus*
  One or more of the following cognitive (or cortical) disturbances:
    Aphasia (language disturbance)
    Apraxia (impaired ability to carry out motor activities despite intact motor function)
    Agnosia (failure to recognize or identify objects despite intact sensory function)
    Disturbance in executive functioning (planning, organization, abstraction)
Part 2: The cognitive deficits must cause significant impairment in social or occupational functioning and represent a decline from a previous level of functioning

---

  - **Language skills commonly affected; motor skills typically spared**
  - **Vascular dementia is associated with a stepwise, sudden progression of decline in cognitive function**
    - In this population, the medical history typically uncovers other risk factors for vascular disease
    - Abnormal motor signs are common, including facial masking, rigidity, an extensor plantar reflex, and gait disturbances
  - **Dementia with Lewy bodies is commonly associated with fluctuations in alertness or cognition, visual hallucinations, and features of parkinsonism**

Diagnosis

- Diagnostic criteria for dementia are listed in Box 63-4
- Assessment of neurocognitive functioning
  - The mini-mental status examination (MMSE), mini-cog, or another similar test may be used to provide a quantitative assessment of cognitive impairment and to provide a baseline for comparison over time
    - Age and education level affect score on MMSE
    - For English-speaking individuals with at least an eighth-grade education, a score less than 24 in the appropriate clinical setting suggests the presence of dementia
  - Functional status can also be assessed with standardized tests such as a functional activities questionnaire, which assess high-level activities (e.g., writing checks and balancing a checkbook, organizing tax records, shopping for groceries)
  - Formal neurocognitive testing is recommended when there is sufficient concern for the diagnosis of dementia and in particular in individuals with a coexisting mood disorder
- Laboratory examination in the patient with suspected dementia (Box 63-5)
  - Increasing evidence has linked the apolipoprotein E ε4 allele with an increased risk of developing Alzheimer disease
  - Until more medical evidence is available, routine testing of the apolipoprotein E genotype in the evaluation of the demented patient is not recommended

BOX 63-5	*Laboratory Evaluation of the Patient with Dementia**

Complete blood count
Electrolytes
Blood urea nitrogen
Creatinine
Liver enzymes
Calcium
Thyroid-stimulating hormone
Rapid plasma reagin
HIV
Vitamin B_{12}

*Some clinicians would add homocysteine and methylmalonic acid to this list.

- Testing for syphilis recommended if there is a history of prior infection, risk factors for syphilis, or the individual lives in an area with high prevalence of syphilis
- Neuroimaging is now recommended by the American Academy of Neurology in the evaluation of all patients with dementia, though not all authorities agree with this approach and its cost-effectiveness has not been demonstrated
  - Often performed to exclude identifiable causes such as tumors, mass lesions, subdural hematoma, or normal-pressure hydrocephalus

Management

- **Overall goals of therapy are to identify and treat reversible causes of dementia and to improve quality of life and maximize functional performance**
  - Caregiver and family education and counseling improve quality of life and delay the need for nursing home placement by as much as 1 year
- Symptomatic therapy focuses on treating cognitive impairment, mood disturbances, and behavioral disturbances
  - **Pharmacotherapy for cognitive impairment limited; all share mechanism of cholinergic augmentation by inhibiting cholinesterase**
    - Examples include tacrine, donepezil, rivastigmine, and galantamine
    - Best experience is in use in patients with mild to moderate Alzheimer disease; no role in patients with severe Alzheimer disease

- **Modest improvement in cognitive functioning may be demonstrable on neurocognitive testing, but improvement is often not evident to caregiver or clinician and does not prevent the progression of disease**
- The role of estrogen, nonsteroidal anti-inflammatory drugs, and 3-hydroxy-3-methylglutaryl coenzyme A (HMG-CoA) reductase inhibitors in the prevention and development of Alzheimer disease has not been defined
- **Mood impairment, most commonly depression, should be anticipated and treated in the patient with dementia**
  - Selective serotonin reuptake inhibitors are preferred. The anticholinergic side effects of tricyclic antidepressants should be avoided.
- Behavioral therapy should be added if the patient becomes agitated or psychotic (seen in 50% of demented patients)
  - Haloperidol has been the drug of choice for behavioral issues that cannot be managed with redirection alone and pose an important risk to the individual or caregiver
    - Some use newer generation antipsychotics that may have fewer extrapyramidal side effects (e.g., risperidone, olanzapine, and quetiapine), but at greater cost and without demonstration of enhanced efficacy
  - Benzodiazepines can worsen confusion and should be avoided

REVIEW QUESTIONS

For review questions, please go to www.expertconsult.com.

SUGGESTED READINGS

Boustani M, Peterson B, Hanson L, et al: Screening for dementia in primary care: a summary of the evidence for the U.S. Preventive Services Task Force, *Ann Intern Med* 138:927–937, 2003.

Cobbs EL, Duthie EH, Murphy JB, editors: *Geriatrics review syllabus: a core curriculum in geriatric medicine*, ed 5, Malden, MA, 2002, Blackwell.

Courtney C, Farrell D, Gray R, et al: Long-term donepezil treatment in 565 patients with Alzheimer's disease (AD2000 Collaborative Group): randomised double-blind trial, *Lancet* 363:2105–2115, 2004.

Executive summary of the American Geriatrics Society, British Geriatrics Society, and American Academy of Orthopaedic Surgeons: Clinical practice guideline: the prevention of falls in older persons, *J Am Geriatr Soc* 49:664–672, 2001.

63

Selected Topics in Women's Health

WENDY L. BENNETT, MD, MPH; and REDONDA G. MILLER, MD, MBA

Internists provide care for women of all ages and often are faced with a variety of disorders specific to women. Familiarity with gynecologic disorders is crucial. In addition, pregnant women may have medical complications that require close evaluation and monitoring by the internist. This chapter covers many of these important issues, including cervical cancer screening, contraception, and medical complications of pregnancy.

Cervical Cancer Screening and Treatment

Basic Information

- Cervical cancer is prevalent, with 16,000 new cases reported each year in the United States. Early detection through the Papanicolaou (Pap) smear has greatly reduced mortality.
- **Risk factors for cervical cancer**
  - **Human papillomavirus (HPV)**
  - **Smoking**
  - **Multiple sexual partners**
  - **Early age of first intercourse**
  - **History of other sexually transmitted diseases (STDs)**
  - **Human immunodeficiency virus (HIV) infection (see Chapter 12)**
  - **Other immunocompromised state**
- **Cervical cancer and its precursors are caused by oncogenic serotypes of HPV**
  - HPV exposure is already common and becoming more prevalent in humans
  - HPV serotypes 16, 18, 33, 35, and 39 confer highest risk and are often associated with high-grade neoplasia and invasive cancer
  - HPV serotypes 6, 11, and 42 are more often associated with low-risk lesions and condylomata
  - Cervical cancer in the absence of heterosexual activity is extremely rare, probably because sperm assist HPV infection of cervical epithelium
  - Testing for high-risk HPV DNA enhances the sensitivity of cervical cytology screening
- HPV vaccine (Gardasil)
  - Directed against HPV 16 and 18 serotypes (two most common oncogenic strains), as well as serotypes 6 and 11

- Vaccine effective at decreasing HPV 16/18–related high-grade cervical intraepithelial neoplasia (CIN) and carcinoma *in situ*
- Series of three injections at 0, 2, and 6 months
- Recommended for women younger than 26 years of age, and is most effective in women never exposed to HPV
- Avoid in pregnancy

Clinical Presentation

- The cervical epithelium most often affected by malignant transformation is where the columnar cells of the endocervical canal are undergoing transformation into the squamous cells of the exocervix (called the "transformation zone") (Fig. 64-1)
- Most women with precursors to cervical cancer are asymptomatic
- Invasive cervical cancer becomes symptomatic at a late stage
  - Abnormal bleeding (menorrhagia, postcoitally, or intermenstrual) may occur early in the disease
  - Late-stage symptoms are usually caused by local spread and may include pelvic, leg, or back pain; pedal edema; rectal bleeding; or hematuria
- Physical examination may show evidence of the following:
  - HPV infection: Condylomata acuminata (verrucous-like lesions; Fig. 64-2)
  - Invasive cancer: Induration, friable tissue, ulceration, exophytic (cauliflower-like) lesions

Diagnosis and Evaluation

- **Cervical cytology (the Pap smear) is the screening test of choice; screens for both dysplasia and cancer**
  - Involves exfoliative cytology of the uterine cervix
  - Proven to reduce the incidence of squamous cervical cancer and resultant mortality
  - Sensitivity is approximately 70% to 80%; specificity is 90% to 95%
    - **Proper interpretation of Pap smear is crucial to avoiding unnecessary testing (see following discussion)**
    - **Many lesions regress over time and do not portend a diagnosis of cancer**
    - **Management of abnormal Pap smears differs significantly in women with HIV infection; see Chapter 12 for details**

FIGURE 64-1 Cervix demonstrating abnormal epithelium on the anterior and posterior margins, demonstrating the white discoloration after the application of acetic acid. *(From Oats J, Abraham S: Llewellyn-Jones fundamentals of obstetrics and gynaecology, ed 8, Philadelphia, Mosby, 2004, Fig. 37.6.)*

FIGURE 64-2 Genital warts on the vulva of a woman, which are associated with human papillomavirus. *(From http://en.wikipedia.org/wiki/Genital_warts)*

- Technique
  - Perform before bimanual examination
  - Visualize the entire cervix if possible
  - Remove any discharge carefully before obtaining specimen
  - Small amount of blood is acceptable; large amounts (i.e., menses) preclude adequate testing
  - Must include cells from the transformation zone to be deemed adequate
  - Conventional brush-and-scrape technique
    - Sample obtained with an endocervical spatula and brush (sequentially)

- Scrape exterior cervix before endocervical canal
- Must undergo rapid fixation on slide to avoid air-drying and subsequent artifact
  - Liquid-based sampling (preferred)
    - Specially designed round brush is inserted into the cervix and rotated clockwise five full rotations
    - Entire brush placed into liquid medium
    - Better sensitivity over conventional technique
    - HPV testing may be performed on the same sample (concurrently or retrospectively)
- Pap smear frequency
  - **Pap smear screening should be initiated in all women once sexually active or at age 21 years (whichever is first)**
  - Screen every 2 years in women age 21 to 29 (more frequently in women with HIV, immunosuppression, diethylstilbestrol exposure, history of CIN, or other risk factors)
  - Women over the age of 30 who have had at least three negative smears can be screened every 3 years
  - Women at high risk (see preceding risk factors) require annual Pap smear screening indefinitely, even if they never have an abnormal result
  - In women who have undergone hysterectomy without a cervical remnant, Pap smears are no longer required unless the hysterectomy was performed for cervical cancer
  - Because cervical cancer develops slowly and risk factors decrease with age, it is reasonable to discontinue cervical cancer screening over age 65 in women who have three or more negative cytology test results in a row and no abnormal test results in the past 10 years
- The Bethesda System is used for classification of Pap smear adequacy and results (Table 64-1)
  - Descriptions may include the following
    - Benign cellular changes (e.g., infection)
    - Reactive cellular changes (e.g., inflammation)
    - Epithelial cell changes
  - **Infections found on Pap smear should be treated (i.e., *Candida, Trichomonas*)**
  - Squamous metaplasia is a normal finding
- **Consensus guidelines (2009) for management of abnormal Pap smears** (see Table 64-1)
  - Atypical squamous cells of unknown significance (ASCUS) and atypical glandular cells of unknown significance (AGUS) diagnoses are not normal, but do not meet the criteria for a more serious diagnosis
  - **ASCUS is the most common finding on abnormal Pap smears**
    - **Majority of these women have benign findings on colposcopy**
    - **HPV testing is a helpful option in triaging cases of ASCUS for colposcopy (see Table 64-1)**
      - Test for high-risk subtypes
      - Testing for low-risk subtypes is not helpful in triaging risk of more aggressive disease
  - ASCUS in an immunosuppressed woman should always prompt colposcopy
- Diagnosis is considered secured when Pap result, colposcopy, and biopsy histology are in agreement

64

TABLE 64-1	*The Bethesda Classification of Pap Smear Results and Management Options*	
Pap Smear Result	**Risk of High-Grade Lesion (by Histology)**	**Management Options***
Normal	Essentially none	Continue routine screening

Atypical squamous cells of undetermined significance (ASCUS)	Low	Three options
		  Repeat Pap smear in 4–6 mo
		    If two consecutive repeats are normal, continue yearly screening
		    If ASCUS obtained before two normal repeats, refer for colposcopy
		  or
		  Colposcopy
		    If normal, resume annual Pap screening
		    If abnormal, perform biopsies
		  or
		  DNA testing for human papillomavirus
		    If positive, refer for colposcopy
		    If negative, repeat Pap smear in 1 year

Atypical glandular cells of undetermined significance (AGUS)	More related to endometrial rather than cervical cancer	More aggressive follow-up because AGUS is more commonly related to serious disease than is ASCUS Colposcopy with directed biopsy is recommended Endometrial biopsy usually indicated as well If all normal, repeat Pap in 3–6 mo
Low-grade squamous intraepithelial lesion (LGSIL)	15–30%	Colposcopy and directed biopsies
High-grade squamous intraepithelial lesion (HGSIL)	70–75%	Colposcopy and directed biopsies
Invasive cancer	>99%	Colposcopy and directed biopsies

*See Chapter 12 for a discussion of management of abnormal Papanicolaou (Pap) smears in women with HIV.

- If the results of the Pap, colposcopic appearance, and biopsy histology are in significant disagreement, treatment can still be initiated, if the histology reports the most severe diagnosis
  - If the histology specimen indicates less severe results than Pap diagnosis, consider that the biopsy did not sample the region of the genital tract shedding the cells resulting in the Pap abnormality (sampling error)
    - Should obtain a larger biopsy specimen
    - Options to remove a larger portion of the cervix to include the entire exocervical portion of the transformation zone (identifiable by an applied stain) and part of the endocervical canal include
      - Cold knife conization (CKC) using a scalpel
      - Loop electrosurgical excision procedure (LEEP) using a heated wire loop
      - Laser conization
    - The biopsy sample is then considered adequate if the histologic diagnosis is at least as serious as the Pap diagnosis, and the margins of the biopsy are free of premalignant or malignant transformation

Treatment

- Low-grade squamous intraepithelial lesions (LGSIL) and high-grade squamous intraepithelial lesions (HGSIL) are considered precursors of invasive squamous cell cancer of the cervix
- LGSIL treatment
  - **If LGSIL is confirmed by colposcopy and histology, treatment can be expectant with quarterly Pap smears because the majority revert to normal without treatment**

- After four quarterly Pap smears in a row have been normal, follow-up can be semiannual Pap smears for another year followed by annual testing (assuming all are normal)
  - Alternatively, if the patient prefers, or in older women or in women in whom follow-up may be problematic, treatment with LEEP or cryosurgery can be undertaken
- HGSIL treatment
  - May be treated in a variety of ways, all of which result in its removal from the cervix
  - If a conization procedure is performed in the evaluation, the cytology and histology do not include invasive cancer, and the margins of the cone are free of disease, treatment is considered complete
  - Otherwise, the affected region of the cervix can be removed by LEEP, CKC, laser conization, or cryosurgery (killing the affected cells using liquid nitrogen)
  - Hysterectomy may be appropriate treatment for women with other problems (e.g., severe dysmenorrhea or menorrhagia)
  - Follow-up is then quarterly Pap smears for a year, semiannual Pap smears for another year, and then annual Pap smears (assuming all are normal)
  - Frequent follow-up is also indicated in women after a hysterectomy, in case part of the cervix remains or disease develops in the vaginal epithelium
- Treatment of invasive cervical cancer
  - Staging is first step: Requires pelvic examination, routine labs, chest radiograph, intravenous pyelogram; other studies as deemed necessary
    - Stage I: Confined to the cervix

- Stage II: Extends beyond cervix but not to pelvic sidewall or lower third of vagina
- Stage III: Involves pelvic sidewall or lower third of vagina
- Stage IV: Metastatic disease (beyond pelvis) or involvement of bladder or rectum
  - Treatment based on stage
    - Stage I can usually be treated with hysterectomy with or without radiation
    - Stages II and III are predominantly treated with radiation
    - Stage IV requires radical surgery, usually with radiation, or palliative chemotherapy or radiation
  - Prognosis based on tumor size, stage, and nodal involvement
    - Stage I: 78% overall survival
    - Stage IV: 8% overall survival

Contraception

- Half of all pregnancies are unplanned; contraception is an important primary care issue
- Many different forms of contraception are available to women; choice is often based on personal preference
- **Contraceptive efficacy can be measured by the Pearl index**
  - **The Pearl index is the number of women out of 100 using a particular method likely to be pregnant at the end of a year of usual use (Table 64-2)**
  - Actual failure rates of the techniques listed are higher than the values shown; usually caused by improper use of the method
- Specific types of contraception
  - Abstinence
  - Rhythm method (Fig. 64-3)
  - Barrier methods
    - Condoms
      - Latex sheath that fits snugly over the penis during intercourse
      - **Advantages: Protection from STDs, easily obtained over the counter**
      - Efficacy greatly enhanced by addition of spermicides, which decrease sperm motility (e.g., nonoxynol-9)
    - Diaphragm
      - Rubber dome-shaped cup that fits over the cervix
      - Inserted manually before intercourse
      - Major disadvantages are inconvenience and required fitting by clinician
  - Hormonal
    - Combination oral contraceptives
      - Most commonly used reversible method of contraception
      - Contain both estrogen and progestin in 21 tablets; remaining 7 tablets contain inert ingredients (to bring on withdrawal bleed)
        - **Estrogen: Serves mainly to inhibit ovulation by suppressing pituitary gonadotropin secretion; usually dosed between 20 μg ("low-dose") and 35 μg per tablet**

TABLE 64-2	*Contraceptive Options and Efficacy*	
Technique	**Pearl Index***	**Possible Side Effects**
Attempting conception	80	N/A
Withdrawal	40	None
Rhythm	40	None
Spermicidal suppositories or foam	20	Local irritation Allergic reactions
Condom	20	Skin irritation Latex allergy
Diaphragm	15	Pelvic irritation and discomfort Small increase in urinary tract infections
Intrauterine device	<1	Menorrhagia Dysmenorrhea Increased risk of salpingitis (leading to possible infertility) Uterine perforation
Combination oral contraceptive pills	1–2	Breakthrough bleeding (if occurs longer than 3 mo, deserves evaluation) Amenorrhea (not harmful) Headache, worsening migraines Breast tenderness Increase in blood pressure Increased risk of thromboembolism Increased risk of gallbladder disease
Progesterone-only contraceptive pills	5	Breakthrough or irregular bleeding Loss of bone density with prolonged use
Injected progesterone	<1	Breakthrough bleeding Weight gain Acne Loss of bone density with prolonged use
Female sterilization	<1	Risk of anesthesia

*Pearl index is the number of couples out of 100 using a particular method that are likely to be pregnant at the end of a year of usual use.

- **Progestin: Causes changes in cervical mucus and endometrium that hinder fertility**
  - Many different formulations and combinations exist on the market
    - Choice of prescribed formulation often based on patient or doctor familiarity, cost, availability
    - Monophasic pill: Constant dose of estrogen and progestin in each tablet
    - Phasic pill: Changing dose of progestin (and sometimes estrogen) in the active tablets; usually an escalating dose
  - **Combination oral contraceptives are highly effective; most common reason for failure is noncompliance**
    - **If a woman misses 1 or 2 tablets, she should take 1 tablet immediately on remembering followed by 1 tablet twice daily until missed tablets have been taken**

64

FIGURE 64-3 Periodic abstinence ("rhythm method"), using the mucus (ovulation) method. *(From Oats J, Abraham S: Llewellyn-Jones fundamentals of obstetrics and gynaecology, ed 8, Philadelphia, Mosby, 2004.)*

- **If more than 2 tablets missed, another form of contraception should be used as backup during that cycle**
- Potential benefits: Improvement in dysmenorrhea, premenstrual symptoms, and benign breast disease; decreased risk of pelvic inflammatory disease and ectopic pregnancy; decreased risk of ovarian and endometrial cancer
- Some women experience cessation of menses (not dangerous)
- **Relative contraindications include:**
  - **History of thromboembolic disease, stroke, or active liver disease, history of breast or endometrial cancer, smokers older than 35 years of age**
- Newer progesterone options (available in combination with estrogen)
  - Third-generation oral contraceptives contain newer progestins (i.e., norgestimate)
    - Fewer side effects and may improve acne
    - May also have a slightly higher thrombosis risk
  - Drosperidone
    - Has both antiandrogenic and antimineralocorticoid properties
    - Useful in polycystic ovary syndrome; reduces hirsutism and other clinical symptoms
    - Watch for hyperkalemia
- Other dosing and administration options
  - Continuous use method: May dose oral contraceptive continuously (skipping the 7 placebo pills) to bring on withdrawal bleed every 3 months (or even longer) rather than monthly
    - Convenience for patient
    - Decrease in premenstrual migraines, premenstrual dysphoric disorder
  - Contraceptive patch
    - Apply patch once weekly for 3 weeks, then remove for 1 week
    - Some patients find it more convenient
    - Minor side effect of local irritation in a few
    - Contraindicated in women with weight greater than 200 pounds due to unpredictable absorption

- May confer higher venous thromboembolism risk compared with other hormonal methods.
  - Contraceptive ring
    - Inserted by patient for 3 weeks, then removed for 1 week
    - No need to remove during intercourse, but may remove for up to 3 hours if desired
    - Caution patients to watch for spontaneous expulsion
- "Mini-pill"
  - Contains small doses of progestin only
  - Has 28 tablets of active hormone; no inert tablets
  - Less efficacious and more breakthrough bleeding than with combination pills
  - **Useful for women who cannot tolerate estrogen, lactating women, and older women with cardiovascular risk factors**
- Injected progesterone (e.g., Depo-Provera)
  - Usually administered once every 3 months
  - Higher efficacy than combination oral contraceptive pills, possibly because of better compliance
  - Long-term use has been associated with reversible losses in bone mineral density
- Intrauterine device (IUD; Fig. 64-4)
  - Contraceptive device inserted into the lining of the uterus by a gynecologist
  - Precise mechanism not known but believed to primarily interfere with fertilization
  - Underused option in the United States that confers excellent efficacy and convenience
  - Best candidates are women at low risk for acquiring STD (since infection may require IUD removal) and not planning pregnancy for at least 1 year
  - Options
    - Copper-clad T-shaped IUD: Has an effective duration of 10 years
    - Levonorgestrel-releasing IUD: Inserted every 5 years; high rates of amenorrhea; no loss of bone mineral density

FIGURE 64-4 Copper 375 multiload intrauterine device. *(From Oats J, Abraham S: Llewellyn-Jones fundamentals of obstetrics and gynaecology, ed 8, Philadelphia, Mosby, 2004, Fig. 38.9.)*

- Whereas one third of failures with female sterilization result in an ectopic pregnancy, there is no increased risk of ectopia with the IUD
- Disadvantages: Risk of expulsion, increased risk of pelvic inflammatory disease (greatest risk in first 20 days after insertion), uterine perforation at time of insertion
- **Contraindications: Severe uterine distortion, acute pelvic infection, known pregnancy, unexplained uterine bleeding, current breast cancer, copper allergy (for copper IUD)**
- Special considerations in adolescents, women with prior STDs, immunocompromised women, and women on anticoagulation therapy
- Sterilization
  - Tubal ligation or vasectomy are standard procedures
  - Most effective method of contraception
- **Emergency contraception (the "morning after" pill)**
  - Use of a contraceptive after unprotected intercourse to prevent pregnancy
  - Probably works by inhibiting ovulation, thus is not an abortifacient
  - 75% to 80% effective if used within 72 hours of intercourse
  - Most common form is 0.75 mg of levonorgestrel given within 72 hours of intercourse and repeated once 12 hours later
  - Alternatively, a single dose of 1.5 mg of levonorgestrel is probably equally effective with fewer side effects
  - Patient should expect usual menses within 21 days of treatment
  - Main side effect of hormonal method is nausea and vomiting; consider simultaneous prescription of an antiemetic to take 1 hour before
  - Contraindications: Pregnancy or undiagnosed pathologic genital bleeding

- Consider STD testing and HIV prevention after unprotected intercourse

Medical Issues Related to Pregnancy

HYPERTENSIVE DISORDERS IN PREGNANCY

- Can assume several different forms (Table 64-3)
- **Chronic hypertension**
  - **Definition: Blood pressure greater than 140/90 mm Hg observed before pregnancy or within the first 20 weeks of gestation**
    - Associated with an increased risk of intrauterine growth retardation, cesarean delivery, abruptio placentae, preterm birth, superimposed preeclampsia, and fetal death
    - Antihypertensive drug therapy in pregnancy has not been proven to improve outcomes, and there is concern about impact of blood pressure–lowering drugs on placental perfusion (resulting in decreased fetal growth)
    - Antihypertensive therapy not indicated for mild hypertension in pregnancy (generally defined as less than 150/100 mm Hg), but there is no consensus on optimal threshold. Treatment is usually started to prevent maternal complications, such as stroke.
  - **All antihypertensive medications cross the placenta. Methyldopa is the antihypertensive medication most frequently prescribed during pregnancy and is the drug of choice, but several other agents are considered safe and are better tolerated. There are no data from large trials on medication choice.**
    - Clonidine
    - Calcium channel blockers (long-acting nifedipine is commonly used)
    - Combined α-, β-blockers (labetolol is commonly used next to methyldopa)
    - Hydralazine
    - β-Blockers (associated with fetal growth restriction and inadequate neonatal response to hypoglycemia)
    - Diuretics (associated with fetal growth restriction and fetal distress if started or increased during pregnancy because the lack of uterine or placental autoregulation puts perfusion of the fetus at the mercy of maternal blood volume)
  - **Angiotensin-converting enzyme inhibitors and angiotensin receptor blockers are absolutely contraindicated in pregnancy because of risk of fetal toxicity**
  - Once therapy is started, care should be taken to avoid large drops in maternal blood pressure because uterine, placental, and fetal perfusion will fall in proportion
  - **A reasonable goal is to keep maternal blood pressures in the 140–160/90–100 mm Hg range**
- Preeclampsia and eclampsia
  - **Preeclampsia is defined as triad of hypertension occurring for the first time after 20 weeks' gestation with proteinuria (>300 mg/24 hr) and edema**

64

TABLE 64-3	*Hypertensive Complications of Pregnancy*	
Disorder	**Clinical Manifestations**	**Treatment**
Chronic hypertension	Usually asymptomatic, preexisting hypertension diagnosis, or BP 140/90 mm Hg before the 20th week of pregnancy If severe, may have headache, blurred vision, hematuria, pulmonary edema	Nonpharmacologic treatment if woman is low risk for stroke or cardiovascular complications with short time frame of pregnancy. Methyldopa is drug of choice, if treating. Second-line choices: Labetolol, calcium channel blockers
Gestational hypertension	Transient hypertension (>140/90 mm Hg) at later than 20 weeks' gestation, and if preeclampsia not present, and blood pressure returns to normal by 12 weeks postpartum	Nonpharmacologic treatment preferred, close monitoring

Preeclampsia	Classic triad
	  Hypertension
	  Proteinuria
	  Edema
	"Severe" preeclampsia also may have:
	  Headache
	  Visual disturbances
	  Pulmonary edema
	  Oliguria
	May also see elevated liver enzymes later in course
		Delivery of fetus, if possible, is definitive therapy
		Antepartum
		  Bed rest and observation
		  Frequent fetal ultrasonography and surveillance
		  Antihypertensives of unproven benefit
		Intrapartum
		  Hydration with careful fluid monitoring
		  Seizure prevention: Intravenous magnesium sulfate
		  Hypertension: Intravenous hydralazine, labetalol, or nitroglycerin; sublingual nifedipine
		Postpartum
		  Need to continue magnesium for 24–48 hr

Eclampsia	New-onset seizures or coma in patient with preeclampsia	Similar to preeclampsia

HELLP syndrome	Hemolysis
	Elevated liver enzymes (AST and ALT up to 4000 U/L)
	Low platelet count (as low as 6000/mm^3)
	Other symptoms
	  Epigastric pain
	  Nausea, vomiting
	  Headache
	  Edema
		Delivery is definitive
		Lab values (AST, ALT, platelets) normalize within 5 days postpartum

ALT, alanine aminotransferase; AST, aspartate aminotransferase; BP, blood pressure; HELLP, hemolysis, elevated liver enzymes, and low platelet count. From Report of the National High Blood Pressure Education Program Working Group on High Blood Pressure in Pregnancy, *Am J Obstet Gynecol* 2000; 183:S1-S22.

- "Severe" preeclampsia: Blood pressure greater than 160/110 mm Hg, more than 5 g protein/24 hr, oliguria, retinal hemorrhages or papilledema, headache or visual disturbances, or pulmonary edema
- Preeclampsia occurs in up to 7% of all pregnancies
  - More common in women during first pregnancy, with advanced maternal age, with twin gestation, with a prior history of preeclampsia, or superimposed on chronic hypertension or diabetes
- **Eclampsia is rare and is diagnosed when a patient with preeclampsia develops seizures (not attributable to another cause)**
- Preeclampsia and eclampsia may be related to maternal and fetal morbidity
  - Maternal: Intracranial hemorrhage, abruptio placentae with hemorrhage, renal cortical necrosis
  - Fetal: Intrauterine growth retardation, increased mortality
- Management: Only "cure" is delivery of the fetus
- **Hemolysis, elevated liver enzymes, and low platelet count (HELLP) syndrome**
  - **Variant of preeclampsia (10–15%), in which patients may also develop microangiopathic anemia, thrombocytopenia, or hepatocellular necrosis**
  - Can also develop in pregnant women without preeclampsia

- May occur antepartum (two thirds of patients) and postpartum (one third of patients)
- May be difficult to differentiate from hemolytic uremic syndrome and thrombotic thrombocytopenic purpura
- Unlikely to recur in subsequent pregnancies
- Clinical manifestations and management: see Table 64-3
- Postpartum considerations for postpartum period in patient with hypertensive disorder in pregnancy
  - Women with chronic hypertension may develop postpartum complications, such as heart failure, pulmonary edema, and renal failure, especially if there are underlying comorbid health conditions
  - Oral hypertensive medications may be required after delivery to control blood pressure, particularly for women who were hypertensive prior to pregnancy and who stopped medications during pregnancy

DIABETES MELLITUS IN PREGNANCY

- Most common medical complication of pregnancy, affecting approximately 7% of pregnancies in the United States
- Definitions of diabetes in pregnancy
  - Pregestational diabetes: Type 1 or 2 diabetes diagnosed before or in early pregnancy using standard diagnostic tests and cutoffs

- Gestational diabetes mellitus (GDM): Glucose intolerance detected for the first time in pregnancy
  - Characterized by hyperglycemia and insulin levels insufficient to meet insulin demands; and pregnancy-induced insulin resistance, which normally occurs in late pregnancy, unmasks (likely chronic) defects in pancreatic beta cell defects
  - Risk factors for GDM include maternal obesity, increased maternal age, previous GDM, parity, increased gestational weight gain, short stature, a family history of diabetes
- **Gestational diabetes is associated with an increased risk of developing type 2 diabetes later in life (about 19% by 9 years compared with 2% of women without GDM), so women with a history of GDM should have periodic screening for diabetes and risk reduction counseling (e.g., weight loss)**
- Diabetes in pregnancy is associated with increased perinatal risks of the following:
  - Fetal macrosomia (defined as birth weight greater than 4000 g)
  - Cesarean delivery
  - Shoulder dystocia
  - Other neonatal problems, including respiratory distress syndrome, hypercalcemia, hyperbilirubinemia, and polycythemia
  - Fetal anomalies: Primarily cardiac and skeletal
- If blood glucose values well controlled in pregnancy, shoulder dystocia and macrosomia rates are decreased
- Screening for GDM is either universal or risk factor–based, using a 50-g glucose challenge test between 24 and 28 weeks gestation
  - A positive screen is a serum glucose of 140 mg/dL or greater 1 hour after the oral ingestion of 50 g of hyperosmolar glucose irrespective of prior oral intake
  - If the screen is greater than 200 mg/dL, patient is diagnosed as having GDM
  - If the screen is 140 to 200 mg/dL, a 3-hour glucose tolerance test should be performed (more sensitive and specific)
- Management of diabetes in pregnancy involves maintaining glucose values approaching euglycemia
  - Insulin or an oral agent (sulfonylurea or metformin) is usually started for fasting glucose values consistently above 100 mg/dL or values 2 hours postprandial consistently over 120 mg/dL
  - **Goals of glycemic control are a fasting glucose value of 60 to 80 mg/dL and a 2-hour postprandial value less than 120 mg/dL (1-hour value <140 mg/dL)**

ASTHMA IN PREGNANCY

- Course in pregnancy is unpredictable: Some patients worsen, others improve
- Asthma exacerbations in pregnancy can result in maternal, and thus fetal, hypoxemia, leading to fetal death, prematurity, or low birth weight
- Benefit of continuing pharmacologic therapy for asthma far outweighs the risk
  - Studies show lack of adverse effects for use of albuterol inhaler, or inhaled steroids (budesonide and beclomethasone)
- Some concern about fetal risks associated with frequent use of chronic oral steroids, so prevention of exacerbations is important

THYROID DISEASE IN PREGNANCY

- Increased incidence of thyroid disease during pregnancy (see Chapter 38)
- During pregnancy, serum thyroid-binding globulin concentration increases, and human chorionic gonadotropin stimulates the thyrotropin receptor
- Thyroid medications are generally safe in pregnancy
- Hypothyroidism in pregnancy
  - Natural and synthetic thyroid hormones (thyroxine, triiodothyronine) do not cross the placenta and can be used during pregnancy
  - **Thyroid replacement requirements increase early in the first trimester—monitor aggressively to improve fetal outcomes**
  - **Goal is to maintain thyroid-stimulating hormone level between 1 and 2**
- Hyperthyroidism in pregnancy
  - Control of hyperthyroidism is important because, if poorly controlled, it is associated with adverse fetal outcomes, such as growth restriction and premature birth
  - Antithyroid medications (propylthiouracil and methimazole) do cross the placenta and may be teratogenic; radioiodine is contraindicated
  - **Antithyroid therapy is directed at keeping the maternal serum free thyroxine at the upper limits of normal; risks of treatment need to be discussed**

DEPRESSION IN PREGNANCY

- Treatment of depression in pregnancy with medications is generally safe
- Fluoxetine is considered the safest and most well-studied selective serotonin reuptake inhibitor (SSRI) in pregnancy; avoid paroxetine, which has been associated with congenital heart defects

MEDICATIONS IN PREGNANCY

- No medication is proven to be absolutely safe; therefore, pregnant women should limit medication usage to true needs and minimize usage as much as possible
- **Food and Drug Administration classification of drugs regarding safety in pregnancy is as follows:**
  - Category A: Controlled studies in women fail to demonstrate risk to fetus in first trimester; unlikely to cause fetal harm
  - Category B: Studies of animal reproduction have not demonstrated risk to fetus, but no controlled studies in pregnant women; or animal studies have shown effect, but no controlled studies in pregnant women
  - Category C: Animal studies have revealed adverse effects in fetus; no controlled studies in women; should be given only if potential benefit justifies risk
  - Category D: Evidence for fetal risk, but benefits may be acceptable in pregnant women despite risk
  - Category X: Studies in humans and animals demonstrate significant fetal risk; contraindicated in pregnancy
- Reasonable treatment for common symptoms in pregnancy (Table 64-4)

TABLE 64-4	Generally Considered Safe Drug Therapy for Common Pregnancy Symptoms
Symptom	**Drug**
Acne	Topical clindamycin, erythromycin, or benzoyl peroxide
Allergic rhinitis	Topical glucocorticoids and cromolyn Antihistamines, including loratadine, chlorpheniramine, and diphenhydramine Decongestants (pseudoephedrine)
Cough	Guaifenesin and dextromethorphan
Constipation	Docusate sodium, lactulose, and mineral oil
Nausea	Pyridoxine (vitamin B_6) and doxylamine succinate
Gastrointestinal reflux	Calcium carbonate and ranitidine
Bronchitis	Amoxicillin and azithromycin
Urinary tract infection	Nitrofurantoin
Headache, generalized aches and pains	Acetaminophen
Thrombophlebitis	Heparin

- Drugs contraindicated in pregnancy (Box 64-1)
- Vaccines
  - **"Dead" vaccines (using killed virus or bacterial or viral fragments) are considered safe**
    - Examples: Hepatitis A vaccine, hepatitis B vaccine, influenza (injected), polio (injected), pneumococcal, and meningococcal vaccines
    - In appropriate cases, these are even indicated during pregnancy (e.g., influenza vaccine for all trimesters)
  - **Only one live, attenuated virus vaccine, the oral polio vaccine, is considered safe in pregnancy**
  - Although no reported problems are associated with measles, mumps, and rubella (MMR) vaccine during pregnancy, it is preferred to withhold until postpartum when it is considered safe
  - The varicella-zoster and smallpox vaccines are contraindicated during pregnancy

Menopause

- **Definition of menopause: The permanent cessation of menses following loss of ovarian activity; a clinical diagnosis: 12 months of amenorrhea**
- **Perimenopause is the entire time period from menstrual irregularity to the year after the menopause itself; usual duration 2 to 8 years**
- Average age of menopause is 51 years, with a range of 45 to 55 years; occurs earlier in smokers and nulliparous women
- An elevated follicle-stimulating hormone (FSH) level can provide supporting evidence, but is not useful for routine diagnosis (FSH fluctuates greatly during the perimenopause)

BOX 64-1	Selected Common Medications Contraindicated in Pregnancy

Antihypertensives
ACE inhibitors (birth defects in first trimester, decreased fetal renal perfusion and death if used in second or third trimester)
Angiotensin receptor blockers (same as ACE inhibitors)
Loop diuretics (fetal growth restriction and distress)

Antimicrobials
Tetracyclines (brittle bones and cartilage and yellow teeth)
Fluoroquinolones (arthropathies)

Anticonvulsants
Phenytoin
Carbamazepine
Valproic acid

Other
Warfarin (fetal anomalies and fetal death)
Temazepam

ACE, angiotensin-converting enzyme.

- **FSH may be useful in certain situations: Women with premature menopause, uncharacteristic clinical presentations, or hysterectomized women without classic symptoms**
- Loss of estrogen at the menopause greatly affects women and affects quality of life
  - Vasomotor symptoms (hot flashes) highly prevalent (≥75% of women in the United States); more frequent at night
  - Insomnia, fatigue
  - Genitourinary: Vaginal dryness, incontinence, recurrent urinary tract infections
  - Loss of bone mineral density (3–5% per year during the first 5 years after menopause)
  - Cardiac: Decrease in high-density lipoprotein (HDL), increase in low-density lipoprotein (LDL)
  - Neurologic and psychological: Depressed mood, irritability, decreased libido
- Treatment of hot flashes
  - Layered, cotton clothing
  - Avoidance of known triggers (caffeine, alcohol, warm humid environments, spicy food)
  - Estrogen is by far the most effective therapy (reduces frequency and severity by >90%)
  - Available selective estrogen receptor modulators are not effective for hot flashes
  - Topical estrogen (delivered intravaginally) relieves vaginal mucosal atrophy and subsequent dryness; only one formulation (the estradiol ring) reaches high enough systemic levels to relieve hot flashes and preserve bone density
- **Indications for estrogen therapy or hormone therapy (HT): Moderate to severe vasomotor symptoms**
  - Other benefits: Preservation of bone mineral density, improvements in lipid profile (increased HDL, decreased LDL), possible reduced risk of colorectal cancer (but other disease-specific treatments, such as

TABLE 64-5	*Alternatives to Estrogen for Vasomotor Symptoms*	
Class	**Typical Agents**	**Side Effects**
SSRIs	Paroxetine Venlafaxine Fluoxetine	GI symptoms Decreased libido
α-Adrenergic agents	Clonidine Methyldopa	Fatigue, dizziness Dry mouth Constipation
Gabapentin		Drowsiness, lethargy
Progestins	Medroxyprogesterone acetate (oral, depot, or transdermal)	Breast tenderness Irritability, depression Headaches ? Long-term safety

GI, gastrointestinal; SSRIs, selective serotonin reuptake inhibitors.

bisphosphonates for osteoporosis, are considered to be first line)
- Risks: Results from the Women's Health Initiative demonstrated that HT in an older population of women increased the risk of breast cancer, stroke, venous thromboembolic disease, and heart disease
- **If HT started, lowest dose for shortest duration (preferably <5 years) generally recommended; reassessment for continued need should be done at least yearly**
- Many forms available (oral, transdermal); none definitively shown to be superior
- **If uterus present, must administer progestin with estrogen to avoid increased risk of endometrial cancer**
  - Cycled use if patient desires monthly withdrawal bleeding
  - Continuous use if withdrawal bleeding undesirable (more commonly used in postmenopausal women)
- Vaginal spotting and bleeding may be a nuisance side effect
  - Usually resolves within 6 months

- **If heavy or if first bleeding occurs 6 months after initiating therapy, endometrial biopsy should be performed to rule out hyperplasia or cancer**
- Other therapies for vasomotor symptoms
  - Certain SSRIs, gabapentin, clonidine, and methyldopa have shown efficacy (Table 64-5)
  - In general, these medications reduce frequency and severity of hot flashes by 50% (not as efficacious as estrogen)
  - Herbal therapies (soy products, black cohosh) have low efficacy

REVIEW QUESTIONS

For review questions, please go to www.expertconsult.com.

SUGGESTED READINGS

Abalos E, Duley L, Steyn DW, et al: Antihypertensive drug therapy for mild to moderate hypertension during pregnancy (Cochrane Review), *The Cochrane Library*, vol 2, Oxford, 2001, Update Software.

American College of Obstetricians and Gynecologists (ACOG): *Gestational diabetes. ACOG Practice Bulletin 30*, Washington, DC, 2001, ACOG.

American College of Obstetricians and Gynecologists Committee on Practice Bulletins—Gynecology: ACOG Practice Bulletin no. 109: cervical cytology screening, *Obstet Gynecol* 114:1409–1420, 2009.

Grimes DA, Raymond EG: Emergency contraception, *Ann Intern Med* 137:180–189, 2002.

Herndon EJ, Zieman M: New contraceptive options, *Am Fam Physician* 69:853–860, 2004.

Kronenberg F, Fugh-Berman A: Complementary and alternative medicine for menopausal symptoms: a review of randomized, controlled trials, *Ann Intern Med* 137:805–813, 2002.

North American Menopause Society: Estrogen and progestogen use in postmenopausal women: 2010 position statement of The North American Menopause Society, *Menopause* 17:242, 2010.

Rossouw JE, Anderson GL, Prentice RL, et al: Risks and benefits of estrogen plus progestin in healthy postmenopausal women: principal results from the Women's Health Initiative randomized controlled trial, *JAMA* 288:321, 2002.

Wright TC, Cox JT, Massad LS, et al: 2001 Consensus guidelines for the management of women with cervical cytological abnormalities, *JAMA* 287:2120–2129, 2002.

64

Dermatology for the Internist

MARY SHEU, MD; REBECCA A. KAZIN, MD; and THOMAS B. HABIF, MD

Internal medicine physicians often encounter patients complaining of skin eruptions. Even though some cutaneous diseases may require specialty referral, it is imperative for internists to be able to recognize common dermatologic conditions, serious conditions that may require urgent referral, and cutaneous manifestations that may signify other disease processes.

Common Dermatologic Conditions

ACNE VULGARIS

See Figure 65-1 for an example of acne vulgaris.

Basic Information

- Defined as a chronic inflammation of pilosebaceous units of the face and trunk
- Affects nearly all adolescents with varying severity
- The primary lesion in acne is the microcomedo, which is an accumulation of keratin and sebum within the follicle
- With androgenic stimulation during puberty, sebum production increases, providing the opportunity for *Propionibacterium acnes* to colonize and proliferate within the follicle, resulting in an inflammatory reaction
- Most patients with acne vulgaris do not overproduce androgens; however, they probably have a genetic hyperresponsiveness to androgens
- Acne formation can also be influenced by external factors
  - Oil-based cosmetics
  - Medications (e.g., steroids, phenytoin, lithium)
  - Endocrine disorders (e.g., Cushing disease, polycystic ovary syndrome)
  - Chloracne: Severe acne occurring after exposure to halogenated hydrocarbons (e.g., herbicides, Agent Orange)

Clinical Presentation and Diagnosis

- Closed comedone ("whitehead"): Further accumulation of sebum within a microcomedo
- Open comedone ("blackhead"): Opening of the follicular orifice; follicle is packed with melanin and keratin, exposure to air results in oxidative darkening of sebum
- Inflammatory lesions: Rupture of follicular contents resulting in formation of cysts, papules
- Cutaneous nodules and scarring
- Emotional scarring (often permanent) is quite common; treatment has been shown to improve self-esteem

Treatment

- Comedonal acne
  - Topical retinoids (e.g., tretinoin, adapalene, tazarotene)
  - Salicylic acid
- Mild to moderate inflammatory acne
  - Topical retinoids (e.g., tretinoin, adapaline, tazarotene)
  - Topical benzoyl peroxide, clindamycin, or erythromycin
  - Oral antibiotics (doxycycline, minocycline usually; may also try erythromycin and trimethoprim-sulfamethoxazole)
  - In-office therapies (acne surgery—extraction of comedones; chemical peels with salicylic acid; photodynamic therapy—topical levulan followed by exposure to light source)
- Severe or resistant inflammatory acne
  - Oral antibiotics plus topical retinoids (anti-inflammatory property of antibiotics thought to play major role in action against acne)
  - Hormonal therapy (females only)—oral contraceptives or spironolactone (used as an antiandrogen; warn patients about hyperkalemia and teratogenicity)
  - Isotretinoin
    - Synthetic vitamin A derivative
    - Common side effects include dry skin and hyperlipidemia
    - Rare side effects include pseudotumor cerebri, myalgias, alopecia
    - **Teratogenicity is a concern; therefore, women of childbearing age must be on two reliable means of birth control that should be continued for at least one menstrual period after the drug has been stopped; patients must be registered in the iPLEDGE program registry (*www.ipledgeprogram.com*)**
- In women with treatment-resistant acne, consider an endocrinopathy (e.g., polycystic ovary disease, Cushing disease)

ACNE ROSACEA

See Figure 65-2 for an example of acne rosacea.

Basic Information

- Chronic inflammatory disorder of the face
- Lesions typically last days to weeks and recur
- Seen predominantly in middle-aged and older adults

Clinical Presentation

- Four subtypes; patients may have one or more than one manifestation: (1) erythrotelangiectatic, (2) papulopustular, (3) rhinophyma, (4) ocular
- Earliest lesions include facial erythema and telangiectasias
- Vascular reactivity (flushing) can be triggered by food (caffeine, alcohol, spicy food, hot beverages), environmental exposure (heat and sun), or emotion (stress)

FIGURE 65-1 Acne vulgaris. *(From Bolognia JL, Jorizzo JL, Rapini RP: Dermatology, St. Louis, Mosby, 2003, p 533.)*

TABLE 65-1	Differential Diagnosis of Acne Rosacea
Disease	**Clinical Differences**
Acne vulgaris	Comedones present Flushing not present Younger age group
Carcinoid syndrome	Rare Flushing is fleeting (lasts only seconds)
Systemic lupus erythematosus	Malar rash that spares the nasolabial folds No papules or pustules Systemic symptoms present
Seborrheic dermatitis	No papules or pustules Background erythema and telangiectasias are usually absent Can occur concurrently with rosacea

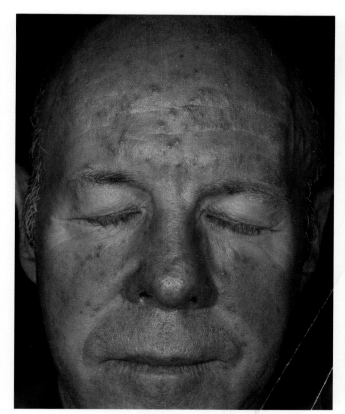

FIGURE 65-2 Rosacea.

- Papules, pustules, cysts, and nodules can develop similarly to acne vulgaris but comedones are not present
- **Eye involvement can cause blepharitis, conjunctivitis, iritis, and keratitis**
- Hyperplasia of the soft tissues and sebaceous glands of the nose (rhinophyma) can be seen in severe cases (usually in men)
- Can easily be confused with a number of other conditions (Table 65-1)

Treatment

- Topical antibiotics (metronidazole), sulfacetamide/sulfur, azelaic acid, or benzoyl peroxide can be tried initially

- Oral antibiotics (e.g., tetracycline, doxycycline, erythromycin, or minocycline; mechanism of action also thought to be anti-inflammatory as in acne vulgaris treatment) or topical tretinoin (or both) can be used in cases that do not respond to the preceding treatments. (Note: Topical retinoids have been reported to worsen telangiectasia in some patients.)
- Light-based therapy including intense pulsed light or pulsed dye laser (a series of treatments improves the flushing and telangiectasia)

ECZEMA

- Defined simply as an inflammation of the epidermis of the skin
- Can be caused by a number of different conditions (Table 65-2; Figs. 65-3 to 65-6)
- Broadly classified into three categories that define the approach to therapy
  - Acute eczema
    - Presentation: Edema, papules, vesicles, bullae, crusting, serous discharge, and scaling can be present
    - Initial treatment: Saline compresses or warm-water bath, followed by medium-strength topical glucocorticoids (e.g., triamcinolone 0.1%) and emollients; use only low-potency steroids (e.g., desonide) for facial lesions; topical tacrolimus or pimecrolimus for maintenance
  - Subacute eczema
    - Presentation: Erythematous, scaling, and pruritic lesions, but no vesicles, bullae, or serous discharge
    - Initial treatment: High-potency corticosteroids (e.g., fluocinonide) and emollients; topical tacrolimus or pimecrolimus for maintenance
  - Chronic eczema
    - Presentation: Scaly thickening of the skin (lichenification); hypo- or hyperpigmentation can occur
    - Treatment: High-potency topical steroids and emollients; topical tacrolimus or pimecrolimus for maintenance
  - Refractory eczema may require systemic therapy (i.e., phototherapy, methotrexate, or rarely a brief course of cyclosporine—appropriate laboratory monitoring required)

65

TABLE 65-2 *Features of Eczematous Eruptions*

Disease	Description	Treatment
Atopic dermatitis (see Fig. 65-3)	Patients usually have a history of allergic rhinitis, asthma, or family history of atopy Lesions often involve flexures of neck, wrist, legs, and arms; hands and face can be involved Secondary staphylococcal infections are common	Topical corticosteroids (medium to high potency) plus emollients Oral antibiotics if there is superinfection Topical nonsteroidal anti-inflammatory agents (e.g., pimecrolimus, tacrolimus)
Allergic contact dermatitis (see Fig. 65-4)	Caused by a delayed hypersensitivity reaction Most commonly caused by plant exposure (e.g., poison ivy, oak, sumac) Can also be caused by jewelry, cosmetics, and occupational exposures Diagnose by history or patch testing (or both)	Removal or avoidance of irritant Topical corticosteroids plus emollients Oral corticosteroids may sometimes be necessary
Irritant contact dermatitis	Caused by harsh cleansers and acids	Same as above
Dyshidrotic eczema (see Fig. 65-5)	Affects fingers, toes, palms, and soles Small (1-mm) vesicles, scaling, fissures Can be quite pruritic	Can be difficult to treat High-potency corticosteroids plus emollients
Seborrheic dermatitis	Epidermal inflammation in areas populated with sebaceous glands (e.g., scalp, face, ears, and chest) Scaling macules and plaques; can develop crusts or fissures *Pityrosporum* yeast may stimulate inflammation Increased incidence in patients with HIV and Parkinson disease	Scalp: Ketoconazole, selenium sulfide, or tar shampoos plus corticosteroid topical solution Face: Low-potency corticosteroids and ketoconazole cream
Stasis dermatitis	Erythematous scaling plaques seen in the lower legs in persons with chronic venous insufficiency Can form ulcers Brown hemosiderin hyperpigmentation may also be present	Dermatitis: Wet dressings, topical corticosteroids, antibiotics (if needed) Ulcer: Wet dressings, leg elevation, compression bandages
Nummular eczema (see Fig. 65-6)	Sharply circumscribed, 1- to 5-cm diameter plaques on the extremities Can resemble tinea corporis but potassium hydroxide prep is negative Secondary staphylococcal infections are common	Topical corticosteroids and emollients Oral antibiotics if there is superinfection Skin should be kept lubricated after treatment to avoid recurrence
Asteotic eczema	Seen in winter in older adults Dry ambient air may predispose to disease Dry, cracked, fissured skin with or without pruritus most commonly seen on the lower legs	Humidify ambient air Tepid baths using oils or oil-based soaps Medium-potency corticosteroid ointment (not cream) plus emollients

FIGURE 65-3 Atopic dermatitis.

FIGURE 65-4 Contact dermatitis: A 2+ positive patch test.

FIGURE 65-5 Dyshidrotic eczema.

FIGURE 65-7 Chronic plaque psoriasis.

FIGURE 65-6 Nummular eczema.

- Subclassification of eczemas can be useful for guiding specific therapy in many instances (see Table 65-2)

PSORIASIS

Basic Information

- A T cell–mediated immune disorder in which CD4$^+$ and CD8$^+$ memory T cells stimulate the hyperproliferation of keratinocytes, causing chronic scaling papules or plaques
  - **Average age of onset is in the third decade of life**
- Disease is characterized by periods of exacerbations and remissions
- Disease can be exacerbated by infections, drugs (e.g., lithium, antimalarials, β-blockers, corticosteroid withdrawal), alcohol, or stress

Clinical Presentation

- Skin disease
  - Chronic plaque psoriasis (Fig. 65-7): Sharply margin-ated, erythematous plaques with silvery-white scale, commonly seen on scalp and extensor surfaces of the knees and elbows
  - Guttate psoriasis (Fig. 65-8)
    - Presents as an acute exanthem over the trunk and proximal extremities
    - Lesions are small (<1 cm) and scaly
    - **Often follows streptococcal pharyngitis or viral infection**
    - May be self-limited, but in some cases may also herald the beginning of chronic psoriasis
  - Erythrodermic and pustular psoriasis are rare; more severe types that can be triggered by tapering of sys-temic corticosteroids
- Nail findings are seen in 30% of patients with psoriasis
  - Nail pitting, onycholysis (separation of nail from nail bed), and subungual hyperkeratosis can occur
- Arthritis can be seen in up to one third of patients and is more common in patients with psoriatic nail disease (see Chapter 42)

Treatment

- Limited chronic plaque psoriasis: Bland emollients with keratolytics, topical corticosteroids, calcipotriene (topi-cal vitamin D derivative), or tazarotene (topical vitamin A derivative)

65

FIGURE 65-8   Guttate psoriasis.

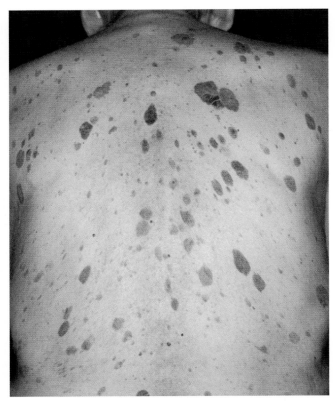

FIGURE 65-9   Seborrheic keratosis.

- Generalized plaque psoriasis: Methotrexate, cyclosporine, acitretin, phototherapy (ultraviolet B radiation), photochemotherapy (psoralen plus ultraviolet A radiation [PUVA]), biologics (e.g., alefacept, etanercept, infliximab, efalizumab)
- Guttate psoriasis: Phototherapy plus emollients and midpotency topical corticosteroids
- Erythrodermic and pustular psoriasis: Methotrexate, cyclosporine, or acitretin (synthetic retinoid); hospitalization may be necessary
- **Systemic corticosteroids should be avoided because tapering predisposes to erythrodermic or pustular psoriasis**

SEBORRHEIC KERATOSIS

Figure 65-9 illustrates seborrheic keratosis.
- Very common benign epidermal growth
- Usually occurs after the age of 30 years
- Start as small papules or plaques with or without pigment
- Grow into fairly large (up to 6 cm) plaques with warty, "stuck on" appearance; variation in pigmentation (e.g., brown, black, gray) can be seen within individual lesions, may contain horn pseudocysts
- Commonly on the face, trunk, and upper extremities (light-exposed areas)
- Lesions may become irritated and resemble atypical pigmented lesions, but do not have a malignant potential
- Once diagnosis is made, therapy is not necessary and considered elective unless the growths are irritated or pruritic
- Lesions can be destroyed with liquid nitrogen, electrocautery, or curettage

FIGURE 65-10   Pityriasis rosea with herald patch.

PITYRIASIS ROSEA

See Figure 65-10 for an example of pityriasis rosea.
- **Self-limited, exanthematous eruption thought to be related to a viral illness**
- Predominantly seen in children and young adults
- Begins with a 2- to 5-cm oval, reddish pink lesion with a fine scale often found on the back or chest (herald patch)
- Similar smaller lesions then develop along the lines of cleavage of the skin (Christmas tree pattern on the back)
- Usually asymptomatic, but occasionally may be pruritic
- Differential diagnosis includes secondary syphilis, drug eruptions, guttate psoriasis, tinea corporis, human immunodeficiency virus (HIV) seroconversion illness

FIGURE 65-11 Erythema nodosum.

FIGURE 65-12 Herpes simplex virus type 1. *(From Bolognia JL, Jorizzo JL, Rapini RP: Dermatology, St. Louis, Mosby, 2003, p 1237.)*

- Usually resolves without treatment in 2 to 3 months; if course is prolonged or pruritus is significant, treatment may include topical steroids or ultraviolet B phototherapy

ERYTHEMA NODOSUM

See Figure 65-11 for an example of erythema nodosum (EN).

Basic Information

- Proposed to be a delayed hypersensitivity reaction to antigens resulting from drugs, infections, or other inflammatory conditions
- More common in women
- Most commonly associated with streptococcal pharyngitis, but a number of other causes have been discovered
  - Sarcoidosis
    - **Löfgren syndrome: Hilar lymphadenopathy, EN, and acute polyarthritis**
  - Tuberculosis, histoplasmosis, coccidioidomycosis
  - Hodgkin lymphoma
  - *Chlamydia* infection
  - Inflammatory bowel disease
  - Behçet disease
  - Medications (e.g., omeprazole, sulfonamides, oral contraceptives, hepatitis B vaccine)

Clinical Presentation

- Erythematous nodules that can develop into bruise-like lesions that can be tender and painful
- **Commonly seen on the lower extremities**

- Palpation of the subcutaneous tissue is often more sensitive than inspection of the rash
- Fever and arthralgias can accompany the eruption even in idiopathic cases

Diagnosis

- Usually made by clinical examination
- When the diagnosis is unclear, deep incisional biopsy (rather than punch biopsy) will show septal panniculitis with no evidence of vasculitis
- Complete blood count, antistreptolysin O titer, urinalysis, throat culture, intradermal tuberculin test, and chest radiograph should be obtained as part of the initial evaluation of a patient with EN

Treatment

- Rash is usually self-limited and improves with treatment of the underlying disease (if known)
- Nonsteroidal anti-inflammatory drugs (NSAIDs), potassium iodide, or systemic corticosteroids may alleviate discomfort

Bacterial Infections of the Skin

See Chapter 15.

Viral Infections of the Skin

HERPES SIMPLEX VIRUS TYPE 1

Figure 65-12 illustrates herpes simplex virus type 1 (HSV-1).
- Transmitted from person to person through oral secretions
- More than 90% of the world's population ages 20 to 40 years is seropositive for HSV-1
- **Characterized by the sudden appearance of multiple grouped vesicles with an erythematous base**
- Infection can occur anywhere in the body but is often asymptomatic
  - Oral cavity
    - Primary infection: Exudative pharyngitis is commonly the primary infection and can be associated with fevers, lymphadenopathy, and myalgias

- Recurrent infections present as vesicles on the lips or in the oral cavity; associated systemic symptoms are usually absent
    - Skin: Any site on the skin, including the fingers (herpetic whitlow), and hips or buttocks
    - Other sites include the eye (see Chapter 66), lungs, liver, and central nervous system (CNS; see Chapter 15)
- **Diagnosis can be made by Tzanck preparation of vesicular fluid, which typically shows multinucleated giant cells; viral culture, immunofluorescence staining, and detection of HSV DNA by polymerase chain reaction may also be useful**
- Treatment of primary infections with oral (or IV) acyclovir may shorten the duration of illness and decrease viral shedding time
- Generalized treatment of all patients with recurrent herpes labialis with acyclovir has not been proven to be beneficial. However, for patients with a distinct prodrome, early administration of oral acyclovir, famciclovir, valacyclovir, or topical penciclovir may be useful.

HERPES SIMPLEX VIRUS TYPE 2

See Chapter 11 for a discussion of herpes simplex virus type 2.

HERPES ZOSTER

Figure 65-13 shows an example of herpes zoster.

Basic Information

- Primary varicella-zoster virus (VZV) infection occurs after inhalation of respiratory droplets and results in a generalized vesicular rash (chickenpox)
- **Primary infection is usually seen in children but can occur in adults and immunocompromised hosts**
- Following primary infection with VZV, latent infection is established in the dorsal root ganglia
- Reactivation of the infection results in a painful, unilateral vesicular rash limited to a restricted dermatomal distribution (herpes zoster, or "shingles")

- At times, neighboring dermatomes can be involved
- Risk factors include advancing age, immune suppression, and Hodgkin disease

Clinical Presentation and Diagnosis

- Localized pain and systemic symptoms, including fever, malaise, and headache, may precede the vesicular rash by several days
- Crusting of the vesicular lesions usually occurs within 10 days, at which time the patient is no longer infectious
- A number of complications can result from infection
    - Postherpetic neuralgia: Persistence of pain more than 30 days after the rash began
    - Herpes zoster ophthalmicus: Can lead to blindness
    - **Ramsay Hunt syndrome (type 2): Ipsilateral facial paralysis caused by involvement of cranial nerve VII, ear pain, vesicles in the auditory canal; can lead to significant hearing loss**
    - Encephalitis/meningitis
    - Motor neuropathy
    - Transverse myelitis: More common in patients with HIV

Treatment

- Acyclovir, valacyclovir, or famciclovir can be used
- Starting therapy within 72 hours of appearance of the rash reduces pain and the incidence of postherpetic neuralgia
- The addition of prednisone may accelerate healing time
- **Postherpetic neuralgia pain can be severe and require treatment with opioids, tricyclic antidepressants, carbamazepine, gabapentin, pregabalin, or topical lidocaine**
- Shingles vaccine now recommended for disease prevention in patients older than 60 years

MOLLUSCUM CONTAGIOSUM

See Figure 65-14 for an example of molluscum contagiosum.
- A disease caused by a poxvirus spread by direct skin-to-skin contact
- Common in young children and in patients with HIV

FIGURE 65-13 Herpes zoster.

FIGURE 65-14 Molluscum contagiosum.

- Lesions are usually small (2–5 mm), flesh-colored or white, umbilicated papules that can occur anywhere on the body except the palms and soles
- Diagnosis is made by clinical presentation or by histologic examination of a biopsied lesion
- Lesions are self-limited in immunocompetent hosts; curettage, cryotherapy, or laser therapy can be used, if needed; topical immune modulators (e.g., imiquimod) may also be effective
- In HIV patients, lesions can be long-lasting and extensive; there may be some improvement from treatment with antiretroviral therapy

Fungal Infections of the Skin

DERMATOPHYTOSIS

See Figure 65-15 for an example of dermaphytosis.
- **Caused by a group of fungi that penetrate the stratum corneum of the skin, hair, and nails**
- Symptoms usually consist of pruritus and burning
- Transmission is usually through direct contact
- Microscopic examination of the lesion with the addition of 1 or 2 drops of potassium hydroxide (KOH prep) usually reveals rod-shaped hyphae with branching
- Classification is based on location of the lesions (Table 65-3)

YEAST INFECTIONS

- Tinea versicolor (Fig. 65-16)
  - Recurrent superficial infection caused by *Pityrosporum orbiculare* (*Malassezia furfur*)
  - Most often seen in young adults
  - More commonly presents during warm, humid weather
  - Lesions are round and scaly; they can be hypopigmented, hyperpigmented, or erythematous
  - Occur predominantly on the trunk

- **Diagnosis is made by KOH prep showing pseudohyphae and spores ("spaghetti and meatballs")**
  - Treatment is with topical antifungals, ketoconazole shampoo, selenium sulfide solution, or oral antifungals (e.g., fluconazole, itraconazole); griseofulvin is not effective
  - Patients experiencing frequent recurrences may benefit from prophylactic treatment with selenium sulfide solution, applied every 3 weeks; or oral ketoconazole, once per month
- Mucocutaneous candidiasis
  - Infection generally involving moist skin sites or mucosal surfaces
  - Most cases caused by *Candida albicans*
  - Predisposing factors include increased moisture at the site of the infection, diabetes, antibiotic therapy, and immunosuppression (e.g., HIV)
  - Infection seen at a number of different sites
    - Oral cavity: Whitish plaques on erythematous base (thrush)
    - Vulvovaginitis: Thick, creamy vaginal discharge with erythema of the vaginal skin and mucous membrane
    - Balanitis: Erosions, scaling, erythema along the penis
    - Diaper candidiasis: Erythema and edema caused by incontinence of urine or stool in the elderly
    - Interdigital candidiasis: Erythema and fissuring between the fingers
    - Intertriginous candidiasis: Erythema, edema, pustule formation beneath the breasts, in the groin, or around the scrotum
    - Paronychial candidiasis: Edema and erythema of the nail folds; creamy discharge may be present
    - Angular cheilitis: Fissures and erythema of the angles of the mouth
- Chronic mucocutaneous candidiasis

65

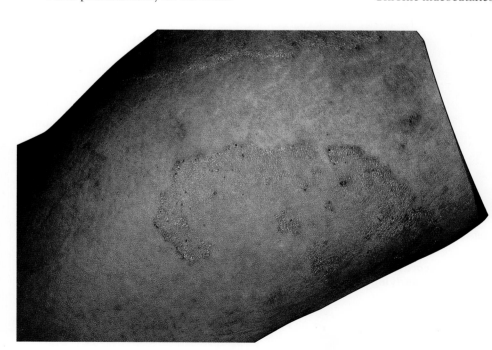

FIGURE 65-15 Dermatophytosis. *(From Bolognia JL, Jorizzo JL, Rapini RP: Dermatology, St. Louis, Mosby, 2003, Fig. 2-8.)*

TABLE 65-3	Dermatophyte Infections	
Disease	**Description**	**Treatment**
Tinea capitis	Usually occurs in children but can be seen in adults Commonly caused by *Trichophyton tonsurans* Starts as an erythematous, scaly patch on the scalp with broken-off hairs Can cause kerion formation (inflammatory pustular plaques with scarring) and permanent patches of hair loss	Topical antifungals usually not effective Griseofulvin is the treatment of choice Oral itraconazole and terbinafine can also be used Kerion treatment may require the addition of selenium sulfide shampoos and oral antistaphylococcal antibiotics
Tinea corporis ("ringworm")	Annular, scaling, papular lesions with an area of central clearing on the trunk, limbs, or face The presence of multiple lesions may be a sign of underlying immunosuppression	Topical antifungals (e.g., terbinafine) are usually effective Oral griseofulvin can be used in severe cases
Tinea cruris	Predominantly seen in men Associated with physical activity and sweating ("jock itch") Can occur with tinea pedis Semicircular erythematous, scaly lesion that begins on the thigh and can extend to the perineal area and buttocks Typically does not involve the scrotum	Topical antifungals (e.g., terbinafine) are usually effective Oral griseofulvin can be used in severe cases Groin area should be kept clean and dry to avoid recurrences Treat tinea pedis (if present)
Tinea pedis ("athlete's foot")	Lesions can range from having mild erythema and scale to maceration and bullae between the toes and on the soles of the feet Can be a point of entry of bacteria, causing cellulitis	Topical antifungals (e.g., terbinafine) are usually effective Oral terbinafine or itraconazole can be used in resistant cases
Tinea unguium (onychomycosis)	Signs include white discoloration, crumbly debris from beneath the nail, and thickening of the nail	Topical therapy is generally ineffective Oral terbinafine or itraconazole for 6–12 wk is the most effective treatment Ciclopirox nail lacquer is effective in <10% of patients

FIGURE 65-16   Tinea versicolor.

- **Characterized by recurrent, severe mucocutaneous candidal infections caused by an underlying T-cell defect**
- Usually presents in childhood
- Suspect HIV in adult patients presenting with this syndrome

- Treatment is with topical antifungal agents; long-term therapy may be necessary in patients with chronic disease

Infestations of the Skin

SCABIES

- Caused by infestation with the mite *Sarcoptes scabei*
- Transmission is from person to person by direct contact, although cases of transmission from clothing and bed linens have occurred
- In young adults, transmission commonly occurs during sexual contact
- **Intractable pruritus that is worse at night is the most prominent symptom**
- The primary lesion is usually a small, erythematous papule or vesicle that may be difficult to find
- Thread-like linear ridges that range from 2 to 15 mm in length (burrows) are pathognomonic for the disease
- **Vesicles, papules, and burrows are most commonly found on the hands, wrists, penis, nipples, axillae, and gluteal cleft; usually spares the scalp**
- The term *Norwegian scabies* describes an extensive scabies infestation involving the hands and feet, and elsewhere, with asymptomatic thick crusting. There is thick, subungual, keratotic material and nail dystrophy. It occurs in people with neurologic or mental disorders (especially Down syndrome), senile dementia, nutritional disorders, infectious diseases, leukemia, and immunosuppression (e.g., patients with AIDS).
- Diagnosis can be presumed on clinical grounds or be confirmed by microscopic examination of the lesion by scraping and applying 2 drops of mineral oil prior to covering with a coverslip. Identification of the mite, eggs, or feces confirms the diagnosis.

FIGURE 65-17 Pediculosis capitis. *(From Bolognia JL, Jorizzo JL, Rapini RP: Dermatology, St. Louis, Mosby, 2003, p 1325.)*

- **Treatment with permethrin cream over the entire body (washed off after 12 hours and repeated 1 week later) is usually effective**
- Family members and close contacts must also be treated
- Clothing and linens should be laundered
- Oral ivermectin may be considered to treat difficult cases and the elderly

PEDICULOSIS (LICE)

See Figure 65-17.
- Infestation with the human louse (*Pediculus humanus*)
- Characterized by the location of the infestation
  - Pediculosis capitis (head lice)
    - Can be transmitted by hats and brushes
    - Epidemics can occur in schools
  - Pediculosis pubis (pubic lice, crabs)
    - Most commonly occurs in young adults
    - Usually transmitted during sexual contact
  - Pediculosis corporis: Seen in patients with poor hygiene with exposure to others with poor hygiene
- Predominant symptom is itching
- Diagnosed by visualization of nits attached to hair shafts or identification of the louse (usually by microscopy)
- **Treatment is with pyrethrin, permethrin, malthion, or lindane shampoos or lotions. Treatment should be followed by combing to remove all visible nits.**
- Ivermectin is also effective and may be used in cases resistant to topical medication

Benign, Premalignant, and Malignant Neoplasms of the Skin

65

MOLES

- Common moles (melanocytic nevi) are seen in everyone
  - They are small (<6 mm), tan or brown macules or papules
  - Develop in childhood, peak in early adulthood, and decline thereafter
- Atypical moles (dysplastic nevi; Fig. 65-18)
  - Are often larger (>6 mm) than common moles
  - Have irregular borders and variegated color
  - Surface may be complex and variable, with both macular and papular components; a characteristic presentation is a pigmented papule surrounded by a macular collar of pigmentation ("fried-egg lesion")
  - Can continue to appear after age 35 years, in contrast with common moles
  - Associated with an increased risk of melanoma
  - Biopsy often necessary to rule out melanoma
  - Familial atypical mole and melanoma (FAMM) syndrome (dysplastic nevus syndrome)
    - Patients have a large number of melanocytic nevi, often more than 50, some of which are atypical and often variable in size; and a positive family history of melanoma in one or more first- or second-degree relatives

FIGURE 65-18   Atypical nevi. *(From Bolognia JL, Jorizzo JL, Rapini RP: Dermatology, St. Louis, Mosby, 2003, p 1779.)*

FIGURE 65-19   **A** and **B**, Superficial spreading melanomas.

- Atypical lesions begin during puberty; melanoma often presents before the age of 40 years
- **Lifetime risk of melanoma approaches 100% for those people with atypical moles from families with two or more first-degree relatives who have cutaneous melanoma**
- Patients need to perform monthly self-examinations
- Referral to a dermatologist is often necessary so that appropriate photographs and biopsies can be done at regular intervals (every 3–12 months)
- Evaluation of a mole
  - All pigmented skin lesions should be examined for the following features (ABCDEs):
    - **A**symmetry
    - **B**order irregularity
    - **C**olor variegation—variable degrees of black, brown, tan, or blue
    - **D**iameter greater than 6 mm
    - **E**volution—change in appearance or symptoms
  - Excisional biopsy should be considered for any lesion considered to be melanoma

MELANOMA

See Figure 65-19 for examples of melanoma.

Basic Information

- Sixth most common cancer in the United States, causing over 7000 deaths per year
- Affects whites more than African Americans
- Diagnosis most commonly made in the sixth decade of life
- Incidence in the United States is rising
- Risk factors (Box 65-1)
- Melanoma subtypes

BOX 65-1	*Risk Factors for the Development of Melanoma*

Sun exposure
Blond or red hair
Freckling on the upper back
Blistering sunburns in childhood
White race
Family history of melanoma
Therapy with psoralen and ultraviolet A radiation (PUVA) for psoriasis
Changing pigmented mole
Many (>50) common moles
Atypical mole
History of basal cell carcinoma or squamous cell carcinoma of the skin
Immunosuppression (e.g., after organ transplantation)
History of treated melanoma

- Superficial spreading melanoma
  - Most common type
  - Deeply pigmented macules or papules usually greater than 6 mm in diameter; usually displays one of the ABCDE criteria (see section on Moles)
- Nodular melanoma
  - Dark black, tan, or brown (rarely amelanotic) dome-shaped papule or nodule
  - Typically do not present with the ABCDEs, making diagnosis difficult
- Acral lentiginous melanoma
  - **Most common type found in African Americans and Asians**
  - Presents in palms, soles, or nail beds

- Hutchinson's sign: Pigmented streak in nail with extension onto the nail-fold skin
- Lentigo maligna melanoma
  - Involves sun-exposed skin (usually the face)
  - Irregular pigmented macule that can develop papules within
  - One of the ABCDEs is typically present

Clinical Presentation

- Most melanomas exhibit one of the ABCDEs or have recently changed in size, shape, or color
- Bleeding, inflammation, or a sensory change at the site of the lesion should also suggest the possibility of malignancy
- In patients with numerous moles, an individual lesion that appears different from the others should be thoroughly evaluated
- Metastasis can occur (typically to the brain, liver, or lung)

Diagnosis

- Suggested by the clinical appearance
- Excisional biopsy of the lesion providing full-thickness skin sample that extends to the subcutaneous fat is the preferred diagnostic method
- **Staging is primarily based on tumor thickness**
- The presence of ulceration is the next most important histologic determinant of prognosis
- Sentinel lymph node biopsy is used for staging information in melanomas greater than 1.0 mm in depth
- Chest radiograph, liver function tests, and lactate dehydrogenase levels should also be obtained
- Scanning is indicated if metastatic disease is suggested

Treatment

- Excision with adequate margins is the treatment of choice for tumors without evidence of metastasis
- Elective lymph node dissection for patients with clinically enlarged lymph nodes and no evidence of distant disease
- Adjuvant chemotherapy may be employed for more advanced disease

BASAL CELL CARCINOMA

Figure 65-20 provides an example of basal cell carcinoma (BCC).

- **Risk factors include inability to tan, intermittent sun exposure, cumulative sun exposure, fair skin, and older age**
- Usually develop on the head and neck
- A patient typically complains of a red, peeling, eroded or bleeding lesion that may improve and then recur
- Subtypes of BCC
  - Nodular ulcerative
    - Most common type
    - Presents as a well-circumscribed pearly papule with telangiectasias; may ulcerate
  - Superficial
    - Well-circumscribed, erythematous, scaly patch
    - Resembles tinea, psoriasis, or dermatitis
    - Often occurs on non–sun-exposed skin
  - Sclerotic
    - Whitish plaque with sclerosis or fibrosis on palpation

FIGURE 65-20 Basal cell carcinoma.

- Pigmented
  - Similar to nodular but are pigmented
  - Most common form seen in darker skinned individuals
- Metastatic disease is very rare
- Diagnosis is made by clinical appearance or biopsy specimen
- Standard treatment options include electrodesiccation and curettage, surgical excision, radiation
- Superficial BCC may respond to topical treatment with the immune modulator imiquimod
- Mohs' micrographic surgery is used for sclerosing BCC and other BCC with poorly defined clinical margins; for tumors in areas of potentially high recurrence, such as the nose or eyelid; and for very large primary tumors and recurrent BCC

ACTINIC KERATOSIS

Figure 65-21 illustrates actinic keratosis.
- Premalignant lesions that develop on sun-exposed skin, usually in people older than 40 years
- **Low but significant risk of transformation to squamous cell carcinoma (SCC)**
- Fair-skinned individuals are more susceptible to developing actinic keratosis
- Present as erythematous, 2- to 8-mm macules with a whitish scale; or as hyperkeratotic plaques on the face, scalp, back of the hands, arms, chest, upper back, and lower legs

65

FIGURE 65-21 Actinic keratosis.

FIGURE 65-22 Squamous cell carcinoma. *(From Bolognia JL, Jorizzo JL, Rapini RP: Dermatology, St. Louis, Mosby, 2003, p 1682.)*

- Diagnosis is usually made by clinical appearance; lesions suggestive of SCC should be biopsied
- There is no way to determine which lesions will progress to SCC
- Patients who are immunosuppressed (especially transplantation patients) are at high risk for the development of SCC from actinic keratosis
- Current treatment modalities include the following:
  - Cryotherapy with liquid nitrogen or surgical curettage is effective for individual lesions
  - Topical 5-fluorouracil, imiquimod, and photodynamic therapy (topical aminolevulinic acid followed by exposure to a blue light source) may be useful in patients with multiple lesions
  - Excision or electrodesiccation and curettage should be performed for thicker or resistant lesions

SQUAMOUS CELL CARCINOMA

See Figure 65-22 for an example of SCC.
- More than half of cases arise from transformation of actinic keratoses
- Chronic exposure to ultraviolet sunlight and increasing age are the more important risk factors
- **Very common in patients after organ transplantation**
- In patients with chronic lymphocytic leukemia, the development of multiple SCCs may indicate deterioration of the leukemia
- Presents as an erythematous papule, nodule, or plaque with a hyperkeratotic scale; ulceration may also occur
- Clinical variants

- Bowen disease (SCC *in situ*): Reddish brown plaque that may have pigment or hyperkeratosis; has been associated with chemical exposures and human papillomavirus infection (SCC of the anogenital skin)
- Keratoacanthoma: Hyperkeratotic nodule with a keratin plug; grows rapidly (over 3–6 weeks); most spontaneously regress
- Cutaneous horns: Columns of hyperkeratosis on an erythematous base; can grow within an SCC
- 5% to 10% metastasize
- Surgical excision is the treatment of choice

CUTANEOUS T-CELL LYMPHOMA

- Presents as erythematous, scaly plaques resembling psoriasis or eczema on sun-protected sites (i.e., buttock and covered areas of trunk and limbs); most common subtype is mycosis fungoides
- Fulminant lesions may be preceded by months to years by nonspecific scaly lesions that have been diagnosed as other dermatoses
- Significant pruritus, fever, and lymphadenopathy can be present
- **Sézary syndrome (Fig. 65-23) is a leukemic variant characterized by generalized erythroderma, lymphadenopathy, pruritus, and leukocytosis with atypical T cells (Sézary cells) in the peripheral blood**
- Patients can be treated with topical nitrogen mustard, phototherapy, topical or oral retinoids, or radiation therapy

Cutaneous Drug Reactions

Basic Information

- Occur in up to 3% of hospitalized patients
- Antibiotics are responsible for most reactions
- Drug-induced skin eruptions can take many forms (the most common and significant ones are discussed in the following section)

FIGURE 65-23   Sézary's syndrome.

FIGURE 65-24   Lichen planus.

URTICARIA AND ANGIODEMA

See Chapter 68.

HYPERSENSITIVITY VASCULITIS

- Most commonly implicated drugs include penicillins, cephalosporins, sulfonamides, allopurinol, and phenytoin
- **Clinical findings include palpable purpura, petechiae, fever, arthralgias, and lymphadenopathy that usually begin within 10 days of the initial drug exposure**
- The sedimentation rate may be elevated; complement levels may be low
- Discontinuation of the drug should lead to resolution of symptoms within weeks; systemic corticosteroids may be necessary in severe cases

LICHEN PLANUS

See Figure 65-24 for an example of lichen planus.

- **Can be drug induced, related to liver disease (e.g., hepatitis C), or idiopathic**
- Implicated drugs include β-blockers, methyldopa, penicillamine, quinidine and quinine, NSAIDs, angiotensin-converting enzyme inhibitors, sulfonylurea agents, carbamazepine, gold, and lithium
- Most lesions occur on the skin or mucous membranes
  - Skin lesions
    - Pruritic, violaceous, polygonal, flat-topped papules with white lacy lines (Wickham striae)
    - Most common site is the flexor aspect of the wrists
  - Mucous membranes
    - Most common presentation
    - Milky-white papules with white lacework on the buccal mucosa

EXANTHEMS

- **The most common acute drug-induced eruption, accounting for 75% of cases**
- Rash is generalized, pruritic, macular, and papular
- In some cases, exfoliative erythroderma can occur and can be an early sign for the development of toxic epidermal necrolysis (see following discussion)
- Onset of the rash is usually within 2 weeks of beginning drug therapy
- In patients who have been sensitized to the drug (by prior use), the rash typically develops within the first 3 days of therapy
- The most commonly implicated drugs include penicillins, cephalosporins, sulfonamides, quinidine, allopurinol, isoniazid, carbamazepine, and phenytoin
- Cessation of the drug usually leads to resolution of the rash; symptomatic treatment with topical corticosteroids, topical antipruritics, or oral antihistamines can be used

65

FIGURE 65-25 Erythema multiforme.

- Patients with chronic disease may have an increased risk of oral SCC
- Withdrawal of the medication should lead to resolution of the lesions
- In cases that are not drug-induced, topical corticosteroids are first-line therapy
- Resistant disease can be treated with systemic corticosteroids, retinoid therapy, or phototherapy

ERYTHEMA MULTIFORME

See Figure 65-25 for an example of erythema multiforme (EM).
- Cell-mediated cytotoxic skin reaction triggered by infection (usually HSV or *Mycoplasma*) or drugs (e.g., sulfonamides, anticonvulsants, penicillins, or NSAIDs)
- Two basic forms of disease
  - EM major
    - Affects more than one mucosal surface (usually conjunctiva and oral mucosa)
    - Typical or raised atypical target lesions
    - Epidermal detachment involving less than 10% of body surface
    - Lesions usually located on the extremities or face
    - Usually associated with drugs
  - EM minor
    - Most are preceded by an HSV infection (a small percentage associated with *Mycoplasma pneumoniae*)
    - Limited or no mucous membrane involvement
    - Bullae and systemic symptoms are seen in some cases
    - Target lesions favor hands, feet, arms, and legs
    - Chronic suppressive acyclovir therapy prevents HSV and EM recurrences

STEVENS-JOHNSON SYNDROME AND TOXIC EPIDERMAL NECROLYSIS

- A spectrum of disease characterized by epidermal necrosis and mucous membrane involvement
- **Stevens-Johnson syndrome (SJS) involves less than 10% of the epidermis, whereas toxic epidermal necrolysis (TEN) involves over 30% of the epidermis. Involvement of 10% to 30% is considered SJS-TEN overlap.**
- Most commonly implicated drugs are sulfonamides, anticonvulsants, allopurinol, penicillins, and NSAIDs

- Lesions usually appear within a few days after the initiation of drug therapy; a prodrome of fever, malaise, and arthralgias can be present
- Skin lesions
  - Begin as tender erythematous macules, followed by formation of blisters that become confluent; the epidermis then begins to slough, leaving areas that resemble burns
  - Nikolsky's sign (separation of the outer layer of the epidermis from the basal layer with minimal pressure applied to the skin) may be present
- Mucous membranes
  - At least two mucosal surfaces are involved
- Erythema and sloughing of the lips, buccal mucosa, conjunctiva, or anogenital area can occur
- Complications of the disease include acute renal failure, fluid and electrolyte imbalances, GI hemorrhage, and sepsis
- **Treatment of TEN involves discontinuation of the offending agent, transfer to a burn unit, possible IV immunoglobulin, not corticosteroids**
- Death occurs in 40% of patients with TEN
- Patients with SJS may benefit from oral corticosteroids

HYPERSENSITIVITY SYNDROME

- Fever, rash, and lymphadenopathy occurring 2 to 6 weeks after initiation of drug therapy
- **Phenytoin, carbamazepine, phenobarbital, and sulfonamides are most commonly implicated**
- Erythematous papules and pustules or bullae are the typical skin manifestations
- Hepatitis and eosinophilia can also be seen
- Prompt withdrawal of the medication usually results in full recovery

Autoimmune Blistering Disorders

Basic Information

- Blisters are fluid-filled skin lesions; small (<0.5 cm) blisters are called vesicles, whereas larger ones are referred to as bullae
- Most acquired forms of disease are autoimmune
- The unifying pathologic abnormality resulting in fluid-filled cavity formation is separation of skin at some level
- One method of classifying these diseases is by their level of tissue disadhesion; some diseases separate within the level of the epidermis, whereas others separate below the epidermis (Table 65-4)

Clinical Presentation, Diagnosis, and Treatment

See Table 65-4.

Cutaneous Manifestations of Internal Disease

CARDIOVASCULAR DISEASE

- LEOPARD syndrome: Generalized **l**entigines (brown macules), **e**lectrocardiogram abnormalities, **o**cular hypertelorism, **p**ulmonic stenosis, **a**bnormal genitalia, **r**etardation of growth (dwarfism), and **d**eafness

TABLE 65-4 Autoimmune Blistering Diseases

Disease	Basic Information	Clinical Presentation	Diagnosis	Treatment
Subepidermal Blistering Diseases				
Bullous pemphigoid (BP) (Fig. 65-26)	Most common type Typically affects older adults Usually chronic and recurrent Most cases are idiopathic, related to drugs (e.g., diuretics, neuroleptics)	Starts as urticarial eruptions and evolves into crops of tense blisters with urticarial bases The edges of the blister do not extend with gentle manual pressure Often involve the axillae, groin, medial aspects of the thighs, lower legs, and flexor aspects of the forearm Cicatricial pemphigoid is a variant that involves the oral cavity, nasopharynx, or conjunctiva	Skin biopsy showing subepidermal blister with inflammatory cells (including eosinophils) Direct immunofluorescence (DIF) shows linear deposition of IgG and C3 in the epidermal-dermal junction (basement membrane zone)	Disease in some patients is self-limited Corticosteroids (topical or oral) can significantly improve symptoms High risk of complications because of systemic steroid therapy Immunosuppressives may be used
Epidermolysis bullosa acquisita	May be associated with inflammatory bowel disease, rheumatoid arthritis, and SLE	Blisters and erosions induced by minor trauma on the hands and feet Mucosal lesions can be present	Histology is similar to BP DIF shows IgG at the basement membrane zone NaCl-split skin technique applied to biopsy specimen shows IgG on the dermal side (as opposed to the epidermal side in BP)	Supportive therapy Does not usually respond to immunosuppressives
Dermatitis herpetiformis (Fig. 65-27)	Usually occurs between ages 20 and 50 yr Almost all patients have some degree of gluten-sensitive enteropathy (similar to celiac disease) Also associated with a number of other autoimmune disorders Linear IgA dermatosis is a variant associated with medications (e.g., NSAIDs, vancomycin) and not gluten-sensitive enteropathy	Clusters of pruritic, grouped vesicles on the elbows, knees, buttocks, or scalp Mucous membranes usually spared except in cases of linear IgA dermatosis Small bowel lymphoma in a small number of patients	Histology reveals a subepidermal vesicle with neutrophils and eosinophils in the dermal papillae DIF shows granular IgA deposits at the basement membrane zone	Steroids not helpful Improvement seen with gluten-free diet Dapsone is the treatment of choice
Intraepidermal Blistering Diseases				
Pemphigus vulgaris (PV)	Usually occurs between the ages of 30 and 60 yr Has been associated with myasthenia gravis and thymoma	Begins with painful, nonhealing ulceration of the oral cavity Bullous lesions on the skin usually present months later Bullae are flaccid and rupture easily Pressure placed on the bulla leads to lateral extension of the blister (unlike BP) Nikolsky's sign* is positive when done on normal-appearing skin	Histologically there is intraepithelial acantholysis (separation of keratinocytes) Basement membrane is intact DIF reveals deposition of IgG and C3 at the epidermal cell surface Serum antidesmoglein antibodies	Fatal if not treated High-dose systemic corticosteroids initially Long-term steroid use may be needed Adjuvant immunosuppressives can help decrease steroid dose
Drug-induced pemphigus	Associated with penicillamine and captopril	Same as PV or PF	Same as PV or PF	Discontinuation of the drug
Mixed Subepidermal and Intraepidermal Blistering Disease				
Paraneoplastic pemphigus	Associated with lymphomas	Large, tense, bullous lesions on skin Oral and conjunctival involvement can be severe	DIF shows IgG in the intraepidermal layer and C3 involvement of the subepidermal layer	Difficult Steroids are attempted

Ig, immunoglobulin; NSAIDs, nonsteroidal anti-inflammatory drugs; PF, pemphigus foliaceus; SLE, systemic lupus erythematosus.
*Nikolsky's sign, separation of the outer layer of the epidermis from the basal layer with application of minimal pressure to the skin.

65

FIGURE 65-26 Bullous pemphigoid.

FIGURE 65-27 Dermatitis herpetiformis.

- LAMB syndrome: Generalized **l**entigines, **a**trial myxoma, **m**ucocutaneous myxomas, **b**lue nevi
- Pseudoxanthoma elasticum
  - Peau d'orange pattern of clusters of yellow papules found on the neck, axillae, or other body folds
  - Associated with peripheral vascular disease, stroke, myocardial infarctions, retinal hemorrhages, and GI hemorrhage
- Ehlers-Danlos syndrome
  - Defects in collagen biosynthesis result in hypermobility of joints and hyperelasticity of the skin
  - Associated with abdominal aortic aneurysm and GI hemorrhage

PULMONARY DISEASE

- Sarcoidosis (Fig. 65-28; see also Chapter 20)
  - **Lupus pernio: Violaceous plaques on the nose, cheeks, and ears**

FIGURE 65-28 **A** to **C**, Cutaneous sarcoidosis. *(From Bolognia JL, Jorizzo JL, Rapini RP: Dermatology, St. Louis, Mosby, 2003, p 1457.)*

- Pathology reveals noncaseating granulomas
- Course is chronic and requires treatment with intralesional steroids, antimalarials, or methotrexate
- A number of other cutaneous diseases are seen with sarocoidosis, including EN (see preceding discussion)
- Yellow nail syndrome: Yellow nails, lymphedema, pleural effusions

ENDOCRINE DISEASE

- Diabetes mellitus (DM)
  - Acanthosis nigricans (Fig. 65-29)

FIGURE 65-29 Acanthosis nigricans.

FIGURE 65-30 Necrobiosis lipoidica.

- Hyperpigmented velvety patches seen predominantly in skin folds such as the axillae, neck, and groin
- Associated with insulin resistance (type 2 DM)
- **Also associated with other endocrinopathies (e.g., acromegaly, Cushing syndrome, polycystic ovary, thyroid disease) and GI malignancies**
- Necrobiosis lipoidica diabeticorum (Fig. 65-30)
  - Multicolored plaques with atrophic centers found on the anterior and lateral aspects of the legs
- Granuloma annulare
  - Skin-colored or erythematous fine papules that exhibit an annular arrangement
  - Seen on the hands, feet, arms, or legs
  - Diffuse form of granuloma annulare can be associated with diabetes
- Stiff hand syndrome
  - Seen in type 1 diabetes
  - Scleroderma-like tightening of the skin over the hands with limited joint mobility
  - Associated with nephropathy and retinopathy
- Scleredema
  - Induration of the skin of the posterior neck and back
  - Usually seen in men with poorly controlled type 2 diabetes
- Diabetic dermopathy
  - Hyperpigmented atrophic macules on anterior shins, from trauma
- Bulla diabeticorum
  - Bullae on anterior shins
- Hyperthyroidism
  - Thinning of hair
  - Onycholysis—separation of the nail from the nail bed
  - Pretibial myxedema (if Graves disease)—edematous plaques primarily on anterior shins, can also get periorbital myxedema

- Vitiligo (Fig. 65-31)
  - Depigmentation of skin, with white macules covering small or large amounts of the body surface
  - Can affect the hair and mucous membranes
  - **May be associated with autoimmune disorders (e.g., thyroid disease, type 1 diabetes, pernicious anemia, and adrenal insufficiency)**
- Hypothyroidism
  - Dull, coarse hair with slow growth
  - Loss of lateral third of eyebrows
  - Dry skin, brittle nails

GASTROINTESTINAL AND LIVER DISEASE
- Inflammatory bowel disease
  - Aphthous stomatitis
  - Pyoderma gangrenosum (Fig. 65-32)
    - Rapidly progressing blue-red ulcers with irregular borders and purulent drainage
    - Can occur at sites of trauma (pathergy)
    - Also seen with inflammatory bowel disease, myeloproliferative disorders, rheumatoid arthritis, and chronic hepatitis; 50% of cases are idiopathic
  - EN (see preceding discussion)
  - Cutaneous Crohn disease
    - Skin lesions with noncaseating granulomas on histology
    - Can take many forms
  - Sweet syndrome
    - Multiple erythematous nodules, most commonly on the head, neck, and upper extremities but can occur anywhere

65

FIGURE 65-31 Vitiligo.

FIGURE 65-32 Pyoderma gangrenosum.

- May be associated with fever, arthritis, arthralgias, myalgias, ocular symptoms, neutrophilic pulmonary alveolitis, sterile osteomyelitis, acute renal failure, aseptic meningitis, and transient involvement of the kidney, liver, and pancreas
- Also may be associated with infections, malignancy, autoimmune disorders, and pregnancy

FIGURE 65-33 Porphyria cutanea tarda.

- Celiac disease (gluten-sensitive enteropathy)
  - Aphthous stomatitis
  - Dermatitis herpetiformis (see Table 65-4 and Fig. 65-27)
- Hepatitis C infection
  - Porphyria cutanea tarda (Fig. 65-33)
    - Patients may present with fragile skin, vesicles, or bullae (usually on the dorsum of the hands) after minor trauma or sun exposure
    - Hypertrichosis, scleroderma-like induration, hyper-pigmentation, and hypopigmentation can all occur as well
    - Also associated with alcohol and drugs (e.g., estrogens)
    - Diagnosis is made by showing elevated uroporphyrin levels
    - Patients who have been diagnosed should be screened for hepatitis C
  - Cryoglobulinemia (see Chapter 44)
  - Lichen planus
  - Pruritus
- Peutz-Jeghers syndrome (Fig. 65-34)
  - **Pigmented macules (freckles) on the lips, oral mucosa, palms, soles, fingers, and toes**
  - Associated with small bowel hamartomas
- Hereditary hemorrhagic telangiectasia (Osler-Weber-Rendu disease)
  - Characterized by telangiectasias on the skin, lungs, GI tract, and CNS
  - Can cause life-threatening bleeding from noncutaneous sites

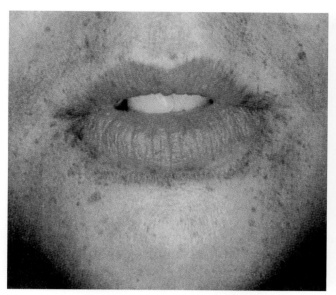

FIGURE 65-34   Peutz-Jeghers syndrome.

HEMATOLOGIC DISEASE

- Mastocytosis
  - Cutaneous and visceral infiltration of mast cells
  - **Urticaria pigmentosa: Reddish brown macules and papules that can urticate on stroking (Darier's sign)**
  - Can cause pruritus, flushing, diarrhea, abdominal pain, and wheezing
  - Diagnosis is made by demonstration of mast cell infiltration on skin biopsy specimen

RENAL DISEASE

- Fabry disease
  - X-linked disorder resulting in deposition of glycosphingolipids in body tissues
  - Causes angiokeratomas (purple papules) on the trunk, extremities, palms, soles, and mucous membranes
  - Also results in paresthesias, renal failure, and cardiovascular disease
- Calciphylaxis (Fig. 65-35)
  - Localized areas of skin necrosis caused by vascular calcification
  - Seen in patients with end-stage renal disease
  - Parathyroidectomy may result in healing
- Nephrogenic systemic fibrosis
  - Thickening and hardening of the skin overlying extremities and trunk due to fibrosis of the dermis
  - Fibrosis can also affect deeper structures, including muscle, fascia, lungs, and heart
  - Seen exclusively in patients with kidney disease
  - **Associated with administration of gadolinium contrast medium for magnetic resonance imaging**
    - Risk is thought to be about 5% after gadolinium exposure in a patient with end-stage renal disease
    - Disease is usually chronic and unremitting
    - No effective treatment at this time

FIGURE 65-35   Calciphylaxis. *(From Bolognia JL, Jorizzo JL, Rapini RP: Dermatology, St. Louis, Mosby, 2003, p 694.)*

65

FIGURE 65-36   Neurofibromatosis. *(From Bolognia JL, Jorizzo JL, Rapini RP: Dermatology, St. Louis, Mosby, 2003, p 855.)*

NEUROLOGIC DISEASE

- Neurofibromatosis (Fig. 65-36)
  - Autosomal dominant disease characterized by soft, tan-colored nodules that arise from peripheral nerves
    - Cutaneous lesions develop before puberty and increase with age
    - Predominantly involves the trunk
    - Can be associated with severe pruritus
  - **Café-au-lait spots (pigmented patches), axillary freckling, and Lisch nodules (pigmented iris hamartomas) are also seen in most patients**

TABLE 65-5	*Dermatologic Manifestations of Oncologic Disease (Paraneoplastic Syndromes)*	
Skin Disorder	**Oncologic Disease(s)**	**Description**
Acanthosis nigricans	Gastric cancer Colon cancer	Velvety hyperpigmentation in axillae, groin, neck Also associated with endocrinopathies (see text)
Acquired ichthyosis	Hodgkin lymphoma Breast, lung, bladder carcinoma	Generalized scaling of the skin, including palms and soles
Bazex syndrome	Squamous cell carcinoma of the pharynx and esophagus Hodgkin lymphoma	Psoriasiform lesions on the hands, feet, ears, and nose
Necrolytic migratory erythema	Glucagonoma	Weeping, eczematous lesions around the mouth, intertriginous areas, flexures, and perigenital area Weight loss, diarrhea, and glossitis also present
Paget disease	Breast: Intraductal carcinoma	Breast: Erythematous eczematous, and scaly lesions around the nipple
	Extramammary: Adnexal cancers, genitourinary cancers, gastrointestinal cancers	Extramammary: Erythematous plaques around the vulva, scrotum, or perianal area
Sweet syndrome	Acute myelogenous leukemia	Acute onset of violaceous/erythematous papules or plaques usually on the face, neck, and upper extremities Fever, arthritis, leukocytosis may be present
Tylosis	Esophageal carcinoma	Inherited disorder presenting with yellow, smooth thickening of the palms and soles (palmar-plantar hyperkeratosis)
Tripe palm	Gastric cancer Bronchogenic carcinoma	Velvety thickening of the palms that leads to accentuation of palmar creases

- Tuberous sclerosis
  - Autosomal dominant disease characterized by skin lesions, mental retardation, seizures, and angiomyolipomas of the kidneys
  - Skin lesions include "adenoma sebaceum" (skin-colored facial papules that are angiofibromas), ash-leaf macules (hypopigmented macules), shagreen patch (connective tissue nevus), and periungual and subungual fibromas

ONCOLOGIC DISEASE

See Table 65-5 for a summary of the dermatologic manifestations of oncologic disease.

RHEUMATOLOGIC DISEASE

- Vasculitis
  - Livedo reticularis (Fig. 65-37)
    - Mottled, blue-purple discoloration in a net-like pattern usually on legs or arms
    - **Can be idiopathic or associated with vasculitis, syphilis, tuberculosis, atheroemboli, or drugs (e.g., amantadine, quinine)**
  - Purpura
    - Caused by extravasation of blood cells into the dermis
    - Nonpalpable purpura and petechiae
      - Primarily caused by thrombocytopenia, disorders of hyperglobulinemia, or disorders of capillary fragility (e.g., amyloidosis, Ehlers-Danlos syndrome, scurvy)

FIGURE 65-37 Livedo reticularis. *(From Bolognia JL, Jorizzo JL, Rapini RP: Dermatology, St. Louis, Mosby, 2003, p 1652.)*

FIGURE 65-38   Palpable purpura.

- Palpable purpura (Fig. 65-38)
  - Seen in vasculitic disorders, embolic disorders (e.g., cholesterol emboli, atrial myxoma, endocarditis), and coagulopathies (e.g., antiphospholipid syndrome)

ITCHING (PRURITUS) IN THE ABSENCE OF A RASH

- Commonly caused by xerosis or xerotic dermatitis ("winter itch")
- Many skin disorders have pruritus as a major finding (atopic dermatitis, infestations such as scabies)
- Localized pruritus without evidence of a rash—nostalgia paresthetica (usually located on the upper back)
  - May be a sign of systemic disease (generalized, chronic and progressive)
  - Biliary/hepatic disease (primary biliary cirrhosis, hepatitis)
  - Renal disease (end-stage renal disease)
  - Lymphoma (Hodgkin lymphoma)
  - Polycythemia vera, myelodysplasia, essential thrombocythemia
  - Thyroid disorder
  - Mastocytosis
  - Hypereosinophilic syndrome
  - Diabetes
  - HIV
- Psychogenic pruritus
- Pregnancy-related pruritus

REVIEW QUESTIONS

For review questions, please go to www.expertconsult.com.

SUGGESTED READINGS

Bershad SV: In the clinic: acne, *Ann Intern Med* 149: ITC1-1–ITC1-16, 2008.

Bieber T: Atopic dermatitis, *N Engl J Med* 358:1483–1494, 2008.

Habif TB: *Clinical dermatology*, ed 5, St. Louis, 2010, Mosby.

Harr T, French LE: Severe cutaneous adverse reactions: acute generalized exanthematous pustulosis, toxic epidermal necrolysis and Stevens-Johnson syndrome, *Med Clin North Am* 94:727–742, 2010.

Kazin RA, Lowitt NR, Lowitt MH: Update in dermatology, *Ann Intern Med* 135:124–132, 2001.

Nainani N, Panesar M: Nephrogenic systemic fibrosis, *Am J Nephrol* 29:1–9, 2009.

65

Ophthalmology for the Internist

JAMES P. DUNN, MD

Although most patients with underlying eye disorders are seen regularly by their ophthalmologists, it is imperative that internists recognize ophthalmologic emergencies, ocular manifestations of systemic diseases, and common causes of diminished visual acuity. Timely management and appropriate referral can serve to minimize potential visual loss and other ocular morbidity.

Review of Anatomy and Function

Figure 66-1 shows the cross-sectional anatomy of the eyelids and globe.
- Eyelids
  - Protect the eye
- Conjunctiva
  - Provides lubrication
  - Immunologic functions (conjunctival-associated lymphoid tissue)
- Cornea
  - Most important refractile component of vision
- Anterior chamber and angle
  - Filtration of the aqueous humor through trabecular meshwork
- Lens
  - Responsible for accommodation (focusing for near tasks)
- Uvea (iris, ciliary body, choroid)
  - Produces aqueous humor (ciliary body)
  - Nourishes outer retina
- Retina
  - Converts light to electrical impulses in first stage of visual processing
  - Macula (central retina) much more critical than peripheral retina; the fovea is the center of the macula and subserves central visual acuity
- Optic nerve
  - Connects retinal nerve fibers (~1 million per eye) to the brain
  - The optic disk is nasal to the fovea and is the only visible part of the optic nerve
- Orbit
  - Contains extraocular muscles, adipose tissue, nerves, blood vessels, part of optic nerve

Common Causes of Visual Loss

REFRACTIVE ERROR
- Myopia (nearsightedness): Distance vision is blurred because light rays are focused anterior to the fovea
- Hyperopia (farsightedness): Near vision is blurred because light rays are focused posterior to the fovea
  - In children, accommodation of the ciliary body can overcome mild hyperopia but can induce accommodative esotropia ("crossed eyes")
  - In moderate and severe hyperopia, distance vision is also blurred
- Astigmatism
  - Refraction unequal in different parts of eyeball
  - Cylindrical (toric) lens needed to correct vision
- Presbyopia
  - Age-related diminution in near vision
  - Onset usually noticed around ages 40 to 45 years
- Laser *in situ* keratomileusis (LASIK) and photorefractive keratectomy (PRK) are used to alter the corneal surface and correct for some refractive errors

CATARACT
Basic Information
- Opacification of the lens of the eye; morphology includes nuclear sclerosis, posterior subcapsular, and cortical
- Most cataracts are age-related (senescent)
- Other causes include steroid use, trauma, diabetes, family history, uveitis, radiation, poor overall nutrition, Wilson disease (sunflower cataract), and prior ocular surgery (especially pars plana vitrectomy)
- Usually bilateral (except for unilateral trauma) with slow progression

Clinical Presentation and Diagnosis
- Symptoms include blurred vision, glare (especially at night), and difficulty with driving
- **No pain or redness except in cases of lens-induced glaucoma or uveitis**
- On examination, visual acuity is impaired; clouding of the lens can often be appreciated with an

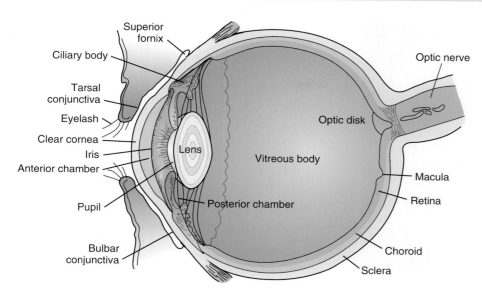

FIGURE 66-1 Cross-sectional anatomy of the eyelids and globe.

ophthalmoscope if slit lamp is unavailable (impairment of normal red reflex or difficulty visualizing optic disk and retina)

Treatment

- If refraction does not improve vision, surgery is the only effective treatment
- **Indications for surgery revolve around functional impairment and difficulty with activities of daily living; Snellen acuity (i.e., vision on eye chart) alone is a poor predictor of visual function (or dysfunction)**
  - Uncommonly, cataract surgery is necessary to allow visualization of internal structures of the eye for diagnostic and treatment purposes (e.g., glaucoma, diabetic retinopathy)
- Standard treatment is phacoemulsification with posterior chamber lens implant (within capsular bag behind the iris)
  - Nearly always performed as outpatient surgery
    - Anesthesia may be general (in children or uncooperative or extremely anxious adults), local (e.g., retrobulbar or peribulbar), or topical/intraocular (most common form of anesthesia)
    - Surgery performed through peripheral clear cornea using topical or intraocular (intracameral) anesthesia allows patients to remain on anticoagulants such as warfarin or aspirin through cataract surgery
  - **Intravenous sedation (e.g., midazolam or propofol) is usually required for surgery, but preoperative laboratory testing in otherwise healthy patients is usually unnecessary**

AGE-RELATED MACULAR DEGENERATION

Basic Information

- Data from the 2005–2008 National Health and Nutrition Examination Survey showed an estimated prevalence of any age-related macular degeneration (AMD) of 6.5% in persons over 40 years and of late AMD of 0.8%;

non-Hispanic blacks over 60 years had a lower incidence of AMD than non-Hispanic whites of the same age (odds ratio 0.37)
- Leading cause of legal blindness in patients age 55 years and older in the United States
- 10% of population older than 43 years and 30% of population age 75 years and older affected to some degree by AMD
- 2% of those older than 65 years have vision of 20/200 or less in at least one eye because of AMD
- By 2020, nearly 3 million Americans will have advanced AMD
- Risk factors include increasing age, family history, cigarette smoking, light iris color
- Likely that different genetic (e.g., variants in complement factor H and complement component 3) and environmental factors influence different forms of AMD
- Two forms of disease
  - Non-neovascular ("dry," atrophic, nonexudative): 90% of cases
    - "Drusen" are deposits of material in the macula that probably represent the accumulation of by-products of photoreceptor metabolism. On ophthalmoscopy, they appear as small, bright yellow objects (Fig. 66-2).
    - "Geographic atrophy" is well-circumscribed area of retinal pigment epithelium or choriocapillaris
  - Neovascular ("wet," exudative): Less common, more rapidly progressive
    - Choroidal neovascularization causes pigment epithelial detachment and photoreceptor damage
    - Hypertension is a risk factor for progression of dry to wet AMD

Clinical Presentation and Diagnosis

- Blurred central vision caused by loss of foveal function
- Distortion of straight lines may be an early presenting complaint
  - Amsler grid has been used to assess progression of disease (Fig. 66-3)

FIGURE 66-2   Drusen in non-neovascular age-related macular degeneration.

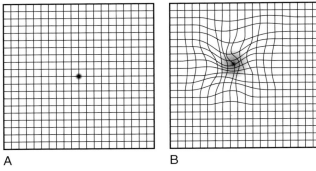

FIGURE 66-3   Amsler grid for monitoring age-related macular degeneration (AMD). **A,** How it would appear normally. **B,** How it might appear to someone with AMD.

- The patient covers one eye and focuses the other eye on the center dot of a hand-held copy of the grid; any new distortion in the lines (metamorphopsia) or blind spots (scotoma) suggests progression of disease
- No pain or redness
- Peripheral vision remains intact

Treatment

- Non-neovascular AMD
  - Antioxidants, zinc supplements, and carotenoids (e.g., lutein) often used, but benefit appears limited to the nonexudative form
  - A combination of zinc, vitamins C and E, and beta-carotene may reduce the risk of progression from moderate to severe AMD, but has not been shown to reduce the risk of progression of mild to moderate AMD (and has no effect on development or worsening of cataracts)
- Neovascular AMD
  - Anti–vascular endothelial growth factor (VEGF) agents (bevacizumab, ranibizumab) injected intraocularly (usually monthly) can stabilize AMD and often improve vision; the two drugs are comparably

effective, and bevacizumab is much less expensive, although systemic adverse effects may be less with ranibizumab
  - Argon laser photocoagulation in some cases, but vision loss still severe
  - Less destructive laser treatments (photodynamic therapy) and intravitreous corticosteroids limited to adjunctive role (e.g., with anti-VEGF agents)
  - Surgery to remove membrane or "translocate" the macula rarely effective
  - Referral to low-vision specialist is highly recommended

Prevention

- Sunglasses or hats to block ultraviolet light possibly helpful
- Control of blood pressure to reduce risk of wet AMD may also be useful
- Cessation of smoking strongly encouraged

Screening

- Comprehensive examination by ophthalmologist recommended every 2 to 4 years for patients ages 40 to 64 years and every 1 to 2 years for patients age 65 years and older

PRIMARY OPEN-ANGLE GLAUCOMA

Basic Information

- Most common type of glaucoma
- Some forms strongly associated with genetic factors (e.g., alterations in myocilin gene)
- Second-leading cause of legal blindness in United States (and leading cause of legal blindness among African Americans)
  - Incidence
    - Estimated 44.7 million people worldwide, and 2.79 million Americans affected in 2010
    - Primary open-angle glaucoma (POAG) undiagnosed in 50% of whites and 75% of African Americans
  - Definition
    - Slowly progressive optic neuropathy characterized by optic disk cupping
    - Trabecular meshwork is blocked by excess glycosaminoglycan production, decreasing aqueous outflow, but not clinically visible
    - **Elevated intraocular pressure (IOP) and elevated cup-to-disk ratio are risk factors, but not diagnostic of POAG by themselves**
    - Other risk factors include increasing age, African American or Latino heritage (10.3% cumulative probability for African Americans versus 4.2% for whites), family history, thinner corneas

Clinical Presentation and Diagnosis

- Asymptomatic until late stages, so measurement of visual acuity is not an adequate screening test; a combination of IOP measurement, automated visual field testing, and imaging studies of optic nerve is mandatory
- Central visual loss occurs in end-stage disease
- **No eye pain or redness**
- Rarely causes headache unless IOP is extremely high

TABLE 66-1	Side Effects of Common Ocular Medications
Drug	**Effects**
β-Adrenergic blocking agents	Bronchospasm Bradycardia Hypotension Fatigue, depression Erectile dysfunction
Corticosteroids	Glaucoma Cataracts Corneal infection
Anesthetics	Poor epithelial healing Corneal melting (with chronic use)
Aminoglycosides	Toxic or allergic keratoconjunctivitis
α-Agonists	Hypotension Dry mouth Dizziness
Oral carbonic anhydrase inhibitors	Fatigue, depression Hypokalemia Acidosis Nausea Aplastic anemia (rare)

- Direct ophthalmoscopy may reveal an enlarged optic cup (cup-to-disk ratio of ≥0.5 is suggestive)
- Screening asymptomatic patients
  - Recommended every 2 to 4 years for patients ages 40 to 64 years, every 1 to 2 years for patients older than 65 years
  - Begin before age 40 years in African Americans

Treatment
- Medical
  - Prostaglandin analogues
  - Aqueous suppressants (topical β-blockers, topical or oral carbonic anhydrase inhibitors)
    - Side effects of oral carbonic anhydrase inhibitors render them poor long-term treatment options
  - Adrenergic agonists (brimonidine, epinephrine derivatives)
  - Cholinergic agonists (e.g., pilocarpine) now used infrequently because of side effects
  - Need to be aware of potential systemic effects of medications (Table 66-1)
- Laser therapy (argon laser trabeculoplasty, selective laser trabeculoplasty)
  - Easy to perform with low risk
  - Effect may only be temporary
- Surgical therapy
  - Trabeculectomy
  - Tube shunt surgery
  - Canaloplasty

NARROW-ANGLE GLAUCOMA
Basic Information
- One-tenth as common as open-angle glaucoma in the United States
- Seen in Asians more commonly than whites or African Americans

Clinical Presentation
- **Manifests with pain, redness, halos, and decreased visual acuity because of rapid elevation in eye pressure**
- Headache, nausea, and vomiting are commonly present
- Attack may be precipitated by mydriatic, sympathomimetic, and hypnotic medications

Treatment
- Requires urgent referral to ophthalmologist for laser iridotomy (and prophylactic laser in opposite eye)

DIABETIC RETINOPATHY
Basic Information
- Leading cause of blindness in patients ages 20 to 60 years in the United States
- 4.1 million adults older than 40 years of age have diabetic retinopathy
- **Risk of retinopathy directly related to duration of diabetes in both type 1 and type 2 patients**
  - After 20 years of diabetes, more than 60% of patients with type 2 disease and nearly all patients with type 1 disease have some degree of retinopathy
  - Among diabetics older than 40 years of age, prevalence rates for diabetic retinopathy and sight-threatening retinopathy are 40.3% and 8.2%, respectively
- Level of glycemic control very important
  - Once retinopathy is present, degree of glucose control is a better predictor of progression to more serious disease than is duration of disease
  - Intensive therapy reduces onset and slows progression of retinopathy
  - Gestational diabetes is not associated with development of retinopathy, but pregnancy may exacerbate preexisting retinopathy

Clinical Presentation and Diagnosis
- Screening recommendations
  - Yearly dilated funduscopic examination for all diabetics
  - More frequent examinations if retinopathy is present
- Nonproliferative ("background," "preproliferative") retinopathy
  - Cotton-wool spots, microaneurysms, intraretinal hemorrhages, lipid ("hard") exudates, retinal edema, venous beading, and intraretinal microvascular abnormalities can be seen (Fig. 66-4)
  - 30% of patients blind after 5 years because of ischemia or macular edema
- Proliferative
  - Retinal vascularization caused by elaboration of angiogenic factors
  - 30% of patients blind after 5 years because of vitreous hemorrhage, retinal detachment, or neovascular glaucoma (angle closed by neovascularization)

Treatment
- Optimal control of diabetes, hypertension, and hyperlipidemia is crucial
- Grid laser photocoagulation more effective than intraocular corticosteroids for leaking vessels causing macular edema

66

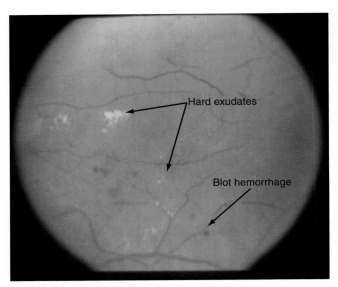

FIGURE 66-4   Nonproliferative diabetic retinopathy.

- Intravitreal injections of VEGF antagonists (bevacizumab, ranibizumab) increasingly used to treat both diabetic macular edema and proliferative diabetic retinopathy
- Panretinal laser photocoagulation proven effective for proliferative retinopathy
  - Most effective when patient has just reached high-risk proliferative diabetic retinopathy or before vision decreases due to macular edema
  - Laser may stabilize vision loss but often does not restore vision
  - Five-year risk of severe visual loss (<5/200) reduced to less than 5% if patients undergo appropriate panretinal photocoagulation for proliferative retinopathy
  - Risk of moderate visual loss (doubling of visual angle) reduced to less than 12% if patients undergo appropriate focal laser therapy for clinically significant macular edema
- Surgical treatment (often combined with laser photocoagulation) necessary to remove vitreous hemorrhage and repair retinal detachments
- Anti-VEGF agents with or without laser more effective than laser alone for diabetic macular edema

CAUSES OF SUDDEN VISUAL LOSS

- Usually monocular
- Can result from a number of different conditions (Box 66-1)

Red Eye

See Table 66-2.

Eye Infections

HERPES SIMPLEX VIRUS

Basic Information and Clinical Presentation

- Major cause of blindness because of keratitis (infection of cornea)

BOX 66-1	*Causes of Sudden Visual Loss*

Transient (Amaurosis Fugax)
Emboli (cholesterol or calcific plaques, cardiac myxoma, platelet-fibrin thrombi)
Vasospasm (migraine, subarachnoid hemorrhage, hypertensive crisis)
Sustained
Optic neuritis (MS, lupus, sarcoidosis)
    Anterior ischemic optic neuropathy
    Arteritic—associated with giant-cell arteritis
Nonarteritic—associated with advancing age, hypertension
Hemorrhage (neovascular AMD, vitreous hemorrhage in diabetes)
Occipital infarct

AMD, age-related macular degeneration; MS, multiple sclerosis.

- Usually caused by herpes simplex virus type 1 (HSV-1)
- **Unilateral redness, with a dendritic pattern on fluorescein staining, is pathognomonic (Fig. 66-5)**
- May recur

Treatment

- Trifluoridine eye drops
- Avoid topical corticosteroids (can cause exacerbation of HSV infection)
- Suppressive oral antiviral therapy (acyclovir 400 mg twice daily or equivalent) may help reduce recurrences

HERPES ZOSTER VIRUS

Basic Information

- Eye can be involved if there is vesicular eruption along any branch of the trigeminal nerve (VI most common)
- Can cause keratitis, uveitis, scleritis, and retinitis

Treatment

- Treat with acyclovir or similar antiviral therapy
  - Most effective if given within 72 hours of outbreak of vesicles

OCULAR COMPLICATIONS OF HIV INFECTION

Basic Information and Clinical Presentation

- Noninfectious retinopathy ("background HIV retinopathy")
  - Occurs in 50% to 100% of patients with CD4 counts less than 200 cells/mm^3
  - Clinical features: Cotton-wool spots, intraretinal hemorrhages
  - Symptoms: None
  - Clinical marker of advanced immunosuppression
  - Need to rule out other causes of retinopathy (e.g., diabetes, hypertension, cytomegalovirus [CMV])
- CMV retinitis
  - **Most common ocular opportunistic infection in AIDS**
  - CD4 count usually less than 50 cells/mm^3

TABLE 66-2	*Differential Diagnosis of the Red Eye*						
	Allergic Conjunctivitis	**Bacterial Conjunctivitis**	**Viral Conjunctivitis**	**Corneal Ulcer**	**Anterior Uveitis**	**Acute Glaucoma**	**Anterior Scleritis**
Symptoms/ findings	Bilateral, itchy eyes	Prominent discharge; no itching or adenopathy	Itching, preauricular adenopathy	Irregular corneal light reflex	Photophobia with ciliary flush	Headache, nausea, vomiting	Pain can be worse at night
Vision	Usually normal	Usually normal	May be impaired	Impaired	Slightly blurred	Decreased	Normal
Discharge	Watery	Mucopurulent	Watery	Tearing or purulent	Tearing	Tearing	None
Pain	None	Minimal	Minimal	Present	Photophobia	Severe	Severe
Pupil size/ shape	Normal	Normal	Normal	Normal	Miotic or irregular	Mid-dilated	Normal
Pupillary responses	Normal	Normal	Normal	Normal	May be nonreactive	Nonreactive	Normal
Redness	Diffuse	Diffuse	Segmental or diffuse	Localized or diffuse	Ciliary flush*	Diffuse with ciliary flush	Local or diffuse
Management/ comments	Eliminate allergen Topical antihistamines or mast cell stabilizers	Topical antibiotics to cover *S. aureus, S. pneumoniae, H. influenzae*	Supportive Avoid close contact with other people for 7–14 days	Associated with trauma, contact lenses, topical steroid use; may require fortified topical antibiotics	Topical corticosteroids† and cycloplegics Systemic work-up usually necessary to assess for rheumatologic disease or sarcoid	Aqueous suppressants Laser Surgical iridectomy	Systemic cortico-steroids or NSAIDs Systemic work-up usually necessary to assess for rheuma-tologic disease or sarcoid

H. *influenzae, Haemophilus influenzae; S. aureus, Staphylococcus aureus; S. pneumoniae, Streptococcus pneumoniae.*
*Ring of injection around the limbus.
†Topical corticosteroids should never be used to treat a red eye without a specific diagnosis because they may cause glaucoma, cataract, or recurrent herpetic keratitis.

66

FIGURE 66-5 Dendritic pattern of herpesvirus keratitis after fluorescein staining. *Inset* shows pattern after passing through cobalt blue filter. *(From Goldman L, Bennett JC, Ausiello D: Cecil textbook of medicine, ed 22, Philadelphia, WB Saunders, 2004, Fig. 465-10.)*

FIGURE 66-6 Cytomegalovirus retinitis in AIDS (note mixed hemorrhage and necrosis with optic nerve infiltration).

- Floaters, flashing lights, blind spots (no pain, discharge, or redness) common
  - 15% to 50% of patients are asymptomatic
  - No external signs of inflammation
- Retinal examination reveals white, fluffy lesions associated with hemorrhage (Fig. 66-6)
- Screen at-risk patients every 4 to 6 months

Treatment

- Systemic
  - Oral valganciclovir (intravenous foscarnet if ganciclovir resistance or intolerance to oral therapy)
  - Reduces morbidity (extraocular disease), mortality, and second-eye involvement

TABLE 66-3	Ocular Manifestations of Rheumatologic Disease	
Condition	**Description**	**Associated Diseases**
Keratoconjunctivitis sicca	Reduced or absent tear production Burning sensation in eye Photophobia may be present Eye(s) may be red Symptoms of dry mouth may also be present and are suggestive of Sjögren syndrome	Primary Sjögren syndrome Secondary Sjögren syndrome 　Rheumatoid arthritis 　Systemic lupus erythematosus 　Polyarteritis nodosa 　Scleroderma
Episcleritis and scleritis	Episcleritis 　Redness of eye usually limited 　Painless Scleritis 　Redness more diffuse 　Painful	Rheumatoid arthritis Systemic lupus erythematosus Wegener granulomatosus Polyarteritis nodosa Relapsing polychondritis Seronegative spondyloarthropathies Inflammatory bowel disease
Uveitis (see Fig. 66-7)	Pain Redness Photophobia Ciliary flush—ring of injection around limbus	Sarcoidosis (bilateral) Seronegative spondyloarthropathies (unilateral) Behçet disease Lyme disease (bilateral) Syphilis
Keratitis	Inflammation of the cornea May lead to ulceration Vision affected	Systemic lupus erythematosus Wegener granulomatosus Polyarteritis nodosa Syphilis
Anterior ischemic optic neuropathy	Sudden loss of vision	Giant-cell arteritis Systemic lupus erythematosus

- Local
  - Ganciclovir implant (with oral valganciclovir for previously listed reasons)
  - Intravitreous ganciclovir or foscarnet injections
- Effect of highly active antiretroviral therapy (HAART)
  - Reduces risk of ocular complications
  - CMV retinitis in less than 5% of patients versus more than 30% in pre-HAART era
  - In patients responsive and adherent to HAART (CD4$^+$ count consistently >100 cells/mm^3), chronic anti-CMV therapy usually not necessary
  - "Immune recovery uveitis" (IRU) occurs in minority of eyes with CMV retinitis in patients responsive to HAART
    - Syndrome of uveitis, vitreitis, macular edema, and epiretinal membrane formation
    - Risk factors for IRU unclear

BACTERIAL AND VIRAL CONJUNCTIVITIS

See Table 66-2.

Disease of the Eyelid

BLEPHARITIS

Basic Information and Clinical Presentation

- Noninfectious lid margin inflammation (bacterial super-infection can occur)
- Symptoms: crusting, irritation, chronic redness
- Common in patients with seborrhea, eczema, and rosacea

Treatment

- Warm compresses, lid scrubs; antibiotic ointment (erythromycin, bacitracin) if superinfection suggested; topical azithromycin drops may be helpful on chronic basis

HORDEOLUM

Basic Information and Clinical Presentation

- Internal hordeolum: Infection of meibomian gland on the conjunctival side of the eyelid
- External hordeolum (stye): Infection of gland and eyelash follicle on skin side of the lid
- *Staphylococcus aureus* is the organism most commonly responsible for infection
- Symptoms: Pain, focal lid erythema; globe unaffected; patients often also have blepharitis

Treatment

- Warm compresses, topical antibiotics (e.g., erythromycin)

CHALAZION

Basic Information and Clinical Presentation

- Focal, noninfectious blockage of meibomian gland
- Symptoms: Nontender swelling of lid (unless superinfected)
- Upper lid more commonly affected
- Commonly associated with acne rosacea

Treatment

- Warm compresses; incision and drainage if chronic and bothersome

BASAL CELL CARCINOMA

Basic Information and Clinical Presentation

- Most common eyelid tumor
- Usually occurs on lower lid or medial canthus

Treatment

- Surgical excision preferred to radiation or cryoablation

FIGURE 66-7 Anterior uveitis with ciliary flush. *(From Henry MM, Thompson JN: Clinical surgery, ed 22, Philadelphia, WB Saunders, 2005, Fig. 36.14.)*

OCULAR SIDE EFFECTS OF SYSTEMIC THERAPY

Basic Information and Clinical Presentation

- Regular ophthalmic screening indicated in patients taking systemic corticosteroids (glaucoma, cataract), antimalarials (retinopathy), and ethambutol (optic neuropathy)
- Bisphosphonates have occasionally been associated with development of scleritis and uveitis

Treatment

- Cessation of drug therapy if possible (e.g., change from oral corticosteroid therapy to steroid-sparing immuno-suppressive therapy)
- Cataract surgery for steroid-induced cataract as necessary
- Topical glaucoma therapy for steroid-induced glaucoma; surgery may be necessary in more severe cases

Eye in Rheumatologic Disease

See Table 66-3. See Figure 66-7 for an example of anterior uveitis.

REVIEW QUESTIONS

For review questions, please go to www.expertconsult.com.

SUGGESTED READINGS

Age-Related Eye Disease Study Group: A randomized, placebo-controlled, clinical trial of high dose supplementation with vitamins C and E and beta-carotene for age-related cataract and vision loss, AREDS report no. 9, *Arch Ophthalmol* 119:1439–1452, 2001.

CATT Research Group, Martin DF, Maguire MG, et al: Ranibizumab and bevacizumab for neovascular age-related macular degeneration, *N Engl J Med* 364:1897–1908, 2011.

Chen Y, Zeng J, Zhao C, et al: Assessing susceptibility to age-related macular degeneration with genetic markers and environmental factors, *Arch Ophthalmol* 129:344–351, 2011.

Congdon N, O'Colmain B, Klaver CC, et al: for the Eye Diseases Prevalence Research Group: Causes and prevalence of visual impairment among adults in the United States, *Arch Ophthalmol* 122:477–485, 2004.

The Diabetes Control and Complications Trial/Epidemiology of Diabetes Interventions and Complications Research Group: Retinopathy and nephropathy in patients with type 1 diabetes 4 years after a trial of intensive therapy, *N Engl J Med* 342:381–389, 2000.

Marmor MF, Kellner U, Lai TY, et al: Revised recommendations on screening for chloroquine and hydroxychloroquine retinopathy, *Ophthalmology* 118:415–422, 2011.

Pokhrel PK, Loftus SA: Ocular emergencies, *Am Fam Physician* 76:829–836, 2007.

Schein OD, Katz J, Bass EB, et al: The value of routine preoperative medical testing before cataract surgery: study of medical testing for cataract surgery, *N Engl J Med* 342:168–175, 2000.

Vogel R, Strahlman E, Rittenhouse KD: Adverse events associated with commonly used glaucoma drugs, *Int Ophthalmol Clin* 39:107–124, 1999.

66

Psychiatry for the Internist

THOMAS W. KOENIG, MD

Psychological and social problems are pervasive in our society. **An estimated 25% of adults experience some form of mental illness at some time in their lives.** This chapter provides the basic framework for diagnosing and treating a number of common conditions, including disorders of mood, anxiety, somatization, and body image. Additionally, issues involving the care of victims of domestic violence will be addressed.

Mood Disorders

DEPRESSION
Basic Information

- Everyone experiences periods in life when he or she feels "depressed"
- Depression is a symptom, not a diagnosis
- "Pathologic depression" refers to a condition that results in limitations to a person's functioning (i.e., social, occupational, or physical)
- **Major depression is seen in up to 15% of all outpatients and inpatients**
- Risk factors for major depressive disorders
  - History of a major depressive disorder in the past
  - Female gender: Major depressive episodes occur in women twice as often as in men
  - Family history of a depressive illness in a first-degree relative
- A number of medical conditions have been associated with depression, including coronary artery disease, stroke, diabetes, HIV, cancer, fibromyalgia, chronic fatigue syndrome, dementia, and other neurodegenerative disorders such as Parkinson disease, and hypothyroidism (including subclinical disease)
  - Treatment of the underlying medical disorder may lead to improvement in the depressive symptoms in many cases
- A number of medications (e.g., β-blockers, glucocorticoids, opioids, and interferon) and illicit substances have also been associated with depression

Clinical Presentation and Diagnosis

- Symptoms vary from patient to patient
- Can coexist with other mental disorders (e.g., anxiety, somatization)
- The evaluation begins with an assessment of functional impairment and inquiry into the presence of a number of symptoms (Box 67-1)
- **Before making the diagnosis of a primary depressive disorder, inquiry should be made into substance abuse, underlying medical disorders, and medication use**

- Depression can be divided into three main groups: Major depression, dysthymia, and atypical depression (see Box 67-1)
  - Grief reactions are normal responses that are not considered depressive disorders, but they may progress to major depressive episodes (Box 67-2)
- **If the diagnosis of major depression is suggested, screening for the possibility of bipolar disorder (see following discussion) is recommended**
- Suicidal or homicidal risk should also be assessed
  - Up to 15% of patients with untreated depression commit suicide
  - Epidemiologic studies reveal increased suicide risk in the following populations:
    - Previous history of suicide attempt
    - Coexisting anxiety or panic disorder
    - Substance abuse
    - Older individuals (age >65 years)
    - Whites or Native Americans
    - Patients living alone (e.g., single, divorced)
    - Patients with a recent stressful life event
    - Family history of completed suicide
  - If suicidal or homicidal ideation is present, an assessment of the patient's plan for such action should be obtained
  - **Patients with an imminent risk of suicide should be immediately referred for emergent psychiatric evaluation**

Treatment

- The first step is an open discussion of and education about depression with the patient in an effort to minimize reluctance to accepting therapy
  - Emphasizing that clinical depression is a medical illness that affects numerous individuals should assist in such discussions
- Psychotherapy
  - Many different types of therapy (e.g., cognitive, behavioral, interpersonal, and group)
  - Effective as the sole mode of therapy for milder presentations of major depression
  - For more severe presentations, medications should be combined with psychotherapy
- Medications
  - A number of antidepressant medications are currently available with roughly equivalent efficacy rates (Table 67-1)
  - Many factors should be considered when choosing a specific antidepressant
    - Patient's previous success with a specific medication
    - Coexisting medical conditions

67

| BOX 67-1 | *Symptoms and Classification of Depression* |

Symptoms of a Depressive Episode

Depressed mood
Markedly diminished interest or pleasure (anhedonia)
Significant weight loss or weight gain
Insomnia or hypersomnia
Mental and physical agitation or slowing
Fatigue or loss of energy
Feelings of worthlessness or guilt
Poor concentration or indecisiveness
Recurrent thoughts of death or suicidal ideation

Major Depressive Disorder

Depressed mood or anhedonia must be present
At least five of the nine symptoms of a depressive episode should be present
Symptoms persist for most of the day, every day, >2 wk
Seasonal affective disorder is a subclassification used when patients present with recurrent depressive episodes at characteristic times of the year

Dysthymic Disorder

Depressed mood >2 yr
Symptoms less severe than with major depression
Anhedonia, low self-esteem, and low energy are commonly present

Atypical Depression*

Most common mood disorder
Symptoms persist for most of the day, every day, >2 wk
Less than five of the nine symptoms of a depressive episode are seen

Adapted from Task Force on DSM-IV: *The diagnostic and statistical manual of mental disorders, fourth edition*, Washington, DC, American Psychiatric Association, 1994.
*Includes the subcategory minor depression.

- Potential drug interactions
- Cost
- Anticipated side effects
- History of response of a family member to a particular agent
- A response is usually seen within 6 to 8 weeks after a therapeutic dose of antidepressant is attained
  - Initially patients may not report any improvement in mood or anhedonia, but questioning may reveal improvement in other symptoms such as energy level, sleep, appetite, anxiety, or ability to concentrate
  - If there has been a partial response to therapy, the medication dosage can be increased, the medication can be changed, psychotherapy can be added, or augmentation therapy can be added (see following discussion)
  - If there is absolutely no response to therapy within 8 weeks, another medication should be chosen
- **The duration of therapy is usually 6 to 12 months. Patients with a history of recurrent major depressive episodes should be considered for maintenance therapy.**

| BOX 67-2 | *Grief and Bereavement Reactions* |

Are considered normal responses to loss of someone of close relationship (usually a spouse)
Usually resolves within a few months of the death
Complicated grief reactions are the persistence of symptoms (e.g., preoccupation with thoughts of the deceased, auditory or visual hallucinations of the deceased, difficulty accepting the death)
The risk of major depression is very high (up to 35%) within the first year of the loss of a loved one
Consider the diagnosis of depression in anyone whose grieving persists for longer than 2–3 mo

- Tapering of medications is usually necessary to prevent or observe for the return of depressive symptoms and withdrawal effect
- Electroconvulsive therapy (ECT)
  - Typically used for severe depression or cases refractory to other therapies
  - Requires general anesthesia
  - Typically requires 6 to 12 treatments over the course of 2 to 4 weeks
  - Patients usually require antidepressant treatment following a course of ECT to prevent relapse
  - Some patients benefit from "maintenance ECT" when medication trials have failed
- Augmentation therapy
  - Considered when there is a partial response to antidepressant therapy
  - A number of medications have been shown to be useful in conjunction with standard antidepressants (e.g., lithium, triiodothyronine, pindolol, and methylphenidate)

BIPOLAR AFFECTIVE DISORDER

Basic Information

- Refers to the occurrence (and recurrence) of manic or hypomanic episodes usually alternating with episodes of depression
- Affects 1% of the population
- First episode usually occurs in the second and third decades of life, and depression is most common as the index episode

Clinical Presentation and Diagnosis

- Mania consists of a persistently elevated, expansive, or irritable mood and three of the following lasting at least 1 week
  - Inflated self-esteem
  - Decreased need for sleep
  - Flight of ideas or racing thoughts
  - Hypertalkativeness, pressured speech
  - Distractibility
  - Psychomotor agitation, hyperactivity, or increased activity
  - Excessive involvement in pleasurable activities (e.g., sexual indiscretions, spending money)
  - May be delusional or experience hallucinations
- Hypomania is considered an abnormal elevation of mood but not to the extent that it seriously impairs functioning

TABLE 67-1	*Antidepressant Medications*		
Drug Class	**Examples**	**Side Effects**	**Comments**
Selective serotonin reuptake inhibitors (SSRIs)	Escitalopram Citalopram Fluoxetine Paroxetine Sertraline Luvoxamine	Nausea, vomiting, diarrhea Sweating Headache Sedation or agitation Sexual dysfunction Serotonin syndrome*	Widely used because of tolerability and ease of use Also effective for cases of anxiety and panic disorder Can raise levels of many drugs including anticonvulsants, digoxin, warfarin, antiarrhythmics, β-blockers
Serotonin/norepinephrine reuptake inhibitor	Venlafaxine Desvenlafaxine Duloxetine	Nausea, vomiting, diarrhea Headache Insomnia Hypertension	Activating rather than sedating so good for "understimulated" patients
Norepinephrine and dopamine reuptake inhibitor	Bupropion	Dry mouth Constipation Dizziness Weight loss Seizures (at high doses)	Also used for smoking cessation Low incidence of sexual dysfunction Activating rather than sedating Avoid in patients with eating or seizure disorders
Norepinephrine and serotonin antagonist	Mirtazapine	Sedation Weight gain Orthostatic hypotension	Low incidence of sexual dysfunction
Serotonin antagonist and reuptake inhibitor	Trazodone	Sedation Orthostatic hypotension Dry mouth Liver damage or failure (nefazodone) Priapism (trazodone)	Low incidence of sexual dysfunction
Norepinephrine/serotonin reuptake inhibitors (tricyclic antidepressants)	Amitriptyline Imipramine Desipramine Nortriptyline	Orthostatic hypotension Dry mouth Blurry vision Constipation Sedation Weight gain Urinary retention Sexual dysfunction Q–T prolongation and arrhythmias	Need to titrate dose and follow blood levels Should avoid in patients with cardiac disease Can be useful in patients with coexisting illnesses such as insomnia, migraine, panic disorder, neuropathic pain disorders
Monoamine oxidase inhibitor	Phenelzine Tranylcypromine Selegiline	Orthostatic hypotension Dry mouth Constipation Sedation Urinary retention Sexual dysfunction Hypertensive crisis with intake of tyramine-rich foods, meperidine, decongestants, SSRIs	Useful for "atypical depression" (hypersomnia, overeating, worsening depression in the evenings, prominent anxiety) Can treat hypertensive crisis with phentolamine

*Serotonin syndrome is a change in mental status, diaphoresis, rigors, hyperreflexia, and tachycardia because of hyperstimulation of brainstem serotonin receptors caused by coadministration of an SSRI and another agent that increases serotonin level.

- Delusions and hallucinations do not occur in hypomania
- Classification of bipolar disorder
  - Type I: Positive history of at least one manic episode, with or without past major depressive episodes
  - Type II: Positive history of at least one episode of major depression and at least one hypomanic episode
- Need to evaluate patient for medical conditions and drug use that may mimic bipolar disorder (e.g., substance abuse, personality disorders, thyrotoxicosis, steroid-induced mania)

Treatment

- Lithium carbonate
  - Most studied mood stabilizer
  - Also has antidepressant effects

- Side effects include GI distress (nausea, vomiting, diarrhea), sedation, weight gain, acne, bradycardia, diabetes insipidus (polyuria, polydipsia, hypernatremia), hypothyroidism, renal insufficiency, and benign leukocytosis
  - **A creatinine level, thyroid function tests, electro-cardiogram, and pregnancy test (if appropriate) should be obtained before beginning therapy**
  - Drug levels must be monitored
- Anticonvulsants (e.g., carbamazepine, valproic acid) can also be effective; lamotrigine shows promise as treatment for bipolar depression
- Antipsychotics (e.g., olanzapine, quetiapine) can be used
- Antidepressants for bipolar depression should be used cautiously as they can precipitate a manic or "mixed" state

- ECT can be helpful during an acute manic episode as well
- Psychotherapy should be employed in addition to pharmacotherapy in virtually all patients

Anxiety Disorders

GENERALIZED ANXIETY DISORDER

Basic Information

- Characterized by excessive anxiety and worry that result in some degree of functional impairment
- Affects women more than men
- Commonly coexists with substance abuse and other psychiatric disorders (e.g., depression, obsessive-compulsive disorder)

Clinical Presentation and Diagnosis

- Excessive, extreme anxiety and worry for more days than not, for at least 6 months
- The patient's worry is difficult or impossible to manage or control and out of proportion to the likelihood of negative events
- Three or more of the following must also occur:
  - Restlessness
  - Easy fatigability
  - Poor concentration
  - Muscle tension
  - Sleep difficulties
  - Irritability or edginess

Treatment

- Antidepressant medications (e.g., selective serotonin reuptake inhibitors [SSRIs], tricyclic antidepressants, and dual reuptake inhibitors) can all be effective
- Benzodiazepines can be useful for short-term therapy until antidepressants have taken effect
  - Avoid short-acting agents (e.g., alprazolam) because of the high incidence of dependence
- Buspirone
- Counseling or psychotherapy can be effective as sole therapy or in conjunction with medications

PANIC DISORDER

Basic Information

- Common problem seen in primary care
- Affects 4% to 6% of the population
- **Most patients present with unexplained somatic complaints (e.g., chest pain, abdominal pain, dizziness, fatigue) rather than the complaint of fear or anxiety**
  - Results in high use of health care resources from doctor visits, laboratory testing, hospitalization, and specialty referrals
- Seen more commonly in patients with mitral valve prolapse, asthma, and migraine headaches

Clinical Presentation and Diagnosis

- Presents with the abrupt onset of intense fear that may manifest with the sudden onset of somatic or cognitive symptoms

BOX 67-3	*Criteria for the Diagnosis of Panic Disorder*

A discrete period of intense fear or discomfort during which four or more of the following occur, reaching a peak within 10 min:
- Palpitations
- Diaphoresis
- Shakiness or trembling
- Shortness of breath
- Sensation of choking
- Chest pain or discomfort
- Nausea or abdominal distress
- Dizziness or lightheadedness
- Depersonalization (being detached from oneself) or derealization (feelings of unreality)
- Fear of losing control
- Fear of dying
- Paresthesias
- Hot flashes

Adapted from Task Force on DSM-IV: *The diagnostic and statistical manual of mental disorders, fourth edition,* Washington, DC, American Psychiatric Association, 1994.

- The *Diagnostic and Statistical Manual of Mental Disorders, Fourth Edition* (DSM-IV) criteria for diagnosing a panic attack are presented in Box 67-3
- Attacks commonly occur after a significant life stress
- Often coexists with other psychiatric conditions (e.g., agoraphobia, major depression, personality disorders, post-traumatic stress disorder, and somatization disorders)
- Need to consider the presence of an underlying medical disorder that may mimic panic disorder (e.g., angina, arrhythmias, pheochromocytoma, thyroid disorders, and temporal lobe epilepsy)

Treatment

- **For mild cases that are infrequent and related to stressors, supportive psychotherapy and relaxation techniques may be the only necessary interventions**
- For more severe cases, with or without phobic tendencies, cognitive behavioral therapy or medications are useful
  - Cognitive behavioral therapy designed to modify maladaptive behavior is equivalent or superior to therapy with medications
  - Effective medications include SSRIs, tricyclic antidepressants, and monoamine oxidase (MAO) inhibitors
- Treatment should be continued for at least 12 months
  - Tapering of medications can be tried thereafter
  - There is a high rate of recurrence after discontinuation of therapy
- For acute treatment of panic attacks, benzodiazepines (e.g., lorazepam) are useful in the short term but carry the risk of dependence when used long term

OBSESSIVE-COMPULSIVE DISORDER

- Occurs in 3% of the population
- Diagnosed in patients with either obsessions or compulsions
  - Obsessions: Recurrent thoughts, images, or impulses that cause marked anxiety and are perceived as being senseless or intrusive

67

- Examples include the fear of contamination or fear of harm
  - Compulsions: Ritualistic behaviors or mental acts that are done in response to an obsession to decrease anxiety or avoid a feared consequence
    - Examples include excessive hand washing, skin picking, or hair pulling (trichotillomania)
- Has a significant negative effect on activities of daily living, social functioning, occupational functioning, and overall quality of life
- Treatment is psychotherapy with or without medications
  - Effective medications include SSRIs (e.g., paroxetine, fluvoxamine, fluoxetine, sertraline) or clomipramine

PHOBIAS

- One of the most common psychiatric conditions
- Divided into three basic categories
  - Specific phobia
    - Fear of objects (e.g., insects, snakes) or situations (e.g., heights, flying, drawing of blood)
    - Usually responds to behavior therapy (systematic desensitization)
    - Benzodiazepines or β-blockers can be used in some cases
  - Social phobia
    - Fear of social situations (e.g., public speaking)
    - Treated with psychotherapy and medications
    - SSRIs are considered first-line therapy
    - Benzodiazepines and MAO inhibitors are also effective
    - β-Blockers may be particularly useful in cases of performance anxiety where somatic sensations (e.g., palpitations) can be troubling
  - Agoraphobia
    - Fear or anxiety over being in a place or situation from which escape might be difficult (e.g., being alone when away from home, being in crowds)
    - Often occurs with panic disorder
    - Treatment is similar to that of panic disorder (see preceding discussion)

POST-TRAUMATIC STRESS DISORDER

- Severe response to a traumatic event that involved the risk of serious injury or death to the patient or someone close to the patient
- Characterized by intrusive recollections of the traumatic event, avoidance of any situations or activities associated with the event, increased arousal, and emotional detachment
- Results in significant functional impairment
- Because of the complexity of the disorder, most patients should be referred to a psychiatrist
- Treatment is with psychotherapy and medications (SSRIs)
- Recovery is expected within 1 year in one third of patients and within 10 years in two thirds of patients

SOMATOFORM DISORDERS

Basic Information

- Refers to the manifestation of psychological distress as unexplained physical symptoms

TABLE 67-2 Somatoform Disorders

Disorder	Description
Somatization disorder	History of seeking treatment for multiple physical complaints before age 30 yr, resulting in significant functional impairment More common in women Symptoms cannot be explained by an underlying medical condition At some point during the disorder, should have complained of pain at four different sites: two gastrointestinal symptoms, one sexual symptom, one neurologic symptom
Undifferentiated somatoform disorder	One or more unexplained physical complaints lasting ≥6 mo Results in significant functional impairment Not caused by another mental disorder
Conversion disorder	One or more unexplained symptoms suggesting deficits in normal neurologic function Presentation follows the patient's view of the disease rather than neurophysiology Examples include amnesia, aphonia, blindness, paralysis, paresthesias, seizures
Hypochondriasis	Misinterpretation of bodily symptoms as a serious underlying disease Preoccupation exists despite appropriate medical evaluation and reassurance Disturbance lasts for >6 mo Usually presents in the third decade of life
Pain disorder	Unexplained or amplified complaints of pain Presents in fourth or fifth decade of life Specific psychological factors can often be related to the onset of the pain
Body dysmorphic disorder	Preoccupation with an imagined or exaggerated defect in appearance Onset is usually in the second or third decade of life
Factitious disorder	Intentional feigning or induction of physical signs or symptoms to assume the sick role Can lead to multiple hospitalizations (chronic factitious disorder or Munchausen syndrome) Secondary gain not evident
Malingering	Intentional feigning or induction of physical signs or symptoms for secondary gain (e.g., compensation for injuries)

- Patients may be aware or unaware of this tendency
- **Leads to high use of medical resources through unnecessary testing, referrals, and procedures**
- Commonly coexists with other psychiatric disorders (e.g., anxiety, depression)
- Somatoform disorders are subdivided into a number of categories by the DSM-IV (Table 67-2)

Clinical Presentation

See Table 67-2.

BOX 67-4 Medical Complications of Eating Disorders

Dental erosions (Fig. 67-1)

Enlarged parotid glands

Hair loss and brittle nails

Calluses over the knuckles (Russell's sign) caused by induction of vomiting

Neurologic disease—seizures, myopathy, neuropathy, cognitive difficulties

Cardiac disease—bradycardia, arrhythmias, congestive heart failure, ECG abnormalities

Gastrointestinal disease—dysmotility, esophagitis, gallstones, Mallory-Weiss tears, superior mesenteric artery syndrome

Endocrinologic disease—amenorrhea, osteoporosis, sick euthyroid syndrome, growth retardation, infertility

Hematologic—anemia, leukopenia, thrombocytopenia

Electrolyte abnormalities—hypokalemia, metabolic alkalosis (in patients who purge), hyponatremia

ECG, electrocardiographic.

FIGURE 67-1 Advanced perimolysis of the maxillary incisors in which the pulp chambers of the teeth are visible due to acid erosion from chronic vomiting. *(From Stefanac S, Nesbit S: Treatment planning for dentistry, ed 2, St. Louis, Elsevier Mosby, 2007, Fig. 15-9.)*

Diagnosis

- Based largely on clinical presentation
- A thorough history and physical examination should be done to help establish a rapport with the patient and to identify coexisting psychiatric disorders and potentially overlooked medical conditions
- A review of previous patient records is invaluable in avoiding repeat testing and overuse of resources

Treatment

- No specific therapy is uniformly effective
- Should be treated as a chronic illness
  - **Regular office visits should be scheduled, rather than urgent visits for new complaints**
- Recognizing the disorder as a medical problem rather than a condition that is "all in your head" is imperative in developing a trusting relationship
- Avoid extensive medical testing and complicated medical regimens

EATING DISORDERS

Basic Information

- Affect over 2 million people in the United States with an overwhelming female predominance
- Usually manifest in late childhood, adolescence, or early adulthood
- Associated with a number of potential medical complications (Box 67-4)

Clinical Presentation and Diagnosis

- Three major disorders are described:
  - Anorexia nervosa
    - Refusal to maintain weight within a normal range for height and age
    - Intense fear of weight gain and becoming fat
    - Disturbance in body image or denial of seriousness of current body weight
    - Absence of at least three consecutive menstrual cycles
  - Bulimia nervosa
    - Episodes of out-of-control binge eating with compensatory purging (vomiting, laxative abuse) or nonpurging (excessive exercise, strict dieting or fasting) behavior to prevent weight gain
    - Binging and compensatory behavior occurs at least twice per week for 3 months
    - Self-evaluation is unduly influenced by body weight and shape
  - Binge-eating disorder (BED)
    - Not yet formally recognized as an independent psychiatric illness but is associated with numerous other psychiatric disorders
    - More common than anorexia or bulimia
    - Defined by episodes of consumption of large amounts of food in discrete amounts of time with a lack of control over eating. On average, episodes should occur twice per week for at least 6 months. No inappropriate compensatory behaviors should be present (i.e., purging, excessive exercise, fasting).
    - **Patients can be obese, overweight, or have normal weight**

Treatment

- Requires a multidisciplinary approach with a mental health specialist, medical provider (to help treat potential complications), and dietitian
- Goal is for weight gain of 0.5 to 1 pound per week in outpatients
- Refeeding syndrome
  - Seen in patients with severe anorexia nervosa within 2 to 3 weeks of refeeding
  - **Manifests as cardiac abnormalities and delirium primarily caused by hypophosphatemia and other electrolyte abnormalities; significant third-spacing of fluid**
- Psychotherapy is the treatment of choice
  - The addition of SSRIs (fluoxetine) or other antidepressants is effective for bulimia nervosa
  - Antidepressants may be helpful in patients with anorexia nervosa to prevent recurrences of illness or to treat comorbid depressive illness but do not significantly contribute to acute disease management

BOX 67-5	*Historical Clues Suggestive of Domestic Violence*

Chronic abdominal or pelvic pain
Chronic headaches
Chronic fatigue
Depression and anxiety
Frequent emergency room visits
Frequent physician visits with vague somatic complaints
History of sexually transmitted diseases
Recurrent, inconsistently explained injuries
Substance abuse

- Treatment for BED consists primarily of psychotherapy. Behavioral weight loss therapy may be used in overweight individuals. Pharmacotherapy with SSRIs may also be useful.

DOMESTIC VIOLENCE

Basic Information

- Defined as ongoing physical, psychological, or sexual abuse in the home, associated with isolation, limited personal freedom, and limited access to resources (e.g., economic resources)
- An estimated 2 million people (usually women) are victims of abuse each year, resulting in over 2000 deaths
- Found in patients of all races, socioeconomic backgrounds, and ages
- Elder abuse
  - Refers to a subset of patients older than age 65 years who are subject to physical abuse, sexual abuse, neglect, or financial abuse
  - Associated with increased mortality
- Children who are victimized by sexual or physical abuse are more prone to be victims of domestic violence in adulthood

Clinical Presentation and Diagnosis

- A number of signs and symptoms are suggestive of domestic violence (Box 67-5)
- Injuries and bruising typically occur on the abdomen, genitalia, around the neck (from attempted strangulation), or around the breasts

- **The abuser may refuse to leave the examining room during the history and physical examination and may try to speak on behalf of the victim**

Diagnosis

- Most cases go unrecognized by physicians
- The key to identification is inquiry
  - Direct questions such as, "Has your partner ever punched or kicked you?" or "Are you afraid of your partner?" are more effective than general ones such as "Do you feel you are being abused?"
  - Questions about sexual and emotional abuse should also be included

Treatment

- Physicians need to identify local resources for dealing with domestic violence
  - Hospital social workers and local domestic violence hotlines can assist in this process
  - The National Domestic Violence Hotline (1-800-799-SAFE) can also assist in providing information about local resources
- If there is an imminent threat to life, immediate referral should be strongly encouraged
- Documentation should be specific and thorough with photographs or sketches of injuries (if present)
- Reporting
  - Only a few states require mandatory reporting of abuse against legally competent adult women
  - Abuse involving children, including children witnessing their parent being abused, should be reported to the local Department of Social Services
  - Elder abuse should be reported to the local elder abuse hotline or adult protective services

REVIEW QUESTIONS

For review questions, please go to www.expertconsult.com.

SUGGESTED READINGS

Gale C, Davidson O: Generalised anxiety disorder, *BMJ* 334:579–581, 2007.
McHugh PR, Slavney PR: *The perspectives of psychiatry*, ed 2, Baltimore, 1998, Johns Hopkins University Press.
Task Force on DSM-IV: *Diagnostic and statistical manual of mental disorders, fourth edition*, Washington, DC, 1994, American Psychiatric Association.
Toohey JS: Domestic violence and rape, *Med Clin North Am* 92:1239–1252, 2008.
Treasure J, Claudino AM, Zucker M: Eating disorders, *Lancet* 375:583–593, 2010.

Allergy and Immunology for the Internist

TAO ZHENG, MD; and SARBJIT S. SAINI, MD

The immune system is normally balanced to protect against foreign proteins and other allergens. Reaction to extrinsic or intrinsic antigens, however, can result in a cascade of events with clinical symptoms ranging from mild (pruritis, rhinorrhea) to severe (respiratory distress, vascular collapse, death).

Basic Information

- Allergens: Proteins of appropriate size that, after inhalation, injection (e.g., drug, venom), or ingestion, provoke an immunoglobulin E (IgE) antibody response and clinical symptoms in sensitive individuals. Common aeroallergens include trees, grasses, and molds, as well as animals (e.g., domesticated pets, rodents), dust mites, and cockroaches.
- **Acute-phase reaction: Allergic response that begins within minutes of allergen exposure; symptoms include pruritis and hives (skin), wheezing (lungs), rhinorrhea and sneezing (nose), erythema, and tearing of eyes**
  - Allergen cross-links specific IgE bound to the surface of mast cells and basophils
  - After surface IgE is cross-linked, mast cells and basophils release mediators such as histamine (stored in cytoplasmic granules) and leukotrienes/prostaglandins (rapidly synthesized from arachidonic acid)
- **Late-phase reaction: Occurs 4 to 12 hours after acute phase and initial allergen exposure; symptoms are similar to acute-phase reaction and mirror the inflammation seen in asthma and chronic allergic rhinitis**
  - Pathogenesis includes leukocyte (eosinophil, T-helper type 2 cell [Th2 cell]) infiltration into tissues, which release Th2 cytokines (interleukin [IL]-4, IL-5, and IL-13) and chemokines (chemoattractant cytokines)
  - Histamine levels also increase

Clinical Presentation of Allergic Reactions

- **Anaphylaxis: An IgE-related response after exposure to antigen, resulting in the rapid onset of systemic symptoms, including pallor, pruritis, dyspnea, wheezing, weakness, urticaria, erythema, flushing, cyanosis, angioedema, diarrhea, nausea, vomiting, abdominal cramping, and hypotension; some present with a biphasic illness, beginning with early abdominal symptoms before respiratory symptoms or vascular collapse set in; may be fatal because of upper airway obstruction or cardiovascular collapse**

- Mechanism: Mast cell and basophil mediators released by allergen binding IgE; mediators released include elevated serum β-tryptase level, histamine, platelet activating factor, prostaglandin D_2, leukotrienes, and cytokines (e.g., tumor necrosis factor-α and IL-1); non–IgE-mediated factors include C3a and C5a
- Causes of anaphylaxis
  - Foods (especially nuts, shellfish, eggs, and milk)
  - Exercise (generally in people with an allergic background)
  - Medications (see following discussion)
  - Insect bites (for which immunotherapy >97% protective)
  - Latex
- Idiopathic anaphylaxis: 30% to 40% of all recurrent anaphylaxis (a diagnosis of exclusion)
- Diagnosis of anaphylaxis is supported by the measurement of elevated serum tryptase (usually peaks in the first 2 hours)
- **Cornerstone of treatment is avoidance of allergens;** treatment of an episode of anaphylaxis includes immediate treatment with epinephrine, followed by oxygen, antihistamines, corticosteroids, and β-agonists (as needed) for support; **patients with a history of anaphylaxis should be prescribed and carry an autoinjectable form of epinephrine**
- Anaphylactoid reaction: A non–IgE-triggered process that clinically resembles anaphylaxis; may be caused by aspirin and nonsteroidal anti-inflammatory drugs (NSAIDs), radiocontrast agents, and, rarely, opiate drugs
  - Symptoms from aspirin and NSAIDs include rhinoconjunctivitis, urticaria, bronchospasm, angioedema, and laryngeal edema; treatment is avoidance or aspirin desensitization
  - Symptoms from radiocontrast agents include the spectrum of symptoms seen with anaphylaxis
    - **Despite common belief, there is no relationship of radiocontrast allergy with allergy to fish, shellfish, or iodine**
    - A typical pretreatment regimen includes prednisone (50 mg, administered at 13 hours, 7 hours, and 1 hour before procedure) and diphenhydramine (IM or PO) 1 hour before procedure
- Urticaria and angioedema
  - **Urticaria (Fig. 68-1) is characterized by well-circumscribed wheals from involvement of the upper layer of the dermis; wheals are**

FIGURE 68-1 Urticaria with characteristic wheals surrounded by an erythematous flare. *(From Forbes CD, Jackson WF: Color atlas and text of clinical medicine, ed 3, St. Louis, Mosby, 2003, Fig. 2.39.)*

FIGURE 68-2 Angioedema commonly involves the lip. *(From Habif TP: Clinical dermatology: a color guide to diagnosis and therapy, ed 4, Philadelphia, Mosby, 2004, Fig. 6-6.)*

erythematous, with blanched centers, are pruritic, and may occur anywhere on the body; usually result from a type 1 hypersensitivity reaction

- Lifetime risk of a single episode of acute urticaria is very high (i.e., one in four adults)
- **Urticaria lasting more than 6 weeks is labeled *chronic* urticaria; most are idiopathic**
  - Biopsy of persistent lesions (>72 hours) should be done to exclude vasculitis
- **Angioedema (Fig. 68-2) is characterized by the acute development of swelling and edema of submucosal or subcutaneous tissue in the skin, mucous membrane, and GI tract;** symptoms are based on tissue involved; typically nonpruritic
  - Occurs with urticaria in approximately 50% of chronic cases
  - 10% of chronic cases have angioedema alone and 40% urticaria alone
  - Hereditary angioedema also occurs without urticaria (Table 68-1)

- Differential causes of urticaria or angioedema
  - Drugs (e.g., angiotensin-converting enzyme inhibitors)
  - Thyroid disorders
  - Autoimmune disorders (e.g., vasculitis)
  - Infections (e.g., viral, including hepatitis, and parasitic)
  - Food
  - Malignancy
  - Cryoglobulins
  - Physical triggers of urticaria may also exist, including cold, heat, pressure, and exercise
- Mechanism unknown; may involve chronic mast cell degranulation; a subset of patients will have antibodies against IgE or the IgE receptor
- **Cornerstone of treatment is antihistamines;** may add histamine$_2$ blocker or tricyclic antidepressant (e.g., doxepin) for severe cases; short-term oral corticosteroids are also used for severe eruptions

Clinical Presentation of Allergic and Immune-Related Diseases

- **Allergic rhinitis: Allergen-induced inflammation of the lining of the nose characterized by nasal congestion, rhinorrhea, sneezing, itch, and postnasal drainage; the most common adult allergic disease (15% of U.S. population)**
  - Overlap of symptoms with viral upper respiratory tract infection, nasal polyposis, nonallergic rhinitis with eosinophilia, and hormonally related nasal congestion (pregnancy, oral contraceptives, hypothyroidism)
  - Medications may also cause symptoms confused with allergic rhinitis (e.g., cocaine and β-blockers)
    - **Rhinitis medicamentosa: Overuse of over-the-counter topical nasal decongestants (vasoconstrictors)**
  - Other causes of symptoms that overlap with allergic rhinitis include vasomotor rhinitis (nasal congestion brought on by irritants such as cigarette smoke and cold air) and anatomic abnormalities (e.g., cerebrospinal fluid leak, deviated septum)
- **Drug allergy: Most adverse drug reactions (ADRs) do not have an immunologic basis** (<10% of all ADRs are immunologically based); the mechanism of many drug reactions is unknown
  - Most drugs are small molecules that cannot act as an antigen unless modified
  - Drugs may act as a hapten, in which the drug or its metabolite combine with a larger carrier protein and can thereby become immunogenic
    - Prior exposure is needed to generate an IgE antibody response
  - Time of onset from drug initiation assists in identifying allergic-type reactions
    - Immediate (<1 hour): Pruritis, urticaria, rhinitis, wheezing, anaphylaxis
    - Accelerated (1–72 hours): Urticaria
    - Late (>72 hours): Maculopapular eruption (Fig. 68-3), drug fever, hemolytic anemia, serum sickness, nephritis, leukopenia, exfoliative dermatitis, Stevens-Johnson syndrome (Fig. 68-4)

TABLE 68-1	*Allergic Skin Diseases*			
Disease	**Clinical Presentation**	**Pathogenesis**	**Diagnosis**	**Treatment**
Hereditary angioedema (HAE–C1-INH)	Autosomal dominant Recurrent swelling of face, airway, GI tract, extremities Bowel edema may result in severe abdominal pain that resolves spontaneously Trauma may trigger symptoms Urticaria uncommon	Absence or reduced level of C1 esterase inhibitor (C1-INH) (85%) Dysfunctional C1-INH (15%)	Clinical presentation Absence or reduced level of C1-INH plus low C4 levels (caused by chronic complement consumption) C4 levels low even if symptoms absent	Synthetic androgens (e.g., danazol, stanazol) induce inhibitor synthesis Purified C1-INH concentrate also available Kallikrein inhibitors
Hereditary angioedema (HAE-FXII)	Missense mutaion in the factor XII (FXII) gene Autosomal dominant Estrogens have a great influence, but highly variable Occurs mainly in women Facial swelling is a cardinal symptom Triggers: acute trauma, estrogens, blockers of the renin-angiotensin system	Activation of the kallikrein-kinin system and the overproduction of bradykinin seem to be involved in the pathophysiology of angioedema attacks of HAE-FXII	Personal history (recurrent angioedema attacks and no urticaria) Genetic tests positive for FXII mutation p.Thr309Lys or p.Thr309Arg C1 esterase inhibitor: normal or slightly decreased	The same drugs are effective or partially effective as those in HAE–C1-INH C1-INH concentrate may be effective for acute attacks Prophylaxis: Danazol, stanazol, and/or kallikrein inhibitors and bradykinin antagonists
Acquired angioedema	Same as above, with onset later in life	Autoantibodies develop to C1-INH Suggests underlying malignancy (leukemia, lymphoma)	C4 levels low Low C1q levels distinguish this from hereditary form	Treat underlying disease
Allergic contact dermatitis	Vesicular eruption with well-demarcated borders on exposed skin area Common causes include poison ivy, nickel, carrier substances in topical medications (e.g., thimerosal)	T cells activated, release interferon-γ Macrophages then activated	Patch testing of suspected substance	Avoid offending agent Topical steroids Oral steroid taper
Atopic dermatitis (AD)	Dry, scaling skin with pruritis Commonly involves head and face Antecubital and popliteal fossae, nape of neck commonly involved in adults	One third of patients with AD have genetic skin barrier defect (filaggrin mutation) Commonly an inherited pattern of elevated IgE, eosinophilia, and evidence of IgE sensitization to antigens	Patients often have positive family history Associated with asthma and allergic rhinitis Associated with dry skin Serum IgE often elevated	Topical corticosteroids to involved area Antihistamines Topical FK506 used for more severe reactions Antistaphylococcal antibiotics
Chronic idiopathic urticaria	Recurrent urticaria or angioedema for >6 wk	Unknown May be related autoantibodies to IgE receptor	Exclusion of drugs or other diseases	$H_1 \pm H_2$ blockers Leukotriene receptor antagonists Steroids

GI, gastrointestinal; H_1, histamine$_1$; H_2, histamine$_2$; IgE, immunoglobulin E.

- **Penicillins and cephalosporins are the most common causes of immunologically based ADRs, typically acting as haptens;** cross-reactivity with cephalosporins is 6% to 30% (second- and third-generation cephalosporins are less likely to cross-react); carbapenems (i.e., imipenem) cross-react with minor determinants of penicillin [PCN], whereas monobactams (i.e., aztreonam) can be safely administered to PCN-allergic patients
  - Other ADRs from PCN include antibody-mediated hemolytic anemia and thrombocytopenia; immune complex disease (characterized by fever, rash, glomerulonephritis, and lymphadenopathy); cell-mediated contact dermatitis (with topical preparations); maculopapular rash seen in 5% to 13% of patients administered amoxicillin (incidence is increased with coincident Epstein-Barr virus and cytomegalovirus)
    - Basis of rash with amoxicillin is unknown; can often treat through the rash with close monitoring
- **Sulfonamides are the second most common antibiotic class to cause drug reactions, usually via a T cell–mediated reaction; seen commonly in patients with HIV**

FIGURE 68-3 A maculopapular eruption in a patient treated with co-trimoxazole. *(From Forbes CD, Jackson WF: Color atlas and text of clinical medicine, ed 3, St. Louis, Mosby, 2003, Fig. 2.147.)*

FIGURE 68-4 Stevens-Johnson syndrome with mucocutaneous facial lesions. *(From Forbes CD, Jackson WF: Color atlas and text of clinical medicine, ed 3, St. Louis, Mosby, 2003, Fig. 2.49.)*

FIGURE 68-5 Allergic contact dermatitis caused by an ankle bracelet. *(From Adkinson NF, Yunginger JW, Busse WW, et al: Middleton's allergy: principles and practice, ed 6, St. Louis, Mosby, 2003, Plate 25.)*

FIGURE 68-6 Acute atopic dermatitis with excoriated lesions. *(From Adkinson NF, Junginger JW, Busse WW, et al: Middleton's allergy: principles and practice, ed 6, St. Louis, Mosby, 2003, Plate 19.)*

- Immunodeficiency syndromes: Include immunoglobulin deficiencies, T-cell and B-cell deficiencies, as well as neutrophil and complement disorders
- Eosinophilia syndromes
  - Churg-Strauss vasculitis: A granulomatous vasculitis involving multiple organ systems, predominantly the lungs
    - Patients present with severe asthma in the setting of systemic illness (fevers, malaise, weight loss), accompanied by pronounced eosinophilia
    - Fleeting pulmonary infiltrates commonly seen on chest radiography
    - Skin rash may also be seen; sinus involvement also has been described

- Allergic skin diseases: Include hereditary and acquired angioedema, allergic contact dermatitis (Fig. 68-5), and atopic dermatitis (Fig. 68-6; see Table 68-1)

TABLE 68-2	Selected Immunodeficiency Syndromes		
Disease	**Clinical Presentation**	**Diagnosis**	**Treatment**
Common variable immunodeficiency	Recurrent sinopulmonary infections Parasitic GI infections seen (esp. *Giardia*) Autoimmune diseases and malignancy risk increased	Quantitative immunoglobulin levels Plasma cells are absent Poor humoral response to immunizations T-cell dysfunction	Antibiotics IV immunoglobulin (IgG) every 3–4 wk subQ immunoglobulin (IgG) weekly
Selective IgA deficiency	The most common primary immunodeficiency (1:600) Recurrent sinopulmonary infections Asthma and atopic dermatitis more common, as are rheumatoid arthritis and lupus Anaphylaxis to blood or blood product transfusion	Low to absent IgA levels IgG and IgM levels normal	Antibiotics Avoid transfusion of blood or blood products unless donor is also IgA deficient
Adult T-cell deficiencies	Opportunistic infections (similar to HIV)	Exclude HIV Wiskott-Aldrich syndrome, a subtype, is associated with thrombocytopenia, small platelets, and eczema	Antimicrobials Wiskott-Aldrich syndrome is treated by bone marrow transplantation
Complement disorders	Early complement component deficiencies: Autoimmune disease C5–C8 deficiencies: Recurrent meningococcal or gonococcal infections	Assay of complement levels	Antibiotic

IgA, immunoglobulin A; IgG, immunoglobulin G; IgM, immunoglobulin M.

- Hypereosinophilic syndrome
  - Systemic disorder characterized by dysfunction of several organs in the setting of persistent eosinophilia (>1500 cells/mL for at least 6 months)
  - Diagnosis involves exclusion of other causes of eosinophilia
  - Cardiac involvement is major cause of mortality
  - Recently identified genetic mutation (platelet-derived growth factor receptor alfa [FIP1L1-PDGFRA]) in some cases

Diagnosis

- Diagnosis of allergic rhinitis
  - **Clinical presentation and historical features are often sufficient for treatment**
  - Skin testing: Search for specific IgE to allergens; antihistamines must be avoided before skin testing
  - **Radioallergosorbent test (RAST): Detects the presence of allergen-specific IgE in a subject's serum by *in vitro* assay**
    - **An alternative to skin testing if patient must continue antihistamines but less sensitive than puncture skin tests**
- Diagnosis of PCN and related β-lactam antibiotic allergy
  - Skin test is performed with major and minor determinants to detect the presence of specific IgE; **skin test does not predict non–IgE-dependent reactions**
  - 80% to 90% of PCN "allergic" patients are not truly allergic because they lack specific IgE
  - Because most PCN- or β-lactam–allergic patients do not have an IgE-dependent reaction, and skin testing only tests for IgE-dependent reactions, a negative skin test does not exclude a reaction to penicillin or β-lactam antibiotic
  - Stevens-Johnson syndrome and exfoliative dermatitis are absolute contraindications for PCN use

- **Diagnosis of allergic skin diseases is often done based on the clinical presentation;** confirmation may be done with serum markers or skin testing (see Table 68-1)
- Diagnosis of immunodeficiency syndromes requires quantitative immunoglobulin levels or other serologic markers (Table 68-2)
- Diagnosis of eosinophilia syndromes
  - Churg-Strauss vasculitis is diagnosed by biopsy demonstrating granulomatous vasculitis with extravascular eosinophilic infiltration in the patient with a compatible clinical presentation
  - Hypereosinophilic syndrome is diagnosed by organ biopsy demonstrating eosinophils and tissue damage in the patient with persistent eosinophilia (>1500 eosinophils/μL for at least 6 months) when other causes of eosinophilia have been excluded

Treatment

- **Allergic rhinitis**
  - **Treatment should follow a three-tiered approach**
    - Avoidance or reduction of identified allergen triggers
    - Medications (Table 68-3)
      - Topical ocular agents may be used for coexisting allergic conjunctivitis
      - Leukotriene receptor antagonists are also approved in allergic rhinitis
    - Allergen-specific immunotherapy: Used in patients with severe allergic rhinitis who are intolerant of or refractory to medications
      - Mechanism of action unknown, appears to involve shift to T-helper type 1 (Th1) cell response to allergen and increased numbers of regulatory T cells

68

TABLE 68-3	*Pharmacotherapy for Allergic Rhinitis*				
Class	**Example**	**Action**	**Symptoms Treated**	**Comments**
First-generation antihistamines	Diphenhydramine	Block H_1 receptor	Sneezing Rhinorrhea Pruritis	Sedation major side effect; limits use
Second-/third-generation antihistamines	Fexofenadine Cetirizine Loratadine	Block H_1 receptor	Sneezing Rhinorrhea Pruritis	Do not cross blood-brain barrier, thus less sedating
Topical or oral decongestants	Pseudoephedrine	Stimulate α-adrenergic receptors to result in vasoconstriction	Congestion	CNS stimulation most common side effect Elevate blood pressure Phenylpropanolamine discontinued because it increases risk of CVA
Intranasal mast cell stabilizers	Cromolyn	Stabilize mast cell membranes, preventing release of histamine, slow-reacting substance of anaphylaxis (SRS-A)	Sneezing Rhinorrhea Congestion	Best used before exposure to allergen Require frequent dosing
Intranasal corticosteroids	Fluticasone	Reduce mast cell numbers in local tissues; inhibits cytokine synthesis	Sneezing Rhinorrhea Congestion Pruritis	Require 1 wk of use before clinical response

CNS, central nervous system; CVA, cerebrovascular; H_1, histamine₁.

- Treatment risks anaphylaxis; 20 to 30 minutes of observation required after injection
  - Maintenance dosing may be continued for 3 to 5 years
- Drug allergy
  - Treat with unrelated drug class if possible
  - **If no alternative antibiotic is available, desensitization may be tried for IgE-mediated hypersensitivity**
    - Can be administered either orally or intravenously with increasing doses of drug
    - Theory is that it prevents anaphylaxis by favoring univalent haptens that do not cross-link IgE and hence do not activate mast cells
    - **Duration of effect is limited to single treatment episode; must maintain uninterrupted treatment for duration of therapy**
    - **Future drug courses will require repeating the entire process**
- Allergic skin diseases: Treatment varies based on the underlying disorder (see Table 68-1)
- Immunodeficiency syndromes: Treatment includes antibiotics for infection, with other treatment based on the underlying disorder
- Eosinophilia syndromes
  - Churg-Strauss vasculitis: High-dose steroids and cyclophosphamide

- Hypereosinophilic syndrome
  - Corticosteroids
  - Hydroxyurea
  - Alfa-interferon
  - Potentially monoclonal anti–IL-5
  - Imatinib mesylate (Gleevec) used in cases with FIP-1–like mutation

REVIEW QUESTIONS

For review questions, please go to www.expertconsult.com.

SUGGESTED READINGS

Joint Task Force on Practice Parameters; American Academy of Allergy, Asthma, and Immunology; American College of Allergy, Asthma, and Immunology; the Joint Council of Allergy, Asthma, and Immunology: The diagnosis and management of anaphylaxis, *J Allergy Clin Immunol* 101(Pt 2):S465–S528, 1998.

Middleton R, Reed S, Ellis B, et al: *Allergy principle and practice*, ed 6, St. Louis, 2003, Mosby.

Shearer WT, Li JT: Primer on allergic and immunologic diseases, *J Allergy Clin Immunol* 111:S441–S778, 2003.

Sicherer SH, Leung DY: Advances in allergic skin disease, anaphylaxis, and hypersensitivity reactions to foods, drugs, and insects in 2010, *J Allergy Clin Immunol* 127:326–335, 2011.

Simons FE, Frew AJ, Ansotegui IJ: Risk assessment in anaphylaxis: current and future approaches, *J Allergy Clin Immunol* 120(Suppl 1):S2–S24, 2007.

Genetics for the Internist

HOWARD LEVY, MD, PhD

Although even the most common disorders attributable to mutation in a single gene are individually rare, when considered collectively, they constitute a major health burden. Genetic diseases affect people of all ages and ancestries and manifest symptoms in every organ system. With the completion of the Human Genome Project and additional advances in complex disease genetics, there is growing recognition of genetic factors in common, everyday conditions encountered in internal medicine. Although cures for genetic disorders are rare, recognition and understanding of genetic factors in disease can improve detection and management of many conditions and prevent or reduce morbidity and mortality.

Basic Genetics Concepts

- Chromosomes
  - Each cell nucleus contains 46 chromosomes
    - 22 pairs of autosomes
    - 1 pair of sex chromosomes (X/Y)
  - In females, one of the two X chromosomes is permanently inactivated in each cell
    - X-inactivation is random and occurs early in embryonic development
    - Both of a woman's X chromosomes are expressed, but only one or the other in any single cell
    - Therefore, women may have some clinical manifestations of an X-linked disorder
- Genes are carried on chromosomes and thus occur in pairs
  - There are approximately 25,000 pairs of genes
  - Each member of a pair of genes is called an *allele*
  - 37 additional genes are carried on a small mitochondrial chromosome, whose inheritance and behavior are very different from that of the 46 nuclear chromosomes
- DNA variation
  - Polymorphism: Alteration in DNA sequence that does not affect the function of the gene and typically has no clinical consequences
  - **Mutation: Alteration in DNA sequence that changes gene function and potentially has clinical manifestations**
  - Alteration of a gene in a germ cell or zygote ultimately will be present in all cells of the resulting person, including his or her germline (the next generation of eggs or sperm), and thus can be inherited
  - Alteration of a gene in a somatic cell may result in clinical manifestations in all or part of an individual, but it will not be present in the germline and cannot be inherited

- Cancer cells accumulate multiple genetic changes that directly affect their behavior and response to therapy, but those changes are not transmitted to future generations
- One or both alleles of a gene may carry an alteration (mutation or polymorphism)
  - **Homozygosity: Both alleles are the same (either normal or altered)**
  - **Heterozygosity: One allele is normal and the other is altered**

Inheritance Patterns

- Multifactorial inheritance: Most of the common diseases and conditions seen by an internist are multifactorial, resulting from a complex interaction of genetic and environmental factors
  - **The relative contribution of genes and environment can vary, but both are important in virtually all medical conditions (Fig. 69-1)**
  - Examples
    - Mutation of a single gene may be the known cause, but environmental factors affect specific clinical outcome(s) (e.g., crises and other manifestations in sickle cell anemia)
    - An environmental exposure may be the known cause, but genetic factors affect the ultimate clinical outcome (e.g., resistance to HIV infection as a result of mutation of the CCR5 cell surface receptor)
    - Several genetic and environmental risk factors may be known to have major effects on a condition (e.g., thromboembolic disease; Fig. 69-2)
    - For most conditions, multiple genetic and environmental factors each contribute relatively small components of risk, and the complete spectrum of risk factors has yet to be fully elucidated
  - Characteristics of multifactorial inheritance
    - Males and females may be equally likely to be affected, or there may be skewing of the sex ratio
    - The condition may cluster in families with greater genetic and/or environmental risk, may appear to skip generations, and may seem to occur at random
    - No single gene inheritance pattern is obvious
    - **Estimation of risk to family members is largely empirical but increases with the number of affected relatives, closer degree of relation, and severity**

Single-gene

Examples
Cystic fibrosis
Sickle cell anemia
Hemochromatosis

Multifactorial

Examples
Diabetes mellitus
Coronary artery disease
Mental illness
Obstructive lung disease
Cancer

Environmental

Examples
HIV infection/AIDS
Sepsis
Trauma and response to it

Genetic factors

Environmental factors

FIGURE 69-1   All medical conditions have at least some genetic and environmental components. Most conditions are multifactorial, with varying mixes of both. Clinical expression of a single-gene disorder is subject to environmental effects. Response to infection or trauma depends in part on genetic susceptibility and capacity for recovery.

FIGURE 69-2   Thromboembolic disease as an example of a multifactorial condition. Several known genetic and environmental risk factors have been identified. Typically more than one risk factor is necessary to manifest the condition. Note that several risk factors are themselves multifactorial—both genetic and environmental factors contribute to cancer, inflammation, anticardiolipin antibody syndrome, hyperhomocysteinemia, and obesity.

Environmental

• Trauma
• Surgery
• Stasis
• Smoking
• Estrogen

• Cancer
• Inflammation
• Anticardiolipin antibody
• Elevated homocysteine
• Obesity

Genetic

• Protein C deficiency
• Protein S deficiency
• Antithrombin deficiency
• Factor V Leiden
• Prothrombin G20210A

BOX 69-1	*Red Flags Suggestive of Increased Genetic Risk for a Multifactorial Condition*

Multiple affected relatives

Closely related affected relatives

Younger-than-expected age of onset

Occurrence in the less commonly affected sex

Multiple primary occurrences of the same or a related condition in an individual

Unusually severe manifestations

Other exceptions to usual epidemiology:
  Histopathology
  Anatomic location

- Box 69-1 lists red flags that should prompt consideration of increased genetic predisposition to a specific disease
- **Single-gene (Mendelian) inheritance: Applies when a trait or condition results from alteration of one or both alleles of a single gene**
  - One member of each pair of chromosomes (and thus genes) is passed along in each egg or sperm cell
  - An altered allele can be inherited from either parent (or both if they are both carriers)
  - DNA polymorphisms and mutations do not have to be inherited from either parent; they can occur as new errors in an egg or sperm cell
  - See Table 69-1 for characteristics of autosomal dominant, autosomal recessive, and X-linked inheritance patterns
  - See Table 69-2 for examples of some Mendelian disorders
- **Mitochondrial inheritance (see Table 69-1): Applies when a trait or condition results from alteration of the mitochondrial DNA**
  - Each mitochondrion carries multiple copies of its chromosome, and each cell contains many mitochondria
  - **Heteroplasmy—the relative proportion of normal and abnormal mitochondria within individual cells, tissues, and organs—affects the severity and distribution of clinical manifestations**
    - Significant genetic variation exists within and between individual mitochondria in a single cell as well as between individual cells, tissues, and organs
    - Heteroplasmy can vary over time within a single person and even in different tissues within a single person

TABLE 69-1 Inheritance Patterns

	Autosomal Dominant	Autosomal Recessive	X-Linked	Mitochondrial
Definition	Heterozygosity for mutation of a single gene is sufficient to cause the condition (unless the gene is on the X or mitochondrial chromosome)	Homozygosity for mutation of a single gene is necessary to cause the condition (unless the gene is on the X or mitochondrial chromosome) Carriers (heterozygotes) usually have no clinical manifestations	The condition results from mutation of a single gene located on the X chromosome Also called "sex-linked," because of characteristic inheritance patterns in men and women	Mutation of a gene contained on the mitochondrial chromosome causes the condition Most mitochondrial proteins are encoded on nuclear genes, and therefore follow autosomal or X-linked inheritance patterns
Distribution in the family	Multiple generations affected	One or more siblings affected, but (usually) only in one generation	Multiple generations affected May appear to skip generations when transmitted by a carrier female Affected males are related to each other through one or more carrier females	Multiple generations affected
Parents of an affected	Usually one or the other affected Sometimes neither affected	Usually both are carriers Usually neither affected	Mothers often carriers Fathers of affected sons are *never* affected	Mothers almost always affected Fathers never affected
Siblings of an affected	50% chance of being affected (unless neither parent affected)	25% chance of being affected 50% chance of being a carrier	Brothers have 50% chance of being affected Sisters have 50% chance of being a carrier	All are affected
Children of an affected	50% chance of being affected	All are carriers Can be affected only if the other parent is a carrier	Sons of affected fathers are *never* affected (always inherit father's Y and mother's X chromosomes) Daughters of affected fathers are *always* carriers (always inherit father's X chromosome) Sons of carrier mothers have 50% chance of being affected Daughters of carrier mothers have 50% chance of being a carrier	All children of affected mothers are affected No children of affected fathers are affected
Sex ratio	Males and females equally likely to be affected	Males and females equally likely to be affected	Almost all affected patients are male	Males and females equally likely to be affected
Other comments	Reduced penetrance and variable expression are common	Parental consanguinity is sometimes present Relatively high prevalence of some recessive conditions due to "heterozygote advantage," in which carriers have a survival advantage (e.g., carriers of sickle cell anemia are relatively resistant to malaria)	Male-to-male transmission does not occur Carrier females may have mild clinical manifestations	Heteroplasmy often results in variable expression, complicating recognition of some affected relatives

69

- **Mitochondria are inherited almost exclusively through the egg; sperm mitochondria only rarely are incorporated into a fertilized egg**
- Clinical manifestations of mitochondrial mutations vary but are primarily neuromuscular
- Central nervous system: encephalopathy, seizures, dementia, migraine, stroke-like episodes, ataxia, spasticity
- Peripheral nervous system: ptosis, external ophthalmoplegia, sensorineural deafness, optic atrophy,

TABLE 69-2	Some Representative Single-Gene Disorders
Condition	**Some Clinical Considerations**
Autosomal Dominant	
Marfan syndrome	Joint laxity; characteristic skeletal features; myopia and/or lens dislocation; aortic aneurysm/dissection
Neurofibromatosis type 1	Benign and occasionally malignant nerve sheath tumors; hypertension
Polycystic kidney disease	Renal, hepatic, and splenic cysts; renal failure; nephrolithiasis; hypertension; cerebral berry aneurysms occur in ~10% and correlate with specific mutations, so family history predicts risk of aneurysm
Hereditary breast and ovarian cancer	Breast and ovarian cancer; other associated cancers
Hereditary nonpolyposis colon cancer	Colon and other associated cancers
Familial adenomatous polyposis	Colon and other associated cancers; characteristic benign ocular manifestations; fully penetrant—100% chance of cancer
Multiple endocrine neoplasia syndromes	Benign and malignant endocrine tumors; benign tumors frequently hormonally active
Achondroplasia	Most common cause of dwarfism
Autosomal Recessive	
Hemochromatosis	Iron overload; cardiac, hepatic, endocrine, and joint complications; low clinical penetrance
Sickle cell anemia	Hemoglobinopathy; painful and degenerative ischemic complications; certain infections; more common in descendents of traditional malarial regions (especially Africa)
Cystic fibrosis	Defective ion transport; sinopulmonary, pancreatic, intestinal, and fertility complications; especially common in Northern Europeans; different specific mutations more common with different ancestry
α- and β-Thalassemia	Hemoglobinopathy; anemia; α more common in Chinese and Southeast Asians; β more common in Mediterranean peoples
Tay-Sachs disease	Neurodegenerative condition due to metabolic enzyme deficiency; common in Ashkenazi Jews and French Canadians, but disease itself is now rare in those populations due to effective screening programs
X-Linked	
Fragile X syndrome	Mental retardation; characteristic facial features; joint laxity
Hemophilia A	Classic hemophilia, due to factor VIII deficiency; bleeding diathesis; variable expression
Duchenne/Becker muscular dystrophy	Most common cause of muscular dystrophy; Becker less severe than Duchenne, but same gene

pigmentary retinopathy, peripheral neuropathy, autonomic neuropathy
- Skeletal muscle: proximal myopathy, weakness, hypotonia
- Cardiomyopathy
- Diabetes mellitus
- Susceptibility to aminoglycoside-induced ototoxicity
- **Chromosomal inheritance: Applies when all or part of a chromosome is duplicated or deleted**
  - Numerical abnormalities
    - An entire chromosome is missing or duplicated
      - Most examples are incompatible with life and result in early miscarriage
      - **Typically not inherited or passed along to future generations**
    - Monosomy of the X chromosome (45 chromosomes, only one X) causes Turner syndrome
      - 99% end in miscarriage
      - Always female
      - Short stature, characteristic physical features, but normal intelligence
      - Most are infertile

- Trisomy 21 (47 chromosomes, three copies of #21) causes Down syndrome, characterized by mental retardation, short stature, cardiac defects, and other malformations
- An extra copy of the X chromosome has milder manifestations, including tall stature and mild mental retardation
- An extra copy of the Y chromosome usually has no clinical effect; contrary to older reports, this condition does not cause violent behavior or greater likelihood of incarceration
- Structural abnormalities
  - Deletions or duplications of large segments of a chromosome
    - Clinical manifestations may include mental retardation, growth retardation, and malformations
    - May be inherited from a parent with a balanced rearrangement (see following discussion), but affected patients with large deletions or duplications usually do not reproduce
  - Microdeletions, or contiguous gene syndromes, involve loss of a short segment of a chromosome and affect only a few genes

- Clinical manifestations vary depending upon the specific genes involved
- Many are compatible with a normal life span and fertility
- Can occur as a new genetic change or can be inherited in an autosomal dominant pattern
  - Balanced rearrangements occur when segments are exchanged between two or more chromosomes, but no material is deleted or duplicated
    - May have no clinical manifestations
    - May cause symptoms by disrupting a gene
    - May cause symptoms by creation of a new abnormal gene (e.g., the Philadelphia chromosome in chronic myelogenous leukemia is a translocation that joins portions of two genes, producing a hybrid that contributes to unregulated growth)

Complications of Inheritance Patterns

- **Variable expression: Any feature of a condition may vary greatly from one patient to the next, including age of onset, severity and frequency of manifestations, and organ and tissue distribution of manifestations**
  - Variation occurs not only between unrelated individuals but also among members of the same family who all carry the same mutation
  - Environmental factors and small effects from other genetic changes contribute to variable expression
  - Distinguished from multifactorial inheritance because the condition is clearly caused by mutation in one or both alleles of a single gene
  - **An individual may carry and transmit a disease-causing mutation, even if the expression is so mild that it goes unrecognized**
  - Sex-limited expression is an example of variable expression and is due to physiologic differences between the sexes
    - Sex-limited expression is distinct from X-linked inheritance because the likelihood of inheriting or transmitting a mutation is independent of sex or degree of clinical expression
    - Daughters of a man carrying an autosomal dominant mutation predisposing to breast cancer are at increased risk for breast cancer, even though their father is unlikely to manifest breast cancer himself
  - See Box 69-2 for examples of variable and sex-limited expression
- **Reduced penetrance: Some genetic conditions fail to manifest any clinical features in a portion of people carrying the mutant allele(s)**
  - May occur in any type of inheritance
  - Distinguished from variable expression by the complete absence of any clinical manifestations
  - Likelihood of inheriting or transmitting a mutation depends only on the mode of inheritance (dominant, recessive, etc.), regardless of whether the individual manifests any clinical features
    - Daughters of a woman carrying an autosomal dominant mutation predisposing to breast/ovarian cancer are at increased risk for the associated cancers, even if their mother never develops any cancer herself

---

BOX 69-2 | *Examples of Variable and Sex-Limited Expression*

Frequency and severity of crises are different in every patient with sickle cell anemia

Presence or absence of berry aneurysms in polycystic kidney disease tends to be consistent within a family, but age of onset and severity of hypertension and/or renal failure are quite variable

Severity, age of onset, and progression of skeletal, ocular, cardiovascular, and other complications in Marfan syndrome are highly variable, both within and between families

Some variation in pulmonary, gastrointestinal, pancreatic, and other manifestations in cystic fibrosis may be attributed to the specific mutation (thus consistent within families), but most of the variation is independent of the specific mutation

Prostate cancer cannot occur in a female

Ovarian cancer cannot occur in a male

Breast cancer is much less likely to occur, but not impossible, in a male

Females with hereditary hemochromatosis tend to have milder and later onset of symptoms than males because of menstrual blood loss

---

- **Anticipation: Some genetic conditions become more severe or onset at an earlier age in successive generations**
  - The most common mutational mechanism is expansion of trinucleotide (or triplet) repeats within a gene, which can increase in successive generations as a result of errors in DNA replication
    - Expansion beyond a threshold results in altered gene function and clinical manifestations
    - Severity increases and age of onset decreases in proportion to the length of the repeat
  - Most diseases in this category are adult- or late childhood-onset conditions that primarily affect the nervous system
    - Huntington disease: Adult-onset chorea, dysarthria, dysphagia, cognitive dysfunction, and psychosis
    - Fragile X syndrome: Classic presentation is childhood-onset mental retardation, characteristic facial features and joint laxity, but shorter trinucleotide expansions result in adult-onset ataxia, tremor, and cognitive dysfunction
- Imprinting: Some parts of the genome are chemically tagged (imprinted) to mark whether they were inherited through the egg or sperm; an imprinted gene is expressed only from the maternal or paternal allele
  - Inheritance of a mutation follows the traditional 50:50 pattern, but clinical expression depends on the parent of origin
    - Mutations in the silenced (inactive) parental allele have no clinical effect
    - Mutations in the active parental allele will be clinically expressed
  - **The sex of the parent who passes along the mutation is the critical factor, not the sex of the child who inherits the mutation**

69

Genetic Testing

- **Although "genetic testing" is usually thought of as direct analysis of DNA, family history and virtually any test or procedure may yield a result with direct or indirect genetic implications**
- Risk assessment and full discussion of the potential risks and benefits (i.e., genetics counseling) should precede DNA testing and many other forms of genetic testing
  - Consultation with a genetics counselor or medical geneticist is often appropriate
  - With adequate experience and training, an internist or subspecialist can perform pretest counseling
- Benefits of DNA testing
  - Can help to confirm a clinical diagnosis
  - Can establish a specific genetic cause for a disorder
  - Can help predict natural history and guide management
  - Can identify carriers of recessive mutations
  - Can facilitate presymptomatic or predictive testing in relatives, subject to variation in actual clinical expression and penetrance
  - DNA test results are generally independent of environmental factors and do not change over the life span; therefore, no need to repeat unless laboratory error is suspected
- **Limitations of DNA testing**
  - **False negatives: A negative (or normal) DNA test usually does not completely rule out disease**
    - Most DNA tests have less than 100% sensitivity (i.e., not all potential mutations in a gene can be detected by most tests)
    - Multiple different genes may cause or contribute to a condition; thus the wrong gene may have been tested
    - The individual family member who underwent testing may coincidentally have a sporadic, non-genetic cause of the disease in the family; another relative might have a detectable mutation; this is of greatest concern for common diseases, such as breast cancer
  - **False positives: A positive (or abnormal) DNA test does not always rule in disease**
    - **Polymorphisms: Some DNA variations cause no clinical manifestations**
    - Reduced penetrance and variable expression complicate prediction of clinical manifestations based solely on DNA test results
- Determining who should undergo DNA testing
  - When trying to establish, confirm, or further elucidate a genetic diagnosis, a clinically affected person is the most appropriate choice to undergo testing (rather than a person who is at risk but not yet manifesting any symptoms or signs)
  - **For predictive, presymptomatic, or carrier testing in an unaffected person, the closest or most severely affected relative should be tested first to establish what genetic mutation(s) is(are) present in that specific family and to facilitate appropriately selected DNA testing in at-risk relatives**

- For predictive, presymptomatic, or carrier testing in an unaffected person if the specific mutation(s) within the family is(are) unknown
  - A negative test in a clinically unaffected individual may be a false negative and not accurately predict protection from disease (e.g., the actual disease-causing mutation may be in a gene other than the one tested)
  - A positive test in a clinically unaffected individual may be a false positive and not accurately predict disease (e.g., the DNA change may represent a meaningless polymorphism, unrelated to the affected relative's disease)
- If an affected relative has been tested and the specific mutation(s) in the family is(are) known
  - A negative DNA test in an unaffected relative means he or she did not inherit the known genetic mutation and is at average risk for the disease based on his or her other risk factors (high negative predictive value)
  - A positive DNA test in an unaffected relative means he or she did inherit the known genetic mutation and is at increased risk for the disease, but the positive predictive value for actual clinical manifestations depends on the variability and penetrance of the disease
- If an affected relative is unavailable or has negative test results, predictive or carrier testing in an unaffected person can still be performed, but positive predictive value and negative predictive value will be reduced
- Ethical and social considerations regarding genetic testing and diagnoses
  - Potential issues for an affected individual
    - Stigmatization and isolation from the family or society
    - Anxiety
    - Guilt related to potentially transmitting a disease or risk to his or her offspring
    - Employment and/or insurance (both life and health) discrimination; some legal protections exist, and abuses are relatively rare, but this is a significant potential concern
    - Privacy; others gaining access to genetic diagnoses and test results
    - Results may reveal that biologic relationships are not the same as social relationships (most commonly that one's father is not who it was thought to be)
  - Additional potential issues for relatives of an affected individual
    - Right to know that they are at increased risk for a genetic condition
    - Right to not know that they are at increased risk for a genetic condition
      - Example: An adult at risk for Huntington disease who elects not to undergo predictive genetic testing; if his or her child has a positive predictive genetic test, then he or she almost certainly carries the same genetic mutation
  - Duty to warn: In some cases, the physician or patient may have a duty to warn relatives of an affected patient of their risk for certain diseases, even if the relatives are not patients of that physician
  - Survivor guilt related to learning that one does not have the same genetic disease or risk as a sibling, parent, or child

- Predictive or presymptomatic testing of children or adolescents for adult-onset conditions is almost always inappropriate because obtaining such knowledge is irreversible
  - It is preferable to wait until adulthood when the risks and benefits of testing can be evaluated by the individual at risk
  - If the disease onsets in childhood, or effective childhood interventions to reduce or prevent disease are available, then such testing may be appropriate (e.g., familial adenomatous polyposis, in which onset, screening, and management all begin in childhood; see below)
  - Diagnostic genetic testing of a symptomatic child is not subject to this concern, but still raises all of the other issues listed in this section

Select Clinical Examples

HEREDITARY BREAST AND OVARIAN CANCER

Basic Information

- Most breast cancer is multifactorial
- Approximately 5% to 10% of all breast cancer is hereditary
- Most (60–80%) of hereditary breast cancer is due to mutations in the *BRCA1* and *BRCA2* genes, accounting for approximately 3% of all breast cancer
  - Inheritance is autosomal dominant with reduced penetrance and variable expression
- Other known genetic causes include
  - Cowden syndrome: Associated with thyroid, skin, and GI hamartomas and cancers
  - Li-Fraumeni syndrome: Associated with sarcomas
- Male breast cancer is suspicious for hereditary breast cancer
- **Men are equally likely as women to transmit a hereditary breast cancer mutation to their children, even if they do not manifest breast cancer themselves; a paternal family history of breast and/or ovarian cancer is as significant as a maternal family history**

Clinical Presentation of *BRCA1* and *BRCA2* Mutations

- Breast cancer can occur as young as 30 years old
- Lifetime risk of breast cancer for women is 40% to 85%
- Lifetime risk of ovarian cancer is 16% to 60%
- Other associated cancers include peritoneal, prostate, and pancreas

Diagnosis and Evaluation

- Genetic testing should be preceded by genetic risk assessment and counseling, usually available through a genetics, oncology, or cancer genetics consultation
- Clinical testing of the *BRCA1* and *BRCA2* genes is available, but sensitivity is less than 100%
- If a *BRCA1* or *BRCA2* mutation is identified in a family, relatives at risk need only be tested for that specific mutation

- Testing for some other genetic causes of hereditary breast cancer is also available and is best managed by a specialist
- Negative DNA testing in an unaffected person with strong family history has low negative predictive value if the specific genetic etiology in the family has not been identified

Treatment

- All first-degree relatives should be informed of their increased risk and offered genetics counseling
- Therapeutic response of identified cancer is similar to sporadic breast or ovarian cancer
- Bilateral mastectomy at the time of initial breast cancer diagnosis may be appropriate

Prevention

- Breast cancer screening (breast self-examination, clinical breast examination, and radiologic imaging) should begin 10 years earlier than standard population screening (25 years old, rather than 35 years old) or 10 years earlier than the earliest age of onset in an affected relative, whichever is younger
- Breast magnetic resonance imaging (MRI) has much higher sensitivity than mammography or ultrasound, and is increasingly being recommended as part of annual breast imaging
- Bilateral prophylactic mastectomy reduces (but does not eliminate) the risk of breast cancer
- Annual or semiannual ovarian cancer screening with pelvic examination, transvaginal ultrasound, and serum cancer antigen 125 (CA 125) testing beginning at age 35 years may improve detection and survival
- Bilateral prophylactic salpingo-oophorectomy reduces (but does not eliminate) the risk of breast and ovarian cancer in patients with known or suspected *BRCA1* or *BRCA2* mutation, but it does not reduce the risk of peritoneal carcinoma
- For men with known or suspected *BRCA1* or *BRCA2* mutation, consider beginning prostate cancer screening 10 years earlier than standard population screening

HEREDITARY COLON CANCER

- Approximately 10% of all colon cancer is attributable to single-gene syndromes
- Hereditary nonpolyposis colon cancer (HNPCC) and familial adenomatous polyposis (FAP) are the most common causes; see individual sections that follow
- An additional 30% of all colon cancer occurs in individuals with a family history of colon cancer, consistent with multifactorial inheritance
- Patients with a family history of hereditary multifactorial colon cancer should begin colon cancer screening 10 years earlier than the youngest age of onset in the family or at age 40 years, whichever is younger; colonoscopy should be repeated every 3 to 5 years

HEREDITARY NONPOLYPOSIS COLON CANCER SYNDROME

Basic Information

- HNPCC accounts for approximately 3% of all colon cancer

69

- Also known as Lynch syndrome
- Due to mutation in one of several DNA mismatch repair genes
- Autosomal dominant predisposition to multiple cancers with variable expression and reduced penetrance

Clinical Presentation

- **Average age of cancer onset (colon or other) is mid-40s**
- Often poorly differentiated and more aggressive than sporadic colon adenocarcinoma
- **Most colon cancers (two thirds) occur in proximal (ascending) colon, in contrast to sporadic colon cancer predominantly occurring more distally**
- Lifetime risk of colon cancer is approximately 80%
- Lifetime risk of endometrial cancer is 20% to 60%
- Other associated tumors include stomach or small bowel adenocarcinoma, transitional cell carcinoma of the proximal ureter, sebaceous skin neoplasms, glioblastoma multiforme, and hepatobiliary and ovarian cancer

Diagnosis and Evaluation

- See Box 69-3 for clinical diagnostic criteria that suggest HNPCC
- When clinically suspected, test tumor tissue for microsatellite instability (MSI) and/or immunohistochemistry (IHC)
  - Microsatellites are regions of highly repetitive DNA
  - In tumor tissue with faulty DNA mismatch repair (i.e., in HNPCC), these regions demonstrate variable length (instability)
  - MSI within tumor tissue is highly predictive of HNPCC
  - IHC showing absence of one or more mismatch repair proteins within tumor tissue is also highly predictive of HNPCC

BOX 69-3 | *Clinical Criteria to Suspect Hereditary Nonpolyposis Colorectal Cancer (HNPCC)*

Amsterdam II Criteria

All of (mnemonic "3-2-1"):
   3 or more family members with HNPCC-associated cancer, each a first-degree relative of at least one other affected relative
   2 successive generations affected
   1 or more cancer(s) onset before age 50 yr

Sensitivity ~75–80%

Specificity ~50–60%

Bethesda Criteria

Any one of:
   Positive Amsterdam II criteria
   Two independent HNPCC-related cancers
   Colon or endometrial cancer onset before age 50 yr
   Colonic adenoma onset before age 40 yr
   Colon cancer at any age, plus a first-degree relative with either an HNPCC-related cancer onset before age 50 yr or colonic adenoma before age 40 yr
   Signet-ring cell–type colon cancer onset before age 50 yr

Sensitivity ~95%

Specificity ~25%

- If MSI is high (strongly positive) and/or IHC is abnormal, proceed to DNA testing of mismatch repair genes
  - Genetic testing should be preceded by genetic risk assessment and counseling, usually available through a genetics, oncology, or cancer genetics consultation
  - Sensitivity of DNA testing is less than 100%

Treatment

- All first-degree relatives should be informed of their increased risk and offered genetics counseling
- HNPCC-associated colon cancer prognosis may be better than for sporadic colon cancer
- Total colectomy is preferred over partial colectomy in HNPCC patients with colon cancer

Prevention

- Colonoscopy every 1 to 2 years beginning at age 20 to 25 years, or 10 years earlier than the earliest age of colon cancer diagnosis in the family, whichever is earlier
- Consider annual transvaginal ultrasound, endometrial biopsy, and serum CA 125 measurement, beginning at age 30 to 35 years, or 10 years earlier than the earliest age of cancer diagnosis in the family, whichever is earlier
- **Prophylactic colectomy is not recommended because colon cancer screening is effective**
- Prophylactic hysterectomy and oophorectomy is an option
- Consider periodic upper endoscopy to screen for duodenal tumors
- Consider annual urine cytology starting around age 30 to screen for urinary tract cancer

FAMILIAL ADENOMATOUS POLYPOSIS

Figure 69-3 shows an example of FAP

Basic Information

- FAP accounts for approximately 1% of all colon cancer
- Due to mutation in *APC*, a tumor suppressor gene
- Autosomal dominant predisposition to colonic adenomas, which evolve into cancer
- **Expression is variable, but penetrance is complete (100%) for colonic adenomas and cancer**

FIGURE 69-3 Familial adenomatous polyposis in an 18-year-old woman. The mucosal surface is carpeted by innumerable polypoid adenomas. *(From Kumar V, Fausto N, Abbas A: Robbins and Cotran pathologic basis of disease, ed 7, Philadelphia, WB Saunders, 2004, Fig. 17.59.)*

Clinical Presentation

- Hundreds to thousands of colonic adenomas
- Average age of polyp onset is 16 years
- Average age of colon cancer is 39 years
- Other manifestations include gastric and small bowel polyps (~5–10% malignant), osteomas (never malignant), papillary thyroid cancer, hepatoblastoma, benign skin lesions (epidermoid cysts, fibromas, desmoid tumors), and extra or missing teeth
- **Congenital hypertrophy of the retinal pigment epithelium (CHRPE) occurs in 70% to 80%**
  - **Benign pigmented retinal hamartomas**
  - **When bilateral, highly suggestive of FAP, and thus a useful clinical diagnostic tool**
- Attenuated FAP (aFAP) is a milder presentation resulting from mutations in the same gene
  - Usually fewer than 100 adenomas, average is about 30
  - Average age of cancer onset is mid-50s
  - Other manifestations of FAP also occur at reduced frequency

Diagnosis and Evaluation

- Genetic testing should be preceded by genetic risk assessment and counseling, usually available through a genetics, oncology, or cancer genetics consultation
- Among patients with typical clinical manifestations, *APC* gene analysis has a mutation detection rate of 80% to 90%

Treatment and Prevention

- First-degree relatives should be informed of their increased risk and offered genetics counseling
- Annual lower endoscopy beginning at age 10 to 12 years
- **Colectomy when there are 20 to 30 adenomas or when polyp histology is advanced; this is usually adolescence or very early adulthood**
- Postcolectomy lower endoscopic surveillance is still necessary
- Nonsteroidal anti-inflammatory drugs and cyclooxygenase-2 inhibitors reduce the rate of adenoma formation and may help to delay colectomy from adolescence to young adulthood
- Endoscopic and radiologic visualization of the stomach and small bowel every 1 to 3 years beginning when colonic polyps are found
- Annual thyroid palpation (± annual thyroid ultrasound)

HEREDITARY HEMOCHROMATOSIS DUE TO *HFE* MUTATIONS

Basic Information

- Homozygous mutation of the *HFE* gene is the most common cause of iron overload in white patients
- Other genetic and environmental causes of hemochromatosis and iron overload exist
- ***HFE* hemochromatosis is the most common autosomal recessive single-gene disorder among adults**
  - 1:200 to 1:400 white individuals has two mutant alleles (genetically affected)
  - 1:10 (10%) white individuals have one mutant allele (unaffected carrier)

- **The high carrier frequency results in pseudodominant inheritance**
  - 100% chance that a genetically affected person passes along a mutant allele to the offspring
  - 10% chance that a white spouse is a carrier
  - 50% chance that a carrier spouse passes along a mutant allele to the offspring
  - 1:20 (100% × 10% × 50% = 5%) chance that a child of a genetically affected person with a white partner will also be genetically affected
- Only two specific mutations are clearly associated with clinical disease: *C282Y* and *H63D*
  - Homozygosity for the *C282Y* mutation accounts for approximately 90% of clinically manifest cases of hereditary hemochromatosis
  - Compound heterozygosity, with one *C282Y* allele and one *H63D* allele, accounts for most of the rest
  - Homozygosity for the *H63D* mutation almost never causes clinical symptoms
  - Other variations of *HFE* are common, but likely represent benign polymorphisms

Clinical Presentation

- Manifestations are due to increased GI iron absorption and storage in multiple organs, especially liver, skin, pancreas, joints, heart, testes, and pituitary
  - Nonspecific symptoms include abdominal pain, weakness, fatigue, lethargy, and weight loss
  - Transaminase elevation and/or hepatomegaly may or may not occur
  - Cirrhosis, portal hypertension, and liver failure may occur late in the disease
  - Hepatocellular carcinoma occurs only in the setting of cirrhosis
  - Arthralgia is common, especially in the hands, but other joints may be involved
  - Hypogonadism may be central (pituitary) or peripheral (testicular)
  - Bronze-colored hyperpigmentation, insulin-resistant or insulin-dependent diabetes mellitus, cardiomyopathy, and arrhythmia are late manifestations
- Variable and sex-limited expression
  - *C282Y* homozygotes are more severely affected than compound heterozygotes
  - Men generally have earlier onset (in their 40s and 50s) and more severe disease than women (perimenopausal or postmenopausal onset)
- Reduced penetrance
  - Estimates vary widely (<1% to >70%), depending on genotype, method of patient ascertainment, and how clinical disease is defined
  - Even with elevated iron levels, there may be no clinical signs or symptoms

Diagnosis and Evaluation

See Figure 69-4 for an evaluation algorithm for suspected hemochromatosis.

- Increased transferrin saturation on two independent assays is the most sensitive and specific blood test for iron overload but does not establish the specific cause
  - Traditional thresholds are 60% for men and 50% for women

69

- A lower threshold of 45% has higher sensitivity but lower specificity
- Increased serum ferritin is common but is not specific for iron overload
- **DNA testing is used only to confirm the diagnosis in affected individuals and to facilitate evaluation of at-risk relatives**
  - The presence of only one mutant allele establishes carrier status but is insufficient to confirm a diagnosis of hereditary hemochromatosis
  - False-positive or false-negative analysis for C282Y and H63D is unlikely
- Quantitative phlebotomy and liver biopsy can help establish the diagnosis in equivocal situations but are rarely needed
  - Older affected patients usually can tolerate removal of 4 g or more of iron via phlebotomy (8 L of blood over 16 treatments) without developing anemia
  - Younger affected patients with smaller total iron stores may become iron depleted earlier

Treatment

- **Iron-depletion therapy is appropriate only in patients with documented iron overload**
  - **Weekly phlebotomy until serum ferritin is less than 50 ng/mL**

- If anemia occurs, decrease frequency of phlebotomy (and potentially reconsider the diagnosis)
- **Maintenance phlebotomy about two to six times per year to keep ferritin level less than 50 ng/mL and transferrin saturation less than 50%**
- Untreated patients with HFE mutations and normal iron studies should have transferrin saturation and serum ferritin checked every 1 to 5 years
- Dietary restrictions: Avoid iron supplements, vitamin C, alcohol, and uncooked seafood
- If cirrhosis is present, screen for hepatocellular carcinoma every 6 to 12 months
- Prognosis
  - **Phlebotomy improves liver disease and may partially reverse cirrhosis but does not reduce the risk of hepatocellular carcinoma once cirrhosis has occurred**
  - Phlebotomy usually reverses cardiac complications and nonspecific symptoms (abdominal pain, weakness, fatigue, lethargy, and weight loss)
  - **Endocrine deficiencies and arthralgia usually do not improve with phlebotomy**

Prevention

- All first-degree relatives of an affected patient should be offered DNA testing
  - Siblings have a 25% chance of being affected and a 50% chance of being carriers

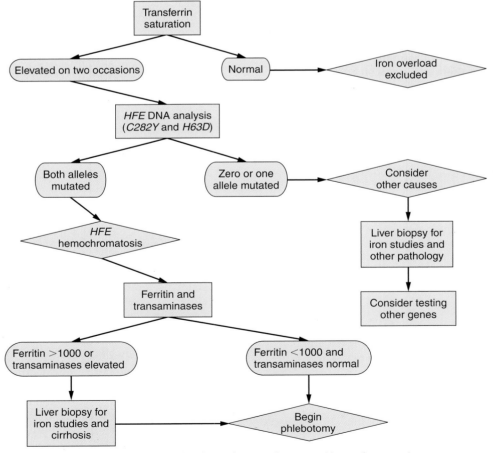

FIGURE 69-4 Algorithm for evaluation of suspected hemochromatosis.

- Both parents are likely to at least be carriers but may be affected
- All children must at least be carriers but may be affected if the other parent is a carrier

NEUROFIBROMATOSIS TYPE 1

Basic Information

- **Autosomal dominant syndrome resulting in focal overgrowth of multiple tissues, especially (but not exclusively) those derived from the neural crest**

- One of the most common dominant single-gene disorders, affecting approximately 1 in 3000 people worldwide
- Results from mutation of the neurofibromatosis type 1 (*NF1*) gene, whose protein product, neurofibromin, functions as a tumor suppressor and regulator of cellular growth and differentiation

Clinical Presentation

- **Penetrance is complete (100%), but clinical expression is quite variable**
- Skin (Fig. 69-5A to C)

FIGURE 69-5 Some clinical features of neurofibromatosis type 1. **A,** Café-au-lait macules. **B,** Axillary freckling. There is also a small café-au-lait macule (*arrowhead*) and a dermal neurofibroma (*arrow*). **C,** Dermal neurofibromas. **D,** Lisch nodules. *(From Habif TP: Clinical dermatology: a color guide to diagnosis and therapy, ed 4, Philadelphia, Mosby, 2004, Figs. 26-11A, 26-11B, 26-12, and 26-13A.)*

69

- Café-au-lait macules occur in the first year of life and increase in size and number throughout childhood
- Axillary or inguinal freckling
- Benign dermal neurofibromas (soft, fleshy nerve or nerve sheath–associated tumors) gradually increase in number and size throughout life but especially rapidly during puberty and pregnancy
- Plexiform neurofibromas (diffuse amorphous nerve sheath tumors) occur in up to 50% of patients, enlarge over time, and may cause significant morbidity
- Ocular
  - Lisch nodules are benign iris hamartomas present in nearly all patients by adulthood (see Fig. 69-5D)
  - Optic gliomas occur in approximately 15% of patients, but only half cause clinical manifestations (proptosis, strabismus, optic nerve pallor, reduced visual acuity, or vision loss)
- Skeletal manifestations include scoliosis, sphenoid dysplasia, and rarely long bone cortical thinning or bowing
  - Pathologic fracture of thinned distal tibia is common and heals poorly, if at all, resulting in pseudarthrosis (creation of a "pseudo-joint")
- Hypertension is more frequent than in the general population
  - Occurs at any age, including childhood
  - Usually essential hypertension
  - Sometimes due to NF1 vasculopathy: Renal artery stenosis, aortic coarctation, narrowing of any other artery
- Malignancy
  - Malignant peripheral nerve sheath tumor develops from a plexiform neurofibroma in about 10% of patients
  - Pheochromocytoma, rhabdomyoma, neuroblastoma, and childhood leukemia may occur
- Unidentified bright objects are T2 hyperintensities on cerebral MRI that occur anywhere in the brain in about 60% of patients and are of no apparent clinical consequence; they often regress or disappear by adulthood
- Premature death is primarily associated with malignancy and vasculopathy; average life span is about 15 years shorter than the general population

Diagnosis and Evaluation

- See Box 69-4 for clinical diagnostic criteria
- Genetic testing can detect *NF1* mutations in about 95% of affected patients but is almost never needed clinically
  - Can be used to establish the diagnosis in young children not yet meeting clinical diagnostic criteria
  - Useful for prenatal diagnosis if the affected parent's specific mutation is known
- Evaluation and monitoring
  - Annual physical examination seeking typical manifestations
  - Blood pressure measurement at every visit
  - Ophthalmologic examination annually in children, less frequently in adults (seeking Lisch nodules and optic glioma)
  - Routine cerebral MRI is not recommended because optic nerve or intracranial lesions that require monitoring or intervention will cause clinical manifestations

---

BOX 69-4	*Neurofibromatosis Type 1 (NF1) Clinical Criteria*

Two or more of the following are required to establish a diagnosis of NF1:

> 6 or more café-au-lait macules (each >5 mm in children or >15 mm after puberty)
>
> 2 or more neurofibromas of any type or one plexiform neurofibroma
>
> Axillary or inguinal freckling
>
> Optic glioma
>
> 2 or more Lisch nodules (iris hamartomas)
>
> Characteristic osseous lesion (sphenoid dysplasia or thinning of long bone cortex with or without pseudarthrosis)
>
> An affected first-degree relative as defined by these diagnostic criteria

Treatment

- Secondary causes of hypertension should be considered at any age, especially renovascular hypertension, pheochromocytoma, and aortic coarctation
- NF1 vasculopathy should be considered in any ischemic condition, including acute coronary and cerebrovascular syndromes
- Plastic surgery or neurosurgery intervention for problematic dermal or plexiform neurofibromas
- Sudden rapid growth or pain in a previously stable plexiform neurofibroma is suspicious for malignant transformation
- Optic gliomas and other intracerebral tumors tend to be slow growing and occasionally regress spontaneously; serial assessment of tumor size and clinical manifestations before therapeutic intervention is appropriate

Prevention

- All first-degree relatives of an affected patient should be evaluated, including slit-lamp examination for Lisch nodules
  - One or the other parent is affected (or at least mosaic—some of the cells in the body are mutated) around 50% of the time; the remaining 50% represent new mutation, with neither parent affected
  - If neither parent is affected, the patient's siblings have a very low chance of being affected (there is a small chance that a parent has germline mosaicism—some of the eggs or sperm carry the mutation without any somatic features of neurofibromatosis)
  - If a parent is affected, each of the patient's siblings has a 50% chance of being affected
  - Each child of an affected person has a 50% chance of being affected

REVIEW QUESTIONS

For review questions, please go to www.expertconsult.com.

SUGGESTED READINGS

Adams PC: Hemochromatosis, *Clin Liver Dis* 8:735–753, 2004.
Beutler E: Hemochromatosis: genetics and pathophysiology, *Annu Rev Med* 57:331–347, 2006.

Galiatsatos P, Foulkes WD: Familial adenomatous polyposis, *Am J Gastroenterol* 101:385–398, 2006.

GeneTests: Medical genetics information resource, Seattle, 1993–2006, University of Washington. Available at: www.genetests.org.

Korf BR: Principles of genetics: overview of the paradigm of genetic contribution to health and disease. In Goldman L, Bennett JC, Ausiello D, editors: *Cecil textbook of medicine*, ed 22, Philadelphia, 2004, WB Saunders.

Mecklin J-P, Järvinen HJ: Surveillance in Lynch syndrome, *Fam Cancer* 4:267–271, 2005.

Vasen HFA: Clinical description of the Lynch syndrome (hereditary nonpolyposis colorectal cancer [HNPCC]), *Fam Cancer* 4:219–225, 2005.

Viskochil D: Neurofibromatosis type 1. In Cassidy SB, Allanson JE, editors: *Management of genetic syndromes*, ed 2, Hoboken, NJ, 2005, John Wiley.

69

Complementary and Alternative Medicine

BIMAL H. ASHAR, MD, MBA

Over the past two decades, the use of healing modalities outside the realm of Western allopathic medicine has increased dramatically. This movement has been a patient-driven phenomenon that has incited the need for physicians to expand their knowledge base beyond principles and concepts taught in medical school to solidify physician-patient relationships and protect patients from potential harm. This chapter provides a basic overview of the field of complementary and alternative medicine (CAM) and describes a few specific popular modalities.

Overview

Definitions

- Alternative medicine: Approaches not routinely used by conventional practitioners
- **Complementary medicine: Use of unconventional modalities as adjuncts to established Western medicine**
- Integrative medicine: Combination of conventional and complementary methods for preventing and treating disease

Classification

- There is no one universally accepted classification system for all of CAM
- **Most modalities are used to enhance the body's natural defenses in preventing and treating disease**
- The National Center for Complementary and Alternative Medicine of the National Institutes of Health has developed a classification system designed primarily to facilitate research efforts (Fig. 70-1)

Alternative Medical Systems

ACUPUNCTURE

Background

- One modality used in traditional Chinese medicine
- Many different types (e.g., auricular, five elements, hand, traditional Chinese)
- Involves the insertion of fine needles into the skin to restore the balance of life energy, or qi (pronounced "chee")
  - **A block in the flow of qi can lead to an imbalance of flow of energy through channels in the body (meridians) and lead to disease**

- Accurate needle placement along these meridians corrects the imbalance and treats the disorder
- Heating of the needles with mugwort (moxibustion), electrical stimulation, or manual twisting of the needles may be used to achieve the desired response

Mechanism of Action

- No unifying mechanism currently exists
- Acupuncture needling has been shown to effect the release of endorphins and neurohormones and alter blood flow

Efficacy

- Data for most conditions are inconclusive
- Studies support the use of acupuncture for the following:
  - Postoperative and chemotherapy-induced nausea and vomiting
  - Chronic low back pain: Equivalent to but not superior to other therapies; American College of Physicians guideline suggests that it may be useful
  - Lateral epicondylitis
  - Osteoarthritis of the knee
  - Tension headaches and migraine prophylaxis
- Data do not support its use for smoking cessation and tinnitus

Safety

- **Overall considered safe with the use of sterile needles by trained practitioners**
- Most common side effects include pain at the insertion site, localized bleeding, tiredness, and vasovagal syncope
- Rare case reports of pneumothorax, organ puncture, and hepatitis B

HOMEOPATHY

Background

- Homeopathy is based around two concepts
  - "Law of similars" suggests that substances that cause symptoms in healthy subjects can cure those symptoms in patients who are sick (e.g., digoxin is used to treat some arrhythmias that it is capable of causing)
  - "Principle of serial dilutions" suggests that medications can have a biologic effect even if diluted to levels at which the original substance is undetectable (a so-called homeopathic dose)

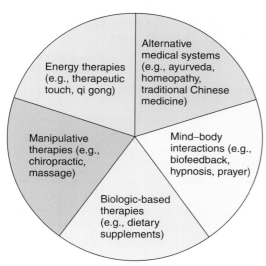

FIGURE 70-1 National Institutes of Health/National Center for Complementary and Alternative Medicine classification of complementary and alternative medicine practices.

- Focuses on subjective symptoms rather than disease diagnoses
- Most commonly used to treat allergy, hypertension, otitis media, arthritis, and headache
- Most homeopathic remedies are sold over-the-counter

Mechanism of Action

- No clear mechanism identified
- Scientific implausibility of the homeopathic dose makes acceptance into mainstream medicine difficult

Efficacy

- Few good studies available
- Systematic reviews have suggested that homeopathy is superior to placebo, but data supporting the use for any particular condition are limited

Safety

- Serious adverse reactions are rare because there is little to no active ingredient in the preparation
- **"Aggravation reactions" are worsening of symptoms shortly after a remedy is started and are not considered side effects by homeopaths**
- Risk of adulteration exists because there is no requirement for finished product testing
- Potential for harm exists when homeopathic physicians recommend against conventional medications and/or immunizations

Manipulative Therapies

CHIROPRACTIC

Background

- Used by up to 20% of the U.S. adult population
- Most commonly used for low back pain, neck pain, and various musculoskeletal conditions

- Basic principles
  - Spinal cord and nervous system are at the center of general well-being
  - Malalignments of vertebrae (subluxations) cause and perpetuate disease
  - Correction of the subluxations (usually via spinal manipulation) restores physiologic balance and allows the body to restore health
- Many chiropractors use massage, heat, and trigger-point injections as adjuncts to therapy

Mechanism of Action

- The mechanism of action is unknown

Efficacy

- **More effective than sham therapy for acute and chronic low back pain—equivalent to other modalities (e.g., physical therapy, analgesics, back exercises)**
- Data on efficacy for neck pain, shoulder pain, headaches, and other conditions are quite limited
- Patient satisfaction seems to be high with this manual approach to treatment

Safety

- Low back manipulation is considered safe, although there are rare reports of cauda equina syndrome after therapy
- Most common side effects include tiredness, headache, and localized pain that are self-limited
- Reports of carotid artery dissection, vertebrobasilar vascular accidents, vertebral fracture, and tracheal rupture with cervical manipulation do exist
- **Contraindications to chiropractic therapy include coagulopathy, osteoporosis, spinal tumors or infection, and spinal instability. It should also be avoided in patients with rheumatoid arthritis.**

MASSAGE THERAPY

Background

- Involves manipulation of soft tissues
- Many different types (e.g., Swedish, deep-tissue, shiatsu)
- Goal is to affect the flow of energy through the body and restore balance and health
- Primarily used for relaxation and stress relief but also used for treatment of back or neck pain, fibromyalgia, headaches, etc.

Efficacy and Safety

- Useful for stress reduction, although duration and intensity of response are variable
- **Recent data suggest that it is a useful, cost-effective measure in the treatment of chronic low back pain**
- **May reduce anxiety and pain in cancer patients**
- No clear data to support its use for other specific conditions
- Generally considered safe, although caution should be used in patients with coagulopathies, especially with deep-tissue techniques

70

Dietary Supplements

Overview

- Most widely used CAM modality
- Regulation in the United States
  - Before 1994, regulated as foods with required premarket testing for safety and efficacy
  - In 1994, the Dietary Supplement Health and Education Act (DSHEA) was enacted. It served to do the following:
    - Expand the definition of dietary supplements to include vitamins, amino acids, herbs, and other botanicals
    - Eliminate the need for companies to prove safety or efficacy before marketing their products
    - Place the burden of proof on the Food and Drug Administration (FDA) to show that a particular product is unsafe to keep it from the marketplace (e.g., ephedra ban took 7 years of data gathering)
    - Allow companies to make claims of "structure or function" (e.g., "for prostate health"), but not allow them to claim that their product was "intended to diagnose, treat, cure, or prevent any specific disease" (e.g., "for the prevention of prostate cancer")
- General issues surrounding dietary supplement safety
  - No product standardization exists (e.g., not all gingko biloba has the same active ingredients)
  - Active ingredient is often unknown, making standardization impossible
  - Potential for misidentification of herbs
  - Potential for adulteration of products with drugs or heavy metals
  - Few published data exist on the efficacy, safety, and potential for drug interactions with most dietary supplements
    - The FDA issued the Dietary Supplement Current Good Manufacturing Practices rule in 2007, which was designed to give consumers greater confidence that the dietary supplement they use has been manufactured to ensure its identity, purity, strength, and composition

Supplement Use for Selected Conditions

- Anxiety, insomnia
  - Kava kava
    - Used by natives of the South Pacific for many years. Superior to placebo for short-term treatment of anxiety but no data on long-term use.
    - Side effects include gastrointestinal upset and rash
    - Reports of idiosyncratic fulminant hepatic failure have led to its ban in parts of Europe but it is still available in the United States
    - **Avoid with other anxiolytics or alcohol**
  - Valerian
    - Primarily used for insomnia
    - Very limited short-term data to support its use
    - Avoid with other anxiolytics
- Depression
  - SAMe (S-adenosylmethionine)
    - A metabolic intermediary thought vital for cellular functioning

TABLE 70-1	**Potential Drug Interactions with St. John's Wort**	
Drug	**Effect**	**Potential Clinical Complication**
Cyclosporine	Decreased drug levels	Transplant graft rejection
Digoxin	Decreased drug levels	Improper rate control or CHF exacerbation
Oral contraceptives	Decreased drug effectiveness	Unplanned pregnancies
Protease inhibitors	Decreased drug levels	Increase in HIV viral load
Theophylline	Decreased drug levels	Asthma/COPD exacerbation
Selective serotonin reuptake inhibitors	Serotonin excess	Serotonin syndrome—confusion, agitation, diaphoresis, tremor, rhabdomyolysis
Warfarin	Decreased drug effectiveness	Reduced INR value

CHF, congestive heart failure; COPD, chronic obstructive pulmonary disease; HIV human immunodeficiency virus; INR, international normalized ratio.

- Small studies suggest utility for treating depression, but most of these were done with parenteral formulations
- **Oral bioavailability is poor**
- Considered safe but there is concern for interactions with tricyclic antidepressants
  - St. John's wort (*Hypericum perforatum*)
    - Most commonly prescribed antidepressant in Germany
    - Data suggest that it is superior to placebo for treatment of major depression and may be equivalent to many standard antidepressants
    - Generally well tolerated
    - Great concern over drug-herb interactions (Table 70-1) because of its effect on the cytochrome P450 system
- Dementia
  - Ginkgo biloba
    - Thought to have a number of biologic effects, including increasing blood flow, inhibiting platelet-activating factor, altering neuronal metabolism, and working as an antioxidant
    - No clear evidence to support its use for cognitive impairment or dementia
    - **No evidence that it is effective for the prevention of memory loss or dementia**
    - Side effects are usually rare and mild and include headaches and gastrointestinal discomfort
    - Case reports of spontaneous bleeding and seizures exist
    - May decrease the plasma concentrations of omeprazole, ritonavir, and tolbutamide
    - Because of its potential antiplatelet effects, it should be avoided in patients taking warfarin
- Hypercholesterolemia
  - Fish oil

TABLE 70-2	*Popular Dietary Supplements Used for the Treatment of Menopausal Symptoms*		
Supplement	**Potential Toxicity**	**Potential Drug Interactions**	**Comments**
Black cohosh (*Cimicifuga racemosa*)	Gastrointestinal discomfort Case reports of liver failure	None known	May be effective for short-term use (<6 mo)
Dong quai (*Angelica sinensis*)	Rash	Increased international normalized ratio (INR) in patients taking warfarin	No clinical evidence of efficacy
Red clover (*Trifolium pretense*)	Generally well tolerated	Theoretical risk of interaction with warfarin and tamoxifen	Is a source of isoflavones No clear efficacy in data
Soy isoflavones	Constipation, bloating, nausea, rash	Potential decreased INR in patients on warfarin; theoretical risk of competition with tamoxifen	Most studies have not shown a benefit

- A source of omega-3 fatty acids (i.e., eicosapentaenoic acid, docosahexaenoic acid)
- **Lowers triglycerides in a dose-dependent manner (30% reduction at doses of 2–4 g/day)**
- Can raise low-density lipoprotein (LDL) levels by 5% to 10% at high doses
- Little effect on high-density lipoprotein levels
- Data have shown decrease in cardiovascular mortality in patients with coronary disease
- No current randomized controlled trials have shown reduced mortality in primary prevention
- American Heart Association has recommended the consumption of 2 to 4 g per day of fish oil capsules for patients who need to lower triglycerides
- An FDA-approved fish oil capsule (Lovaza) is now available by prescription
- Side effects include fishy aftertaste and gastrointestinal upset
- Theoretical risk of bleeding at high doses due to antiplatelet effects
- Garlic (*Allium sativum*)
  - True active ingredient is unknown
  - May decrease total cholesterol and LDL in the short term
  - No data on impact on cardiovascular mortality
  - Side effects include bad breath, body odor, and gastrointestinal upset
  - Case reports of bleeding and interactions with warfarin exist
  - Has been shown to decrease saquinivir (protease inhibitor) levels
- Menopausal symptoms (Table 70-2)
- Osteoarthritis
  - Glucosamine sulfate and chondroitin sulfate
    - Theoretically support cartilage and connective tissue formation
    - May also have anti-inflammatory properties
    - Conflicting data exist on their use for symptomatic and functional benefits for patients with osteoarthritis of the knees or hips. Studies are also conflicting regarding their ability to slow the progression of joint-space narrowing.
    - Treatment effect may not be seen for up to 12 weeks
    - Generally well tolerated
    - No known drug interactions

- Prostatic hyperplasia
  - Saw palmetto (*Serenoa repens*)
    - Mechanism of action unknown
    - Conflicting data on its efficacy for improving urologic symptoms and urinary flow measures; most larger recent trials have been negative
    - No data to suggest that it prevents the complications of prostatic hyperplasia (i.e., acute urinary retention) or the development of prostate cancer
    - Generally well tolerated
    - No effect on prostate-specific antigen levels
- Probiotics
  - Microorganisms that have properties beneficial to the host
    - Examples include *Lactobacillus*, *Bifidobacterium*, *Streptococcus salivarius*, and *Saccharomyces boulardii*
    - Thought to work by preventing invasion by pathogenic bacteria and improving intestinal barrier function; may also play a role in perception of pain
    - **Data are limited, but some studies suggest that probiotics may be useful in the care of patients with acute infectious arthritis, inflammatory bowel disease, irritable bowel syndrome, antibiotic-associated diarrhea, chronic liver disease, and allergic disorders**
    - Avoid in seriously ill or immunocompromised patients

REVIEW QUESTIONS

For review questions, please go to www.expertconsult.com.

SUGGESTED READINGS

Ashar BH: Complementary and alternative medicine. In Dale DC, Federman DG, editors: *ACP medicine*, New York, 2007, WebMD.

Ashar BH, Rowland-Seymour A: Advising patients who use dietary supplements, *Am J Med* 121:91–97, 2008.

Ernst E: Acupuncture—a critical analysis, *J Intern Med* 259:125–137, 2006.

Furlan AD, Imamura M, Dryden T, Irvin E: Massage for low-back pain, *Cochrane Database Syst Rev* 4:CD001929, 2008.

Izzo AA, Ernst E: Interactions between herbal medicines and prescribed drugs: an updated systematic review, *Drugs* 69:1777–1798, 2009.

Jonas W, Levin JS: *Essentials of complementary and alternative medicine*, Philadelphia, Lippincott, 1999, Williams & Wilkins.

70

Substance Use Disorders

AMINA A. CHAUDHRY, MD, MPH

Substance use disorders are a worldwide public health problem and are associated with significant personal morbidity and mortality, enormous public health burden, numerous adverse societal consequences, and high costs. In the United States in 2009, over 22 million persons age 12 or older were classified with substance abuse or dependence in the past year. Societal economic costs from lost productivity, medical expenses, motor-vehicle accidents, domestic violence, and drug-related crime have been estimated at more than $180 billion for alcohol abuse and more than $180 billion for drug abuse per year. The problem of substance abuse spans all racial and socioeconomic strata and continues to grow. Despite the high prevalence of substance use disorders in the United States, the vast majority of individuals who need treatment do not receive it. The *Diagnostic and Statistical Manual of Mental Disorders* outlines accepted criteria for a spectrum of substance-related disorders based on the substances used and the severity of the disorder. Substances can be a drug of abuse, a medication, or a toxin.

Basic Information

- **Definitions: Two groups of disorders exist: Substance use disorders and substance-induced disorders**
  - Key features and diagnostic criteria for substance use disorders are listed in Box 71-1 and Box 71-2, respectively
    - **Substance abuse is characterized by continued use of a substance despite evidence of harm, either physically, legally, socially, or in employment**
    - **Substance dependence also includes the manifestations of tolerance, withdrawal, and typically extreme behavioral changes in response to compulsive cravings for the substance**
      - Patients with substance dependence have often tried unsuccessfully to cut down or abstain
    - ***Tolerance* is defined as either an individual requiring an increasing amount of a substance to achieve a desired effect or the same amount of a substance producing a decreased specific effect**
      - The development of tolerance and withdrawal, by themselves, do not indicate the presence of substance dependence
      - The psychological dependence on a substance must also be present for this diagnosis to apply
  - **The substance-induced disorders range from substance intoxication to substance withdrawal,** **substance-induced delirium, dementia, psychosis, mood or anxiety disorders, sexual dysfunction, and sleep disorder**
    - **The hallmarks of substance intoxication are reversible, clinically significant behavioral or psychological changes that develop during or shortly after the ingestion of a substance**
    - ***Substance withdrawal* involves characteristic physiologic and cognitive impairments as a result of the cessation of, or significant decrease in, the amount of a substance typically used continuously over a prolonged period**
      - Once withdrawal develops, most individuals will want to ingest the substance again to relieve the withdrawal symptoms
      - Substances with a recognized withdrawal state include alcohol, amphetamines, cocaine, nicotine, opioids, sedatives, hypnotics, and anxiolytics
- Common drugs of abuse
  - Marijuana: Peripheral and central nervous system (CNS) depressant through the cannabinoid receptor system
  - Benzodiazepines: CNS depressants that have anxiolytic and hypnotic effects
  - Opioids: Potent analgesics, including heroin and prescription opioids
  - Alcohol: CNS depressant that rapidly equilibrates between blood and tissues
  - Nicotine: Peripheral and central cholinergic agonist that paradoxically produces both stimulatory and relaxing effects
  - Cocaine: Peripheral and central stimulant with anesthetic and potent vasoconstrictive activity and average duration of action ranging from 20 to 90 minutes depending on route of administration.
  - Methamphetamine: Stimulant similar to cocaine in mechanism of action but with duration of action of 8 to 24 hours and a half-life of 12 hours

BOX 71-1	*Key Features of Substance Use Disorders*

Substance use disorders include substance abuse and the more severe substance dependence

Although tolerance and withdrawal may be present, the key feature of substance dependence is the psychological dependence on a particular substance

- Club drugs: Numerous drugs, mostly serotoninergic agonists
  - LSD (lysergic acid diethylamide)
  - "Ecstasy" or MDMA (methylene-dioxymethamphetamine)
  - "Love drug" or MDA (methylene-dioxyphenylaminopropane)
  - GHB (γ-hydroxybutyrate): A short-acting, γ-aminobutyric acid (GABA)–like aqueous solution with CNS sedating effects
- Anabolic steroids: Performance-enhancing, tissue-building compounds with concomitant androgenic effects
- Inhalants: Include volatile solvents (e.g., adhesives, aerosols, solvents, propellant gases) nitrites, and anesthetics; highly lipophilic
- Epidemiology
  - Prevalence and incidence of substance use disorders
    - In the United States, alcohol and tobacco are the most commonly taken substances among persons age 12 and older
      - In 2009, 18.7 million people age 12 or older (7.4% of the population) met the criteria for an alcohol use disorder (abuse or dependence)
    - The prevalence of cigarette smoking and nicotine dependence among adults has declined in the 21st century
      - The Centers for Disease Control and Prevention estimates that 46 million people, or 20.6% of all adults (age 18 years and older), in the United States smoke cigarettes. Cigarette smoking is more common among men than women.
      - Cigarette smoking is the leading cause of preventable death in the United States, resulting in an estimated 443,000 premature deaths and $193 billion in direct health-care expenditures and productivity losses each year

- Marijuana is the most commonly used illegal substance among Americans, with 16.7 million age 12 or older reporting past month use in 2009
- Nonmedical use of prescription drugs is the second highest category of drug use. The number of persons who used prescription psychotherapeutics nonmedically in the previous month was 7 million (2.8% of the population) in 2009. Prescription pain relievers are the most commonly used.
- The prevalence of alcohol and drug use disorders is highest among young adults ages 18 to 25
- **Alcohol- and drug-related disorders are more common among men than women**
- Risk factors for the development of substance use disorders (Fig. 71-1)
  - **Genetics may explain approximately 50% of the propensity to develop a substance use disorder**
  - **Other host factors include premorbid depression, anxiety disorders, and borderline and antisocial personality disorders**
    - Alcohol dependence is most likely an antecedent to the development of depression rather than a result of self-medication of a mood disorder
  - **Marital stability seems to have a protective effect**
  - Educational level
    - Youths who drop out of high school are at higher risk for developing alcohol and drug dependence later in life
    - Drug use during adolescence and young adulthood is also a predictor for not completing high school
  - Environmental factors
    - More frequent in populations in which drug use is more socially acceptable
    - Associated with community and family disorganization

71

BOX 71-2 *Diagnostic Criteria: Substance Use Disorders*

Substance Abuse:

A. A maladaptive pattern of substance use leading to clinically significant impairment or distress, as manifested by one (or more) of the following, occurring within a 12-month period:
  a. Recurrent substance use resulting in a failure to fulfill major role obligations at work, school, or home
  b. Recurrent substance use in situations in which it is physically hazardous
  c. Recurrent substance-related legal problems
  d. Continued substance use despite having persistent or recurrent social or interpersonal problems caused by or exacerbated by the effects of the substance

B. The symptoms have never met the criteria for Substance Dependence for this class of substance.

Substance Dependence:

A. A maladaptive pattern of substance use, leading to clinically significant impairment or distress, as manifested by three (or more) of the following, occurring at any time in the same 12-month period:

1. Tolerance, as defined by either of the following:
  a. a need for markedly increased amounts of the substance to achieve intoxication or desired effect
  b. markedly diminished effect with continued use of the same amount of the substance
2. Withdrawal, as manifested by either of the following:
  a. the characteristic withdrawal syndrome for the substance
  b. the same (or a closely related) substance is taken to relieve or avoid withdrawal symptoms
3. The substance is often taken in larger amounts or over a longer period than was intended
4. There is a persistent desire or unsuccessful efforts to cut down or control substance use
5. A great deal of time is spent in activities necessary to obtain the substance, use the substance, or recover from its effects
6. Important social, occupational, or recreational activities are given up or reduced because of substance use
7. The substance use is continued despite knowledge of having a persistent or recurrent physical or psychological problem that is likely to have been caused or exacerbated by the substance

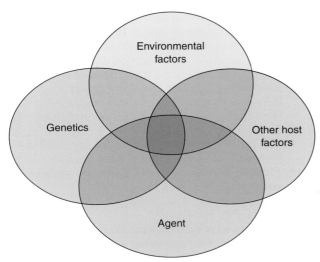

FIGURE 71-1 Risk factors for the development of substance use disorders.

- Peer influence impacts the initiation and ongoing use of alcohol and drugs, particularly among adolescents and young adults
  - **The absence of employment and particular jobs or work settings (bartenders, anesthesiologists) may also carry risk**
  - Agent factors
    - **Agents that quickly reach the brain, such as lipophilic substances that are injected intravenously, have a higher addictive potential**
    - Substances that are effective for self-medication, such as heroin or opioids for pain, may help explain addiction to certain drugs
    - Easily accessible substances obtained at low cost tend to have a higher abuse potential
- **Common physiologic mechanisms of action**
  - **Drugs of abuse and alcohol share a common final pathway: The dopamine reward pathway**
  - **In the early stages of drug use, reward pathway activation causes euphoria and intense pleasure**
  - **With repeated use, reward pathway activation results in diminished responses and the development of long-lasting memories linked to drug-using experiences**
  - These changes are responsible for the development of tolerance, psychological dependence, and the relapse that can happen after years of abstinence

Clinical Presentation

- **Warning signs in the office setting**
  - Sudden change in behavior (e.g., sudden job loss, financial difficulty, or family problem)
  - History of two or more non–sports-related traumas in an adult
  - Sexual dysfunction
  - Intoxicated behavior secondary to active use (inebriated, agitated, extremely lethargic)
  - Family concerns about patient
  - History of "driving under the influence" (DUI) or other substance-related arrest

- **Overdose complications**
  - Alcohol
    - Symptoms consist of somnolence, bradycardia, coma, and eventual death
    - Symptoms vary with blood alcohol concentration (BAC)
      - Cognitive and behavioral changes occur at BAC of 20 to 30 mg/dL
      - Legal intoxication is at BAC of 80 to 100 mg/dL
      - Death can occur at BAC of 300 to 400 mg/dL
    - Treatment is supportive with close monitoring of electrolytes and for evidence of alcohol withdrawal as the BAC decreases
  - Stimulants such as cocaine and methamphetamine
    - Overdose may result in seizures, arrhythmias, and death
    - Treatment is supportive and management of any medical complications that arise
  - Opioids
    - Symptoms include respiratory depression with shallow respirations, miosis, bradycardia, decreased level of consciousness, coma, and eventual death
    - Treatment is with intravenous (IV) naloxone 0.4 to 2 mg immediately. May be administered intramuscularly or subcutaneously if no venous access. Repeat every 2 to 3 minutes as needed. Naloxone may also be administered intranasally.
      - May require frequent additional doses of naloxone over the first 24 hours because this medication may clear before the effects of the opioids have diminished sufficiently, particularly in the case of long-acting prescription opioids
      - If no reponse after 10 mg, consider diagnoses other than opioid toxicity
- **Withdrawal syndromes**
  - **Alcohol withdrawal, which may be life-threatening, typically occurs in several stages (Table 71-1)**
  - Withdrawal from stimulants, including cocaine and methamphetamine
    - Symptoms typically are mild and include depression, anxiety, hypersomnolence, anhedonia, difficulty concentrating, increased appetite, and increased drug cravings
    - Acute hospitalization is almost never warranted solely for cocaine withdrawal. Severe depressive or psychiatric symptoms may be an exception.
  - **Opioid withdrawal typically occurs in two phases**
    - Acute physiologic withdrawal: Generally not life-threatening, but may be in people with underlying cardiac conditions or other medical illness
    - Protracted withdrawal phase
      - May involve insomnia, decreased blood pressure and heart rate, and persistent drug cravings
      - May last up to 6 to 12 months
  - **Marijuana withdrawal is increasingly being recognized as a clinical syndrome most commonly manifesting with irritability, anxiety, restlessness, and appetite and sleep disturbances**

TABLE 71-1	*Stages of Alcohol Withdrawal*			
	Autonomic Dysfunction →	**Withdrawal Seizures →**	**Alcoholic Hallucinosis →**	**Delirium Tremens**
Symptoms	Tremors Mild elevations in blood pressure and heart rate	Generalized motor seizures singly or in episodic bursts	Hallucinations (visual, auditory, tactile) with generally normal vital signs Patient is otherwise oriented	Severe autonomic dysregulation Confusion Auditory, visual, or tactile hallucinations
Time course	Begins within 5–10 hr	Begins within 8–24 hr	Begins within 12–24 hr	Begins within 48–96 hr
Treatment	Frequent assessments Symptom-driven doses of benzodiazepines	Treat seizure with parenteral benzodiazepines Other antiepileptics minimally effective	Frequent assessments Symptom-driven doses of benzodiazepines Close monitoring	Frequent parenteral doses of benzodiazepines or continuous drip Close monitoring

- **Secondary medical complications**
  - Complications from substance use in general
    - Trauma
    - Infectious diseases such as HIV/AIDS, sexually transmitted infections, hepatitis B and C
    - Renal complications such as acute tubular necrosis from rhabdomyolysis
    - Altered mental status with delirium
    - Malnutrition in general or specific vitamin B complex deficiency
    - Poor adherence to medical appointments and recommended treatments
  - Complications from injection drug use
    - Endocarditis, often with septic emboli
    - Cellulitis and deep tissue infections
    - Thrombophlebitis
    - Foreign-body granulomatosis, often called "talc lung" from talc or other fillers used in drug tablets
    - Secondary amyloidosis
    - Emphysema and bullous lung disease
    - Pulmonary hypertension
  - Complications from alcohol
    - Cardiovascular: Arrhythmias with atrial fibrillation or "holiday heart" being the most common, hypertension, dilated cardiomyopathy
    - GI: Esophagitis, esophageal varices, gastritis, pancreatitis, alcoholic hepatitis, cirrhosis, GI bleeding
    - Endocrine: Testicular atrophy, amenorrhea
    - Hematologic: Macrocytic anemia, thrombocytopenia, leukopenia
    - Electrolyte derangements (hypokalemia, hypomagnesemia, hypophosphatemia)
    - Neurologic: Peripheral neuropathy, alcoholic myopathy
      - **Wernicke encephalopathy, a medical emergency, is a confusional state of abrupt onset caused by thiamine deficiency**
        - Characterized by a triad of confusion, ataxia, and oculomotor dysfunction (usually cranial nerve VI palsy leading to ophthalmoplegia)
        - The diagnosis is made clinically, although necrosis and atrophy of mamillary bodies are visible on brain magnetic resonance imaging (MRI) in 80% of cases
        - Treatment is immediate administration of IV thiamine, admission for observation and continued IV thiamine therapy, and long-term oral supplementation on an outpatient basis
        - **Symptoms may be precipitated or worsened by administration of glucose before thiamine**
        - Patients usually improve over hours to days
      - **Korsakoff amnestic syndrome refers to profound memory impairment for ongoing events with a marked inability to retain new information**
        - Occurs often late in the course of chronic alcohol dependence
        - Usually seen after an episode of Wernicke encephalopathy
        - **Both anterograde and retrograde memory are affected, although long-term memory is usually preserved**
        - **Patients often appear apathetic, unconcerned, or unaware of their illness and may confabulate**
        - Treatment with thiamine is usually ineffective, and recovery of memory is often poor
      - **Alcoholic cerebellar degeneration is a syndrome characterized by gait abnormalities, including complaints of weakness, unsteadiness, or incoordination, with wide-based ataxic gait and abnormal heel-knee-shin test**
        - Occasionally patients may also have tremors or incoordination of the upper extremities, dysarthria, or blurred vision
        - Onset of symptoms can be progressive over weeks to months, but acute worsening of mild symptoms may occur
        - Head MRI may show evidence of cerebellar atrophy
        - Treatment consists of abstinence from alcohol and nutritional supplementation, but gait abnormalities may persist
  - Complications from stimulants (cocaine and methamphetamine)
    - Cardiovascular: Arrhythmias and sudden death; severe, sometimes malignant, hypertension; myocarditis; cardiomyopathy
      - Myocardial infarction that is usually caused by vasospasm; cocaine may also accelerate atherosclerosis

71

■ Treatment consists of aspirin, benzodiazepines to reduce blood pressure and heart rate, and nitrates or calcium channel blockers to decrease vasospasm and prevent arrhythmias

- **Avoid β-blockers because they enhance cocaine-induced vasoconstriction, allow unopposed α activity, and may decrease survival**

■ Neurologic: Seizure, cerebrovascular accidents, intracranial hemorrhage, migraine headache, vasculitis, acute lead poisoning from methamphetamine use

■ Psychiatric: Psychosis, auditory hallucinations, paranoia, extreme violent behavior from methamphetamine use

■ Renal: Rhabdomyolysis

■ Gastrointestinal: Bowel ischemia leading to infarction and perforation

■ Pulmonary: Alveolar hemorrhage and infarction; pulmonary edema

● Complications from heroin

■ Renal: Focal, segmental glomerulosclerosis that may progress to renal failure

■ Pulmonary: Pulmonary edema

■ Endocrine: Amenorrhea, hypogonadism and erectile dysfunction, euthyroid increase in thyroxine-binding globulin concentration

Screening, Diagnosis and Evaluation

● **Screening for substance use and substance use disorders**
  ● History should include family history of alcohol or drug use disorders, presence of co-occurring psychiatric disorders, employment and family status, history of experimenting with or using illicit drugs
    ■ For alcohol consumption, the **National Institute on Alcohol Abuse and Alcoholism** has defined maximum limits, based on epidemiologic data that suggest that those who exceed these amounts are at increased risk for alcohol-related problems such as injury, social and legal problems, and illness
    ■ **The maximum drinking limits are defined as no more than 3 drinks in 1 day AND no more than 7 drinks per week for healthy women and healthy men over age 65, and no more than 4 drinks in 1 day AND no more than 14 drinks per week for healthy men up to age 65**
    ■ One standard drink equals 12 oz regular beer, or 5 oz wine, or 1.5 oz distilled spirits
    ■ **Lower limits or abstinence** may be medically indicated
  ● Screening instruments
    ■ **AUDIT: The Alcohol Use Disorders Identification Test**
      ▪ A 10-item questionnaire developed by the World Health Organization specifically for identifying unhealthy alcohol use and disorders of alcohol use in primary care
      ▪ Has been extensively validated across populations and languages
    ■ **AUDIT-C: An abbreviated version of the AUDIT using only the first three questions; also performs well when the longer version is not feasible (Box 71-3)**

BOX 71-3   *AUDIT-C Questionnaire*

Question 1: How often did you have a drink containing alcohol in the past year?
 a. Never
 b. Monthly or less
 c. 2–4 times/month
 d. 2–3 times/week
 e. 4 or more times/week

Question 2: How many drinks did you have on a typical day when you were drinking in the past year?
 a. 1 or 2
 b. 3 or 4
 c. 5 or 6
 d. 7 to 9
 e. 10 or more

Question 3: How often did you have six or more drinks on one occasion in the past year?
 a. Never
 b. Less than monthly
 c. Monthly
 d. Weekly
 e. Daily or almost daily

(a = 0 points; b = 1 point; c = 2 points; d = 3 points; e = 4 points)

In men, a total score of 4 or more is considered positive. In women, a total score of 3 or more is considered positive.

BOX 71-4   *CAGE Questions to Screen for Substance Abuse*

C: Have you ever tried to **cut down** on your alcohol or drug use?

A: Do you get **annoyed** when people comment about your drinking or drug use?

G: Do you feel **guilty** about things you have done while drinking or using drugs?

E: Do you need an **eye-opener** to get started in the morning?

● **CAGE Questionnaire: Can be used to screen for alcohol dependence (Box 71-4)**
  ■ The more affirmative answers, the more likely the person is alcohol dependent. Two or more affirmative answers on the CAGE is considered a positive result; however, answering any affirmative responses merits further evaluation for alcohol-related disorders.
  ■ Has been adapted to assess for drug use as well
● **Assessment of severity of substance use and substance use disorders should be comprehensive and thorough (Box 71-5)**
● **Physical findings**
  ● Alcohol dependence: Secondary medical complications caused by use of the substance
    ■ Abdominal discomfort and/or hemoccult-positive stool

BOX 71-5	*Assessment Questions to Identify Severity of Substance Use Disorder*

Duration of use or age at first use

Route of administration

Measurement of frequency and quantity of use

Timing of last use

Past history of blackouts, delirium tremens, withdrawal seizures, and/or hospitalizations for alcohol or drug withdrawal

Past legal problems because of use

Past treatment history and treatment impact on use

Duration of longest, continuous time clean and how achieved

Review of systems for physiologic consequences of substance use

- Findings consistent with liver disease, such as jaundice, palmar erythema, caput medusa, ascites, bruising, encephalopathy
  - Peripheral neuropathy
- Smoked or snorted cocaine: Atrophy or perforation of nasal septum; acute respiratory wheezing; digit burns; nervous picking at skin (formication); and agitation
- Methamphetamine
  - Acute: Hyperthermia, hyperventilation, delusions, and paranoia
  - Chronic: Poor dentition from bruxism, decreased saliva production, inadequate dental hygiene, skin findings such as burns or excoriations caused by formication
- Opioids
  - Intranasal or oral opioid use: Shallow breathing; lethargy, "pinpoint pupils" or miosis, and acute respiratory wheezing
  - Injection drug use: New and old needle track marks, healed and new abscesses
- **Laboratory testing**
  - **Toxicology screens**
    - Alcohol: With acute alcohol intoxication, blood alcohol concentration should be measured
    - Cocaine: Urine tests for cocaine and metabolites
      - Positive for cocaine for less than 48 hours
      - Cocaine is rapidly metabolized into its major metabolite, benzoylecgonine, usually within hours; however, benzoylecgonine may be present in urine for up to 60 hours after single use but may persist much longer after the cessation of heavy cocaine
      - Cocaine and alcohol interact to form another active metabolite, cocaethylene
      - Substances used to "cut" the drugs (quinine and quinidine) may be positive for up to 10 days
    - **Opioids: Heroin is metabolized to morphine and will result in a morphine-positive urine test result**
      - Typical opiate assays do not cross-react with oxycodone or hydrocodone. Thus, oxycodone and hydrocodone will not show up as morphine-positive on urine toxicology testing; these must be tested for separately.
      - Poppy seeds and certain fluoroquinolone antibiotics may cause false-positive results

- Hematology testing
  - Elevated mean corpuscular volume may be seen in chronic alcohol exposure
  - Acute alcohol consumption may cause pancytopenia, particularly thrombocytopenia
- Hepatic panel
  - Alcohol has direct toxic effects on the liver, resulting in abnormalities in several liver enzymes
    - γ-Glutamyl transpeptidase levels may be elevated, often greater than 1000 units/L
    - Aspartate transaminotransferase is typically elevated to a greater degree than alanine transaminotransferase, but neither increases to levels above 500 units/L
    - Serum bilirubin levels and prothrombin time may be abnormal in acute alcoholic hepatitis
- Chemistries
  - Abrupt cessation of alcohol consumption may result in an anion gap ketoacidosis secondary to poor nutrition and alcohol-induced increased lipolysis with decreased gluconeogenesis
  - Hypomagnesemia is common with chronic alcohol use and often is accompanied by hypokalemia and hypophosphatemia

Treatment

- **Treatment of acute withdrawal and detoxification**
  - **Alcohol: Mainstay is benzodiazepines to prevent alcohol withdrawal seizures and delirium tremens (DTs)**
    - In patients with liver disease, lorazepam and oxazepam are the benzodiazepines of choice
    - Dosing should be symptom driven, with frequent assessments for worsening or improvement of symptoms
    - Patients should also receive thiamine and folate, followed by dextrose-containing fluids
  - **Cocaine: Treatment is mostly supportive and typically does not require acute inpatient care; be alert, however, for other substance use and severe depression, which may necessitate hospitalization**
  - **Opioids: Symptoms are most effectively relieved with administration of either a long-acting full opioid agonist such as methadone or a partial opioid agonist such as buprenorphine**
    - Clonidine may decrease the autonomic dysfunction associated with opioid withdrawal but will not treat many of the other symptoms
    - Dicyclomine may relieve abdominal cramping, and ibuprofen or other nonsteroidal anti-inflammatory drugs may treat the generalized myalgias and joint pains
    - Methocarbamol can ease muscle spasms
- **Assessment of motivation and interest in long-term treatment**
  - **Assess stage of readiness for change**
    - **Precontemplative: Patient has not yet considered stopping substance use; may not think substance use is a problem**
    - **Contemplative: Patient is thinking about cessation**

71

- **Determination: Patient has decided to stop substance use but is not yet taking action to quit**
- **Action: Patient is actively goal setting, problem solving, and trying to quit**
- **Maintenance: Patient has successfully quit and is working on relapse prevention**
- **Relapse: Can occur at any point through this process; goal is then to get back to action stage**

- Nonpharmacologic interventions
  - A brief intervention by a physician in an office takes about 5 to 10 minutes to complete and takes advantage of the unique role in the patient-physician relationship to effect change
    - Consists of assessment, feedback to the patient, and referrals or recommendations
    - Studies demonstrate that it reduces levels of unhealthy alcohol use in the primary care setting. However, it has not been found to reduce drinking among those with alcohol dependence in primary care, or to reduce drinking among hospitalized patients.
    - **The FRAMES algorithm is useful in a primary care office (Box 71-6)**
  - Specialized substance abuse treatment programs are able to perform more comprehensive assessment, evaluation, and treatment
    - Provide more intensive substance abuse treatment
    - Group and individual addiction counseling
    - May offer psychiatric or medical care, but often do not
  - Community support programs and self-help groups are common
    - Many, such as Alcoholics Anonymous and Narcotics Anonymous, are based on 12-step approach
    - "Rational Recovery" uses a cognitive behavioral approach and may be an alternative for patients who are uncomfortable with the spiritual approach
- **Pharmacologic therapies**
  - All pharmacologic therapies for substance use disorders are most effective in combination with counseling or active self-help group participation
  - Alcohol
    - **Disulfiram acts as a deterrent to continued alcohol intake**
      - **Usual daily doses range from 250 to 500 mg**
      - **Patients develop severe flushing, shortness of breath, dizziness, nausea, vomiting, and abdominal pain, often with significant volume depletion if alcohol is consumed concomitantly**
      - Should be avoided in pregnant women and in patients with severe liver disease or medical comorbidities
      - Advise patients to avoid foods and beauty products that contain alcohol
    - **Acamprosate is thought to affect GABA and excitatory glutamate neurotransmission in the CNS to decrease alcohol cravings**
      - Results from numerous clinical trials demonstrate modest reductions in number of drinking days compared with placebo
    - **Naltrexone, an opioid antagonist, is modestly effective in preventing relapse to heavy drinking by diminishing cravings for alcohol**
      - Thought to act by decreasing some of the reinforcing effects of alcohol that may occur through opioid neurotransmission
      - Avoid the medication in patients with severe liver disease, pregnant patients, and those on chronic opioids
      - Available in oral form (daily dosing) and an extended-release formulation for intramuscular injection (monthly)
  - Opioids
    - **Methadone is a full opioid agonist at the μ opioid receptor with a duration of action for opioid dependence treatment of 24 hours**
      - Available for opioid dependence maintenance; treatment occurs in regulated, specialized treatment centers where patients are observed taking the medication unless they have earned privileges to take home individual doses
      - In combination with counseling, methadone reduces illicit drug use by 50% to 70%; keeps patients in treatment; reduces HIV and hepatitis C seroconversion; may reduce crime and improves health-related quality of life for patients
      - About 50% of patients relapse to heroin use within 1 year of stopping methadone treatment
      - Therapeutic doses typically range between 60 and 100 mg, but individualized dosing is key, and therapeutic doses vary
    - **Buprenorphine is a partial opioid agonist at the μ opioid receptor with a higher affinity and a much slower dissociation rate compared with full opioid agonists**
      - **May be dosed once daily or every other day**
      - Because of its partial agonist properties, buprenorphine has a ceiling beyond which increasing the dose will not result in any further opioid effects
      - Available in a parenteral formulation, a transdermal patch, and sublingual formulations (buprenorphine and buprenorphine/naloxone); only the sublingual forms are Food and Drug Administration approved for treatment of opioid dependence
      - **Office-based physicians can prescribe sublingual buprenorphine to treat opioid-dependent patients**

BOX 71-7 *Key Steps in Relapse Prevention*

Establish a supportive patient-physician relationship
Schedule regular follow-up
Mobilize family support
Facilitate involvement in self-help and community groups
Help patients recognize and cope with relapse triggers and cravings
Facilitate positive lifestyle changes
Manage depression, anxiety, pain, and other comorbid conditions
Consider pharmacotherapy
Collaborate with addiction treatment specialists, if available

- The combination tablet (buprenorphine/naloxone) contains naloxone, which may decrease the abuse and diversion potential of the medication because IV administration of crushed tablets may cause withdrawal
- **Buprenorphine may precipitate withdrawal in patients who have recently taken full-agonist opioids**
- **Naltrexone, an opioid antagonist approved for the treatment of opioid dependence, effectively blocks heroin effects.** However, its use is limited, as treatment retention is relatively low in oral naltrexone treatment. An extended-release formulation for monthly intramuscular injection was recently approved for treatment of opioid dependence. Patients must be free of opioids at the initiation of treatment.
- Cocaine: Currently no effective pharmacologic agents exist for treatment of cocaine abuse or dependence

- **Relapse prevention (Box 71-7)**
  - Relapse is a common part of recovery
  - 50% to 80% of patients return to substance use within their first year of recovery. Most of these patients relapse within the first 3 months after stopping alcohol or drug use.
  - 60% of those with lifetime substance use disorders eventually do achieve sustained abstinence
  - Factors associated with sustaining abstinence include self-efficacy, vocational engagement, income, having friends that are abstinent, and social and spiritual support
  - Additionally, longer periods of abstinence are associated with sustained abstinence

- Relapse rates for addiction resemble those of exacerbations of other chronic diseases such as diabetes, hypertension, and asthma
- As a chronic, relapsing condition, preventing relapse is a key component of long-term management of substance use disorders

REVIEW QUESTIONS

For review questions, please go to www.expertconsult.com.

SUGGESTED READINGS

American Psychiatric Association: *Diagnostic and statistical manual of mental disorders, ed 4, text revision*, Washington, DC, 2000, American Psychiatric Association.
Anton RF, O'Malley SS, Ciraulo DA, et al: Combined pharmacotherapies and behavioral interventions for alcohol dependence: the COMBINE study: a randomized controlled trial, JAMA 295:2003–2017, 2006.
Buchsbaum DG, Buchanan RG, Centor RM, et al: Screening for alcohol abuse using CAGE scores and likelihood ratios, Ann Intern Med 115:774–777, 1991.
Bush K, Kivlahan DR, McDonell MB, et al: The AUDIT alcohol consumption questions (AUDIT-C): an effective brief screening test for problem drinking, Arch Intern Med 158:1789–1795, 1998.
Dawson DA, Grant BF, Stinson FS, Zhou Y: Effectiveness of the derived Alcohol Use Disorders Identification Test (AUDIT-C) in screening for alcohol use disorders and risk drinking in the US general population, Alcoholism Clin Exp Res 29:844–854, 2005.
Dennis ML, Foss MA, Scott CK: An eight-year perspective on the relationship between the duration of abstinence and other aspects of recovery, Evaluation Rev 31:585–612, 2007.
Fudala PJ, Bridge TP, Herbert S, et al: for the Buprenorphine/Naloxone Collaborative Study GroupOffice-based treatment of opiate addiction with a sublingual-tablet formulation of buprenorphine and naloxone, N Engl J Med 349:949–958, 2003.
Kaner EFS, Dickinson HO, Beyer FR, et al: Effectiveness of brief alcohol interventions in primary care populations, Cochrane Database Syst Rev 2:CD004148, 2007.
Mattick RP, Kimber J, Breen C, Davoli M: Buprenorphine maintenance versus placebo or methadone maintenance for opioid dependence, Cochrane Database Syst Rev 2:CD002207, 2008.
Mattick RP, Breen C, Kimber J, Davoli M: Methadone maintenance therapy versus no opioid replacement therapy for opioid dependence, Cochrane Database Syst Rev 3:CD002209, 2009.
Office of National Drug Control Policy: The economic costs of drug abuse in the United States, 1992–2002 (Publication No. 207303), Washington, DC, 2004, Executive Office of the President.
Ries R, Fiellin D, Miller S, et al editors: Principles of addiction medicine, ed 4, Chevy Chase, MD, 2009, American Society of Addiction Medicine.
Substance Abuse and Mental Health Services Administration: Results from the 2009 National Survey on Drug Use and Health: volume I. summary of national findings (Office of Applied Studies, NSDUH Series H-38A, HHS Publication No. SMA 10–4856Findings), Rockville, MD, 2010, Substance Abuse and Mental Health Services Administration.
World Health Organization (WHO): The Alcohol Use Disorders Identification Test: guidelines for use in primary care (WHO/MSD/MSB/01.6a), Geneva, WHO, 2001. (Available at: http://whqlibdoc.who.int/hq/2001/WHO_MSD_MSB_01.6a.pdf; accessed April 26, 2011.)

71

Preoperative Evaluation

STEPHEN D. SISSON, MD

Preoperative evaluation is a common task for the internist. The primary objective of the preoperative evaluation is **to assess the patient's medical readiness for surgery.** Every operative procedure carries some level of risk; clinical judgment, accompanied by appropriate testing, is needed to define risk. The preoperative evaluation **includes three steps: clinical risk assessment, functional assessment, and surgery-specific risk assessment.** These assessments determine whether or not to proceed with surgery or to obtain cardiac testing before proceeding with surgery. Mounting evidence has demonstrated **the beneficial impact of β-blockers on cardiovascular outcomes** in some, but not all, patients undergoing noncardiac surgery.

Clinical Risk Assessment

- Clinical risk assessment is the first step in the preoperative evaluation; in this assessment, clinical predictors of increased risk are identified. The presence of certain conditions, termed *active cardiac conditions* (Table 72-1), should lead to the postponement of elective surgery until they are resolved.
  - Cardiovascular disease is commonly associated with increased operative risk
    - **The five areas of potential cardiovascular risk include ischemic cardiovascular disease, congestive heart failure (CHF), valvular heart disease, hypertension, and arrhythmia**
    - Prior **history of myocardial infarction (MI),** especially within the **past month,** is associated **with increased operative risk;** acute MI is an "active cardiac condition" that should delay elective surgery for at least 1 month
      - Stable angina that is mild (i.e., class I or II angina) is not a contraindication to surgery. Unstable angina and class III or IV angina are considered "active cardiac conditions" that should delay surgery until they are resolved.
    - In the absence of MI, surgery should also be postponed following percutaneous coronary intervention as follows:
      - Balloon angioplasty: Delay surgery 2 to 4 weeks following angioplasty; ideally complete surgery before 8 weeks following angioplasty
      - Bare metal intracoronary stent: delay surgery 4 to 6 weeks following stent placement
      - Drug-eluting intracoronary stent: Delay surgery 1 year following stent placement

- In all cases, aspirin should be continued perioperatively, if possible
    - **Cardiac catheterization does not have a role in perioperative risk assessment;** performing cardiac catheterization solely to evaluate a person for elective surgery should not be done
    - **Similarly, performing cardiac revascularization procedures specifically to prepare a patient with known coronary artery disease for elective surgery has not been shown to be of benefit and should not be done**
  - CHF is associated with increased perioperative risk, especially if uncontrolled. **Decompensated CHF is another active cardiac condition that is a contraindication to elective surgery**.
  - Valvular heart disease is poorly tolerated during surgery because of fluid shifts; **severe aortic stenosis** (defined as aortic valve area <1 cm or mean pressure gradient >40 mm Hg) is another active cardiac condition that should delay elective surgery until addressed
    - Similarly, symptomatic **mitral stenosis is an active cardiac condition**
    - Patients with prosthetic heart valves, prior infective endocarditis, intracardiac shunts, and/or prosthetic patches, as well as cardiac transplantation patients with cardiac valvulopathy, should receive endocarditis prophylaxis when undergoing certain dental procedures or respiratory tract procedures
  - Hypertension has not been demonstrated to affect surgery, but general consensus has been to control hypertension so that diastolic pressure is maintained at less than 110 mm Hg
    - **β-Blockers are the drug of choice for perioperative hypertension**
  - Arrhythmias may be poorly tolerated with surgery
    - **Supraventricular arrhythmias** should be **rate-controlled** before surgery
    - Ventricular arrhythmias should prompt evaluation by a cardiologist to recommend perioperative management
  - First degree and Mobitz I heart block are well tolerated during surgery. **Mobitz II and third degree heart block require intraoperative pacing.**
- Pulmonary disease is also associated with perioperative risk. **Pulmonary complications** (e.g., atelectasis, pneumonia) are the **leading cause of perioperative morbidity.**

TABLE 72-1	Clinical Risk and Elective Surgery
Active Cardiac Conditions (should Postpone or Cancel Surgery Until Resolved)	**Clinical Risk Factors (should be Included in Preoperative Risk Assessment)**

Unstable coronary syndromes:
   Unstable angina
   Class III or IV angina
   Recent (i.e., ≤30 days) myocardial infarction
 Decompensated heart failure
 Significant arrhythmia
   Supraventricular tachyarrhythmias with heart rate >100 bpm
   High-grade atrioventricular block
   Mobitz II atrioventricular block
   Symptomatic ventricular arrhythmias
   Symptomatic bradycardia
 Severe valvular disease
   Severe aortic stenosis (i.e., mean pressure gradient >40 mm Hg or aortic valve area <1 cm, or symptomatic)
   Symptomatic mitral stenosis (i.e., progressive dyspnea on exertion, exertional syncope, or heart failure)
	History of heart disease
	 History of compensated or prior heart failure
	 History of cerebrovascular disease
	 Diabetes mellitus (or specifically, anyone treated with insulin)
	 Renal insufficiency (defined as serum creatinine >2 mg/dL)

TABLE 72-2	METs and Physical Activity	
1 MET	**≥4 METs**	**>10 METs**
Take care of self Eat, dress, use toilet Walk indoors around house Walk 1–2 blocks on level ground at 2–3 mph Dusting/washing dishes (some classify this as 1–4 METs)	Climb 1 flight stairs or walk up a hill Walk on level ground at 4 mph Run a short distance Scrubbing floors, moving heavy furniture Golf, bowl, dance, doubles tennis, throw baseball or football	Participate in strenuous sports including: singles tennis, football, basketball, skiing

METs, metabolic equivalents.

- Patients with chronic pulmonary disease should have local or epidural anesthesia whenever possible
- Preoperative pulmonary testing is controversial; the American College of Physicians recommends against preoperative spirometry or chest radiography, except in patients with chronic obstructive pulmonary disease (COPD) or asthma
  - Serum albumin less than 3.5 g/dL is a marker for increased pulmonary complications
  - **Forced expiratory volume in 1 second (FEV$_1$) less than 1.5 L** is associated with **increased** risk of **pulmonary complications**
  - An **FEV$_1$ less than 1 L** is associated with **prolonged intubation** and should prompt consultation with a pulmonologist
- Other **diseases that are associated with increased operative risk** include cerebrovascular disease, **diabetes mellitus,** and **renal insufficiency** (defined as creatinine >2 mg/dL) (see Table 72-1)
- **Patients should delay surgery in the presence of active infection**
- If **corticosteroids** have been administered for at least **2 weeks** in the year preceding surgery, **stress-dose corticosteroids should be administered perioperatively**

Functional Assessment

- Surgery creates a stress on the cardiovascular system, which may unmask subclinical cardiovascular disease, especially in someone who is physically deconditioned

- Functional status assessment is a means of quantifying the physical conditioning of a patient who is about to undergo surgery
  - Functional status is standardized into units of metabolic equivalents, referred to as METs
  - METs can be correlated with routine daily activities, allowing the physician to perform a functional status assessment by inquiring about those activities a patient is able to perform without developing limiting dyspnea or chest pain
  - The **inability** to perform at least **4 METs** of activity without symptoms is consistent with **poor functional status** and is associated with **increased operative risk**
  - If the patient **is unable to perform physical activity** (e.g., a patient who cannot walk because of severe degenerative arthritis), **assume that patient cannot perform 4 METs** and has poor functional status
- The amount of METs associated with common physical activities is summarized in Table 72-2

Surgery-Specific Risk Assessment

- Overall risks
  - For all surgeries, perioperative mortality is 0.3%
    - Most perioperative deaths (55%) occur in **the first 48 hours postoperatively**
    - Of perioperative deaths, 35% occur in the operating room, and 10% of deaths occur during anesthesia induction
    - **Pulmonary complications are the most common perioperative complications**
    - **Cardiac complications are the most common cause of perioperative death**
    - Perioperative MIs usually occur by postoperative day 3
    - Of perioperative MIs, 50% are fatal
  - Procedure-associated risk
    - Surgery-specific risk is determined by the operative procedure planned
      - **Low-risk** procedures are associated with a less than **1%** risk of death

72

TABLE 72-3	*Surgery-Specific Risk*	
Low Risk (<1%)	**Intermediate Risk (<5%)**	**High-Risk Vascular (>5%)**
Endoscopic procedures	Carotid endarterectomy	Peripheral vascular surgery
Superficial procedures	Endovascular abdominal aortic aneurysm repair	Aortic/major vascular surgery
Cataract surgery	Head and neck surgery	
Breast surgery	Intraperitoneal surgery	
Ambulatory surgery	Intrathoracic surgery	
	Orthopedic surgery	
	Prostate surgery	

- Intermediate-risk procedures are associated with a 1% to 5% risk of death
- **High-risk** procedures are associated with a **greater than 5%** risk of death
- Emergency surgery is considered very high risk
- A summary of surgery-specific risks is provided in Table 72-3

Summarizing Preoperative Risk

- Preoperative risk is summarized by **combining clinical risk, functional status, and surgery-specific risk**
  - Patients with an active cardiac condition should not undergo elective surgery until the active cardiac condition has been treated
  - Patients with no clinical risk factors can proceed to surgery without noninvasive cardiac testing
  - Patients with good functional status can proceed to surgery without noninvasive cardiac testing
  - Patients undergoing low-risk surgical procedures can proceed to surgery without noninvasive cardiac testing
  - Patients with one or two clinical risk factors undergoing intermediate-risk or vascular surgery or with poor or unknown functional status should be treated with perioperative β-blockers or consider noninvasive cardiac testing
  - Patients with three or more clinical risk factors should be managed similarly, unless undergoing vascular surgery, in which case they should undergo noninvasive cardiac testing

Instructions to the Patient

- Medication adjustments
  - **Check serum levels of all medications** that are monitored with serum levels preoperatively and adjust doses accordingly
  - **Antihypertensives are continued** on the morning of surgery **with the exception** of diuretics, angiotensin-converting enzyme inhibitors, and angiotensin receptor blockers, which are held the morning of surgery
  - Diabetes medications are adjusted as follows:
    - **Oral hypoglycemics are held on the day of surgery**

- **Metformin,** with its risk of lactic acidosis, is **held 2 days preoperatively**
- **Regular insulin and rapid-acting insulins are held on the day of surgery**
- **Glargine** insulin and **NPH** insulin doses are reduced by one half to one third
- **Hydroxymethylglutaryl coenzyme A reductase inhibitors are continued** on the day of surgery and may reduce risk of a cardiac event
- Sedatives, hypnotics, and other central nervous system–active medications are held on the day of surgery
- **Aspirin is held 1 week before surgery;** although the effect on platelets of other nonsteroidal anti-inflammatory drugs is less pronounced than aspirin, they are typically held 1 week before surgery
- Other idiosyncratic reactions include the following:
  - **Lithium:** May cause myocardial suppression and is **held the day of surgery**
  - **Tetracycline:** May cause renal failure if administered with methoxyflurane (anesthetic) and **is held the day of surgery**
  - Neuroleptics may enhance neuromuscular blocking agents; if given, anesthetist may need to adjust neuromuscular blockade during surgery
  - All herbal remedies (e.g., St. John's wort and ginkgo biloba) should be discontinued prior to surgery
- New symptom monitoring
  - Patients should be reminded to contact the internist or surgeon if a febrile illness, chest pain, or new medical symptoms develop between the preoperative assessment and surgery
- Preoperative testing
  - Although routine preoperative testing is often performed, there are few data to support its use. Surgeons typically will make specific requests based on the type of surgical procedure.
  - The following preoperative testing is commonplace:
    - For patients 65 years and older: Electrolytes, glucose, creatinine, and complete blood count (CBC)
    - Electrocardiography: For men older than 40 years, women older than 50 years
    - Chest radiography: Consider in patients with chest complaints or greater than 10 pack-years of tobacco use (this recommendation is in flux)
    - CBC: Consider in menstruating women
    - Glucose: Consider in younger African American patients
    - Prothrombin time/partial thromboplastin time: Consider in patients with liver disease, malignancy, patients receiving anticoagulants, or patients having neurosurgery
    - Urinalysis: For prosthetic joint placement
- Role of β-blockers
  - The role of **perioperative β-blocker administration** in a selected population has demonstrated **a reduced risk of perioperative MI and death.** The benefit persists for at least 2 years postoperatively.
  - Studies have demonstrated that perioperative β-blockers (specifically **cardioselective β-blockers** such as atenolol, metoprolol, or bisoprolol) were well tolerated, including in those with COPD

TABLE 72-4	*Recommendations for Perioperative β-Blockers*
Strength of Recommendation	**Recommendation**
Strongest	β-Blockers should be continued in patients undergoing surgery who are receiving β-blockers for other indications β-Blockers should be given to patients undergoing vascular surgery who have ischemia on preoperative testing
Intermediate	β-Blockers probably recommended for patients undergoing vascular surgery in whom preoperative assessment identifies CAD, or in patients with high cardiac risk, as defined by the presence of >1 clinical risk factor (i.e., known cardiac disease, diabetes, renal insufficiency, cerebrovascular disease, prior CHF) β-Blockers are probably recommended for patients in whom preoperative assessment identifies CHD or high cardiac risk as defined by >1 clinical risk factor and who are undergoing intermediate-risk or vascular surgery
Low	β-Blockers may be considered for patients who are undergoing intermediate or high-risk procedures in whom preoperative assessment identifies intermediate cardiac risk as defined by the presence of a single clinical risk factor β-Blockers may be considered in patients undergoing vascular surgery with low cardiac risk who are not currently on β-blockers

CAD, coronary artery disease; CHD, congenital heart disease; CHF, congestive heart failure.

- **Mortality may be reduced by 50%** in patients treated appropriately with **perioperative β-blockers,** but mortality may also increase when perioperative β-blockers are used inappropriately
  - American College of Cardiology/American Heart Association recommendations on use of perioperative β-blockers are listed in Table 72-4

REVIEW QUESTIONS

For review questions, please go to www.expertconsult.com.

SUGGESTED READINGS

ACC/AHA writing committee. 2009: ACCF/AHA focused update on perioperative beta blockade incorporated into the ACC/AHA 2007 guidelines on perioperative cardiovascular evaluation and care for noncardiac surgery: A report of the American College of Cardiology Foundation/American Heart Association task force on practice guidelines, *Circulation* 120:e169–e276, 2009.

Fleisher LA, Beckman JA, Brown KA, et al: ACC/AHA 2007 guidelines on perioperative cardiovascular evaluation and care for noncardiac surgery, *Circulation* 116:418–499, 2007.

Fleisher LA, Beckman JA, Brown KA, et al: ACC/AHA 2006 guideline update on perioperative cardiovascular evaluation for noncardiac surgery: focused update on perioperative beta-blocker therapy, *J Am Coll Cardiol* 47:2343–2355, 2006.

Ford MK, Beattie WS, Wijeysundera DN: Systematic review: prediction of perioperative cardiac complications and mortality by the Revised Cardiac Risk Index, *Ann Intern Med* 152:26–35, 2010.

Wilson W, Taubert KA, Gewitz M, et al: Prevention of infective endocarditis: guidelines from the American Heart Association, *Circulation* 116:1736–1754, 2007.

72

Immunization and Prevention

BIMAL H. ASHAR, MD, MBA

Immunizations and screening for designated pathologic conditions are the cornerstones of preventive medicine. Several major medical societies have published guidelines for these practices, which vary in several of their recommendations. The following is an overview of the necessary immunizations and side effect profiles as well as other health maintenance screening guidelines.

Immunization

- General concepts
  - Active versus passive
    - Active immunization involves administration of antigen to induce an antibody response
    - Passive immunization involves administration of an exogenous antibody (temporary protection against a disease)
      - Usually done by infusion of human immunoglobulin (e.g., hepatitis A, tetanus)
  - Types of active immunization (i.e., vaccination)
    - Live, attenuated
      - Usually confers lifelong immunity
      - **Should not be given to immunocompromised patients**
      - Examples: Measles, mumps, and rubella (MMR); varicella-zoster (chickenpox); shingles, influenza (intranasal)
    - Inactivated (killed) whole pathogen
      - Examples: Influenza (flu shot), hepatitis A, rabies
    - Fractional protein-based
      - Examples: Hepatitis B, tetanus
    - Polysaccharide
      - Examples: *Pneumococcus, Meningococcus, Haemophilus influenzae*
  - Principles of administration
    - Live vaccines should either be given together or at least 4 weeks apart
    - **It is not necessary to restart an interrupted vaccine series (except oral typhoid)**
    - Live vaccines should not be given with immunoglobulin or blood products
    - Common patient misconceptions about vaccination
      - **Many vaccines cause a local reaction and fever that lasts 24 to 48 hours. This does not contraindicate using the vaccine again and should not be considered an allergic response.**
      - Mild acute illness (or recent illness) or the current use of antibiotics does not contraindicate the use of vaccines
      - Family history of adverse reaction to a vaccine does not contraindicate the use of vaccines
- Individual vaccines (see also Fig. 73-1)
  - Influenza
    - Vaccine characteristics
      - New formulation created each year for different strain
      - Ideally given in October or November, but can be given as late as February
      - Needs to be given annually
      - **60% to 80% effective in preventing disease, but 95% effective in preventing complications**
      - Two types: Live, attenuated influenza vaccine (LAIV) can be used in healthy individuals ages 2 to 49 years; trivalent inactivated influenza vaccine (TIV) should be used for all others
    - Indications
      - The Advisory Committee on Immunization Practices (ACIP) recommends annual influenza vaccination for all people age 6 months and older
      - Data show improved economic outcomes for inoculating healthy working young adults
    - Adverse reactions: TIV
      - Local reaction 15% to 20%; soreness at the site
      - Low-grade fever
      - Myalgias
    - Adverse reactions: LAIV
      - Runny nose, sore throat
      - Headache
      - Cough
    - Contraindications
      - Egg allergy
      - History of severe postvaccine reaction or Guillain-Barré syndrome within 6 weeks of influenza vaccine administration
  - *Pneumococcus*
    - Vaccine characteristics
      - Polysaccharide vaccine made from 23 strains (90% of strains causing the morbidity of *Pneumococcus*)
    - Indications
      - Age 65 years or older
      - Immunocompetent adults less than 65 years of age with certain chronic conditions/risks (i.e., diabetes, chronic heart disease, chronic liver disease, alcoholism, chronic lung disease, cerebrospinal fluid leaks, cochlear implant, cigarette smoking)

VACCINE ▼ AGE GROUP ▶	19–26 years	27–49 years	50–59 years	60–64 years	≥65 years
Influenza[1],*	1 dose annually				
Tetanus, diphtheria, pertussis (Td/Tdap)[2],*	Substitute 1-time dose of Tdap for Td booster; then boost with Td every 10 years				Td booster every 10 years
Varicella[3],*	2 doses				
Human papillomavirus (HPV)[4],*	3 doses (females)				
Zoster[5]				1 dose	
Measles, mumps, rubella (MMR)[6],*	1 or 2 doses		1 dose		
Pneumococcal (polysaccharide)[7,8]	1 or 2 doses				1 dose
Meningococcal[9],*	1 or more doses				
Hepatitis A[10],*	2 doses				
Hepatitis B[11],*	3 doses				

* Covered by the Vaccine Injury Compensation Program

[shaded] For all persons in this category who meet the age requirements and who lack evidence of immunity (e.g., lack documentation of vaccination or have no evidence of previous infection)

[shaded] Recommended if some other risk factor is present (e.g., based on medical, occupational, lifestyle, or other indications)

[blank] No recommendation

FIGURE 73-1 Recommended adult vaccination schedule. *(From the Centers for Disease Control Advisory Committee on Immunization Practices. Document and footnotes available at:* http://www.cdc.gov/vaccines/recs/schedules/downloads/adult/mmwr-adult-schedule.pdf*)*

- Immunocompromised patients less than 65 years of age (including patients with malignancies, chronic renal disease, human immunodeficiency virus [HIV], and conditions requiring immunosuppressive drugs)
- Persons with anatomic or functional asplenia
- Revaccination
  - ACIP does not recommend routine revaccination for most people
  - Revaccination recommended 5 years after initial administration for immunocompromised patients and those with functional or anatomic asplenia
  - Those patients who received pneumococcal vaccine before age 65 years for any indication should receive another dose of the vaccine at age 65 years or later if at least 5 years have passed since their previous dose
  - If patient is unsure if he or she has received the pneumococcal vaccine before, it is okay to revaccinate regardless of the time interval
  - **It is currently not recommended to vaccinate any individual more than twice**
- Tetanus (tetanus, diphtheria [Td])
  - Vaccine characteristics
    - Fractional protein-based toxoid
    - Administer primary adult series if no history of vaccination: three-shot series at 0, 1, and then 6 to 12 months
    - Recommended every 10 years unless patient has not had one Tdap (tetanus, diphtheria, acellular pertussis) booster as an adult (see below)

- Important to revaccinate elderly patients because the elderly and children are the at-risk populations for the illness
- Treatment of exposure (i.e., dirty wound)
  - Administer Td vaccine if last shot was 5 or more years before, or begin primary series if never given
  - Administer tetanus immune globulin if Td never given (okay to give with first Td vaccine)
- Pertussis (Tdap)
  - An estimated 17,000 cases of pertussis were reported in the United States in 2009
  - ACIP now recommends that a single dose of Tdap be given to
    - All adults ages 19 to 64 regardless of the interval since last tetanus shot
    - Adults 65 and older who anticipate having close contact with an infant less than 12 months of age regardless of the interval since last tetanus shot
  - For other adults age 65 years and older, a single dose of Tdap vaccine may be given instead of Td vaccine, in persons who have not previously received Tdap
  - After single dose of Tdap given, resume 10-year vaccination schedule with Td (see above)
- Hepatitis A
  - Vaccine characteristics
    - Inactivated whole-virus vaccine (killed)
    - Given as two-shot series at least 6 months apart
    - First dose should be given at least a month before anticipated exposure

73

- Unknown if booster doses are required; immune response appears to last at least 10 years
  - Indications
    - Men who have sex with men
    - Intravenous (IV) drug users
    - Patients with chronic liver disease
    - Travelers to endemic areas
    - People who work with the virus or with primates
    - Recipients of clotting factors
    - Note that heterosexual promiscuity and health-care workers are not indications
  - Postexposure prophylaxis
    - For healthy persons ages 12 months to 40 years, single-antigen hepatitis A vaccine at the age-appropriate dose is preferred to hepatitis A immune globulin
    - For persons greater than 40 years of age, hepatitis A immune globulin is preferred
- Hepatitis B
  - Vaccine characteristics
    - Recombinant subunit (protein-based) vaccine
    - Three-shot series at 0, 1, and 6 months
    - Test for hepatitis B surface antibody (anti-HBs) 1 to 2 months after third shot in health-care workers, hemodialysis patients, immunocompromised patients (including HIV), and sex partners of persons with hepatitis B infection
    - **Nonresponders after three doses should be revaccinated**
    - High risk of nonresponder in dialysis patients, elderly, obese, smokers, and males
    - Use high dose (40 μg versus 10–20 μg standard dose) for dialysis patients and nonresponders after three standard doses
  - Indications
    - Men who have sex with men
    - Multiple sex partners
    - IV drug users
    - Patients with chronic liver disease
    - Patients with HIV
    - Long-term travelers to endemic areas
    - Contacts of patients with hepatitis B
    - Health-care workers
    - Institutionalized developmentally disabled patients
    - Hemodialysis patients
    - Regular recipients of blood products (e.g., hemophiliacs)
    - Now recommended for all adolescents
- Human papillomavirus (HPV) vaccine
  - Vaccine characteristics
    - Two vaccines currently approved (quadrivalent and bivalent)
    - Three-shot series at 0, 2, and 6 months used for both vaccines
    - Quadrivalent vaccine (HPV4) efficacious in preventing infection from HPV types 6, 11, 16, and 18
    - Bivalent vaccine (HPV2) efficacious in preventing infection from HPV types 16 and 18
    - **About 70% of cervical cancers are caused by HPV-16 and HPV-18**

- Indications
  - Currently approved for use in girls/women ages 9 to 26 years to prevent genital warts, precancerous lesions, and cervical cancer
  - Vaccine should ideally be given before the onset of sexual activity so current targeted group is girls ages 11 to 12 years
  - Recommended for sexually active women younger than age 27 years, but may be less efficacious in preventing disease
  - Need to continue screening Papanicolaou smears even in women who received the vaccine
  - HPV4 has been approved in males and may be given to males ages 9 through 26 years to reduce their likelihood of acquiring genital warts; however, data supporting its use are currently less compelling
- Contraindications
  - Hypersensitivity to yeast
  - Patients with a moderate to severe acute illness
- Measles, mumps, and rubella (MMR)
  - Vaccine characteristics
    - Live, attenuated vaccine
    - Given in two doses: typically at 0 and at 1 to 2 months
    - **Do not give to patients who are pregnant or trying to get pregnant or to severely immunocompromised patients**
    - May suppress a tuberculosis test (purified protein derivative [PPD]) response for 4 to 6 weeks
  - Indications
    - Patients vaccinated between 1957 and 1968 received a killed vaccine that is not effective, so they are not immune; if in an at-risk group, they need revaccination
    - Patients born before 1957 are considered immune
    - Women of childbearing age (if rubella titer is negative)
    - College students (if measles titer is negative)
    - Travelers (if measles titer is negative)
    - Health-care workers (if measles titer is negative)
- Varicella-zoster (chickenpox)
  - Vaccine characteristics
    - Live, attenuated vaccine
    - Given in two doses: one each at 0 and 1 month
    - **Diffuse varicella-like rash can occur in up to 5% of patients; transmission from a patient with the vaccine rash to immunocompromised children has been reported; patients should be advised not to have contact with immunosuppressed patients until rash is gone**
  - Indications
    - All adults without evidence of immunity (Box 73-1)
    - Consider testing for immunity in health-care workers, teachers and day care workers, contacts of chronically ill patients, immunocompromised patients, and pregnant women
  - Contraindications
    - HIV-positive and immunocompromised controversial; ACIP recommends for mild HIV in children and adults (CD4$^+$ count >200 cells/mm^3)

| BOX 73-1 | *Evidence of Immunity to Varicella for Adults* |

Documentation of two-dose vaccine series
Laboratory evidence of immunity
Birth in the United States before 1980*
Verification of history of chickenpox by a health-care provider[†]
Verification of a history of herpes zoster by a health-care provider

*Birth before 1980 not considered adequate evidence for health-care workers, pregnant women, and immunocompromised patients.
[†]Self-report of disease is not sufficient.

- Pregnancy (woman should avoid pregnancy for 1 month after vaccination)
- Avoid in patients with malignancy and severe immunocompromised states (including medication-induced immune compromise)
- Varicella-zoster immune globulin (VZIG) can be given postexposure in patients who cannot receive the varicella-zoster vaccine (may be effective when given up to 4 days postexposure)
- Herpes zoster (shingles) vaccine
  - Vaccine characteristics
    - Live, attenuated vaccine
    - About 50% to 60% effective in preventing shingles; about 60% to 70% effective in preventing postherpetic neuralgia
    - Given as a single shot; no revaccination currently recommended
  - Indications
    - ACIP currently recommends vaccination for all patients 60 years and older
    - Vaccine recently approved by Food and Drug Administration for adults 50 to 59 years
    - **Not necessary to ask about history of chickenpox or to conduct serologic testing for varicella-zoster immunity**
    - Patients who have a history of a shingles episode in the past can be vaccinated unless contraindications exist
  - Contraindications
    - History of anaphylaxis to vaccine components (e.g., gelatin, neomycin)
    - Anyone with acquired, primary, or medication-induced immunodeficiency
    - Should not be given concomitantly with pneumococcal vaccine due to decreased varicella-zoster virus antibody response
- Meningococcal vaccine
  - Vaccine characteristics
    - Polysaccharide-based vaccine
    - Active against *Neisseria meningitidis* groups A, C, Y, and W-135
    - Does not protect against group B, the most common one in United States
  - Indications
    - ACIP recommends vaccinating all adolescents at age 11 to 12 years, with a booster at age 16

- Patients with complement deficiency, asplenia, and adolescents with HIV should have a two-shot primary series separated by 2 months
- Rabies vaccine (pre-exposure)
  - Vaccine characteristics/background
    - Bats, skunks, raccoons, dogs, and cats can transmit disease
    - If given as pre-exposure prophylaxis, three doses given
    - If given after bite, four doses of vaccine plus rabies immune globulin should be given
  - Indications for pre-exposure prophylaxis
    - Veterinarians, animal handlers
    - Travelers who will likely come in contact with animals in parts of the world where rabies is common
- Polio vaccine
  - Live oral poliovirus vaccine (OPV) no longer recommended
  - Unvaccinated adults should get the enhanced inactivated poliovirus vaccine (eIPV) in three doses at 0, 1 to 2, and 6 to 12 months, particularly if they may be traveling to endemic areas (South Asia, sub-Saharan Africa)
- *Haemophilus influenzae* type B vaccine
  - Indications
    - Usually given in childhood
    - Patients should be revaccinated after bone marrow transplantation and given the first dose before splenectomy (if possible)
- Other vaccines
  - Yellow fever and typhoid vaccines for travelers to endemic areas only
  - Bacille Calmette-Guérin (BCG)
    - Not widely used in the United States but may be given to children born in other countries to prevent tuberculosis
    - Important to realize that it may cause a positive PPD test
- Special populations (Fig. 73-2)
  - HIV
    - Only live, attenuated vaccines are contraindicated in patients with severe immunosuppression (CD4$^+$ count <200 cells/mm^3)
    - Flu vaccine had been thought to raise HIV viral load, but recent data show safety; it should be given annually to HIV patients
    - Should receive flu and pneumococcal vaccines; consider hepatitis A and B
  - Multiple sclerosis
- No evidence of a risk from vaccination in multiple sclerosis patients despite concerns in 1990s; they should be vaccinated without reservation
  - Bone marrow transplant recipients
    - Need to be reimmunized with primary series
    - Killed vaccines should be given 12 to 24 months post-transplantation
    - Live vaccines should be given 24 months post-transplantation assuming no graft-versus-host disease or immunosuppressant drugs

INDICATION ▶ VACCINE ▼	Pregnancy	Immuno-compromising conditions (excluding human immuno-deficiency virus [HIV])[3,5,6,13]	HIV infection[3,6,12,13] CD4+ T lymphocyte count <200 cells/µL	≥200 cells/µL	Diabetes, heart disease, chronic lung disease, chronic alcoholism	Asplenia[12] (including elective splenectomy and persistent complement component deficiencies)	Chronic liver disease	Kidney failure, end-stage renal disease, receipt of hemodialysis	Health-care personnel
Influenza[1,*]	1 dose TIV annually								[1 dose TIV or LAIV annually]
Tetanus, diphtheria, pertussis (Td/Tdap)[2,*]	Td	Substitute 1-time dose of Tdap for Td booster; then boost with Td every 10 years							
Varicella[3,*]	Contraindicated		2 doses						
Human papillomavirus (HPV)[4,*]		3 doses through age 26 years							
Zoster[5]	Contraindicated			1 dose					
Measles, mumps, rubella[6,*]	Contraindicated		1 or 2 doses						
Pneumococcal (polysaccharide)[7,8]	1 or 2 doses								
Meningococcal[9,*]	1 or more doses								
Hepatitis A[10,*]	2 doses								
Hepatitis B[11,*]	3 doses								

* Covered by the Vaccine Injury Compensation Program

▢ For all persons in this category who meet the age requirements and who lack evidence of immunity (e.g., lack documentation of vaccination or have no evidence of previous infection)

▢ Recommended if some other risk factor is present (e.g., on the basis of medical, occupational, lifestyle, or other indications)

▢ No recommendation

FIGURE 73-2 Immunization schedule for special adult populations. (LAIV, live, attenuated influenza vaccine; TIV, inactivated influenza vaccine.) *(From the Centers for Disease Control Advisory Committee on Immunization Practices. Document and footnotes available at:* http://www.cdc.gov/vaccines/recs/schedules/downloads/adult/mmwr-adult-schedule.pdf*)*

Screening

- General principles
  - Recommendations for screening vary widely
    - U.S. Preventive Services Task Force (USPSTF)
      - Government-sponsored group whose mission is to make recommendations on which preventive services should be part of routine primary care
      - Cost-effectiveness does play a role in recommendations made
      - The USPSTF has a grading system for its recommendations (Table 73-1)
    - Specialty societies (e.g., the American Cancer Society [ACS], American Urologic Association [AUA], American Thyroid Association, and American College of Physicians [ACP])
      - Often make recommendations and develop independent guidelines for screening
      - Cost-effectiveness may or may not play a role in guidelines
  - Screening tests are generally a form of secondary prevention
    - **Primary prevention: Intervention designed to avert disease before it develops** (e.g., nutritional counseling)

TABLE 73-1	U.S. Preventive Services Task Force Grading System
Grade	**Description**
A	Service recommended. Net benefit is thought to be substantial
B	Service recommended. Net benefit is thought to be moderate to substantial
C	Not routinely recommended. There may be some individuals for which service is appropriate
D	Not recommended. Data show no benefit or potential for harm
I	Current evidence insufficient to make a recommendation for or against the service

- **Secondary prevention: Intervention aimed at early detection of disease** (e.g., mammography)
- **Tertiary prevention: Preventing complications of a symptomatic disease** (e.g., hepatitis B vaccine in hepatitis C patients)
- An ideal screening test is one that does the following:
  - Screens for a disease that has high morbidity and mortality
  - Is sensitive with a confirmatory test available, inexpensive, and noninvasive

- Screens for a disease that has a long premorbid phase during which intervention can affect outcome

Cancer Screening

BREAST CANCER

- Mammography
  - USPSTF recommends screening mammograms every 2 years for women ages 50 to 74; starting before age 50 should be determined on a case-by-case basis
  - Other groups recommend more frequent testing; annual mammography for patients older than 40
  - No clear data on screening for women ≥75 years of age, but life expectancy and comorbid diseases should be taken into consideration
- Clinical breast examination (CBE) and self-breast examination (SBE)
  - USPSTF recommends against teaching SBE
  - CBE has not been shown to reduce mortality either alone or in combination with mammography
  - Many groups still recommend both of these
- Genetic testing
  - Indicated for women whose family history is associated with an increased risk of BRCA1 or BRCA2 mutation
  - Patients should be referred for genetic counseling and testing
- Chemoprevention
  - Should discuss use of tamoxifen or raloxifene in women at high risk for breast cancer
  - Can estimate risk with the use of online tools (e.g., the National Cancer Institute's Breast Cancer Risk Assessment Tool, http://cancer.gov/bcrisktool/)
  - Need to weigh risks of medications (i.e., venous thrombosis, uterine cancer) against benefits of prevention

COLORECTAL CANCER

- Screening options (by the USPSTF)
  - Annual high-sensitivity fecal occult blood testing (FOBT)
    - Chemical FOBT has been shown to reduce colon cancer mortality by 15% to 20%
    - Immunologic FOBT results in fewer false positives but long-term data are currently limited
  - Flexible sigmoidoscopy every 5 years plus high-sensitivity FOBT every 3 years
  - Colonoscopy every 10 years
  - Computed tomographic colonography and fecal DNA may be useful tools in the near future but currently not recommended
- Timing
  - Start screening at age 50 years in individuals at average risk
  - Net benefit of screening between the ages of 76 to 85 years is small but should be individualized
  - Absolutely stop screening in adults older than 85 years (harm outweighs benefits)
- High-risk patients may need colonoscopy earlier than age 50 years or more frequently than every 10 years
  - Familial polyposis

- Strong family history (first-degree relative younger than 60 years)
- History of adenomatous polyps
- History of inflammatory bowel disease

PROSTATE CANCER

- Prostate-specific antigen (PSA)
  - USPSTF recently released a new guideline against routine screening; however this is currently being reviewed
  - ACP just recommends discussion of pros and cons between physician and patient
  - AUA recommends beginning screening at age 40 years
  - **USPSTF recommends against screening men older than age 75 years since harms outweigh benefits**
- Digital rectal examination
  - Insufficient evidence to recommend routine screening per USPSTF
  - ACS and AUA recommend same guidelines as for PSA

CERVICAL CANCER

- Papanicolaou test (Pap smear)
  - Perform on all sexually active women older than 21 years with a cervix (or within 3 years of onset of sexual activity)
  - If no risk factors (e.g., HIV, recurrent sexually transmitted diseases [STDs], multiple partners, abnormal Pap in past), can perform every 3 years (per both USPSTF and ACP)
  - ACS agrees but recommends three annual negative Pap smears before doing 3-year intervals. If no history of abnormal Pap and no risk factors, can stop after age 65
  - If no or distant history of last Pap smear, the test should be performed regardless of age
  - USPSTF recommends against Pap smears in women who underwent hysterectomy for benign disease (e.g., fibroids)
- HPV testing
  - USPSTF found insufficient evidence for or against testing for HPV
  - The American College of Obstetricians and Gynecologists suggests HPV testing in addition to Pap smear as an option for women older than 30 years; if both are negative, no need to repeat the Pap for at least 3 more years

OVARIAN CANCER

- **Screening not recommended for individuals at average risk; tests (cancer antigen 125 and ultrasound) are inaccurate with very low positive predictive value**
- Routine pelvic examinations done for ovarian cancer screening are not recommended (except by the ACS)

LUNG CANCER

- Currently, chest radiograph, sputum cytology, and low-dose computed tomography (CT) are not recommended for early detection in smokers
  - Low-dose CT scans are being studied as a screening tool in high-risk patients and may prove beneficial

Screening for Infectious Diseases

- HIV
  - USPSTF strongly recommends screening patients at increased risk
    - Recent history of STD
    - Men who have sex with men
    - Past or present IV drug users
    - Women or men whose sex partners have been HIV-positive, IV drug users, bisexuals, or those who have multiple partners without protection
    - History of receiving blood products between 1978 and 1985
  - USPSTF also recommends screening all pregnant women
  - Centers for Disease Control and Prevention (CDC) recommends screening all individuals between the ages of 13 and 64 years
  - All patients should be counseled on how to prevent HIV transmission
- STDs (USPSTF recommendations)
  - Hepatitis B: Routine screening not recommended except in high-risk individuals or pregnant women
  - Syphilis: Rapid plasma reagin for all pregnant women and high-risk patients (e.g., history of STD or HIV, multiple sex partners)
  - Gonorrhea: Routine screening not recommended but asymptomatic high-risk patients should be screened
  - **Chlamydia: Recommends screening all asymptomatic adolescent sexually active women (24 years or younger) and high-risk adult women; does not recommend routine screening of men or adult women at low risk**
  - Herpes simplex virus: Routine screening is not recommended
- Rubella immunity
  - USPSTF recommends all women of childbearing age be screened for rubella immunity; if nonimmune, they should receive the MMR vaccine
- Tuberculosis screening
  - Routine screening not necessary
  - CDC recommends screening in high-risk patients such as the following:
    - Chronic disease (e.g., diabetes, renal failure, HIV)
    - Recent emigrants from Africa, Asia, and Latin America
    - Health-care workers and anyone in close contact with a patient with known tuberculosis
    - Medically underserved populations
    - Residents of long-term facilities (e.g., jails, nursing homes)
    - Immunosuppressed
    - Alcoholics and IV drug users
  - Frequency of screening is a matter of clinical discretion
  - Two types of tests now available: PPD and interferon-γ release assay blood test
  - Criteria for positive PPD test are as follows:
    - Low-risk patients: 15-mm diameter or greater
    - High-risk patients (any of the previous indications for screening makes a patient at least high risk): 10-mm diameter or greater
    - Very-high-risk patients (HIV infection, abnormal chest film, recent contact with known infected patients): 5-mm diameter or greater
  - Blood test is preferred for patients who have had the BCG vaccine

Screening for Cardiovascular Disease

- Hypertension
  - USPSTF suggests screening for all adults older than age 18, but they do not specify frequency
  - The Seventh Report of the Joint National Committee on Detection, Evaluation, and Treatment of High Blood Pressure (JNC 7) recommends yearly evaluations in everyone with a blood pressure over 120/80 mm Hg and every 2 years in those with pressures lower than 120/80 mm Hg
- Hypercholesterolemia
  - USPSTF recommends screening all men 35 years or older and men and women 20 years and older if they have another risk factor for coronary heart disease
  - USPSTF makes no recommendation for screening women without risk factors
  - National Cholesterol Education Program (NCEP) recommends screening all adults over age 20 years with a lipid profile
  - Ideal frequency of screening has not been established, but NCEP recommends every 5 years if profile is normal
- Coronary heart disease
  - USPSTF recommends against resting electrocardiography, exercise treadmill testing, or coronary calcium scoring for the prediction of coronary disease in low-risk patients
  - USPSTF reports that there is insufficient evidence for or against use of these modalities in adults at increased risk of coronary artery disease
- Abdominal aortic aneurysm (AAA)
  - USPSTF recommends one-time screening for AAA by ultrasound in men ages 65 to 75 years who have ever smoked
  - USPSTF recommends against screening in women
- Aspirin use
  - Use of aspirin for men ages 45 to 79 years is recommended when the potential benefit due to a reduction in myocardial infarctions outweighs the potential harm due to an increase in gastrointestinal hemorrhage
  - Use of aspirin for women ages 55 to 79 years is recommended when the potential benefit of a reduction in ischemic strokes outweighs the potential harm of an increase in gastrointestinal hemorrhage
  - Ideal dose is unclear since beneficial effects are shown for doses ranging from 75 mg to 325 mg

Other Disease Screening

See Table 73-2.

TABLE 73-2	*USPSTF Screening Guidelines for Common Disorders*	
Disorder	**USPSTF Guideline**	**Comments**
Obesity	Screen all patients for obesity by calculating body mass index.	
Type 2 diabetes	Screen for diabetes in patients with blood pressures >135/80 mm Hg.	American Diabetes Association suggests screening everyone older than age 45 yr with a hemoglobin A_{1c}, fasting glucose, or glucose tolerance test every 3 yr
Thyroid disease	Insufficient evidence for or against screening.	American Thyroid Association recommends screening all adults every 5 yr beginning at age 35 yr
Osteoporosis	Screen women >65 yr with a DEXA scan. Start earlier if risk factors exist	National Osteoporosis Foundation has much broader recommendations, including screening all men older than 70 yr
Alcohol abuse	Screen all adults for alcohol misuse and begin counseling.	Screening tools are available at the National Institute on Alcohol Abuse and Alcoholism Web site: *www.niaaa. nih.gov/Publications/AlcoholResearch/*
Depression	Screen all adults	Many different short screening tools available
Smoking	Screen all adults and provide cessation interventions.	
Chronic obstructive pulmonary disease	Screening with spirometry not recommended	American Thoracic Society recommends spirometry for all persons with tobacco exposure

DEXA, dual-energy x-ray absorptiometry; USPSTF, U.S. Preventive Services Task Force.

Psychosocial and Behavioral Screening

- The USPSTF does not make recommendations for or against routine screening for a number of behavioral and situational disorders (other than depression and smoking cessation). However, they do state that clinicians should be aware of them and address these issues when appropriate.
- The following areas of concern may need to be addressed in an individual patient:
  - Depression
  - Eating disorders
  - Contraception and safe sex practices
  - Domestic violence
  - Nutrition
  - Exercise
  - Tobacco cessation
  - Alcohol and drug abuse
  - Injury prevention (e.g., seat belts, firearms, smoke detectors)
  - Advance directives

Periodic Health Examination

- There is significant controversy as to the value of the periodic health examination
  - Evidence suggests increased receipt of preventive services, including Pap smear, cholesterol testing, and FOBT

- There is no definitive evidence on the long-term benefits and effect on morbidity and mortality
- Significant variability in what services should be included in a periodic health examination and how frequently those services should be repeated

REVIEW QUESTIONS
For review questions, please go to www.expertconsult.com.

SUGGESTED READINGS

Advisory Committee on Immunization Practices: Recommended adult immunization schedule: United States, 2011, *Ann Intern Med* 154:168–173, 2011.

Boulware LE, Marinopoulos S, Phillips KA, et al: Systematic review: the value of the periodic health evaluation, *Ann Intern Med* 146:289–300, 2007.

Agency for Healthcare Research and Quality: *The guide to clinical preventive services 2010–11.* Available at:*http://www.ahrq.gov/clinic/pocketgd1011/.*

Petitti DB, Teutsch SM, Barton MB, et al: for the U.SPreventive Services Task Force: Update on the methods of the U.S. Preventive Services Task Force: insufficient evidence, *Ann Intern Med* 150:199–205, 2009.

73

CHAPTER **74**

Clinical Epidemiology

L. EBONY BOULWARE, MD, MPH

Common Terms and Concepts in Research

- Many common terms and concepts derive from the 2 × 2 table (Fig. 74-1)
- Most research questions can be reduced to a 2 × 2 table
- **Prevalence:** The number of **existing cases** of a disease at any given time divided by the total population at that time (see Fig. 74-1)
- **Incidence:** The number of **new cases** of a disease that develop over a specific time divided by the population at risk for developing the disease
  - Prevalence and incidence are related to each other via the duration of disease: **Prevalence = incidence × duration of disease** (P = ID)
  - Example: Before 1972, the prevalence of end-stage renal disease (ESRD) patients was very low (the duration of disease was very short because ESRD patients died at a very high rate without dialysis). After the Medicare dialysis program, the prevalence of ESRD soared (the duration of disease was extended, so prevalence increased).

Validity and Reliability of Diagnostic and Screening Tests

- Sensitivity and specificity: Characteristics of the test that reflect the test's ability to correctly identify disease in any population (see Fig. 74-1)
  - **Sensitivity: The ability of the test to correctly identify persons who have the disease of interest**
    - Example: If a test is able to correctly identify 80 persons (among 100) who have diabetes as having diabetes, the sensitivity of the test is 80/100 (80%)
  - **Specificity: The ability of the test to correctly identify persons who do not have the disease of interest**
    - Example: If a test is able to correctly identify 95 persons (among 100) who do not have diabetes as not having diabetes, the specificity of the test is 95/100 (95%)
- Positive and negative predictive values: The **test result's** likelihood of reflecting disease presence or absence in a specific population (affected by both disease prevalence and specificity of test) (see Fig. 74-1)
  - **Positive predictive value:** The probability that a **positive test in a patient reflects disease**

- Example: If 200 people test positive for diabetes, but only 80 of those people have diabetes, the positive predictive value of a positive test is 80/200 = 40%. Note that positive predictive value increases as prevalence increases; of the preceding group of people, if 100 of the 200 had diabetes, positive predictive value would be 100/200 = 50%.
- **Negative predictive value:** The probability that a **negative test in a patient reflects health (no disease)**
  - Example: If 200 persons test negative for diabetes, but only 40 do not have diabetes, the negative predictive value of the negative test is 40/200 = 20%. Note that negative predictive value increases as prevalence decreases. If 100 of the 200 preceding patients did not have diabetes, negative predictive value would be 100/200 = 50%.

Sources of Error in Measurement, Interpretation, or Analysis

- **Precision:** On repeated measurement of the same sample, **how closely do the results *cluster*?**
  - Precision does not consider how close a result is to truth
  - Precision depends on random error (greater random error results in lower precision; increasing sample size decreases effect of random error)
- **Accuracy: How close to the truth is the result?**
- **Bias: Systematic error,** resulting in decreased accuracy (Table 74-1)
  - Bias is reduced by careful study design
  - Randomization and blinding are powerful tools used in clinical trials to reduce selection and information bias
- **Confounding** (Fig. 74-2)
  - Confounding describes a relationship between an exposure and an outcome of interest that is distorted by a second exposure that is related to both the outcome and the exposure of interest
    - Simply termed, confounding is guilt by association
    - Confounding is a particular problem in observational studies
- Internal and external validity
  - **Internal validity in a study refers to whether the results accurately reflect the connection between exposure and disease within the population being studied**
    - Randomized clinical trials maximize internal validity through randomization, blinding, and placebo control

Sensitivity: Of those with disease, what percent test positive? ("sensitivity is positive in disease, or PID")

$$Sensitivity = a/(a + c)$$

Specificity: Of those without disease, what percent test negative? ("specificity is negative in health, or NIH")

$$Specificity = d/(b + d)$$

Prevalence: The percentage of a population that has a disease

$$Prevalence = (a + c)/(a + b + c + d)$$

Positive predictive value: If the test is positive, what percent will have disease? Markedly increases with increasing prevalence

$$PPV = a/(a + b)$$

Negative predictive value: If the test is negative, what percent will not have the disease? Markedly increases with decreasing prevalence

$$NPV = d/(c + d)$$

Relative risk: Risk of developing disease in those exposed, divided by the risk of developing disease in those not exposed

$$RR = Risk(exp)/Risk(unexp) = (a/[a + b])/(c/[c + d])$$

Attributable risk (AR): The absolute increase in risk of developing disease in those exposed compared to those not exposed. Absolute risk reduction (ARR) is the absolute decrease in risk among those taking a medication compared to those not taking it

$$AR = Risk(exp) - Risk(unexp) = a/(a + b) - c/(c + d)$$
$$ARR = Risk(not\ taking) - Risk(taking) = c/(c + d) - a/(a + b)$$

Number needed to treat: How many individuals will need to be treated to prevent a single event?

$$NNT = 1/ARR$$

Odds ratio: In individuals with disease, what are the odds of having been exposed compared to those who were exposed who do not have disease?

$$OR = Odds\ (exposure\ in\ those\ with\ disease)/Odds$$
$$(exposure\ in\ those\ without\ disease)$$
$$OR = (a/c)/(b/d)$$

FIGURE 74-1 The 2 × 2 table.

- **External validity** (i.e., generalizability)
  - Ability of a study to produce **results that can be applied to a target population (beyond the study participants)**
  - To be externally valid, a study must also be internally valid. A study with restrictive inclusion criteria enhances internal validity at the expense of external validity.

- Analyzing "crossovers" in clinical trials: Intention to treat
  - **Intention to treat is a conservative approach to the analysis of a clinical trial, in which analysis is based on the original assignment of a participant regardless of what assignment the participant actually received in the study**

74

TABLE 74-1 | *Types of Bias*

Type of Bias	Example
Selection bias: When those chosen for a study (or those leaving a study) systematically differ from those not chosen (or those not leaving) with respect to characteristics important to the study question	In a case-control study of pancreatic cancer, controls are chosen from a GI clinic. If the controls from the GI clinic are avoiding coffee because of GI side effects, this will tend to create a false association between coffee drinking and pancreatic cancer, resulting simply from the control group that was chosen.
Information bias: Occurs when individuals of a particular exposure or outcome are systematically erroneously classified as having a different exposure or outcome; for instance, recall bias: When individuals with a particular outcome retrospectively recall an exposure, their memory may be influenced by the event itself	Mothers of infants with a birth defect are more likely to remember taking a medication than other mothers. This will tend to create a false association between the medication use and birth defects.
Lead-time bias: Seen in studies of screening tests, in which identification of disease at an earlier stage will "lengthen" apparent survival, even if prognosis is not improved	A new test for detecting pancreatic cancer is associated with a doubling of survival time. However, the test merely detected the cancer at an earlier, untreatable stage.
Length bias: Seen in studies of screening tests when screening a population will detect those with the longest survival (i.e., less severe disease) more than those with shorter survival (i.e., more severe disease), thus creating the illusion that the screening test prolongs survival when in fact it does not	A new screening test for renal cell cancer is performed every 5 yr. Survival rates in the screened group are 7 yr, as compared with 4 yr in an unscreened group. Those with more aggressive disease die before the screening interval, so that those screened have less aggressive disease.

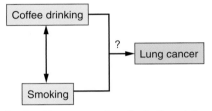

FIGURE 74-2 Smoking as a confounder in the relationship between coffee and lung cancer.

- Example: Randomized clinical trial of medical versus surgical treatment of mild carotid stenosis; if some in the medical arm cross over into the surgical arm, why not analyze them in the surgical group? Suppose most of those who crossed over had transient ischemic attacks: If they are counted in the surgical group, they will enrich (i.e., bias) the surgical arm with those who are more likely to have strokes (i.e., it will make surgery look worse than it really is).
  - When performing analyses using "intention to treat," the preceding crossover will bias the relative risk toward the null (result demonstrating less difference between study groups) but will never bias the association away from the null (result demonstrating more difference between study groups)
  - "As-treated" analysis has potential to bias away from the null

Study Design

- **Observational studies: No intervention performed;** observations made between exposures and outcomes (Table 74-2)
  - Strengths
    - Only way possible to study a number of important research questions (e.g., prognostic effect of disease)

- More likely to reflect real-world situations (external generalizability)
- Less expensive and generally faster to perform than randomized controlled trials
  - Limitations
    - Lower validity
    - More subject to bias and confounding of results
- Experimental studies: The randomized clinical trial (RCT)
  - **RCTs are a true experiment, the purpose of which is to test interventions**
    - Example: Does treating hypertensive patients with antihypertensive therapy reduce cardiovascular events?
  - Strengths
    - The gold standard study design to evaluate therapeutic interventions without bias or confounding
    - Stronger internal validity than cohort studies
  - Limitations
    - Limited to questions of clinical equipoise and clinical benefit
    - The study is run under ideal conditions and therefore most often measures efficacy, not effectiveness: **Efficacy refers to how the intervention performs under ideal conditions. Effectiveness refers to how the intervention performs in the real world.**
    - Generalizability often can be questioned
- Data synthesis studies
  - Qualitative review article: No explicit methods; must trust author's judgment
  - Practice guidelines: Consensus statements; quality varies
  - Decision analysis
    - Create a decision analysis tree, assign probabilities and utilities
    - Calculate the expected value of various decisions
  - Systematic review and meta-analysis

TABLE 74-2	*Types of Observational Studies*		
Name	**Design/Example**	**Strengths**	**Weaknesses**
Case report/series	Observations from clinical practice. *Example:* Case report of seizure associated with cat-scratch disease	Useful for generating hypotheses	Limited use in clinical decision making; no control group; selection bias
Ecologic study	Compare average exposure with average outcome between populations. *Example:* Comparison of mean salt intake and mean blood pressure in United States and Japan	Useful for generating hypotheses; can be used to compare prevalence of disease or exposures in various populations	No individual data; not useful for demonstrating causation
Cross-sectional study	Determine exposure and disease status simultaneously in a representative sample of a population. *Example:* Prevalence of *Chlamydia* antibodies in patients with coronary artery disease	Good initial step in evaluating associations; useful for public health surveys	Causation cannot be determined; temporal relationship not defined; cannot evaluate prognosis
Case-control study (retrospective study)	Identify cases (with disease) and select controls (without disease). Determine exposure status retrospectively in both groups. *Example:* Is history of head trauma greater in Alzheimer's disease patients than in controls?	Lower cost than cohort studies; useful for studying uncommon diseases	Susceptible to recall bias and selection bias; cannot evaluate prevalence, incidence, prognosis; can only determine odds ratio
Cohort study (prospective study)	Prospective study of subgroup in a population that shares a particular characteristic; determine exposure at beginning and ascertain outcomes with follow-up over time. *Example:* Incidence of mesothelioma in steel mill workers who smoke	Studies incidence and prognosis; establishes temporal relationships; strong external validity	Long and costly; limited in studying treatment effects

- Explicit methods to review and possibly pool or combine (meta-analysis) data from multiple studies
- **Beware of meta-analysis of observational studies** (pooled results may reflect bias or confounding in individual studies)
- Publication bias: Positive studies are published more frequently than negative studies and are most often included in systematic reviews, meta-analyses

Measures of Risk Reduction

See also Figure 74-1
- Example: Results of a recently performed RCT demonstrating patients' 5-year risk of death from breast cancer on treatment A versus treatment B are 50% versus 40%, respectively
- **Absolute risk reduction** (absolute improvement provided by treatment B versus treatment A) is 50% − 40% = 10%

- **Relative risk reduction** (improvement provided by treatment B relative to treatment A) is (50% − 40%)/50% = 20%
- **Number needed to treat** (NNT) (number of patients needed to treat with treatment B to prevent one additional death over 5 years compared with what would happen with treatment A [NNT = 1/Absolute risk reduction]) is 1/0.1 = 10

REVIEW QUESTIONS

For review questions, please go to www.expertconsult.com.

SUGGESTED READINGS

Gordis L: *Epidemiology*, Philadelphia, 1996, WB Saunders.
Last JM: *A dictionary of epidemiology*, New York, 1995, Oxford Press.
Sackett DL, Haynes RB, Guyatt GH, et al: *Clinical epidemiology: a basic science for clinical medicine*, Boston, 1991, Little Brown.

74

Medical Ethics

MARK T. HUGHES, MD, MA

Ethics is the systematic study of human actions with respect to good and bad, right and wrong, what should and should not be done, and the character of the individuals involved in the actions. The field of bioethics began about 40 years ago, but medical ethics can be traced back millennia to professional codes and standards of conduct, including the Hippocratic Oath. Clinical bioethics deals with the interface between moral philosophy and health care.

General Principles

- **Respect for autonomy: Self-rule, self-determination**
  - Respect for autonomy is the cornerstone principle for informed consent (allowing the patient to make an informed decision about his or her medical care) and confidentiality (respecting the individual's privacy)
  - Respect for persons acknowledges the patient as an individual and also as a member of various groups. The physician should pay attention to the individual and cultural identification of the patient when determining a treatment plan.
- **Beneficence: Acting in the best interests of the individual**
  - Beneficence is an inherent duty in medicine, in which a vulnerable patient seeks the help from one who professes to be a healer
- **Nonmaleficence: Enjoins the physician not to pursue interventions that are harmful to the patient, especially if the possibility of medical good cannot be achieved (*primum non nocere,* or "first, do no harm")**
  - Nonmaleficence also requires a physician to avoid negligence—not doing what the standard of care dictates in a situation—which can involve intentionally imposing risks of harm that are unreasonable (recklessness) or unintentionally (but carelessly) imposing risk of harm (physician should have known better)
- **Justice: Fairness, similars should be treated similarly**
  - In health-care ethics, one generally considers justice in terms of distributive justice—that is, how scarce resources are distributed
- **Professionalism: The elements of professionalism include expertise and competence, self-regulation, subjugation of self-interest, and an ongoing dialogue with society**
  - In medicine, professionalism is best exemplified in the Hippocratic tradition, in which one takes an oath to uphold certain values with respect to patients and colleagues on entering the profession

- Codes of ethics propagate the standards of the profession. Professional organizations such as the American Medical Association codify what it means to be a responsible physician attentive to the needs of the patient and society.
- Issues in professionalism include commitment to lifelong learning, the power differential between physician and patient, the societal role of physicians to prescribe medications and determine disability, truth telling, communication skills in breaking bad news and engaging in difficult encounters, response to medical errors, physician impairment, reimbursement for services, competition, collegiality within the interdisciplinary team, interpersonal conflict management, conflicts of interest (personal interests influence primary obligation), and conflicts of obligation (e.g., dual role of clinician-researcher)

Selected Issues

- Medical economics: Response to the perceived scarcity of health-care resources, the escalating costs of health care, the increasing number of uninsured and underinsured patients, and the fiduciary responsibilities of the physician caring for patients in the medical marketplace
  - Issues in medical economics include triage of patients for limited intensive care unit beds, drug formularies, denial of services dictated by insurance plans or prescription formularies, gaming the system, pay-for-performance reimbursement standards, physicians as employees, physicians as entrepreneurs, and physicians as stockholders
- Confidentiality: Protection of information shared in confidence between physician and patient, extending also to information systems that need safeguards to ensure privacy
  - Confidentiality is felt to be important to adequately treat the patient (i.e., the patient must feel comfortable disclosing personal information, so that a complete picture of his or her condition can be made)
  - Confidentiality may be breached only if all of the following criteria are met:
    - Identifiable third party at risk of harm
    - A high probability of serious harm exists
    - A likely benefit will result from breaking the confidence
    - All other avenues of disclosing the information (such as encouraging the patient to disclose to the third party) are unavailable

BOX 75-1	*Decision-Making Capacity*

Decision-making capacity (competency): The ability to make health-care decisions

Assessment of decision-making capacity involves the following:

 Ability to communicate a choice and preference
 Ability to understand medical condition
 Ability to understand consequences of condition and treatment(s)
 Judgment not impaired (e.g., through depression or substance abuse)
 Consistency with previously expressed wishes or values
 Ability to reason about medical situation, risks, and benefits
 Making a decision (with some fixity in decision made)

BOX 75-2	*Legal Hierarchy of Surrogate Decision Makers*

1. Health-care agent designated by patient
2. Court-appointed guardian
3. Spouse (or domestic partner in some states)
4. Adult child
5. Parent
6. Sibling
7. Other relative
8. Close friend

- Local jurisdictions may require reporting of private health information for public health considerations (e.g., tracking of infectious diseases)
- Informed consent: The patient should be an active participant in the decision-making process and has the right to accept or refuse medical treatment; involves the following:
  - Disclosure of information: Providing sufficient information on the patient's medical condition, risks, benefits, and options; usual standard is what would be expected by a reasonable person to make a decision
  - Voluntariness: Ensuring that the patient's decision is made free of undue influence, such as coercion, improper persuasion, or manipulation (framing effects when giving information)
  - Comprehension: Confirming that the patient understands what has been disclosed about the proposed test or treatment, and the patient's questions have been answered
  - Decision-making capacity (competency; Box 75-1)
    - Sliding scale notion of competency: Determination of capacity depends on the decision to be made, with complex or riskier decisions requiring a higher threshold in assessing capacity
  - Emancipated minors: Medical decisions for minors require the consent of their parents, guardians, or legally authorized representatives, except when minors are legally emancipated to make their own decisions, either uniformly or for particular medical decisions (e.g., related to reproductive health)
- Surrogate decision-making: **Situation in which a person is selected to make medical decisions on behalf of a patient who does not have the capacity to make his or her own decisions**
  - The surrogate can be preselected by the patient in an advance directive or selected by the medical team based on a hierarchy of relationships established by law (Box 75-2)
    - The morally appropriate surrogate for a particular patient might differ from the person selected by the legal hierarchy, as when a patient has been estranged from his or her family or has a close friend or significant other who knows his or her wishes and values more intimately. The physician in these circumstances should be guided by his or her conscience and legal advice as to whom to select as the surrogate.

- Standards of surrogate decision-making
  - Substituted judgment: Surrogate makes decision based on knowledge of the incompetent patient's previously expressed values and goals
  - Best interests: Surrogate weighs risks and benefits of each option available in given situation for incompetent patient in order to make decision
- **Emergency situations: Physician can act without surrogate consent when an action to save life or prevent significant harm must be taken immediately and cannot wait for the time needed to contact next of kin**

End-of-Life Issues

- Patient Self-Determination Act of 1991: Federal law passed requiring health-care organizations to inform patients that they have the right to make medical decisions and to execute advance directives
- Advance directives: Two types of documents completed by a competent patient in anticipation of one day being unable to speak for himself or herself (Box 75-3)
  - Appointment of health-care agent or proxy (i.e., the durable power of attorney for health care): Naming surrogate with or without explicit instructions about future care
  - Living will: Specifying wishes of medical care when the patient has a terminal medical condition, coma, or persistent vegetative state
  - Sometimes the decisions made by a duly appointed health-care agent seem to differ from the wishes documented in the instructions of a living will or advance directive; careful discussion with the health-care agent should try to resolve the discrepancies; consultation with the ethics committee of the health-care facility may be necessary
- Advance care planning: Places an emphasis on finding out about the "authentic" preferences that reflect the values important to the patient in shaping the goals of care
  - Includes traditional elements of advance directives such as health-care agent appointment and scenario-based decisional preferences
  - Also covers such items as how to deal with medical uncertainty, how surrogates should be guided in making decisions, patient wishes about comfort, how others should treat the patient at the end of

75

BOX 75-3   *Types of Advance Directives*

Durable Power of Attorney for Health Care (Health-Care Agent)

Designated by the patient when competent

Takes effect once patient loses decision-making capacity

Applies even in nonterminal conditions

Most effective when prior discussion has occurred

When activated, designated health-care agent can consent to medical treatments or make decisions to withhold or withdraw treatments

Some states make exceptions regarding health-care agent's authority to make certain decisions about artificial nutrition and hydration, involuntary psychiatric admission, psychosurgery, and sterilization

Living Will

Specifies patient's wishes in event of incapacitation

Applies in terminal condition, persistent vegetative state, coma

Typically advances comfort care approach when death is imminent

Wishes may be too general to provide guidance in particular situations

Must be witnessed by adults unrelated to patient, with no financial conflict of interest

---

life, what loved ones should know about the patient, the patient's thoughts and feelings about the dying process and death, options regarding organ donation, funeral arrangements and what the patient would want at a memorial service, and how the patient would want to be remembered by family and friends

- Do not (attempt to) resuscitate (DNR) orders: Applies only to resuscitation efforts (cardiopulmonary resuscitation, defibrillation, tracheal intubation) in the event of cardiac or pulmonary arrest. Some institutions have moved to the term *allow natural death* (AND) in place of DNR
  - Other measures of concurrent care (monitoring in a critical care setting, vasopressors, chemical antiarrhythmics, electrical cardioversion, external pacemakers, mechanical ventilation for conditions short of pulmonary arrest, artificial nutrition and hydration) require separate consent procedure and are not included within a DNR order
  - "Do not intubate" orders are used by some health-care facilities for patients who would opt against mechanical ventilation under any circumstances
  - Because DNR is a medical order written by a physician, a patient does not sign a DNR. Most states, however, require at least prior discussion with the patient or surrogate, if not a full informed-consent process, before the physician can institute a DNR order. The reasons for writing a DNR order should be documented in the medical record.
  - Generally, states have specific requirements for outpatient DNR orders and for transfer of DNR orders from a chronic nursing facility to a hospital. Typically, a separate form needs to be completed to specify that

the DNR order endures after the hospitalization, and this documentation should be readily available to other health-care providers, such as emergency medical technicians.

- Ordinary versus extraordinary care
  - Ordinary care: Benefits outweigh risks and burdens, such that care is to be pursued at the patient's or surrogate's discretion in an effort to preserve life
  - **Extraordinary care: Risks and burdens outweigh benefits.** If the means to preserve life are excessively burdensome and beyond that expected of a reasonable person, treatment is considered above and beyond the call of duty, and need not be pursued. Extraordinary care has nothing to do with how technologically advanced the treatment is, as even everyday treatments (e.g., antibiotics) can be considered extraordinary if they are overly burdensome.
- **Withholding and withdrawal of treatment:** Because the patient can refuse treatment at any time, no moral distinction is made between withholding and withdrawal of life-sustaining treatment, although emotional and practical distinctions may exist. Sometimes a trial of therapy is indicated to determine if the goals of care can be met.
- **Rule of double effect has four principal conditions:**
  - The act itself must be good or morally neutral
  - While a bad effect from the act may be foreseen, the agent (in this case, the clinician) intends only the good effect
  - The bad effect must not be the means to achieve the good effect
  - The good effect must outweigh the bad effect
- **Futility: When treatment is medically ineffective or not able to achieve the desired goal as set forth by the treatment team, the patient, or the surrogate**
  - Quantitative futility (physiologic futility): Treatment cannot achieve the desired physiologic effect (e.g., restoration of heart rhythm)
    - Most states have laws that recognize that physicians are not obligated to provide treatments that are ineffective or outside the bounds of good medical care
  - Qualitative futility: Treatment is considered futile because certain goals with respect to the patient's quality of life cannot be met. For instance, a surrogate may judge mechanical ventilation to be qualitatively futile in a patient permanently comatose, even though it achieves the physiologic effect of maintaining respiration and ventilation.
    - **The standards for determining qualitative futility ultimately reside with the patient or surrogate**
    - The physician can help in discussing qualitative futility with the patient or surrogate but generally cannot unilaterally forego treatment on the basis of the physician's personal assessment of the patient's quality of life
  - Conflict may arise when there is a dispute between the treatment team and the patient or surrogate regarding whether treatment constitutes futile care
    - Discussion regarding potentially futile treatment should focus on mutually agreed-on goals of care

- If dispute persists despite ongoing dialogue and involvement of ethics consultants, then transfer to another facility or physician should be pursued
  - State laws differ on whether and how physicians can unilaterally forego medical treatment without consent of surrogate
- Euthanasia and physician-assisted suicide
  - Euthanasia: Intentional act to cause the (immediate) death of another person, usually by administration of a lethal drug
    - Illegal in all states
  - Physician-assisted suicide ("Physician aid in dying"): Physician prescribes medication to the patient with instructions on how to commit suicide
    - Legal only in Oregon, Washington State, and Montana
  - The physician should ensure proper palliative care so that patients do not view these as their only options

REVIEW QUESTIONS

For review questions, please go to www.expertconsult.com.

SUGGESTED READINGS

Beauchamp TL, Childress JF: *Principles of biomedical ethics*, ed 6, New York, 2008, Oxford University Press.

Fletcher JC, Lombardo PA, Spencer EM: *Fletcher's introduction to clinical ethics*, ed 3, Frederick, MD, 2005, University Publishing Group.

Jonsen A, Siegler M, Winslade W: *Clinical ethics: a practical approach to ethical decisions in clinical medicine*, ed 7, New York, 2010, McGraw-Hill.

Junkerman CJ, Derse A, Schiedermayer D: *Practical ethics for students, interns, and residents*, ed 3, Frederick, MD, 2008, University Publishing Group.

Pellegrino ED, Thomasma DC: *A philosophical basis of medical practice*, New York, 1981, Oxford University Press.

Sugarman J: *Ethics in primary care*, New York, 2000, McGraw-Hill.

75

INDEX

Note: Page numbers followed by *f* refer to figures; page numbers followed by *t* refer to tables; page numbers followed by *b* refer to boxes.